Mastering Endo-Laparoscopic and Thoracoscopic Surgery

W0082709

Section Editor

Alembert Lee-Ong
Department of Surgery
Manila Doctors Hospital
Manila, Philippines

Section Editor

Emily Rose Nery
Department of Anesthesiology
The Medical City
Pasig, Philippines

Section Editor

Michael Lawenko
De La Salle Medical and Health Sciences
Dasmarinas, Philippines

Section Editor

Eva Lourdes Sta. Clara
Department of Surgery
Cardinal Santos Medical Center
San Juan, Philippines

Section Editor

Marilou B. Fuentes
Department of Surgery
The Medical City
Pasig, Philippines

Section Editor

Siau Wei Tang
Department of Surgery
National University Hospital
Singapore, Singapore

Section Editor

Narendra Agarwal
Department of Thoracic Surgery
Fortis Memorial Research Institute
Gurgaon, Haryana, India

Section Editor

Asim Shabbir
National University Hospital
Singapore, Singapore

Section Editor

Jaideep Rao
Mount Elizabeth Novena Hospital
Singapore, Singapore

Davide Lomanto
William Tzu-Liang Chen
Marilou B. Fuentes
Editors

Mastering Endo-Laparoscopic and Thoracoscopic Surgery

ELSA Manual

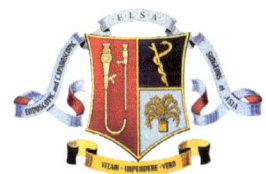

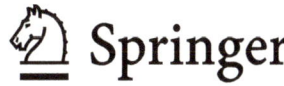

Editors
Davide Lomanto
Department of Surgery
Yong Loo Lin School of Medicine
National University of Singapore
Singapore, Singapore

William Tzu-Liang Chen
Department of Surgery
School of Medicine
China Medical University
Taichung City, Taiwan

Marilou B. Fuentes
Department of Surgery
The Medical City
Pasig, Philippines

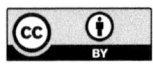

MIS Education Asia

ISBN 978-981-19-3757-6   ISBN 978-981-19-3755-2   (eBook)
https://doi.org/10.1007/978-981-19-3755-2

This Springer imprint is published by the registered company Springer Nature Singapore Pte Ltd. The registered company address is: 152 Beach Road, #21-01/04 Gateway East, Singapore 189721, Singapore

Foreword

Since its breakthroughs in 1990, minimally invasive surgery has changed significantly the practice of general surgery as a result of the increasing number of surgical procedures that can be carried out today with minimal discomfort for the patient. These changes that occurred in the last decades have a great impact also on the way we train and teach the upcoming generations of surgeons, surgical residents and trainees. Today, for all surgical trainees after completing their basic surgical skills, lap training is mandatory to familiarize themselves with the basic and then advanced laparoscopic procedures because it will become an important part of their surgical future procedures. Technologies like imaging systems, monitors and surgical energies that have developed impressively with continuous evolution have not only made surgical procedures safer and faster but also allowed the surgeons to provide better care and improved outcome for the patients. Indeed, all these changes and evolution involved the entire staff of the operating theatre from our anaesthetist colleagues to nurses. Many are involved in the development and dissemination of the minimally invasive procedure, and we hope that this comprehensive manual will be a valuable tool to help the neophytes of all the surgical specialties and those who are involved in MIS daily practice to surmount the learning stage of endo-laparoscopic surgery.

The Endoscopic and Laparoscopic Surgeons of Asia, the ELSA, as society and its members, has been charged with the responsibility to disseminate the knowledge and to assure a proper standard of training, and we are sure that with the experience of our leading experts involved in this manual we will provide a high standard of educational tools for all surgeons and colleagues.

Davide Lomanto
William Tzu-Liang Chen
Marilou B. Fuentes

Preface

In almost a century of surgery, few advances can be compared to the changes brought by the introduction of minimally invasive surgery that represent a true revolution in surgical practice for the greatest benefits offered to the patients. Since the early 1990s, laparoscopic surgery has evolved significantly covering all ranges of procedures from simple appendectomy to liver and kidney transplantation. The obvious success was mainly due to the better outcome and acceptance from patients for the several benefits. Today, some procedures have been completely replaced by laparoscopic approach also changing the way we teach and practice.

In fact, the revolution behind laparoscopic surgery also brings new concepts in training and gaining proficiency; technological advancements were introduced in training programmes like surgical simulators, virtual reality, surgical preplanning, making space for new and more objective training programme with full involvement of the surgical trainees in hands-on practice and skills acquisitions. All tools that are mandatory and necessary are accessible in current surgical training centres to enforce the skills needed for both basic and advanced procedural training. But of course, all these activities must complement also an active clinical practice with proctoring and fellowship.

In a new panorama in surgical education, more online training programmes are taking place either on online dedicated learning platforms or on social media with all the pros and cons.

The decision to publish this manual is mainly to provide to all surgical trainees and all surgeons that want to start endo-laparoscopic surgery a Compendium of core information and knowledge and also pearls and tip to learn and to improve their surgical skills.

This aim is fulfilled with the decision by the Endoscopic and Laparoscopic Surgeons of Asia (ELSA) to make it available as open access for all.

This manual has been an effort of ELSA Experts and is organized in sections in which surgical technical aspects of each procedure is presented and analysed from the procedural point of view. Our aim is to provide information in detail from patient's preparation and OR setup to the surgical steps and managements of complications.

We would like to extend our sincere appreciation to all the section editors, authors our illustrators for their contributions who have been outstanding throughout the editorial process and to our families for their continuous support.

Singapore, Singapore   Davide Lomanto
Taichung City, Taiwan   William Tzu-Liang Chen
Pasig, Philippines   Marilou B. Fuentes

Introduction

The historical development of laparoscopy can be traced back to early 1900s when Georg Kelling from Dresden in Germany, performed a celioscopy by inserting a Nitze cystoscope into the abdomen of a living dog after creating a pneumoperitoneum using air. This was the beginning of laparoscopic era; his study on physiology and anatomy together with the knowledge of using gas to insufflate the abdomen was a pioneering achievement that took laparoscopy forward. Hans Christian Jacobaeus, based on Kelling's experience, performed the first clinical laparoscopy and thoracoscopy in 1910, recognizing the immense diagnostic and therapeutic possibilities of laparoscopic surgery. A century ahead, we are now more technical and technological. With the culmination of technological advances, laparoscopic surgery is ingrained in our surgical practice, and we are able to perform diverse and complex laparoscopic procedures, also termed as minimally invasive surgery.

Laparoscopic surgery is defined by its three main components of image production (light source, laparoscope, rod lens system or today's electronic imaging and camera), pneumoperitoneum—the insufflation of carbon dioxide gas to create space for operation and laparoscopic instruments. With this combination, surgeons could perform diagnostic and some basic gynaecological procedures since the 1960s.

However, a major revolutionary shift in surgical practice and thinking came in 1988 when Philippe Mouret from France performed the first laparoscopic cholecystectomy. Instead of removing the gallbladder through a Kocher's incision, he did it through a few small wounds each not larger than 1 cm. This exciting concept sparked intense developments in instrumentation, innovation in advanced technical procedures, proliferation of training programmes and setting up of laparoscopic centres. We were indeed at the start of a modern surgery era.

Laparoscopic surgery and conventional open surgery are today co-existing and part of repertoire of any surgeons, so all young surgeon in training should develop skills in. This brings us back to the objective of writing this Manual for improvement in training and safety in practice.

Several procedures are totally being replaced by laparoscopic approach like cholecystectomy that has replaced the traditional open approach in all gallbladder disease as the new gold standard because it results in less postoperative pain, less postoperative pulmonary dysfunction, faster return of bowel function, shorter length of hospital stay, faster return to normal activities and work and greater patient satisfaction. These benefits also generally extend to other laparoscopic procedures.

The advantages mentioned, concludes the most obvious difference between laparoscopic and open surgery- that of less surgical trauma to the wound in laparoscopy. The access scar is minimized, leading to less pain, less wound infection and dehiscence with better cosmetic result. In addition, laparoscopy also reduces tissue trauma during dissection, and subsequent blood loss, systemic and immune response and adhesive complications.

From the surgeon's point of view, the projected image on the monitor is a magnified image, resulting in better definition of structures. The smaller wounds take shorter duration to close. And the video-recorded procedure can be used for review and training purposes.

As in all surgical techniques and technologies, minimally invasive surgery also has its limitations and disadvantages. First, one may encounter problems during access into the abdominal cavity, such as iatrogenic injuries to the bowel or major vascular structures. The incidence is about 0.05 to 0.1%. This incidence can be reduced by practising the open technique of introduction, rather than using the "blind" Veress needle technique and blunt-tipped trocars. Second, there may be undesirable side-effects of carbon dioxide pneumoperitoneum, such as hypercarbia (see chapter on physiology of pneumoperitoneum). And third, from the surgeon's perspective, migration from open to laparoscopic skills means that the 3D vision is reduced to monocular 2D vision on the screen, depth perception and field of view is much reduced, and haptics, or the "feel" and tactile sensation of tissues, is limited to gross probing of tissues. However, these limitations, once understood and overcome, have not hampered the development of laparoscopy.

In a way, the surgeon is required to master a new set of skills to perform laparoscopy safely. With training and experience, surgery can be performed at a new standard that benefits patients.

Laparoscopy can now be performed in three main areas of the body—the abdomen, the thorax, and closed spaces. Laparoscopy can be used to resect tissues or to reconstruct tissues.

One can see that laparoscopy is widely applied. It is important, however, to realize that for certain conditions laparoscopy is feasible but does not necessarily replace open techniques. The practice will depend on the expertise available and also on literature evidence that laparoscopy is superior to the open approach.

Surgical training is the core reason for the conception of this training manual. Surgeons in training are taught well-established skills in open surgery. However, learning of laparoscopic skills is now becoming an increasingly important part of the training programme because of the new set of skills that need to be acquired. The main focus is to operate efficiently and minimize surgical errors, i.e. operate safely. Training and constant practice are ways to overcome the learning curve. A case point is the dramatic increase by three- to fivefold in bile duct injuries in the early years when laparoscopic cholecystectomy was performed by inexperienced and poorly trained surgeons; the rate has since dropped to acceptable levels.

Minimally invasive surgery, as it stands today, has been the result of intense and continuous development and innovation on the part of surgeons in techniques, private industries in instrumentation and in no small part by public demands and patient requests. Surgical innovation will and should continue, however, while maintaining a balance of not escalating costs of healthcare delivery.

The progress of MIS will mirror that of developments in instrumentation because technical innovation and expansion into previously "difficult" territories and advanced procedures has reached a plateau. With better and newer instruments, procedures can be performed faster and more effectively, with the potential of reducing operating duration and overall costs.

With progress in information technology (IT), mass data can be exchanged faster along the Internet and 5G technologies, thus enabling more use of broadcasting and teleproctoring to remote areas. Robotic devices have been developed and today several devices are in the market ready to be used for all procedures to assist in surgery and may one day also allow surgeons to operate from remote locations. And interconnectivity of information will streamline the process of surgery.

In conclusion, laparoscopy is a marriage of surgical skills, surgical innovation and technology advancements. Training is at the core of improving surgeons so that patients benefit from the high quality of care given to them.

Davide Lomanto

Contents

Part XX   Colorectal Surgery

Part XXI   Robotic Surgery

Part XXII   Other Laparoscopic Procedures

Editors and Contributors

About the Editors

Davide Lomanto graduated with distinction (Magna cum Laude) in medicine and surgery in 1983 at the University of Rome "La Sapienza", Italy. He completed his training in general surgery in 1992 and his PhD in gastrointestinal surgery in 1990 at the University of Rome "La Sapienza", Italy, where he subsequently became Associate Professor. He spent several periods of time overseas for training in Switzerland, Germany and the USA.

Professor Lomanto is currently Professor of Surgery at the Yong Loo Lin School of Medicine, National University of Singapore; Director of the Minimally Invasive Surgical Centre (MISC) at the National University Hospital (NUH) and Director of the Tan Sri Khoo Teck Puat Advanced Surgery Training Centre (ASTC) at the National University of Singapore. He is also a Senior Consultant in General Surgery and Paediatric Surgery at NUH.

Professor Lomanto has a special interest in minimally invasive surgery, laparoscopic digestive surgery including robotic and obesity surgery and abdominal wall hernia repair. He is a fellow of international surgical societies like SAGES, EAES, ACS and ELSA. He takes part in the organizing of the International Surgical Congress and has been invited to speak and chair in many international conferences. He received more than 15 awards for his scientific studies at international congress. He is a member of the editorial committee and reviewer of several scientific surgical journals.

Professor Lomanto is the Secretary-General and Past-President of the Endoscopic and Laparoscopic Surgeons of ASIA (ELSA), founding member and Advisory President of the Asia Pacific Hernia Society (APHS), founding member and Past-President of the Asia-Pacific Metabolic and Bariatric Surgery Society (APMBSS) and President of the Asia Endoscopic Task Force (AETF). He is Secretary General and Treasurer of the International Federation of Societies of Endoscopic Surgeons (IFSES).

Professor Lomanto has more than 150 publications in international peer-reviewed surgical journals and more than 25 chapters in surgical books. He is editor of 5 surgical books. He has been awarded the honorary membership of the Surgical and Endolaparoscopic Societies of Japan (JSES), India (IAGES), Indonesia (PBEI, PERHERI), Philippines (PCS, PALES), Thailand (RCST), the European Association for Endoscopic Surgery (EAES) and the Royal

College of Surgeons of Edinburgh (FRCS). He is member of the International Committee of the Consortium of American College of Surgeons Accredited Education Institutes (ACS-AEIs). He serves as Managing Editor of Asian Journal of Endoscopic Surgery, Associate Editor of Hernia Journal and international editorial member of Surgical Endoscopy and Asian Journal of Surgery.

Professor Davide Lomanto attained his knighthood on 26 December 2009. He was conferred the prestigious award Ordine della Stella della Solidarieta Italiana by the Italian government for his leadership in clinical service, research and academic recognition as expert in the field of surgery, minimally invasive surgery and robotic surgery.

Marilou B. Fuentes is a consultant and the training officer of the Department of Surgery at The Medical City Hospital, Manila, Philippines. She is a guest faculty at the Ateneo School of Medicine and Public Health. Dr. Fuentes is a fellow of Philippine College of Surgeons, Philippine Society of General Surgeons and Philippine Association of Laparoscopic and Endoscopic Surgeons and a member of Endoscopic and Laparoscopic Surgeons of Asia (ELSA) and Asia Pacific Hernia Society (APHS).

William Tzu-Liang Chen is currently the superintendent of China Medical University Hospital Hsin-Chu. After earning his medical degree in Taiwan, he completed a research fellowship in colorectal surgery at the Cleveland Clinic in Florida. Utilizing his training and clinical experiences, he has made notable contributions to literature regarding cutting-edge techniques of colorectal minimally invasive surgery. Dr. Chen is also a charismatic speaker who has been invited to present at over many international conferences. Along with serving as a clinician and researcher, Dr. Chen is currently an associate professor in the Department of Surgery, School of Medicine at China Medical University, Taichung City, Taiwan.

Editor-in-Chief

Davide Lomanto, PhD, FAMS, FACS, FRCS Minimally Invasive Surgery Centre, National University Hospital, Singapore, Singapore

General Surgery and Minimally Invasive Surgery, Department of Surgery, National University Health System, Singapore, Singapore

Department of Surgery, YLL School of Medicine, National University Singapore, Singapore, Singapore

Editors

William Tzu-Liang Chen Division of Colorectal Surgery, Department of Surgery, China Medical University Hsinchu Hospital, Zhubei City, Hsinchu County, Taiwan

Marilou B. Fuentes, FPCS, FPSGS, FPALES Department of Surgery, The Medical City, Pasig, Manila, Philippines

Section Editors

Narendra Agarwal, MBBS MS, FCPS Department of Thoracic Surgery, Fortis Memorial Research Institute, Gurgaon, India

William Tzu-Liang Chen Division of Colorectal Surgery, Department of Surgery, China Medical University Hsinchu Hospital, Zhubei City, Hsinchu County, Taiwan

Henry Chua, MD, FPSGS, FPCS, FPALES, FACS Section of Minimally Invasive Surgery, Cebu Doctors' University Hospital, Cebu, Philippines

Advanced Minimally Invasive Surgery Fellowship Program, Cebu Doctors' University Hospital, Cebu, Philippines

Advanced Minimally Invasive Surgery, Cebu Doctors' University Hospital, Cebu, Philippines

Eva Lourdes Sta Clara, FPCS, FPSGS, FPALES Training Officer (UMIST) and Training Committee Department of Surgery, Cardinal Santos Medical Center, Manila, Philippines

Department of Surgery, Rizal Medical Center, Manila, Philippines

Department of Surgery, Asian Hospital Medical Center, Manila, Philippines

Department of Surgery, University of Perpetual Help Dalta Medical Center, Manila, Philippines

Marilou B. Fuentes, FPCS, FPSGS, FPALES Department of Surgery, The Medical City, Pasig, Philippines

Faculty of Surgery, Philippine Board of Surgery, Ateneo School of Medicine and Public Health, Manila, Philippines

Rajat Goel, MBBS, MS, DNB, MNAMS, FMIS, FMBS Supreme Superspecialty Hospital, Faridabad, India

Aakash Healthcare Superspeciality Hospital, Dwarka, New Delhi, India

Rakesh Kumar Gupta, MS, FMAS GS & MIS Unit, Department of Surgery, B.P. Koirala Institute of Health Sciences, Dharan, Nepal

Kiyotaka Imamura Minimally Invasive Surgery Center, Yotsuya Medical Cube, Tokyo, Japan

Enrico Lauro General Surgery Division, Santa Maria del Carmine Hospital, Rovereto, Italy

General Surgery Division, St. Maria del Carmine Hospital, Rovereto, Italy

Michael M. Lawenko, MD, FPCS, FPSGS, FPALES De La Salle Medical and Health Sciences Institute, Dasmarinas City, Philippines

Alembert Lee-Ong, FPCS, FPSGS, FPALES Department of Surgery, Manila Doctors Hospital, Manila, Philippines

Philippine Center for Advanced Surgery, San Juan, Philippines

Department of Surgery, Cardinal Santos Medical Center, San Juan, Philippines

Department of Surgery, Quirino Memorial Medical Center, Quezon City, Philippines

Sajid Malik, MBBS, FCPS, MRCS Department of General Surgery, Allama Iqbal Medical College, Jinnah Hospital, Lahore, Pakistan

Emily Rose Nery, DPBA, FPSA, FPSCCM Department of Anesthesiology, The Medical City, Pasig, Philippines

Acute and Critical Care Institute, The Medical City, Pasig, Philippines

Department of Anesthesiology and Perioperative Medicine, Rizal Medical Center, Pasig, Philippines

Jaideep Rao, MBBS, MRCS, MMED, FRCS, FAMS Mount Elizabeth Novena Hospital, Singapore, Singapore

Hrishikesh Salgaonkar, DNB, MRCS Department of Bariatric and Upper GI Surgery, University Hospitals North Midlands, Stoke-on-Trent, UK

Asim Shabbir, MBBS, MRCS, MMed, FCPS (Edin) National University of Singapore, Singapore, Singapore

Siau Wei Tang, BMedSci, BMBS, MMed, MRCS, FRCS Division of General (Breast) Surgery, Department of Surgery, National University Hospital, Singapore, Singapore

Division of Surgical Oncology, National University Cancer Institute, Singapore, Singapore

Le Quan Anh Tuan Department of Hepatobiliary and Pancreatic Surgery, University Medical Center, Minimally Invasive Surgical Training Center, Ho Chi Minh City, Vietnam

Department of General Surgery, University of Medicine and Pharmacy, Ho Chi Minh City, Vietnam

Authors

Arnel Abatayo, MD, FPSGS, FPCS, FPALES Department of Surgery, Chong Hua Hospital Mandaue, Cebu, Philippines

Di Leo Alberto General and Mini-Invasive Surgery, San Camillo Hospital, Rovereto, Italy

Nguyen Hoang Bac Department of Surgery, University of Medicine and Pharmacy, Ho Chi Minh city, Vietnam

Nagammapudur Balaji Department of Bariatric and Upper GI Surgery, University Hospitals North Midlands, Stoke-on-Trent, UK

Alfred Allen Buenafe, FPCS, FPSGS, FPALES Department of Surgery, Rizal Medical Center, Pasig, Philippines

Philippine Center for Advanced Surgery, San Juan, Philippines

Department of Surgery, Cardinal Santos Medical Center, San Juan, Philippines

Department of Surgery, Batangas Medical Center, Batangas, Philippines

Department of Surgery, Asian Hospital and Medical Center, Alabang, Muntinlupa, Philippines

B. Mario Cervantes Minimally Invasive Surgery and Robotic Surgery CMN 20 de Noviembre, ISSSTE CDMX, Mexico city, Mexico

Adam Frankel, MD, PhD, FRACS, FRCSEd Upper Gastro-intestinal and Soft Tissue Unit, Princess Alexandra Hospital, Brisbane, Australia

Brian K. P. Goh, MBBS, MMed, MSc, FRCSEd Department of Hepatopancreatobiliary and Transplant Surgery, Singapore General Hospital and National Cancer Centre Singapore, Singapore Liver Transplant Service, SingHealth Duke-National University of Singapore Transplant Centre, Singapore, Singapore

SingHealth Duke-NUS Liver Transplant Center, Duke-National University of Singapore Medical School, Singapore, Singapore

Emir Guldogan, MD, FEBS Department of Surgery, Liv Hospital, Ankara, Turkey

Pham Minh Hai Department of Hepatobiliary and Pancreatic Surgery, University Medical Center, Ho Chi Minh city, Vietnam

Ming Li Leonard Ho Division of Colorectal Surgery, Department of Surgery, China Medical University Hsinchu Hospital, Zhubei City, Hsinchu County, Taiwan

Chih-Kun Huang Body Science & Metabolic Disorders International Medical Center, China Medical Hospital, Taichung, Taiwan

Andreuccetti Jacopo General Surgery 2, ASST Spedali Civili of Brescia, Brescia, Italy

Cheah Wei Keat, MBBS, FRACS, FAMS, FACS General Surgery, Ng Teng Fong General Hospital, Singapore, Singapore

Division of General Surgery (Thyroid and Endocrine Surgery), Department of Surgery, University Surgical Cluster, National University Hospital, Kent Ridge, Singapore

Farah Khairi General Surgery Services, Alexandra Hospital, Queenstown, Singapore

James Lee Wai Kit Minimally Invasive Surgery Centre, National University Hospital, Singapore, Singapore

Department of Surgery, YLL School of Medicine, National University Singapore, Singapore, Singapore

Koji Kono, MD, PhD Department of Gastrointestinal Tract Surgery, Fukushima Medical University, Fukushima, Japan

Shirin Khor Pui Kwan National University Hospital, Kent Ridge, Singapore

Yeen Chin Leow Colorectal Surgery Unit, Department of Surgery, Hospital Sultanah Bahiyah, Alor Star, Malaysia

Division of Colorectal Surgery, Department of Surgery, China Medical University Hospital, Taichung, Taiwan

Chwee Ming Lim, MBBS, MRCS, MMed Department of Otorhinolaryngology-Head and Neck Surgery, Singapore General Hospital, Singapore, Singapore

Surgery Academic Clinical Programme, Duke-NUS Medical School, Singapore, Singapore

Javier Lopez-Gutierrez, FACS Minimally Invasive Surgery and Gastrointestinal Endoscopy CMN 20 de Noviembre, ISSSTE CDMX, Mexico City, Mexico

Rainier Lutanco, FPCS Department of Surgery, The Medical City, Pasig, Manila, Philippines

Raquel Maia Brazilian College of Gastric Surgeons, Sao Paulo, Brazil

Kanagaraj Marimuthu Department of Bariatric and Upper GI Surgery, University Hospitals North Midlands, Stoke-on-Trent, UK

Abdul Gafoor Mubarak, MD, MBBS, MS, MRCSED, MMED Island Hospital, Penang, Malaysia

Christina H. L. Ng, MBBS, MRCS, MMed Department of Otorhinolaryngology-Head and Neck Surgery, Singapore General Hospital, Singapore, Singapore

Elaine Hui Been Ng Colorectal Surgery Unit, Department of Surgery, Hospital Raja Permaisuri Bainum, Ipoh, Malaysia

Division of Colorectal Surgery, Department of Surgery, China Medical University Hospital, Taichung, Taiwan

Mahir Ozmen, MS, FRCS, FACS, FASMBS Department of Surgery, Medical School, Istinye University, Istanbul, Turkey

Aung Myint Oo, Upper GI, Bariatric and Metabolic Surgery, Department of General Surgery, Tan Tock Seng Hospital, Singapore, Singapore

Victor Gheorghe Radu Medlife, Bucharest, Romania

Vittal Rao Department of Bariatric and Upper GI Surgery, University Hospitals North Midlands, Stoke-on-Trent, UK

Salvatore Rizzo General Surgery Division, Cavalese Hospital, Cavalese, Italy

Vincent Matthew Roble II, MD, FPSGS, FPCS Advanced Minimally Invasive Surgery Fellowship Program, Cebu Doctors' University Hospital, Cebu, Philippines

Advanced Minimally Invasive Surgery, Cebu Doctors' University Hospital, Cebu, Philippines

Giovanni Scudo General Surgery Division, St. Maria del Carmine Hospital, Rovereto, Italy

Alistair Sharples Department of Bariatric and Upper GI Surgery, University Hospitals North Midlands, Stoke-on-Trent, UK

Isaac Seow-En Department of Colorectal Surgery, Singapore General Hospital, Singapore, Singapore

Division of Colorectal Surgery, China Medical University Hospital, Taichung, Taiwan

Rasik Shah, MCh SRCC Children's Hospital, Narayana Health, Mumbai, India

Tuhin Shah, MS, FACS Department of Surgery, Manmohan Memorial Medical College, Kathmandu, Nepal

MISC Department of Surgery, National University Hospital, Kent Ridge, Singapore

Ming-Yin Shen Division of Colorectal Surgery, Department of Surgery, China Medical University Hsinchu Hospital, Zhubei City, Hsinchu County, Taiwan

Mina Ming Yin Shen Division of Colorectal Surgery, Department of Surgery, China Medical University Hsinchu Hospital, Zhubei City, Hsinchu County, Taiwan

B. Mark Smithers, AM, MBBS, FRACS, FRCSEng, FRCSEd Upper Gastro-intestinal and Soft Tissue Unit, Princess Alexandra Hospital, Brisbane, Australia

Academy of Surgery, The University of Queensland, Brisbane, Australia

Jun Liang Teh, MBBS, MMED, ChM (Edin), FRCEsd Ng Teng Fong General Hospital, National University Health System, Singapore, Singapore

Angelica Feliz Versoza-Delgado, MD, DPBS Department of Health Informatics, De La Salle Medical and Health Sciences Institute, Dasmarinas City, Philippines

Danson Yeo, MBBS, MRCS, MMed, FRCSEd Upper Gastrointestinal and Bariatric Surgery, Department of General Surgery, Tan Tock Seng Hospital, Singapore, Singapore

Sujith Wijerathne, MBBS, MRCS, MMed, FRCS, FAMS Minimally Invasive Surgery Centre, National University Hospital Singapore, Singapore, Singapore

General Surgery Services, Alexandra Hospital, Queenstown, Singapore

Department of Surgery, YLL School of Medicine, National University Singapore, Singapore, Singapore

Mika Yamamoto Department of Surgery, Teine Keijinkai Hospital, Sapporo, Japan

George Pei Cheung Yang Hong Kong Hernia Society, Hong Kong, China

Hong Kong Adventist Hospital, Hong Kong, China

Ahmad Ramzi Yusoff, MBBCh, MSurg, MRCS Department of Surgery, Universiti Teknologi MARA, Sungai Buloh, Selangor, Malaysia

Department of Surgery, Universiti Teknologi MARA, Sg. Buloh, Selangor, Malaysia

Part I

Basic Principles

Access, Pneumoperitoneum, and Complications

Eva Lourdes Sta Clara

Creating a pneumoperitoneum, the safe way is one of the first steps a surgeon should learn in doing laparoscopic surgeries. As with any procedure, there is risk of complications which might occur like bleeding, subcutaneous emphysema, vascular injuries, and bowel injuries in accessing the abdomen.

The purpose of this chapter is to discuss the four techniques in establishing pneumoperitoneum namely the Veress needle technique, direct trocar insertion, optical trocar insertion, and open (Hasson's) technique. The choice as to which technique to choose depends on the surgeon's preference, habitus of the patient, and anticipated previous postoperative conditions like adhesions.

Veress Needle Technique

The Veress needle (Fig. 1) was invented by Janos Veress in 1930 as a tool for treating patients with tuberculosis. It was only in 1947,

that Raoul Palmer introduced its use in establishing pneumoperitoneum for laparoscopy [1].

It has an outer cannula with a beveled needle and a spring-loaded inner stylet with a dull tip which retracts as the needle goes through the abdominal wall and pushes forward once it is inside the abdominal cavity to protect the underlying viscera. Its length ranges from 7 to 15 cm with a diameter of 2 mm.

Technique: A small incision is made superior or inferior to the umbilicus just enough for the veress needle to pass through. The patient is then placed in Trendelenburg's position and the abdominal wall is lifted using towel clamps at the sides of the umbilicus to create negative pressure. The needle is then inserted with the tip towards the pelvis to prevent injuries to bowels and vessels. A "give" will be felt once it enters the peri-

E. L. Sta Clara (✉)
Training Officer (UMIST) and Training Committee
Department of Surgery, Cardinal Santos Medical
Center, Manila, Philippines

Department of Surgery, Rizal Medical Center,
Manila, Philippines

Department of Surgery, Asian Hospital Medical
Center, Manila, Philippines

Department of Surgery, University of Perpetual Help
Dalta Medical Center, Manila, Philippines

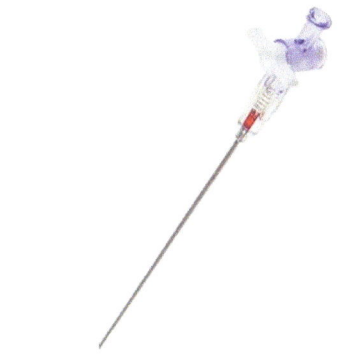

Fig. 1 Veress needle

© The Author(s) 2023
D. Lomanto et al. (eds.), *Mastering Endo-Laparoscopic and Thoracoscopic Surgery*,
https://doi.org/10.1007/978-981-19-3755-2_1

toneal cavity. Avoid moving side to side the needle as this may enlarge a bowel or vessel perforation.

Correct placement of the needle can be verified by injecting saline solution and there should be no resistance. It can also be checked by the sudden escape of air from the abdominal cavity and drop test.

Low flow insufflation of CO_2 is then started until the intraabdominal pressure reaches 13–15 mm Hg. The needle is then replaced with a sharp trocar and the scope is used immediately to verify the correct entry. The other trocars are then inserted under direct vision.

If midline adhesions are anticipated, another location to insert the Veress needle is at Palmer's point. This is located 3 cm below at left subcostal area at the midclavicular line [1]. This is recommended for obese and very thin patients.

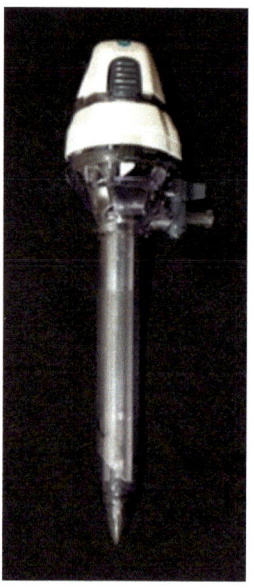

Fig. 2 Hollow trocar with transparent tip

Direct Trocar Insertion

Direct trocar insertion was first described by Dingfelder in 1978. Advocates of this technique prefer this because it excludes the use of a Veress needle thus avoiding double-blind puncture of the abdomen and is the fastest [2]. However, this must be carried out by experienced and skilled surgeons because it is a blind direct insertion. Prerequisites to this technique are adequate skin incision, sharp trocar, and a completely relaxed abdominal wall. The abdominal wall is lifted with towel clamps at the trocar and is inserted in a twisting motion. The trocar is held like a pen to avoid accidentally going too deep and inadvertently perforating bowels or vessels. The scope is then used, and an explorative laparoscopy is then done to check for injuries.

Optical Trocar Insertion

Optical trocars as seen in Fig. 2 have a hollow shaft with a transparent tip. An adequate skin incision is made then a zero-degree telescope is inserted through the trocar as the surgeon inserts the trocar through the abdominal wall in a rotat-

ing movement. The transparent tip allows direct visualization and allows the user to see the different abdominal layers as the trocar goes through the abdomen until the peritoneal cavity is reached.

Open (Hasson) Technique

Open technique was first described by Hasson in 1971. This technique lessens the probability of visceral or vascular injuries which are more commonly encountered in blind techniques [3].

A 2 cm incision is made at the umbilicus or either superior or inferior to the umbilicus. The fascia and the peritoneum are incised, and the peritoneal cavity is entered under direct vision. Finger exploration around the periumbilical area is sometimes done to determine if there are abdominal adhesions. The Hasson's trocar (Fig. 3) is then inserted and anchored with stay sutures at the fascia. The scope is then inserted to verify correct position of the trocar and to look for any injuries. Insufflation of CO_2 is then initiated at low pressure. Rapid expansion of the diaphragm might lead to vagal stimulation and bradyarrhythmias. The open technique is recommended especially for patients with previous abdominal operations.

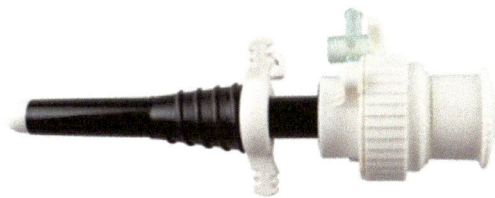

Fig. 3 Hasson's trocar

Pneumoperitoneum

Creation of the pneumoperitoneum and maintenance of it is essential in laparoscopic surgery.
Otherwise, one will not have adequate working
space. The ideal insufflating gas should be cheap,
physiologically inert, colorless, have high blood
solubility, and is nonexplosive. Some of the
insufflating agents are carbon dioxide, nitrous
oxide, helium, and argon. However, the most
used one is carbon dioxide since it is cheap, has
low toxicity, is easily reabsorbed, has a low risk
of gas embolism, and is nonexplosive [4].

Insufflation is achieved by using an insufflator
which delivers carbon dioxide at a flow rate of up to
20 L/min. The insufflator also has an alarm which
sounds when the abdominal pressure exceeds the
predetermined level, which is set at 12–15 mm Hg.
Higher pressures may lead to hypercarbia, acidosis,
and adverse hemodynamic and pulmonary effects.

Complications and Management

As in any procedure, there will always be a risk of
complications, which ranges from 0.05 to 0.2%.
However, this represents about 20–30% of the complications encountered in laparoscopic surgery. This
may be namely bowel injury, vascular injury, and
extraperitoneal gas insufflation. The most common
is extraperitoneal gas insufflation, which can be prevented by inserting the Veress needle perpendicu-
larly and making sure it is in place during the

creation of the pneumoperitoneum. One should suspect that the gas is going extraperitoneally if there is
no obliteration of the liver dull sounds and the CO_2
pressure does not rise. Conversion to open
(Hasson's) technique is advisable if there is difficulty in positioning the Veress needle safely.

Vascular injury has a low incidence rate of
0.04% however this is the most life-threatening
[5]. Immediate surgical intervention is required
and conversion to open laparotomy and subsequent vascular repair is done. The most common
vessels injured during the blind entry of the first
trocar are the following: abdominal aorta, iliac
vessel at the level of the aortic bifurcation, and
inferior vena cava. Vascular injuries usually occur
during uncontrolled forced entry.

Another complication is visceral injury. It has
a 0.13% incidence but the mortality rate can go as
high as 3.6% [6]. Whenever this is suspected it is
crucial to determine immediately the location. A
complete bowel examination is mandatory, and
the injury is sutured via open laparotomy, mini-
laparotomy, or laparoscopy. This can be repaired
based on its severity and the surgeon's choice.

References

1. Palmer R. Safety in laparoscopy. J Repro Med.
   1974;13:1–5.
2. Dingfelder JR. Direct laparoscopic trocar insertion
   without prior pneumoperitoneum. J Reprod Med.
   1978;21:45–7.
3. Hasson HM. A modified instrument and method for
   laparoscopy. Am J Obstet Gynecol. 1971;110:886–7.
4. Neuhaus SJ, Gupta A, Watson DI. Helium and other
   alternative insufflation gases for laparoscopy. Surg
   Endosc. 2014;15:553–60.
5. Molloty et al. Laparoscopic entry: a literature review
   and analysis of technique and complications of primary port entry. Aust N Z J Obstet Gynaecol 2002.
6. der Voort V, EAM H, Gourma DJ. Bowel injury as
   complication of laparoscopy. BJS. 2004;91:1253–8.

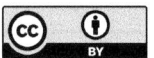

Image Systems in Endo-Laparoscopic Surgery

Michael M. Lawenko
and Angelica Feliz Versoza-Delgado

Introduction

The field of minimally invasive surgery (MIS) has seen tremendous growth and advancement since its advent in the 1980s. New procedures, MIS techniques, and instruments are evolving regularly which makes it important for surgeons to be familiar with these developments. MIS is a technologically dependent specialty and every surgeon is expected to have good background knowledge of new instruments and imaging systems. Endo-laparoscopic surgery is conducted using an array of imaging devices that are all interconnected. Basic components of the image systems in endo-laparoscopy include a telescope connected to a light source and a controller unit. The images are then transmitted through a monitor that allows the surgical team to visualize the operative field. Documentation of the surgical procedure, both real-time and recorded, can be achieved through a video recording hub and/or printer.

Telescope

There are two common types of endoscope: One using standard Rod-lens system and the other is a fully digital scope using a camera chip on the tip of the rigid or flexible endoscope.

The conventional Endoscope is made of surgical stainless steel and contains a series of optical lens comprised of precisely aligned glass lenses and spacers (so-called Rod Lens System). It contains an objective lens, which is located at the distal tip of the rigid endoscope, which determines the viewing angle. The light post at right angles to the shaft allows attachment of the light cable to the telescope. The eyepiece or ocular lens remains outside of the patient's body and is attached to a camera to view the images on a video monitor.

Telescopes or laparoscopes come in various diameters. The 10 mm diameter is the most commonly used scope and provides the greatest light and visual acuity. Other varieties are the 5 mm and 2–3 mm needlescopes which is mostly used in children. Full screen 5 mm laparoscopes capable of providing images comparable to 10 mm systems are now available in the market. Various visualization capabilities such as a 0° forward viewing, 30 or 45° telescope are the varieties (Fig. 1).

Advances in digital endoscopy utilizes a chip on the tip (CMOS or CCD) of a rigid videolaparoscope (e.g., Endoeye Olympus™) or flexible endoscope. There is no longer an interface

M. M. Lawenko (✉)
De La Salle Medical and Health Sciences Institute,
Dasmarinas City, Philippines
e-mail: mmlawenko@dlshsi.edu.ph

A. F. Versoza-Delgado
Department of Health Informatics, De La Salle
Medical and Health Sciences Institute,
Dasmarinas City, Philippines

© The Author(s) 2023
D. Lomanto et al. (eds.), *Mastering Endo-Laparoscopic and Thoracoscopic Surgery*,
https://doi.org/10.1007/978-981-19-3755-2_2

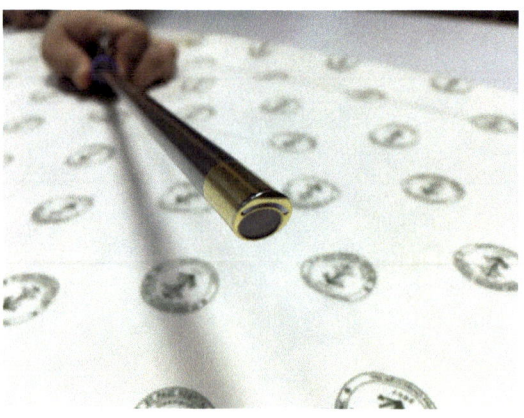

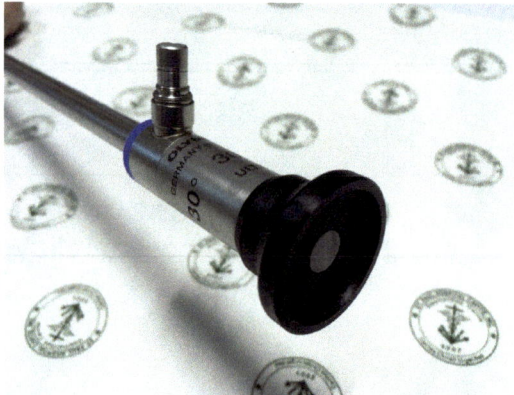

Fig. 1 10 mm forward oblique telescope (30°)

between the camera head and the endoscope, and traditional rod lenses are no longer used. In lieu of this, a distally mounted image sensor with a lens is used. This delivers better resolution and clarity of images. It also offers a focus-free and better ergonomic design. These scopes are also autoclavable.

Light Source

This is critical for visualization of the operative field. A typical light source is composed of a lamp or bulb, a condensing lens, a heat filter, and an intensity-controlled circuit. Light quality is dependent on the type of lamp that is used. Most light sources nowadays use the high-intensity xenon light source which provides white light illumination (Fig. 2). The previous light sources used a quartz halogen bulb, incandescent bulbs, and metal halide vapor arc lamps.

Newer light sources have incorporated the use of LED technology. An LED light source is able to deliver cold, white light that generates virtually no heat. These light sources are energy-efficient and noiseless. Compared to Xenon light sources (Fig. 2), LED light sources offer up to 30,000 h of service life and therefore do not require lamp changes.

Light Cable

Light is transmitted from the lamp to the laparoscope through cables (Fig. 3). The two types of cables are the fiberoptic and the liquid crystal gel cable.

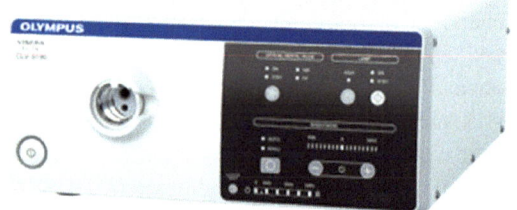

Fig. 2 Xenon light source (Olympus VISERA ELITE™)

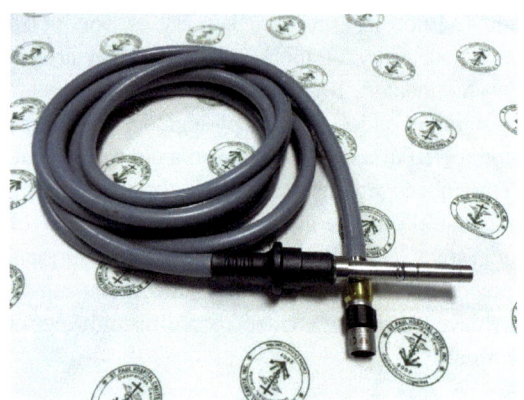

Fig. 3 Fiberoptic light cable

The principle of fiberoptic cables is based on the total internal reflection of light wherein light would enter one end of the fiber after numerous internal reflections and go out through the other end with virtually all its strength intact. Fiberoptic cables are flexible but do not transmit a precise light spectrum. They have a very high quality of optical transmission but are fragile.

Liquid crystal gel cable is composed of a sheath that is filled with a clear gel. These cables are capable of transmitting more light than optic fibers. They can transmit a complete spectrum but are more rigid and fragile. Liquid crystal gel cables require soaking for sterilization and cannot be gas sterilized.

Camera Head (From 2D to 3D Technology)

Since the advent of laparoscopy, technologies in camera systems have quickly evolved. A few decades ago, the main technology utilized in minimal access surgery was the charged coupled device. Now, two new systems are at the cutting edge of surgical video technology: 3D and UHD/4 K. These systems were developed with the goal of providing better imaging and better depth perception.

The traditional camera for endo-laparoscopic surgery (Fig. 4) contains a solid-state silicon chip or the charged coupled device (CCD). This essentially functions as an electric retina and consists of an array of light-sensitive silicon elements. Silicon emits an electrical charge when exposed to light. These charges can be amplified, transmitted, displayed, and recorded. Each silicon element contributes one unit (referred to as a pixel) to the total image. The resolution or clarity of the image depends upon the number of pixels or light receptors on the chip. Standard cameras in endo-

laparoscopic use contains 250,000–380,000 pixels. The single-chip camera has a composite transmission in which three colors of red, blue, and green are compressed into a single chip. The three-chip camera has a separate chip for each color with a high resolution. The clarity of the image eventually displayed or recorded will also depend on the resolution capability of the monitor and the recording medium. The resolution is defined as the number of vertical lines that can be discriminated as separate in three quarters of the width of the monitor screen. Standard consumer-grade video monitors have 350 lines, monitors with about 700 lines are preferred for laparoscopy.

Three-dimensional (3D) cameras have been developed to overcome the lack of depth perception in traditional 2D laparoscopy. In 3D laparoscopy, different images are presented to each of the surgeon's eyes to facilitate stereopsis. This is accomplished using two different technologies: by a single channel laparoscopes with one system of lenses, then using a digital filter to separate the images for each eye; another system utilizes a dual channel laparoscopes with one lens system for each eye, this provides a real and better stereovision (Fig. 5).

In both technologies, it is necessary for the surgeons and the OR Staff to wear passive or active stereoscopic glasses to visualize the 3D Image (Fig. 6a–c).

The eyepieces which may be shutter glasses, head mounted displays/headsets or passive polariz-

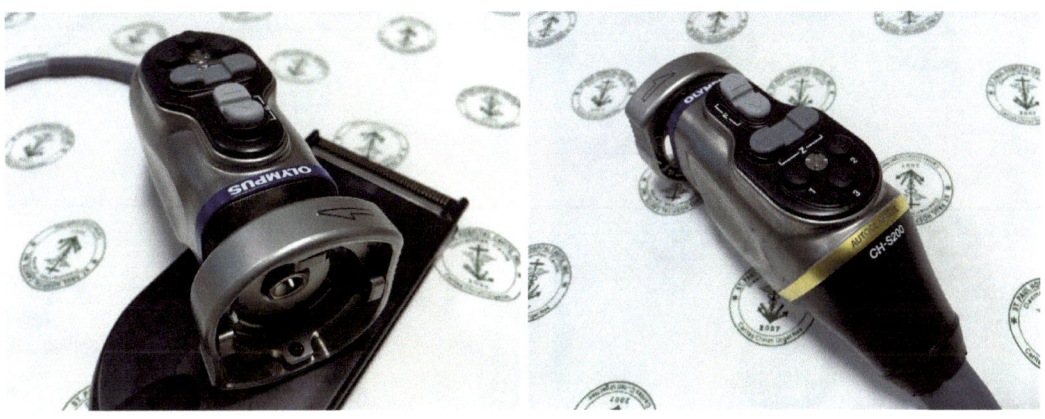

Fig. 4 HD camera head

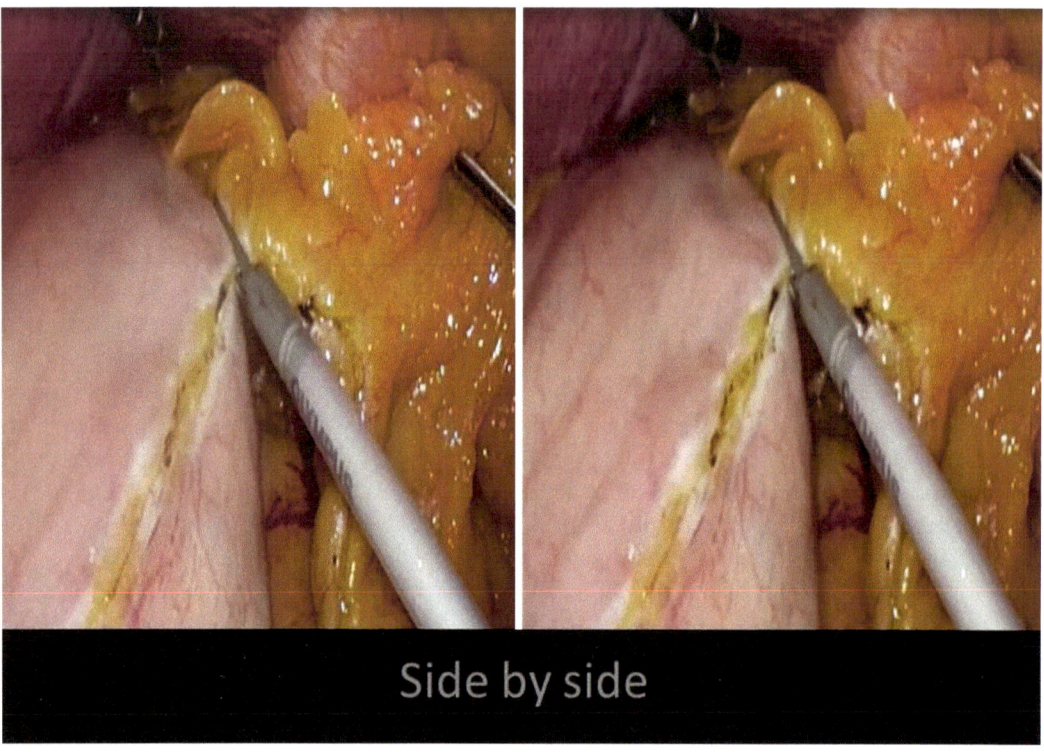

Fig. 5 Dual channel telescope with two images one for each eye

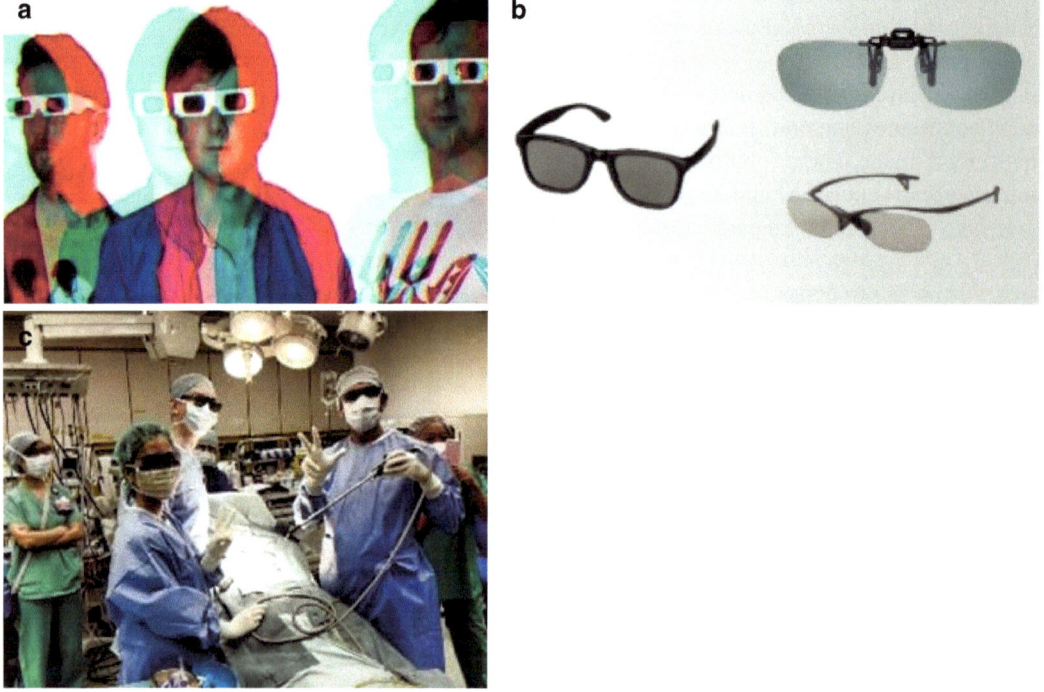

Fig. 6 (**a**) Anaglyph lens (not for medical use), (**b**) Passive polarization lens for medical use, (**c**) OR team wearing passive lenses

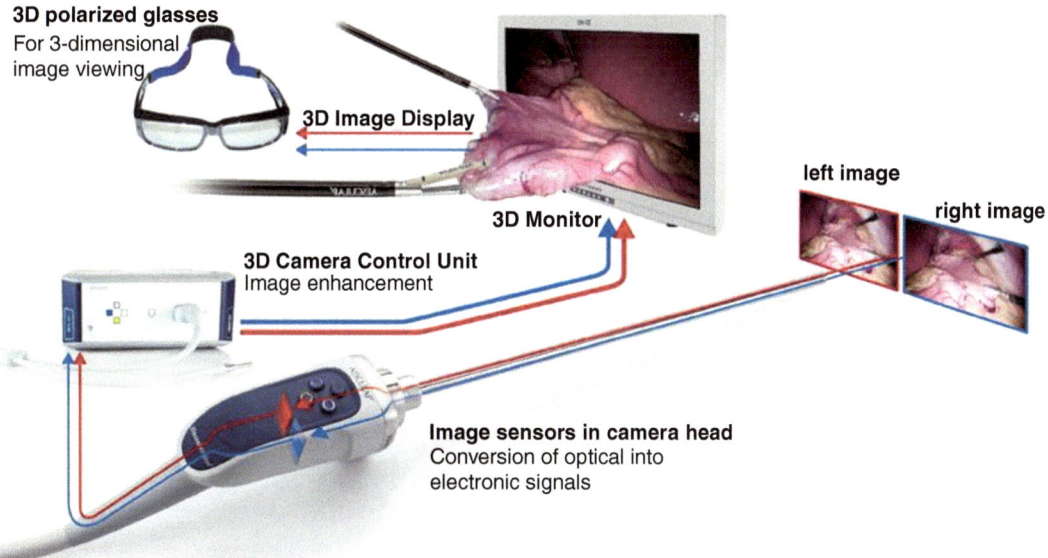

Fig. 7 3D technology in laparoscopy (Aesculap EinsteinVision®)

ing glasses are the most commonly utilized. Disadvantages of 3D laparoscopy involve a higher cost of video systems, need to wear 3D glasses, and eye fatigues even though the evolution of a new 3D system in the last decade have reduced most of the side effects and improved sensibly the quality of the image (Fig. 7). On the other side better accuracy and performance, easier depth judgment, and better identification of structure at different depth levels have been shown in several studies that improve significantly surgical performance, reduce fatigue, and are helpful in demanding tasks like suturing and fine dissection with an overall reduced time for skills acquisition.

Similar to a fixed 0° 3D telescope, there was a development of a flexible tip fiberoptic telescope to overcome the lack of angled vision (Fig. 8).

The challenges of 3D Image adoption and the evolution in imaging for both professional and consumers has also evolved in the medical field with the advent of 4 K technology. After an initial shifting from standard definition to high definition (1920×1080) today more surgeons utilized the 4 K technology in which resolution is 3840×2160 that allow the use of larger monitor (40″–65″ and bigger) with an incredible perception of the fine anatomical details. Fine structure that is used to be blurred in HD become clearer in 4 K and no more pixelation effect on the large

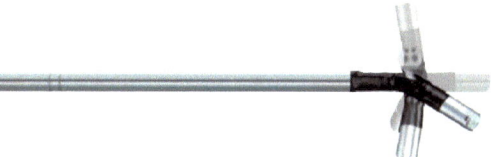

Fig. 8 Flexible tip telescope for angled vision

monitors. This indirectly provides a better depth perception due to improved clarity and light reaction to the anatomic structures.

Certainly, evolution will continue for surgical imaging with 8 K in development and may be further higher resolution to provide an even better visual experience superior to reality.

Controller Unit

The function of the controller unit is to capture and process the video signals taken by the telescope and camera head to the video monitor to provide an accurate visualization of the operative field. It also functions to convert gathered video signals to digital HD images or downgrade it to standard definition (SD) images.

The control unit is attached to the camera head in its front console while connections to the video monitor are at the back panel. Connection to the

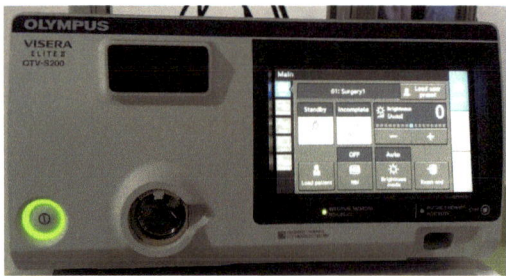

Fig. 9 Video system center unit with both image processor and light source

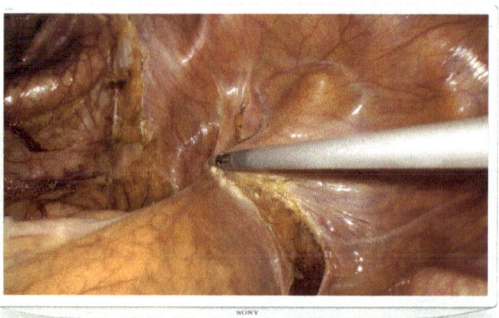

Fig. 10 4 K image quality

video monitor is in the form of digital cables which are the digital video interface (DVI) for the HD image and the serial digital interface (SDI) for the SD image. Newer controller units combine both image processor and light source functions in one unit (Fig. 9).

Video Monitor

High-resolution liquid crystal display (LCD) monitors are suitable for the reproduction of endoscopic image. This is a type of monitor wherein grids of liquid crystals are arranged in RGB (red-green-blue) triads in front of a light source to produce an image. In general, the resolution capability of the monitor should match that of the video camera. Three chip cameras require monitors with 800–900 lines of resolution to realize the improved resolution of the extra chip sensors. Two separate monitors on each side of the table are commonly used for laparoscopic procedures. The use of special video carts for housing the monitor and other video equipment allows greater flexibility and maneuverability.

A larger screen displaying the same number of pixels will have a lower spatial resolution compared to a smaller screen since the resolution is dependent on the pixel density. The advantage of ultra high definition UHD-4 K technology in laparoscopy monitors is it allows the image to be displayed on a larger screen of up to 55 in without compromising the resolution of 4098 × 2160 pixels (Fig. 10). Larger 4 K screens are available

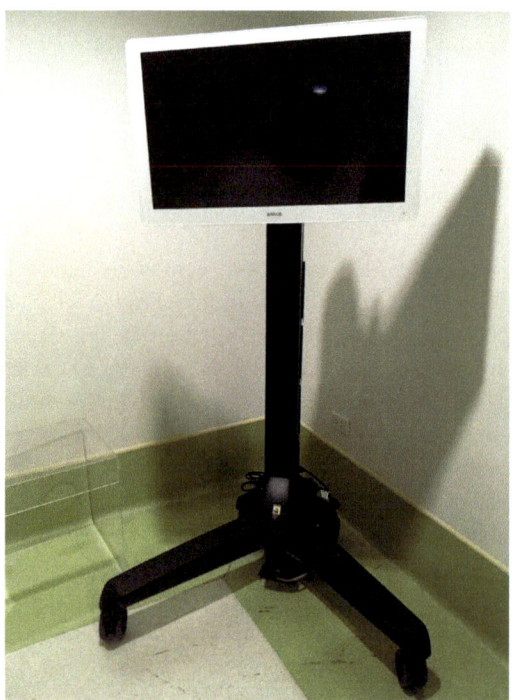

Fig. 11 LED video monitor

in different sizes ranging from 40–55 in. This optimizes the surgeon's performance in minimally invasive surgery. With these features, 4 K systems are being used as an alternative to the passive polarizing 3D display systems.

Some medical-grade monitors are now equipped with LED (light-emitting diode) or OLED (organic light-emitting diode) technology. LED monitors (Fig. 11) also feature a liquid crystal display panel to control where light is displayed on the screen, but the backlighting is produced using more efficient LEDs instead of fluorescent lamps. When used in endo-laparoscopy, these monitors are able to produce an extremely detailed image representation of the operative field. They offer several advantages which include high resolution, excellent image response times, and more precise and faithful color reproduction compared to traditional LCD monitors.

Documentation

A video recorder or a printer can be utilized for documentation during a surgical procedure. Today, both digital videos and images can be captured either on a medium like CD-DVD or digitally like a hard drive, USB, etc. The standard documentation equipment housed in the video card has multiple functions. First, a digitally recorded file can be transferred to an optical media device such as a digital video disc (DVD). Second, video snapshots taken during a procedure can be printed on a digital printer.

Recent technology available for intraoperative documentation provides full HD for still/video images along with two-channel, simultaneous real-time recording. It has the capability of processing records, managing images as well as editing (Fig. 12).

Integrated Operating Room

As surgical equipment continues to modernize, advanced operating theaters (OT) are now using systems integration (Fig. 13). This functionally connects the OT environment including the patient information system, audio, video, surgical lights, and other aspects of building automation. When integrated, all the technology used in the OT can be controlled through a single command console by a single operator. This provides seamless connections between equipment and personnel inside and out of the OT. To improve the space within the OT, devices are mounted on movable arms or carts that can swing around the patient to optimize visualization. These mounts allow proper positioning of the monitors and image systems in relation to the different areas of the patient's body during a surgical procedure. Integration allows not only a centralized control of the different units but also interaction with any external party like Meeting Rooms, Conference Centre, or for any other educational purpose. This avoids unnecessary visitors within the sterile operating field.

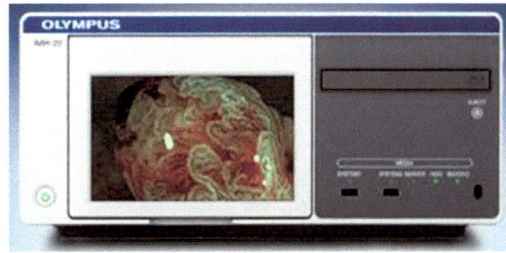

Fig. 12 Image management hub

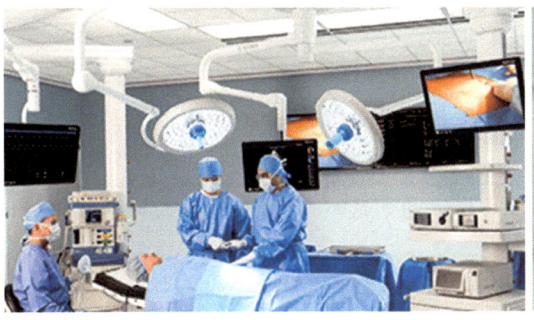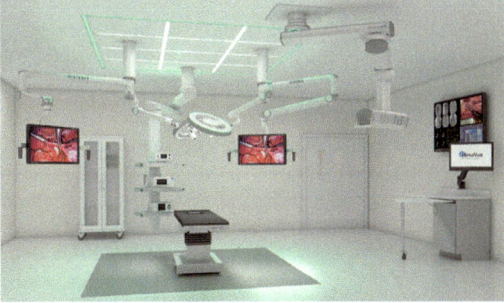

Fig. 13 Example of integrated operating room (Hexavue™ Integration System)

Further Reading

3D Technology in Laparoscopy. https://www.bbraun.com/en/products-and-therapies/laparoscopic-surgery/3d-technology-in-laparoscopy.html.

Destro F, et al. 3D laparoscopic monitors. Med Equip Insights. 2014;5:9–12.

Ohuchida K, et al. New advances in three-dimensional endoscopic surgery. J Gastrointest Dig Syst. 2013;3:152.

Olympus Endoeye. https://www.olympus-europa.com/medical/rmt/media/en/Content/Content-MSD/Documents/Brochures/HD_EndoEye_EN_201303.pdf

Schwab K, et al. Evolution of stereoscopic imaging in surgery and recent advances. World J Gastrointest Endosc. 2017;9:368–77.

Siddharth V, Kant S, Chandrashekhar R, Gupta SK. Integration in operation theater: need of the hour. Int J Res Foundation Hosp Healthc Adm. 2015;3(2):123–8.

Sørensen SMD, et al. Three-Dimesional versus two-dimensional vision in laparoscopy: a systematic review. Surg Endosc. 2016;30:11–23.

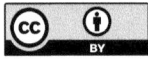

Care and Handling of Laparoscopic Instrumentations

Alembert Lee-Ong and Shirin Khor Pui Kwan

Introduction

Laparoscopic instrumentation ranging from operating telescopes and fiber optic light cables to surgical instruments represents a substantial investment for the operating theater department [1, 2]. The delicate nature of these devices and the high cost involved in the acquisition and subsequently to maintain or repair them when damaged, warrants surgeons, nurses, and reprocessing personnel to handle them carefully and appropriately at all times. Proper care and handling of laparoscopic instrumentation can help to prolong their lifespan and maintain them at an optimal performance level. With the goal of delivering the finest in-patient care, all surgical team members and reprocessing personnel must be familiar with the use of and recommendations for care and handling of all laparoscopic instrumentation.

Care and Handling of Telescopes

The telescope is the most expensive and fragile component of laparoscopic instrumentation. It is also an integral part of the instrumentation, providing image and light through two distinct systems. As such, telescopes must be handled with care from the start to the end of the surgery, and also during the cleaning and sterilization process.

All surfaces of a telescope should be inspected regularly for any scratches, dents, or other flaws. The telescope should also be inspected before each use to assess functional integrity. The eyepiece should be examined to evaluate the clarity of the image from the reflected light. In addition, it is also important to check the optical fibers surrounding the lens train at the tip of the telescope by holding the light post toward a bright light. If the image is discolored or hazy or there is the presence of black dots or shadowed areas, it may be due to improper cleaning, a disinfectant residue, a cracked or broken lens, the presence of internal moisture, or external damage.

When using a metal cannula, the telescope should be inserted gently into the lumen, so as not to break or scratch the lens. At any point of time during use or cleaning and disinfection process, the telescope should not be bent during handling, and avoid placing any heavy instruments on top of the telescope. The telescope also should never be placed near the edge of a sterile trolley or surgical field to prevent it from accidental

A. Lee-Ong (✉)
Department of Surgery, Manila Doctors Hospital, Manila, Philippines

Philippine Center for Advanced Surgery, San Juan, Philippines

Department of Surgery, Cardinal Santos Medical Center, San Juan, Philippines

Department of Surgery, Quirino Memorial Center, Quezon City, Philippines

S. K. P. Kwan
National University Hospital, Kent Ridge, Singapore

© The Author(s) 2023
D. Lomanto et al. (eds.), *Mastering Endo-Laparoscopic and Thoracoscopic Surgery*,
https://doi.org/10.1007/978-981-19-3755-2_3

dropping onto the floor. When transferring the telescope from one point to another, it is best done by gripping the ocular lens in the palm and never by the shaft. Immediately after use, wash the surfaces of the telescope with a soft cloth or sponge using a neutral pH enzymatic solution and a thorough rinse with distilled water to remove any residual cleaning solution.

Care and Handling of Light Cables

Another important component of laparoscopic instrumentation is the use of a light source cable to transmit light through the telescope to view the operative field. Light cables are made of hundreds of glass fibers to transmit the light, and these fibers can be broken if the cable is dropped, kinked, or bent at extreme angles. Following are some general guidelines regarding the care and maintenance of light cables:

- Avoid squeezing, stretching, or sharply bending the cable.
- Grasp the connector piece when inserting or removing the light cord from the light source. Never pull the cable directly when disconnecting it from the light source.
- Avoid puncturing the cable with towel clips, when securing the cables to the surgical drape.
- Do not turn the light source on before connecting the light cable to the telescope to prevent igniting a fire on the surgical drape.
- Inspect the cable for broken fibers before each use.
- Inspect both ends of the cable to ensure they have a clean, reflective, and polished surface.
- Wipe the fiber optic light cable gently to remove all blood and organic materials immediately after use using a mild detergent.

Insulation Care

The majority of laparoscopic instruments have an insulation sheath; this isolates the current flow along the hand instrument from the electrosurgical post to the tip of the instrument where the desired tissue effect is needed. Damage to the insulation results from a combination of physical insult, mechanical degradation, cleaning, temperature cycling from repeated sterilization, and high-voltage corona heating [3–5].

Insulation failures can result in inadvertent electrosurgical injuries by providing alternate pathways for the current; these breaks need not be large, as the current density is inversely proportional to the area size of the break which it passes. A good portion (18%) of these insulation failures have been detected in the segment described as "Zone 2" by Voyles and Tucker; proximal to the segment in view by the monitor but outside of the port cannula and is likely to cause devastating injuries.

Visual inspection of the insulation sheath is suggested before use, after use, and after the processing of the instruments [6]. Some instrument manufacturers have designed the insulation in double layers, the underlying brighter colored layer ease detection of a break in the outer layer. However, only 10% of insulation failures are detected visually.

The use of a current leak or insulation break detector improved break identification, Yaznadi and Krause [3] noted a significant decrease in the prevalence of insulation breaks after an institution established routine testing with such a device.

Cleaning, Disinfecting, and Sterilizing of Laparoscopic Instruments

Reprocessing laparoscopic instruments is one of the toughest challenges to OR personnel today. These instruments are extremely difficult to clean because of their long shaft and complex jaw assemblies, which may trap infectious bioburden and debris. The positive pressure of the CO_2 in the insufflated abdomen may also cause blood and other body fluids to flow up into these channels, and making them difficult or impossible to remove. Many of these instruments cannot be disassembled to facilitate manual cleaning, an ultrasonic cleaning system may be contraindicated due to the small joints and jaws. Nevertheless, for effective sterilization to take place, surgical instruments need to be clean and free from all bioburden. And meticulous cleaning should begin at the point of use and immediately after a surgical procedure.

To assist in the subsequent cleaning process, laparoscopic instruments should be periodically wiped down with a wet sponge and flushed with solutions during surgery to prevent bioburden solidification. The instruments should also be immersed in an enzymatic solution immediately following a procedure to initiate the decontamination procedure. Items in these instruments that can be disassembled should be disassembled to its smallest parts, and those with flush ports should be flushed, before soaking and cleaning. For the cleaning process, a detergent with a neutral pH of 7.0 is recommended and avoids using abrasives, such as steel wool, that could disrupt the surface of the instruments. Instead use appropriate cleaning tools, such as soft bristle brushes, to adequately clean ports, lumens, serrations, fulcrums, box locks, and crevices. Both the external and internal surfaces of the instruments must be cleaned thoroughly if not, they cannot be sterilized. If available, automatic cleaning devices, with port and lumen flusher systems, can be used to assist in completely cleaning the instruments. Contradictory to telescopes and light cables, which should not be routinely cleaned in an ultrasonic device (as the vibration may damage the tiny fiberoptic bundles), laparoscopic instruments can be cleaned using an ultrasonic cleaner, where appropriate.

Following the cleaning process, the devices should be sterilized or high-level disinfected using chemical agents. Glutaraldehyde is one of the most appropriate chemical high-level disinfectants for soaking laparoscopes and accessories because they do not damage rubber, plastics, or lens adhesive. For sterilization, steam, liquid immersion, or plasma are some of the sterilization modalities that can be used. Nevertheless, since the manufacturers are responsible for developing instructions for a process, which will render a properly cleaned instrument sterile while preserving its function, the instruments should be sterilized according to the manufacturers' written instructions.

Conclusion

Proper care and handling of laparoscopic instrumentation can help prevent malfunctions and rapid deterioration, which in turn eliminates costly repairs and replacements. Every member of the surgical team together with the reprocessing personnel must work collaboratively to achieve this important goal, to ensure the delivery of the safest and highest quality of patient care.

References

1. Zucker KA. Surgical laparoscopy. St Louis, Mo: Quality Medical Publishing; 2001.
2. The SAGES manual. New York: Springer-Verlag; 1999.
3. Yazdani A, Krause H. Laparoscopic instrument insulation failure: the hidden hazard. J Minim Invasive Gynecol. 2007;14(2):228–32.
4. Alkatout I, Schollmeyer T, Hawaldar NA, et al. Principles and safety measures of electrosurgery in laparoscopy. JSLS. 2012;16(1):130–9.
5. Montero PN, Robinson TN, Weaver JS, et al. Insulation failure in laparoscopic instruments. Surg Endosc. 2010;24(2):462–5.
6. Voyles CR, Tucker RD. Education and engineering solutions for potential problems with laparoscopic monopolar electrosurgery. Am J Surg. 1992;164(1):57–62.

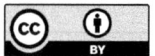

Electrosurgery and Energy Devices

Sajid Malik, Farah Khairi, and Sujith Wijerathne

Energy Devices

Energy and surgery have evolved together so closely that in the modern era, even thinking of doing surgery without energy has become nearly impossible. There are many types of energy devices available to be used today but to use them safely, the knowledge on the principles of surgical energy and safety is important.

During electrosurgery, radiofrequency alternating current is used to raise intra-cellular temperature to achieve vaporization or a combination of desiccation and protein coagulation. And these effects of old electro surgery devices (Fig. 1) have been modified in various energy devices to achieve the desired effects on the tissues such as cutting, coagulation, sealing or approximation of tissue, or a combination of these in new electrosurgery devices (Figs. 2 and 3). The electromagnetic energy is first converted to kinetic energy inside the cells then the kinetic energy gets converted to thermal energy and the desired effect in the tissue is determined by the electrical properties of the equipment being used, type, shape, size, thickness of the tissues as well as the duration of exposure.

Electrosurgical unit (ESU) or electrosurgical generators (Figs. 1, 2, and 3) are an essential part of modern-day surgery and nearly all operation theaters will include at least one of them. It converts alternating current with 50–60 Hz to a radiofrequency output of around 500 KHz. During the use of ESU, the patient or the tissue is included in the circuit.

Most ESUs (Figs. 1 and 2) have two types of outputs. Namely, they are "cut" and "coagulation." Some of the ESUs have a combination of these two that is known as "blend." "Cut" uses low voltage and continuous output from the generator which is characterized by continuous waveform. "Coagulation" uses high voltage and modulated and dampened output from the generator. "Blend" options use a combination of these settings at varying degrees to achieve the desired effect on tissues [1] (Fig. 3). The ESU output will travel through one electrode and enter the patient or the tissues and need to return back to the ESU through a second electrode to complete the circuit.

S. Malik (✉)
Allama Iqbal Medical College, Jinnah Hospital, Lahore, Pakistan

F. Khairi
General Surgery Services, Alexandra Hospital, Queenstown, Singapore

S. Wijerathne
General Surgery Services, Alexandra Hospital, Queenstown, Singapore

General Surgery and Minimally Invasive Surgery, Department of Surgery, National University Health System, Kent Ridge, Singapore

© The Author(s) 2023
D. Lomanto et al. (eds.), *Mastering Endo-Laparoscopic and Thoracoscopic Surgery*, https://doi.org/10.1007/978-981-19-3755-2_4

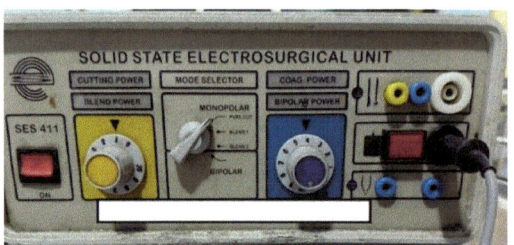

Fig. 1 Old solid state electrosurgical unit

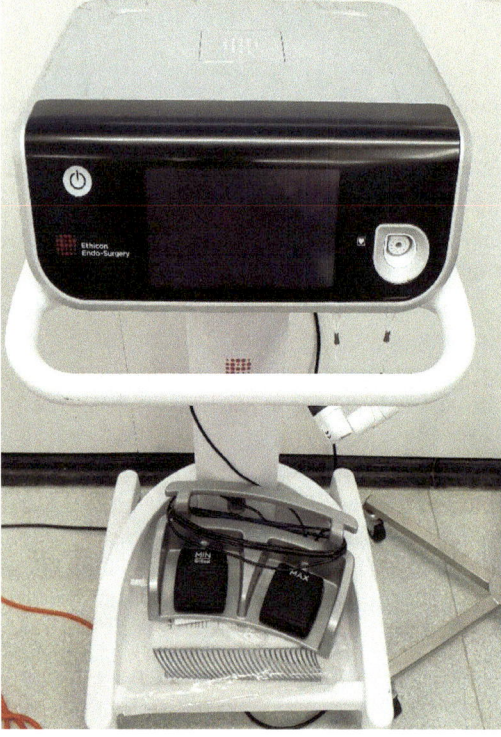

Fig. 2 Ethicon endo-surgery unit-harmonic

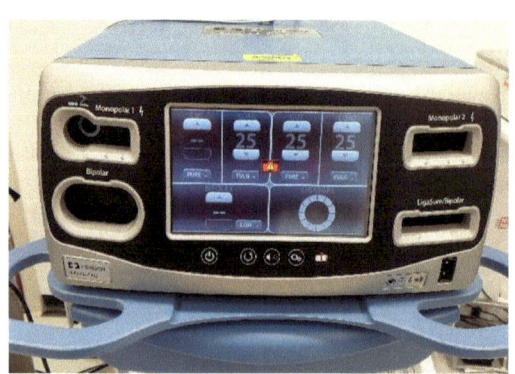

Fig. 3 Modern valleylab FT 10 energy platform

Monopolar Systems

In Monopolar instruments, the surface area of the active electrode is significantly smaller compared to the dispersive electrode in order to achieve the desired effect on the tissues and to prevent injury to the patient at the dispersive electrode end. Therefore, during Monopolar systems, the entire patient becomes part of the circuit. The routine handheld monopolar instrument, Laparoscopic monopolar instrument with hook, and Multi-tined radiofrequency ablation instrument are examples for monopolar systems (Figs. 4, 5, and 6).

During the use of monopolar systems, the active electrode can be held a few millimeters away from the tissue and by using high voltage output from the generator a tissue effect called Fulguration can be achieved. During this process, the high voltage allows ionization of the media in the gap between the electrode and tissue and causes superficial coagulation and carbonization of tissues. A similar principle is used during the Argon beam coagulator that is used to achieve hemostasis without tissue contact. Argon gas is used as the medium between the tissue and the electrode, in this case, to facilitate arcing of the current [1].

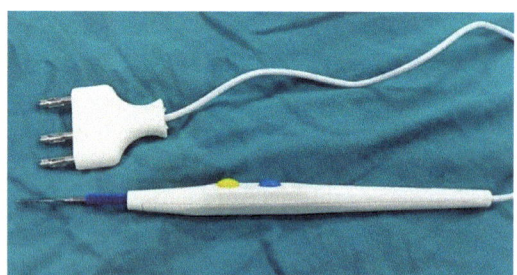

Fig. 4 Monopolar hand control diathermy

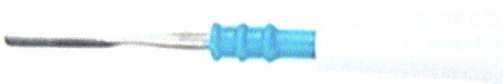

Fig. 5 Monopolar diathermy tip

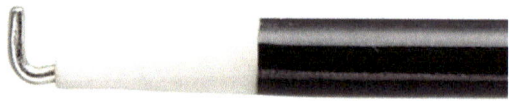

Fig. 6 Laparoscopic monopolar L-hook

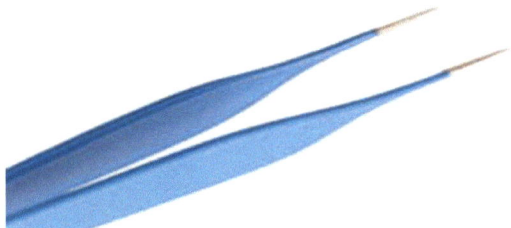

Fig. 7 Bipolar diathermy tip

Bipolar Systems

In bipolar systems, both electrodes are incorporated into the instrument and are at the tissue level. The output from the ESU only goes through the tissues that lie between the two electrodes of the instrument. Bipolar forceps used in both open and laparoscopic surgery are examples of bipolar systems (Fig. 7).

Mechanisms of Electrosurgical Injury

It is important to understand the principles of electrosurgery for early identification and prevention of electrosurgical injury. In relation to the ESU, these injuries can happen anywhere between the active electrode and the dispersive electrodes include the sites of the two electrodes.

At the active electrode site, injuries can happen because of inadvertent activation of the electrode or as a result of direct extension of the desired tissue effect beyond the targeted area which is also known as the lateral thermal spread or damage.

Dispersive electrode should be applied on a clean and dry area of skin and this area should not have excess hair that would result in entrapment of air and also should be away from any metal implants or bony prominences to avoid any thermal injury. Partial detachment of the dispersive electrode can also result in thermal burns but the new ESU has built-in safety systems to detect adequate contact between the dispersive electrode and the application site of the patient.

The other mechanism of injury is due to current diversion. All our active electrodes come with insulation except at its tip to protect the rest of the instrument and the surgeon and to make the surface area of the active electrode smaller to ensure desired tissue effect. This insulation can get damaged due to repeated usage and this can result in diversion of current from the noninsulated areas to adjacent tissues resulting in injuries and this is called insulation failure.

Direct coupling can happen if an active electrode is activated while another metal instrument is in contact with it, resulting in injury to the tissues that the metal instrument touches. Capacitive coupling happens when the circuit is not completed when an active electrode is activated with high voltage output and when using longer instruments with thin insulation in narrow metal trocars. There is a buildup of charge between two conductors that are separated by the insulator that can get discharged to adjacent tissues causing injury. Injury can also happen if the insulation of the wires in the circuit is damaged causing diversion of the current [2].

Advanced Bipolar Devices

The flow of current in a bipolar device is only through the tissue between the two electrodes therefore the tissue effect can be precisely controlled to minimize the lateral thermal injury. In advanced bipolar devices, the ESU is capable of recognizing the impedance in the tissue grasped between the two electrodes or jaws of an instrument while the energy is delivered, and these ESU microprocessors (Fig. 8) are able to then adjust the amount of energy delivered based on the impedance. And this process allows for adequate tissue sealing while minimizing collateral tissue damage.

Most modern advanced bipolar devices are capable of sealing vessels up to 7 mm in diameter. However, the advanced bipolar devices use a mechanical blade hidden within the jaws to cut the sealed tissue once the sealing is complete.

LigaSure™ (Medtronic, USA) and ENSEAL (Ethicon Endo-Surgery, USA) are some of the

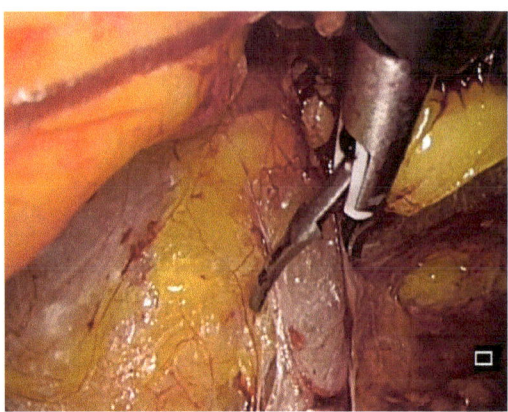

Fig. 8 Laparoscopic advanced ESU bipolar micro bisect

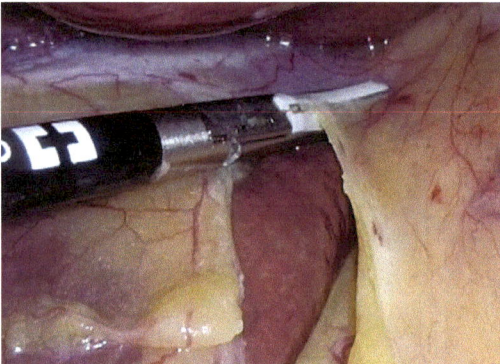

Fig. 9 Laparoscopic advanced bipolar-Ligasure device

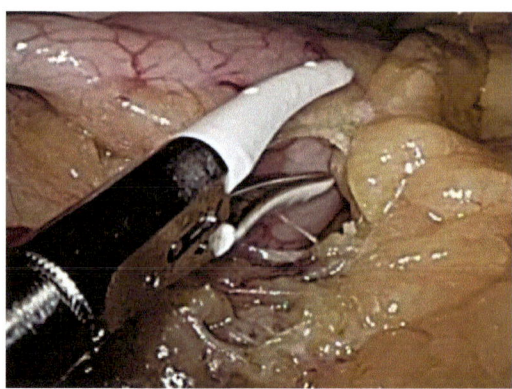

Fig. 10 Ligasure energy device tip insulation

examples of advanced bipolar energy devices that are currently available. Lamberton et al. [3] compared three of the 5 mm bipolar (Ligasure V, Gyrus PK, and Enseal) and an Ultrasonic energy device in a bovine model to check for burst pressure, vessel sealing time, and measurements of lateral thermal spread. They found that the Ligasure device (Figs. 9 and 10) attained consistent seals with burst pressure above 150 mmHg for a majority (80%) of repeated applications while all other devices performed at 50 %. The time needed for vessel sealing was also shortest for Ligasure and longest for EnSeal. The maximal lateral tissue temperature which was measured by a needle thermistor placed 2 mm from the edge of the instrument showed that the ultrasonic energy device had the lowest recorded.

In most other studies comparing similar instruments, the burst pressures were well above physiologic blood pressure and they achieved vessel seals within 8 s [4–10].

Ultrasonic Energy Devices

Ultrasonic energy device systems convert electrical energy into mechanical energy. And these systems use frequencies between 23 and 55 kHz. The tissue effects of these devices include mechanical cutting, desiccation, protein coagulation, cavitation, or a combination of these.

These devices have an ultrasonic transducer usually located in the handle and it is composed of a stack of piezoelectrodes positioned between metal cylinders. Once the transducer is activated then the piezoelectrodes get excited and vibrate the cylinders to an ultra-high frequency which then linearly oscillates. And a metal blade or jaw that is attached to this then oscillates in a linear fashion to achieve the tissue effects [11]. The amount of mechanical energy applied to tissue per unit time is adjusted by varying the length of excursion of the blade or jaw of the device. Usually, the range of excursions can be adjusted between 50 and 100 μm. Based on the excursion range; two settings of function are offered in these instruments. "Max" setting is offered at the maximum excursion where rapid cutting of tissue occurs with less thermal spread, but this option has minimal hemostasis capability. The "Min" setting is where excursion is minimum which results in less efficient cutting and a greater degree of collateral thermal damage and better hemostasis.

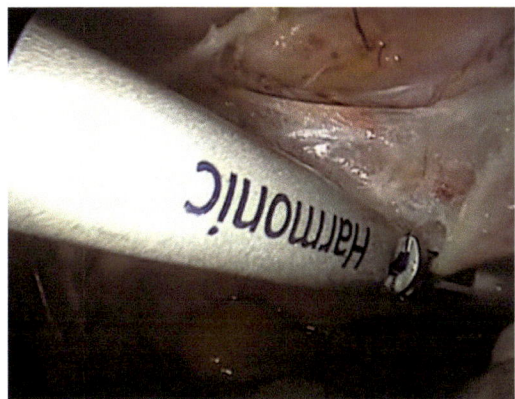

Fig. 11 Laparoscopic advanced bipolar—Harmonic device

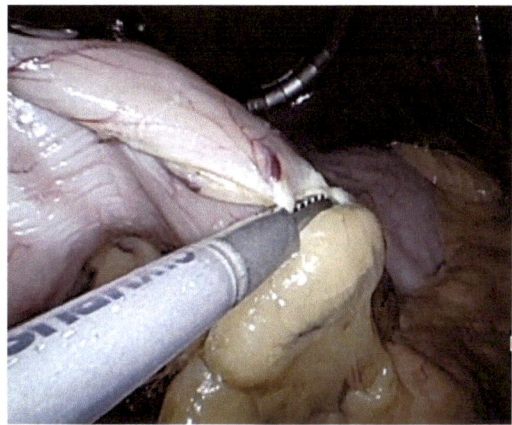

Fig. 12 Laparoscopic advanced bipolar—Thunderbeat device

HARMONIC scalpel (Ethicon Endo-Surgery, USA) and Sonicision™ (Medtronic, USA) are examples of ultrasonic energy devices that are currently available. Sonicision™ (Medtronic, USA) is a cordless ultrasonic device that gives more freedom and maneuverability to the surgeon. HARMONIC ACE® + 7 Shears (Ethicon Endo-Surgery, USA) is the newest version of the HARMONIC scalpel available (Fig. 11).

These are 5 mm instruments and have straight or curved tip configurations. Blade temperatures can go up to 105 °C and the lateral thermal spread can be up to 3 mm. Average arterial burst pressures ranged from 204 mm Hg to 1071 mm Hg while average burst failure rates were 8–39% [12–16].

Newer surgical energy devices like THUNDERBEAT® (Olympus, Japan) have incorporated both advanced bipolar and ultrasonic systems and have shown advantages in achieving faster cutting speeds thereby reducing operation time, reliable 7 mm vessel sealing, precise dissection with fine jaw design, availability of bipolar energy for hemostasis without cutting, minimal thermal spread, fewer instrument exchanges and reduced smoke generation that helps to maintain visibility.

The ultrasonic and bipolar technique of the THUNDERBEAT® (Olympus, Japan) (Figs. 12 and 13) has the potential to surpass the dissection speed of ultrasonic devices with the sealing efficacy of bipolar clamps.

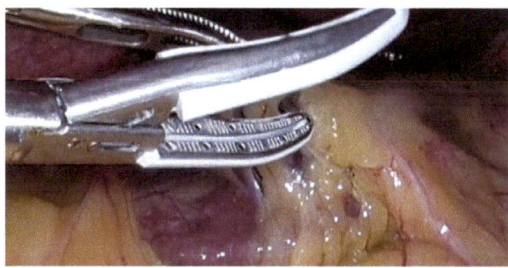

Fig. 13 Thunderbeat tip insulation

However, heat production that is comparable to conventional ultrasonic scissors should be minded for clinical use [17].

References

1. Munro MG. Fundamentals of electrosurgery part I: principles of radiofrequency energy for surgery. In: Feldman LS, Fuchshuber PR, Jones DB, editors. The SAGES manual on the fundamental use of surgical energy (FUSE). New York, NY: Springer; 2012. p. 15–60.
2. Brunt LM. Fundamentals of electrosurgery part II: thermal injury mechanisms and prevention. In: Feldman LS, Fuchshuber PR, Jones DB, editors. The SAGES manual on the fundamental use of surgical energy (FUSE). New YorkNY: Springer; 2012. p. 15–60.
3. Lamberton GR, Hsi RS, Jin DH, et al. Prospective comparison of four laparoscopic vessel ligation devices. J Endourol. 2008;22:2307–12.
4. Person B, Vivas DA, Ruiz D, Talcott M, Coad JE, Wexner SD. Comparison of four energy-based

vascular sealing and cutting instruments: a porcine model. Surg Endosc. 2008;22:534–8.

5. Newcomb WL, Hope WW, Schmeizer TM, et al. Comparison of blood vessel sealing among new electrosurgical and ultrasonic devices. Surg Endosc. 2009;23:90–6.

6. Sutton PA, Awad S, Perkins AC, Lobo DN. Comparison of lateral thermal spread using monopolar and bipolar diathermy, the harmonic scalpel and the ligasure. Br J Surg. 2010;97:428–33.

7. Targarona EM, Balague C, Marin J, et al. Energy sources of laparoscopic colectomy: a prospective randomized comparison of conventional electrosurgery, bipolar compter-controlled electrosurgery and ultrasonic dissection. Operative outcome and costs analysis. Surg Innov. 2005;12(4):339–44.

8. Levy B, Emery L. Randomized trial of suture versus electrosurgical bipolar vessel sealing in vaginal hysterectomy. Obstet Gynecol. 2003;102(1):147–51.

9. Macario A, Dexter F, Sypal J, Cosgriff N, Heniford BT. Operative time and other outcomes of the electrothermal bipolar vessel sealing system (LigaSure) versus other methods for surgical hemostasis: a meta-analysis. Surg Innov. 2008;15(4):284–91.

10. Song C, Tang B, Campbell PA, Cuschieri A. Thermal spread and heat absorbance differences between open and laparoscopic surgeries during energized dissections by electrosurgical instruments. Surg Endosc. 2009;23(11):2480–7.

11. Bittner JG IV, Varela JE, Herron D. Ultrasonic energy systems. In: Feldman LS, Fuchshuber PR, Jones DB, editors. The SAGES manual on the fundamental use of surgical energy (FUSE). New York, NY: Springer; 2012. p. 123–32.

12. Clements RH, Paiepu R. In vivo comparison of the coagulation capability of Sono Surg and harmonic ace on 4 mm and 5 mm arteries. Surg Endosc. 2007;21:2203–6.

13. Gandsas A, Adrales GL. Energy sources. In: Talamini MA, editor. Advanced therapy in minimally invasive surgery. Lewiston, NY: BC Decker; 2006. p. 3–9.

14. Hruby GW, Marruffo FC, Durak E, et al. Evaluation of surgical energy devices for vessel sealing and peripheral energy spread in a porcine model. J Urol. 2007;178:2689–93.

15. Kim FJ, Chammas MF Jr, Gewehr E, et al. Temperature safety profile of laparoscopic devices: harmonic ACE (ACE), Ligasure V (LV), and plasma trisector (PT). Surg Endosc. 2008;22:1464–9.

16. Lamberton GR, His RS, Jin DH, Lindler TU, Jellison FC, Baldwin DD. Prospective comparison of four laparoscopic vessel ligation devices. J Endourol. 2008;22:2307–12.

17. Seehofer D, Mogl M, Boas-Knoop S, et al. Safety and efficacy of new integrated bipolar and ultrasonic scissors compared to conventional laparoscopic 5-mm sealing and cutting instruments. Surg Endosc. 2012;26(9):2541–9.

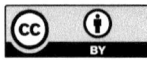

Endo-Laparoscopic Suturing and Knotting: Tips and Tricks

Tuhin Shah

Introduction

During General Surgery training, suturing and knot-tying for open surgery is relatively easy and one of the initial skills to be acquired and mastered. In contrast, similar skills in Minimally Invasive Surgery (MIS) are more challenging to acquire and take an eternity to achieve proficiency. Competence and confidence in laparoscopic suturing allow the surgeon to venture into complex procedures and is an indispensable skill for dealing with intraoperative events.

In open surgery, one has the advantage of binocular vision providing depth perception; however, in MIS, the surgeon encounters various hindrances: indirect visualization, loss of freedom of movement, fixed-port positions, and limited working space. These eliminate three-dimensional view (unless using a 3D video system), restriction of instrument movements and movement about the target, and restricted movement within the workspace. Ergonomics contributes to setting a comfortable and efficient posture for executing the skill; cognizance of elements like azimuth angle, elevation angle, manipulation angle, and triangulation are beneficial. Effect of stress, pressure, and fatigue during MIS procedures contribute to the adverse performance of fine movements in this skill. Thus, endo-laparoscopic suturing is associated with a longer and steeper learning curve compared to that in open surgery [1].

Aside from the knot-tying skill and the type of knot thrown, the braiding, the material, and the size of the suture used influence the security of the knot. The monofilament sutures have a risk of slippage and are less pliable compared to braided sutures. The hydrophilic material (catgut, Dacron, polyglactin, and lactomer) swells on contact with water and theoretically results in a more secure or tighter properly thrown knot. Among sutures of similar material, the larger sized will allow more force to be applied before breaking thus the tightness of a knot using 2–0 suture is double that of one with 3–0 suture.

As a teaching module, there are various options to choose from and Peyton's four-step approach seems the most attractive. It can be used for a better teaching-learning experience. It includes:

1. Demonstration
2. Deconstruction
3. Comprehension
4. Performance

It is practice and repetition which helps acquire the skill and bring finesse to the application of the trained knowledge in the operating room [2]. Hospitals and medical universities

T. Shah (✉)
Department of Surgery, Manmohan Memorial Medical College, Kathmandu, Nepal

MISC Department of Surgery, National University Hospital, Kent Ridge, Singapore

© The Author(s) 2023
D. Lomanto et al. (eds.), *Mastering Endo-Laparoscopic and Thoracoscopic Surgery*,
https://doi.org/10.1007/978-981-19-3755-2_5

need to modify their training curricula to include the basic and advanced suture training courses, skills lab, simulators, and personal video-box assembly and self-training along with regular conduction of outreach programs to further spread the basic skill, knowledge, and awareness.

Equipment and Instruments

- Laparoscope camera with monitor display and light source,
- Laparoscopic needle driver set,
- Laparoscopic grasper and forceps laparoscopic scissors,
- Knot pusher for extracorporeal suturing,
- Trocars–5, 10, 12 mm ports—metallic or plastic.
- Sutures.
- Mayo scissors.
- Artery forceps.
- Measuring tape.

There are different types of needle holders available. Generally, needle holders have jaws that are more powerful and sturdier than other laparoscopic forceps and graspers. They have serrations for better needle grip, a catch for locking and unlocking, and they can be straight or curved and fits in the 5 mm trocars.

General Principles

Setting the Scene. It is a crucial and important step in suturing. It should be like an orchestra and the surgeon needs to put himself in the best ergonomically available condition concerning position, angle, height, choice and placement of instrumentation, light source, choice of suture, and type of knotting among others. A good camera with adequate lighting and a high-definition display can make all the difference that is required for a smooth surgery.

The thickness of the abdominal wall, the position, and the angle of the port placement are vital. Too far or too near will make it difficult to maneu-

ver. If the angle of the port is not in the same direction as the region of surgery then it will cause the surgeon to work against the abdominal wall, especially if it is an obese patient.

Position of the Surgeon. The camera should be positioned between the two instrument ports; this setup matches the normal relationship between the eyes and two hands as in open surgery (Fig. 1a). The surgeon should be in a relaxed stance with the table height matched adequately so that he/she does not have to slouch or strain. The monitor should also be placed at an eye level to prevent neck strain, this is especially important in lengthy surgeries and high-volume centers (Fig. 1b).

Eye-Hand Coordination. Movements made during laparoscopic surgery should be slow and steady compared to open surgery and the movements have to be limited to the field of vision. This is especially true when one is dealing with sutures and instruments like scissors and cautery. Eliminating unnecessary movements and taking choreographed actions during the procedure will help the surgeon and the OR team for more focused and productive output. A formal training course can help to learn these ergonomic skills for better productivity. A high level of concentration is integral to perform even simple needle-driving maneuvers.

Needle Tip and Suture Materials

Different types of needles:

- Straight needle,
- Ski needle, and
- curved needle.

The straight needle is easier to insert and remove from the trocars but is not used frequently. Also, the different angles to be achieved by the straight needle is difficult to achieve comparatively. Ski needles are easier to go through the trocars on the comparison. Straightening the curved needle using the needle drivers/forceps before removal is another tip for easy extraction.

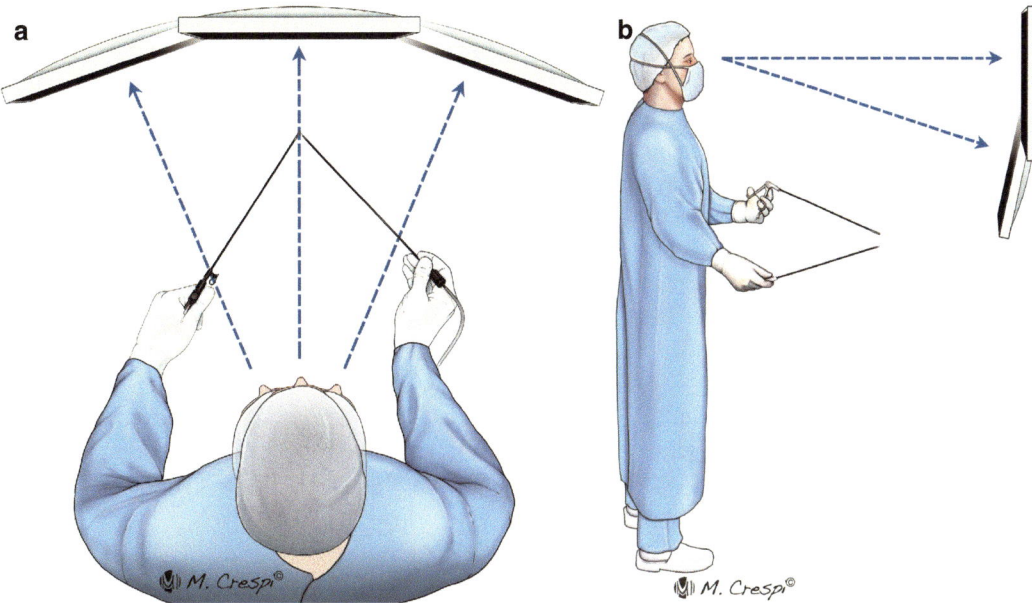

Fig. 1 (**a**) Camera position and (**b**) Surgeon's stance

A needle tip with taper cut penetrates tissues more readily than blunt tip needles hence lesser trauma. Needle size of 2–0 and 3–0 is optimal for laparoscopic use as it allows easy passage and removal in the trocars.

While using just the one 10 mm camera port with a combination of 5 mm ports during surgery, inserting a needle can be done through the 10 mm camera trocar and after suturing, it can be extracted through the 5 mm trocar after straightening the needle. Before inserting the suture, the direction of the 10 mm trocar should be static after confirming the visual field of the camera to a safe area so that even though it is a blind insertion of the needle, it will land safely in the operative field.

Colored sutures are preferred over colorless sutures for better visibility. Traditionally divided into two groups: absorbable and nonabsorbable; braided and monofilament. A suture that swells in contact with water increases its capacity of tying and tightening and can be considered safer, whereas monofilament sutures have a higher risk of slippage when compared to braided sutures. The tightness of a suture knot of a 2/0 thread is double than a 3/0 thread (Fig. 2).

Insertion and Retrieval of the Needle. It should be done only under direct laparoscopic vision. The suture thread should be grasped some

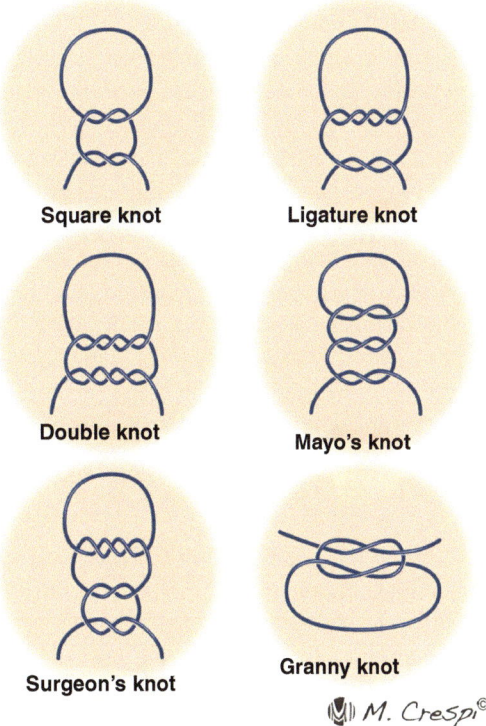

Fig. 2 Types of knot

2–3 cm behind the needle while transferring it in or out through the trocars.

While extracting the needle through metal trocars, there is a chance of the needle to get caught in the diaphragm of the trocar on its exit, which can then snap and/or break the needle. The diaphragm should be kept open manually while extracting the needle. Some may prefer to straighten the needle for easy extraction.

Loading the Needle: Loading depends upon the conditions and also the proximity or otherwise of a smooth serosal surface. There are two processes for loading the needle.

- The dangling pirouette technique.
- The deposit—pick-up technique.

This can be achieved in three ways:

1. First, the thread around 2–3 cm from the needle is held using the dominant hand. Next using the nondominant hand grasp the needle about one-third from the tip. Now the dominant hand is repositioned at two-third from the needle tip—the sweet spot.
2. Lightly grasp the needle at the distal one-third with the nondominant hand. With the dominant hand gently pull the thread—2–3 cm from the needle—towards you or away from you so that angle from the needle can be modified. Now with the dominant hand reposition the grip on the needle at the sweet spot.
3. After laying the suture on a safe surface, using the dominant handgrip the needle lightly at the sweet spot and gently brush with the concavity of the needle on the tissue forward for backward within the 3 o'clock direction till the correct position is attained. The nondominant hand can be used to assist as well.

Loading the needle during laparoscopy is an important skill to master. It should be learned by all surgeons who are interested in pursuing the minimally invasive approach. Suturing and needle handling are crucial. A trainee has to understand and learn how the needle driver works laparoscopically and how to move the needle and the needle drivers effectively through the tissues without causing unnecessary trauma.

The ideal length of a suture for intracorporeal suturing is 10 cm; this length makes the knot-tying maneuver easier. For a continuous suture, the thread should be about 15 cm long, this allows the surgeon a way to accomplish the final knot with enough suture thread in hand.

Techniques of Knot Tying

In the *intracorporeal technique*, the knot is made inside the abdominal cavity using two instruments, these can be two needle holders or forceps.

In the *extracorporeal technique*, the knot is made completely outside the abdominal cavity and then it is pushed inside the abdomen with a knot pusher.

Intracorporeal Knot Tying

The advantage of intracorporeal suturing [3] are:

- The amount of suture that is being drawn through the tissue is limited thus reducing trauma and cut through, and,
- The suture material that is being used can be finer.

Hence, delicate structures like bile ducts and intestines can be sutured using this technique.

Before throwing the knots, it should be checked that the distal end of the suture is no longer than 2–3 cm and in vision so it can be grasped easily. The number of throws depends on the suture used.

Roser Technique

Hold the needle with its concavity bent downwards with the nondominant hand. In this way, the curved and rigid structure of the needle allows the forming of the "C-loop" for the needle holder of the dominant hand to twirl on it. This makes it easy to perform the spirals around the needle holder before grasping the distal end of the suture.

To complete the knot, the needle is dropped in a safe place and the nondominant hand grasps the thread close to the knot to tighten it by moving the hands in opposite directions. Repositioning of the instruments to hold the suture closer to the knot should be done to stay within the visual field to avoid injury to adjacent structures.

The first knot placed is a double spiral/throw. This is followed by again holding the needle with concavity down and repeating the above process to throw single knots and tightening it.

Szabo Technique

The C-loop can also be made with the suture instead of the needle concavity around which the twirls can be made for the knots. The C-loop can be made by just pulling the suture slightly forward or outward with the dominant hand while the distal end is being held by the dominant hand before throwing the spirals.

Alternative Method

Grasping the suture thread 1/2 cm distal to the needle with the dominant hand, then one has just to rotate the instrument to wind the thread around the needle holder. Then forceps are used to grasp the needle end with the other hand while the dominant hand catches the distal end of the suture. The knot is accomplished by pulling on both ends.

Suture Designs

A thread furnished with absorbable terminal clips for anchoring. The clip anchored to the suture thread end functions as an initial knot and a second clip can be applied at the proximal end after suturing is complete to avoid the need for tying knots.

Another is barbed sutures which prevent it from slipping back through the tissues and avoids the need to make knots to secure it in place.

When using a braided thread, a preformed loop can be created simply by piercing the distal end of the suture with the needle, exactly at its middle. Then the needle is pulled through this newly formed loop, to stabilize the suture and continue for continuous suturing.

Or a preformed loop can be made for this purpose (described below).

Extracorporeal Knot Tying

It is important to learn at least one knotting technique and use it when required. The advantage of extracorporeal suturing is the ability to use familiar knotting as in open surgeries which can then be secured using a knot pusher. However, it is not preferred for suturing delicate structures. Extracorporeal slip knots can only be used for free-ending structures, like the appendix, peritoneal tear in TEP, and for ligating transected duct/vessel.

It is of two types:

1. Extracorporeal slip knot
2. Extracorporeal surgeon's knot

There are a lot of methods to make a preformed loop for a slip knot, here a couple of them are described. The length of the suture has to be 45 cm for the creation of the loop for the slip knot.

- Tayside knot: Perform 3–4 windings between the distal and the medial end of the suture, this results in a loop through which the distal suture end is threaded. This generates a new loop through which the distal end of the suture is passed. By pulling on the distal suture end the knot is tightened generating a slipknot.
- The formula for making the Roeder's knot is (1:3:1) "one hitch, three winds, and one locking hitch". First, a loop is made around a post and then a simple knot is made. With the shorter end, three winds are made around both posts and are secured with the last half hitch. The knot is then tightened and checked for sliding. The excess length of the string is trimmed.
- Also, there are commercially available Endoloops which can be used, but with added cost.

Once this preformed loop/Endoloop is inside the abdominal cavity, the structure to be ligated is placed through the loop and the loop is tightened with the knot pusher, and the excess suture cut.

For structures which are not blind-ended (e.g., vessels or cystic duct) the following methods can be used.

- A suture thread is passed under the structure and both ends are taken out. A loop as described above is tied and is then pushed down with knot pusher and tightened.
- Also instead an extracorporeal surgeon's knot can be made and pushed in followed by square knots to secure. This can be used in all instances of laparoscopic suturing however due to the long length of suture chances of cut through and inadvertent injury is higher. For extracorporeal suturing, the suture length has to be at least 75 cm (Fig. 3).
- The granny knot and square knot can be converted into a slip knot by applying tension on the suture ends as demonstrated. And then this can be slipped down using graspers/knot pusher to tighten the knot. This is easier when using monofilament sutures.

There are other options available for stitching apart from the sutures. They are:

- Liga clips and Hemolok clips: They can be used for clipping small and medium-sized vessels/ducts and replaces the need to place sutures and saves time.
- However, they require specific instruments for their deployment.
- Tackers: They are absorbable or nonabsorbable. They are used to fix the mesh in situ and for the closure of the peritoneum.
- But since they are driven into tissues they are associated with some pain postoperatively, can lead to bleeding if it punctures vessels and if used in the path of the nerves then chronic pain.
- Hence should be used with good anatomical knowledge.
- Stapling devices: They can also be used laparoscopically with good outcomes. They can be used for gastrointestinal resection/anastomosis and bile duct resection. Stapling devices borrow the same principle as used in open surgery, but are technically more demanding, with the limited space available and different

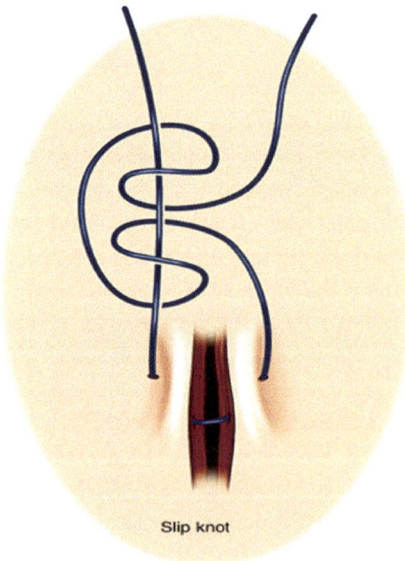

Slip knot

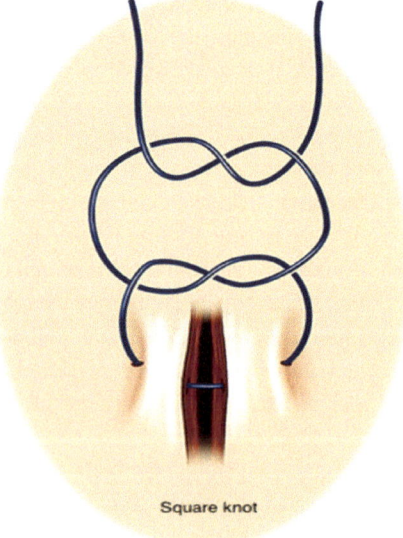

Square knot

M. Crespi©

Fig. 3 Slip and square knot

angles to fire the staples at. They are available as straight and circular devices for anastomotic purposes. The circular device is more complex to use. It is used for endo-laparoscopic anastomosis of the esophagus, rectum, and gastric cuff in bypass surgery. For intra-abdominal insertion of laparoscopic stapling devices, a 12 mm port is required.

• Tissue Glue: Tissue adhesives are also being used in certain conditions like for fixation of hernia mesh in TEP and TAPP. The advantage being that it does not cause chronic pain and can be used on and near the triangle of pain for better fixation when compared to tackers. It is also being used in combination with other techniques as an aid that provides a hemostatic or hydrostatic seal.

Conclusion

Practice and repetition are required to master any skill in surgery and especially in laparoscopy and laparoscopic suturing and knotting.

Performing a suture and a knot in laparoscopy without the necessary experience and practice not only increases the operative time but it also indirectly increases the hospital costs by increasing the consumption of medical supplies, increasing morbidity, increasing the patient recovery period, length of stay, and more importantly decreasing the surgeons productive and functional output during the operation. To improve on this, a trainee can record and analyze their techniques from simulators/skills lab and obtain feedback from colleagues and experienced trainers to perfect them.

Despite modern technology, a laparoscopic surgeon still needs to learn and perform the traditional suturing and knotting techniques as one may never know when and where it will be required and essential. Skills lab and training courses are important for such teaching-learning programs and should be made essential for all teaching institutes as a part of their curricula.

References

1. Chew S, Wattiez A, Chomicki L, editors. Basic laparoscopic techniques and advanced endoscopic suturing: a practical guidebook. World Scientific; 2000.
2. Liceaga A, Fernandes LF, Romeo A, Gagstatter F. Romeo's gladiator rule: knots, stitches and knot tying techniques a tutorial based on a few simple rules; new concepts to teach suturing techniques in laparoscopic surgery. Tuttlingen: Endo-Press; 2013.
3. Croce E, Olmi S. Intracorporeal knot-tying and suturing techniques in laparoscopic surgery: technical details. JSLS. 2000;4(1):17–22.

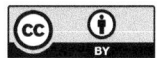

Ergonomics: An Overlooked Training

Tuhin Shah

Introduction

Ergonomics plays an important role in the work environment however it does not receive due attention. Many are unaware of the terminology much less the specifics it contributes to an efficient, safe, and productive workplace.

The term "ergonomics" is derived from the Greek words "ergon" meaning work and "nomos" meaning natural laws or arrangement. Ergonomics can be defined as the scientific study of people at work, in terms of equipment design, workplace layout, working environment, safety, productivity, and training. This depends on many factors including anatomy, physiology, psychology, and engineering. Simply, it can be said that ergonomics is the science of best suiting the worker to his workspace.

Ergonomics may also be referred to as the human factor in certain places. Considering that ergonomics involved in the operative room is vital for increasing efficiency and minimizing the fatigue of the surgical team. Ergonomics is essential in centers with high volume, where long continuous working time and repetitive actions are the norms.

Human errors have been classified in the following categories:

(a) *Mistakes*: The surgeon makes an error because of an incorrect interpretation of the anatomy or situation, e.g., mistaking the CBD for the cystic duct and dividing it.
(b) *Slips*: The surgeon makes the right decision but carries out the wrong action (e.g., presses the "cut" instead of the "coagulation" pedal on the electrocautery).
(c) *Lapses*: The surgeon neglects to perform a procedure or a specific step in a procedure (e.g., forgets to check the integrity of a colonic anastomosis using air insufflation before closing).

There are various factors to consider in the OR during laparoscopic surgery which can ease the access and make working in such a setting productive and well-organized. Though they may seem insignificant initially however incorporating them into the daily workplace will reap benefits over time [1–3].

Straight Line Principle

The visual monitor from the surgery should be adjusted before the surgery to avoid undesirable postures or neck-straining for a prolonged time.

The monitor should be adjusted during the surgery if required depending on the surgical field to keep the visual plane in a straight line.

T. Shah (✉)
Department of Surgery, Manmohan Memorial Medical College, Kathmandu, Nepal

MISC Department of Surgery, National University Hospital, Kent Ridge, Singapore

© The Author(s) 2023
D. Lomanto et al. (eds.), *Mastering Endo-Laparoscopic and Thoracoscopic Surgery*,
https://doi.org/10.1007/978-981-19-3755-2_6

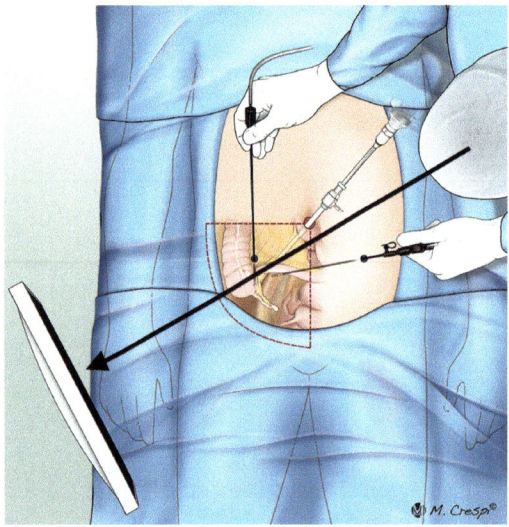

Fig. 1 Straight line principle: the surgeon, the operative field, and the monitor should be in a straight line for maximum efficiency

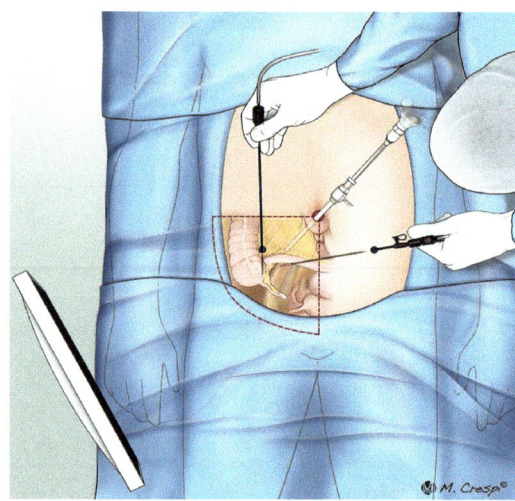

Fig. 2 Triangulation: This is important to avoid fighting and clashing of instruments and easy tiring

In the horizontal plane, the monitor should be straight ahead of the surgeon and in line with the surgical field along with the forearm–instrument motor axis. Additional monitors should be used if the assistants and nurses are standing in a different or opposite to the operating surgeon/operative field to avoid fatigue for the assistants (Fig. 1).

Triangulation

The placement of ports by surgeons is based on individual preference and experience. To facilitate easy instrument handling and to have a good visualization, trocars should be placed in a triangular manner. This is known as triangulation (Fig. 2). The target organ should be about 15 cm from the camera port. The remaining trocars are placed similarly in an arc at 5–7 cm on either side of the camera port. More ports can be placed in the same arc with a gap between instruments to prevent clashing. This allows the instruments to work freely at a 60–90° angle with no clashing and fighting with the other instruments (Fig. 3).

When the endo-laparoscope is situated lateral to the working instruments, it is called "sectorization." This makes it more challenging to work with all lateral ports as the vision is also lateralized, but with practice and use of an angled laparoscope, it can be adapted.

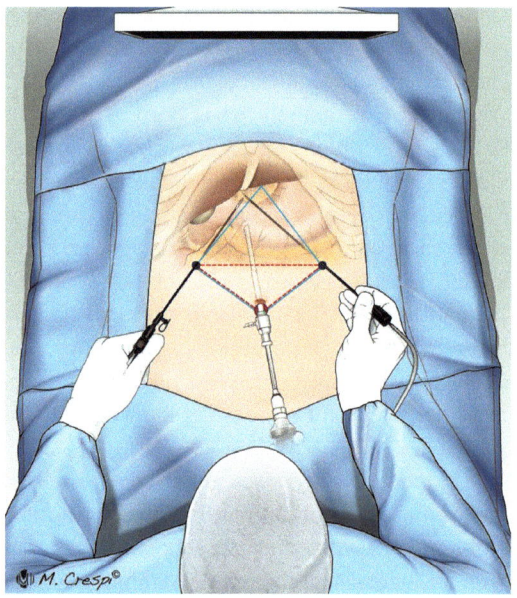

Fig. 3 Baseball diamond concept

Manipulation Angle

The manipulation angle is the angle formed between two working instruments (active and assisting). The ideal manipulation angle is between 45–60° (Fig. 4); a smaller or larger angle is associated with increased maneuvering difficulty and poorer performance. A narrow angle will cause clashing and fighting between instruments, while a larger angle will result in the need to abduct the arms more leading to straining of the shoulder muscles.

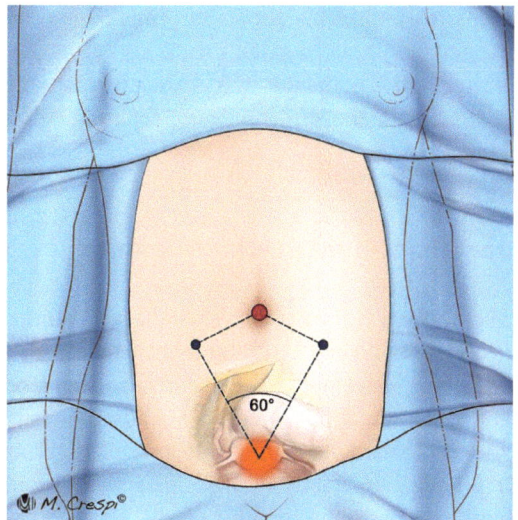

Fig. 4 Ideal manipulation angle

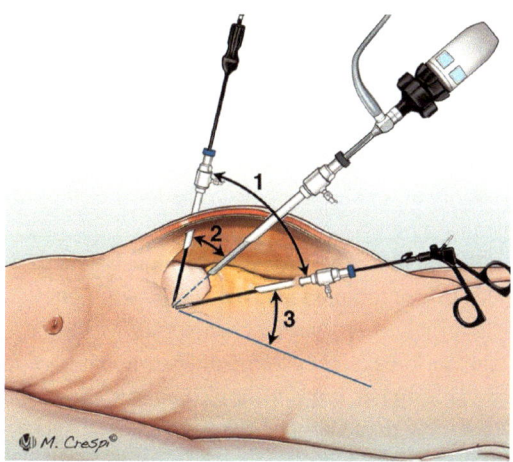

Fig. 5 Manipulation, Elevation, and Azimuth angle shown in a patient. 1. Manipulation angle, 2. Azimuth angle, 3. Elevation angle

Elevation Angle

The elevation angle is the angle between the instrument and the horizontal plane. There is a direct correlation between the manipulation and elevation angles. They should be equal to each other for maximum efficiency. For example, with a manipulation angle of 60°, the corresponding optimal elevation angle, which yields the shortest execution time and optimal performance is also 60° (Fig. 5).

Azimuth Angle

The azimuth angle is the angle between the instrument and the optical axis of the endoscope. The ideal azimuth angle for easy and maximum productivity ranges from 30–45°.

Surgeons' Body Posture

The ideal position for the laparoscopic surgeon is a relaxed stance with the arms slightly abducted, retroverted, and rotated inward at the shoulder level and the elbow should be bent at a 90–120° angle and the neck slightly flexed with a downward gaze. The operating table with clamps on the side for attachments can obstruct the surgeons/assistants from standing in the desired position. These should be organized so that they are at least obstructive position and removed if unnecessary.

Position of Visual Display (Monitor)

The position of the monitor depends on the size of the screen that is being used. However, ideally, the monitor should be 90–200 cm away in the straight line across from the surgeon in a gaze-down view. This is easier to attain by the use of ceiling booms which will help the movement of the monitor in forward/backward as well as up/down direction rather than on a trolley placed on the ground as then the height cannot be adjusted.

It is also beneficial to occasionally relax the body and mind by moving around, looking away from the monitor, and letting go of the instruments. In open surgery, the surgeon unconsciously takes these minibreaks but forgets during laparoscopic operations which are usually more intense with the surgeon/assistants in a more stationary position.

Gaze-Down View

The screen should be positioned lower than the surgeon's eye level to avoid neck extension and straining. The most comfortable viewing direction is approximately 15° below the eye level to avoid the

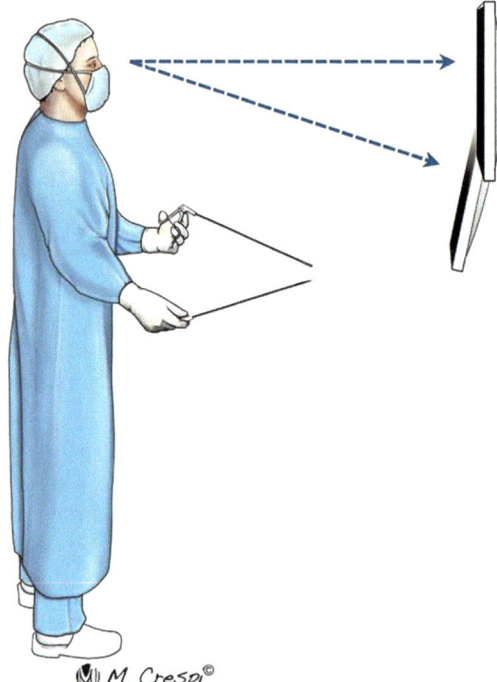

M. Crespi©

Fig. 6 Ideal surgeon stance, ideal monitor and table height during laparoscopy

chin-up position. Viewing distance is dependent on the monitor size. It should be far enough to avoid straining on the eyes usually at 90–200 cm distance (Fig. 6).

Height of Operating Surface (Table)

The operating table must be adapted to the surgeon's height and position. The table's height should be adjusted in such a way that laparoscopic instrument handles are slightly below the level of the surgeon's elbows which should be flexed at a 90–120° angle. This is usually 0.8 times the elbow height of the surgeon.

Foot Pedal Location

Pedals should be placed near the surgeon's foot and lined in the same direction as the instruments, toward the target quadrant and laparo-scopic monitor. This allows surgeons to activate the pedal without twisting their body or the leg. Newer pedals with built-in footrest are preferable as it prevents the surgeon from keeping the foot hanging in the air.

Port Placement and Instruments

The ports should be placed such that the various instruments do not clash with each other. Also while the placement of the ports it should be noted that the ports should lie slightly obliquely pointed toward the target quadrant. This is of importance especially in obese patients to avoid working against the abdominal wall with a poorly inserted trocar.

Instruments should be inserted such that at least half of the instrument is inside the patient. If less than half of the instrument is inserted inside the abdominal wall then excessive motion at the shoulder will be required, which is likely to fatigue the surgeon sooner. After the instruments have been inserted into the ports they should be roughly at, or slightly below, the level of the surgeon's elbows.

When it is necessary to continuously grasp tissues it is recommended to use an instrument that has a lock or ratchet mechanism that will maintain the force, also palming an instrument instead of using finger bows to hold it or using external fixators help in such conditions.

Surgeons and Team Placement

The surgeon can stand on either side or between the legs of the patient depending on the easy access, comfort, and preference to maintain a straight line principle. The assistant/nurse also should stand such that the view of the monitor is not obliquely placed or blocked by another. It is advisable to use multiple monitors to avoid visual obstruction, especially on ceiling booms to be height adjustable depending on the OR team.

Ambient Room Lighting

The OR should have the capacity to be dimmed during laparoscopic surgery to avoid glare and visual discomfort to the surgeon and the operating team. However, it should not be too dark for the assistants/scrub nurses/circulating nurses to pass instruments or hamper movement in the OR.

Scrubs and Footwear

The scrubs used should not be oversized or small to cause a restriction in the movement. The scrubs and the footwear should be light and well ventilated. The scrubs should not have too many pockets or items placed in them to drag down the scrubs to cause discomfort.

Technical Advancement and Clutter of Equipment

With the use of laparoscopy, there are extra instruments and equipment that are required, these take up valuable space hence a laparoscopic OR should be bigger. Also, since all the equipment are numerous and bulkier therefore they should be circulated using trolleys to avoid fatigue and musculoskeletal strain. The tubes and scopes should be organized on and off the operating table so that they do not cross and get tangled. Usually, each team has their method to achieve this and is usually perfected over time. Also, the assistant/nurse can help during the operation to maintain order. The Mayo's trolley should be placed such that it avoids excessive turning and torsion of the scrubbed nurse/assistant while passing the instruments.

Conclusion

With the increasing use of technology in the field of laparoscopy, there are newer physical and mental challenges. This warrants more attention to promote better ergonomics in laparoscopy by encouraging the medical field to promote the principles of ergonomics and to conduct training using these ergonomic guidelines and also by promoting research in this field for a better understanding.

These matters though they seem minor and insignificant however, in the long run, they can lead to medical problems as well as decrease the efficiency of the surgeon/OR team and increase the operative time thus indirectly increasing OR cost, patient recovery time, and admission period.

The most common reason for the inability of ergonomics to be applied optimally is lack of awareness, communication gap, and lack of knowledge about associated medical problems. It is advised to have an active member/team who can communicate the properties and benefits of ergonomics to the rest of the OR for its implementation and smooth movement throughout the OR.

References

1. Mishra RK. Textbook of practical laparoscopic surgery. 2nd ed. New Delhi: Jaypee; 2009.
2. Berguer R. Ergonomics in laparoscopic surgery; 2006. https://doi.org/10.1007/0-387-29050-8_60.
3. Sánchez-Margallo FM, Sánchez-Margallo JA. Ergonomics in laparoscopic surgery. 2017; https://doi.org/10.5772/66170.

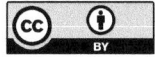

Hemostasis in Laparoscopic Surgery

Ahmad Ramzi Yusoff and Davide Lomanto

Introduction

Hemostasis is the term that refers to the typical response of the vessel to injury by activation of the blood clotting mechanism to limit bleeding. It has been an essential goal in any surgery to maintain hemostasis by restricting the blood loss thus reducing the need for blood transfusion and its complications. Hemostasis is more prudent during laparoscopic surgery where the intervention is performed through small incisions using the camera and specialized instruments, as even minor bleeding may affect visualization, the safety and quality of the procedure, and patient outcome.

In laparoscopy, surgeons can attain a bloodless field with various available methods of hemostasis which requires the timely and appropriate use of technology. Having a sound understanding of each of the numerous forms of hemostasis will ensure proper usage and avoid complications. As a general rule, there are two available methods for hemostasis during laparoscopy, namely standard mechanical hemostasis (ligation, suturing, and electrocautery) and adjunct hemostasis (tissue adhesives and sealants) methods [1]. We provide a broad overview of these two available methods during laparoscopic surgical intervention.

Mechanical Methods of Hemostasis

Direct Pressure

Direct pressure is often possibly the first maneuver employed to achieve hemostasis in laparoscopic surgery. Direct application of blunt laparoscopic equipment, e.g., a 5 mm blunt tip atraumatic grasper to a bleeder point, temporarily stops the blood loss through local tamponade [2]. Direct pressure allows the surgeon time to adequately visualize the area of interest and formulate the next course of action for hemostasis. Applying the direct pressure against a gauze wick or sponge at the bleeding point, which is inserted through a 10 mm port can further enhance the effect of this method (Fig. 1).

With regards to physiology, such maneuver initiates the process of hemostasis through platelet aggregation and fibrin clot formation. Furthermore, it may well be all that is required to halt the bleeding depending on the size of the blood vessels and the patient's coagulation status [2].

Electrosurgical Tools

Electrosurgical tools are often the principal instrument for securing hemostasis after local tamponade. This tool delivers an energy source

A. R. Yusoff (✉)
Department of Surgery, Universiti Teknologi MARA, Sungai Buloh, Selangor, Malaysia

D. Lomanto
Department of Surgery, NUS KTP Advanced Surgery Training Centre and Minimally Invasive Surgical Centre, YLL School of Medicine, National University of Singapore, Kent Ridge, Singapore

D. Lomanto et al. (eds.), *Mastering Endo-Laparoscopic and Thoracoscopic Surgery*,
https://doi.org/10.1007/978-981-19-3755-2_7

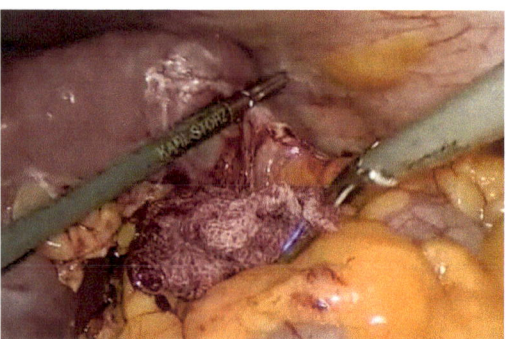

Fig. 1 Using tonsil swab for hemostasis

from an electrosurgical unit (ESU) to the tissue causing thermal destruction and consequently hemostasis. The energy can be achieved either by monopolar or bipolar electrocautery [2]. Details of the physics of ESU, its principle and complications are discussed in another chapter.

- Monopolar Electrocautery
  This form of electrosurgery involves current from an active electrode, predominantly hook, grasping forceps, or scissors that are attached to a monopolar generator, which passes through the patient and returns through a large grounding plate.
- Bipolar Electrocautery
  In this form of electrosurgery, the active electrode is intermittently opposed to the return electrode (usually in a forceps-type arrangement). The electrical current passes between the electrodes to complete the circuit, and the flow of current beyond the surgical field is minimal. The bipolar application thus minimizes the risk of damage to nearby tissue.
- Argon Beam Coagulator
  Argon beam coagulator is a monopolar electrocautery instrument that uses an ionized, argon jet to complete the circuit between the active electrode and the target tissue to "blow-off" the surgical field by surface proteins denaturation and shallow eschar formation. It is sufficient for minor capillary bleeding after dissection, especially that involves solid organ parenchyma. It is however unsuitable for con-

trol of significant bleeding or larger vessels and complications such as argon gas embolism and pneumothorax have been reported from its injudicious use.
- Advanced Bipolar System
  The LigaSure™ vessel sealing system (Valleylab, Boulder, CO) utilizes a form of bipolar current that is locally modified through a feedback control mechanism on the ESU. As the resistance of the tissue changes during desiccation, the generator adjusts the pulsed energy accordingly. Therefore, a high current with low voltages energy is used to melt the collagen and elastin thus creating a seal with a simultaneous hemostatic division of tissue. The LigaSure™ device is recommended for vessels sized <6 mm only [1].
- Ultrasonic Energy
  A piezoelectric harmonic scalpel (Harmonic®, Ethicon US, OH, USA) is a tool that simultaneously excises and coagulates tissue with high-frequency ultrasound. A frequency of 25 kHz induces mechanical vibration at the cellular level resulting in dissection and cavitation as seen in cavitational ultrasonic aspirator (CUSA Technologies, Salt Lake City, UT) [1, 2]. At a higher ultrasound frequency of >55 kHz, this piezoelectric ceramic element expands and contracts rapidly thus generating frictional energy that causes a hidden moving blade to oscillate. This results in mechanical energy that seals blood vessels and transects tissues without passing the current to, or through the patient.

The harmonic scalpel is known to cause less collateral damage, avoid carbonization of the tissue, and reduces local thermal injury. It has been used widely in laparoscopy for tissue dissection and control of local blood vessels. It has two modes of action; lower power causes slower tissue heating and more coagulation effect, while higher power setting causes rapid cutting but is relatively nonhemostatic. However, the use of the harmonic scalpel is limited to vessels of <4 mm in diameter (Fig. 2). Newer generation device may allow sealing of up to <7 mm diameter [1, 2].

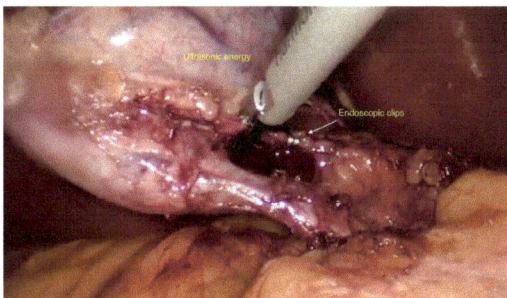

Fig. 2 Application of endoscopic clip system for ligation of cystic artery and use of ultrasonic energy device for transection of the artery

Suturing

Similar to open surgery, tissue approximation by suturing will result in immediate hemostasis if done correctly. Suturing can be achieved either by extracorporeal or intracorporeal methods depending on the surgeon's preference or experience. Although suturing is the most basic in open surgery, it is the most challenging skill required of a laparoscopic surgeon.

- Extracorporeal Suturing
  The surgeon creates the knot outside the body using a series of half-hitch knots that are advanced into the abdomen through a port by using a knot pusher. The suture lengths are usually longer than 70 cm. Care must be exercised during extracorporeal suturing as excessive traction during passing and redelivery of the suture may lead to "sawing" of the tissue.
- Intracorporeal Suturing
  This technique requires skill to manipulate the needle, to pass it from one needle driver to the next, and to execute a series of knots. The required suture length for this type of suturing is usually between 12–17 cm.

Ligation

Occluding the bleeding vessel by suture ligation is an effective way of hemostasis in surgery; however, as for suturing, it may not be handy in laparoscopic surgery for many.

- Simple Ligature
  Again both extracorporeal and intracorporeal methods can be used to execute the ligature.
- Pretied Suture Loops
  Ready-to-use pretied suture loops (Endo-loops) may be particularly useful for surgeons unfamiliar with laparoscopic suturing. Its use however requires the division of a bleeding vessel or vascular pedicle in order to loop the vessel of interest hence its suboptimal choice where the vessels are still intact.

Endoscopic Clip Systems

An endoscopic clip is another method preferred by most surgeons to seal a blood vessel. Both 5 and 10 mm reusable clips and appliers, as well as their disposable counterparts, are available. The only difference is that reusable clips are reloaded after each firing which may potentially delay clipping of a targeted vessel.

- Titanium Clips
  Most mechanical clips using reusable clip applier are made from titanium. However, they tend to slip off during dissection; therefore, multiple applications of at least 2–5 clips seem to be necessary for safe control of vessels (Fig. 2).
- Polymer Ligation Clip System (Hem-o-lock™ clips, Weck, USA).
  This clip system comprises of a self-sealing, hook-like mechanism that "lock" when applied correctly with fewer tendencies to slip off as compared to titanium clips. It is a safer alternative to control even significantly large vessels such as renal vein or artery as it comes in various sizes from the medium, large, and extra-large.

The preferred method of clip system largely depends on the surgeon and also on the anticipated size of the vessels. Before the clip application, it is crucial to visualize both sides of the clip to ensure adequate tissue uptake and prevent inadvertent clipping of nontarget structure. Ischaemic necrosis, perforation, and laceration of surrounding tissues are common complications resulting from inadequate meticulous dissection before clipping a structure and incorrect clip application.

Endoscopic Stapling Devices

This device sometimes referred to as vascular endo stapler (Endo-GIA, Covidien, US; Endopath Flex, Ethicon, US) is ideal in situations where mechanical clips are not large enough to seal large caliber vessels [3]. Stapler height of 2.0–2.5 mm can safely occlude major vessels or vascular pedicles as a newer device utilizes three lines of staples for simultaneous vascular sealing and cutting. However, modern endo staplers are bulky instruments that require 12–18 mm access port to work in a limited space and equipped with a rotating or angulating system hence costly [1]. The firing of stapler requires some training beforehand to avoid stapler "malfunction" as the improper technique may cause insufficient sealing of vessel resulting in life-threatening bleeding.

Tissue Hemostasis Agents

Topical hemostatic agents and tissue sealants or adhesives are available as an adjunct to manage bleeding during open surgery or laparoscopy when conventional hemostatic techniques (mechanical, thermal, and chemical) are inadequate or impractical [1, 4]. Topical hemostats and sealants have become essential tools of laparoscopic surgery due to their ability to reduce bleeding complications. These are especially convenient for diffuse bleeding from the nonanatomic region, bleeding near sensitive structures, e.g., nerve, and bleeding in patients with coagulopathy.

The two main categories of topical hemostatic agents are physical agents, which promote hemostasis using a passive substrate, and biologically active agents, which enhance the coagulation process at the bleeding site [4]. Examples of the commonly used hemostatic agents in laparoscopy are;

Physical Agents or Dry Matrix

Dry physical agents produce a matrix that activates the coagulation cascade and acts as a scaffold for thrombus to form and build up. These agents are easy to use; however, they are less effective if bleeding is brisk.

- Oxidized Regenerated Cellulose
  Oxidized regenerated cellulose (ORC) is a dry, absorbable sterile mesh (Surgicel™) that is derived from cotton cellulose which can be applied directly to an area of bleeding (Fig. 3). Results are optimal if bleeding is minimal (i.e., oozing). ORC is commonly used to control bleeding at vascular anastomotic sites, the cut surfaces of solid organs (Fig. 3), and retroperitoneal or pelvic surfaces after lymphadenectomy [4]. Apart from mechanical effects, cellulosic acid helps hemostasis by blood protein denaturation. Because ORC is pliable, it can be rolled and passed easily through laparoscopic trocars. A single-layer sheet is fully absorbed in approximately 14 days.

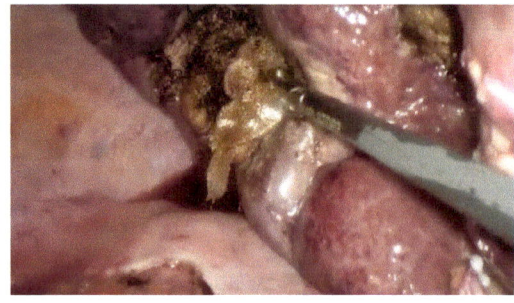

Fig. 3 Hemostasis by application of oxidized regenerated cellulose (Surgicel™) to liver parenchymal surface

- Recently, ORC has been manufactured into a powder form (Surgicel® Powder) that can penetrate the blood to stop bleeding at the source. It comes with a unique endoscopic applicator for use in laparoscopy.
- Gelatin Matrix

  Gelatin (e.g., Gelfoam, Surgifoam™) is a hydrocolloid made from partial acid hydrolysis of porcine-derived collagen that is whipped into foam and then dried. It is available in sponge or powder form. Gelatin sponge absorbs blood or fluid up to 40 times its weight, and when saturated with blood, it expands up to 200% in its dimensions [4].

  The dry sponge is rigid and firm when dry, but became soft and pliable after moistening thus able to be molded into any shape for easy passage through laparoscopic ports. Hemostasis occurs when the sponge is pressed for several minutes at the intended area and left in place. It is completely absorbed after 4–6 weeks.

Biologically Active Agents

These agents are commonly referred to as tissue adhesives or glues promote tissue sealing and support by reproducing the different phases of coagulation. They are suitable for managing diffuse bleeding from oozing surfaces but not from major vascular bleeding. The lack of adequate adhesion strength enables any forceful bleeder to displace the products away from the bleeding tissue. Some of these agents are;

1. Topical Thrombin

   Topical thrombin that is reconstituted from a lyophilized powder is a bovine-derived thrombin component. It can be applied using a sprayer onto an oozing surface or applied with a needle and syringe directly to a specific area of bleeding [3]. Topical thrombin can also be used in conjunction with a bovine gelatin matrix agent (sponge or granules) that provides the thrombin with an immediate scaffold for clot formation (Floseal™, Surgiflo™).

   Recently, human thrombin and recombinant thrombin are available for use and have primarily replaced bovine thrombin.

2. Fibrin Sealant

   Fibrin sealants or glues are typically a mixture of a two-component system; a solution of concentrated fibrinogen and factor XII, and a solution of thrombin and calcium. When the components are mixed immediately before use, a solid fibrin matrix or clot forms [3]. Owing to their liquid nature, they are readily used in laparoscopy which is then applied using a long applicator needle and a dual-lumen adapter.

   Fibrin sealant can control bleeding at vascular anastomotic sites. Use of fibrin glue in conjunction with a gelatin sponge (Tisseel™) is useful to control bleeding from superficial cut surfaces but not from severe vascular bleeding. Human-derived fibrin glue (Crosseal™) meanwhile has a shorter operative time but higher complication rate [1].

3. TachoComb™ or Tachosil™

   Made from dry, equine collagen bovine thrombin, bovine aprotinin, and human fibrinogen, this fleece (TachoComb™, NycomedLinz, Austria) works by mimicking the final steps of the human coagulation process [1, 3]. As the fleece comes in contact with blood or body fluids, it immediately activated and forms a patch and hemostasis ensued. It must be applied correctly to prevent premature activation of the patch. Hence, for laparoscopy, the pre-rolled TachoSil™ is delivered by a special clamp. TachoSil™ (human fibrinogen and equine collagen) forms a dense tissue-like sealant at the surface of the parenchymal lesion or defect within 3–5 min, following constant compression and moisturizing with normal saline, and will be replaced by vital tissue. Therefore, it can be applied even when bleeding is absent and in patients with coagulopathy. After proper application, it is possible to subject the sealed surface to further bipolar coagulation, or suturing without jeopardizing the sealant effect. TachoSil™ has an anti-adhesive property that separates the sealant tissues from other structures nearby.

Choice of Topical Hemostatic Agents

With various types of topical hemostatic agents available, the choice of which to use will depend on the character, amount, and location of bleeding; surgeon preference and cost considerations. Dry matrix agents are less effective when bleeding is brisk; however, fibrin sealant is a more appropriate choice when moderate bleeding is uncontrolled by other measures.

Methods of Prevention of Hemorrhage During Laparoscopy

1. Visualize and identify all structures before division.
2. Avoid blunt avulsion or stripping of adhesions and fat tissues.
3. Safely apply energy to the area to be divided.
4. Preemptive clipping of a structure or dissect generous enough if unsure about its vascularity to allow prompt control if bleeding occurred after division.

Management of Active Hemorrhage During Laparoscopy

1. Avoid panic situation.
2. Avoid random application of energy or clips towards the presumed bleeding point.
3. Visually identify the bleeding without taking away necessary retraction.
4. Suction the area with a suitable suction device and avoid too much irrigation. If pos-

sible, insert a gauze through a 10 mm port site to achieve temporary tamponade (Fig. 1).
5. Apply gentle pressure with an atraumatic grasper to the bleeding point where identified.
6. If the bleeding does not stop with direct identification and pressure, convert to an open procedure.
7. If the bleeding stops with the above measures, ensure that there are enough port sites for adequate instrumentation. Insert extra ports for better visualization and retraction, and possibly for optimal triangulation if suturing is required.
8. Place a mechanical clip on both sides of the area being grasped (Fig. 2).
9. Irrigate and evaluate.
10. If necessary, apply electrical and ultrasonic energy judiciously.

References

1. Klingler CH, Remzi M, Marberger M, Janetschek G. Haemostasis in laparoscopy. Eur Urol. 2006;50(5):948–57.
2. Newman RM, Traverso LW. Principles of laparoscopic hemostasis. The SAGES manual. New York: Springer; 2006. p. 49–59.
3. Vecchio R, Catalano R, Basile F, Spataro C, Caputo M, Intagliata E. Topical hemostasis in laparoscopic surgery. G Chir. 2016;37(6):266.
4. Peralta E. Overview of topical haemostatic agents and tissue adhesives. In Cochran A, UpToDate; 2019. https://www.uptodate.com/contents/overview-of-topical-hemostatic-agents-and-tissue-adhesives. Accessed 1 May 2019.

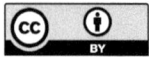

Imaging-Enhancing System

Alembert Lee-Ong and Alfred Allen Buenafe

Visualization is one of the fundamental pillars (including CO_2 insufflation and instrumentation) critical to performing MIS. Initially evolved from direct view through the laparoscope to indirect view on the monitor projected from a camera system. Early advances were geared towards improving the image quality and reproduction of stereoscopic vision. Current advancements involve in part or in combination, the application of optical filters to manipulate specific light spectrums (narrow-band imaging) and the use of fluo-rescent dye (indocyanine green-fluorescent imaging) to see beyond what can be viewed with the naked eye, coupled with the advantage of real-time application. Narrow-band imaging is primarily used in gastrointestinal endoscopy to detect mucosal pathologies, while ICG aid in revealing specific structures beneath tissues and assess tissue perfusion; it is finding interest for application in various MIS procedures.

A. Lee-Ong (✉)
Department of Surgery, Manila Doctors Hospital, Manila, Philippines

Philippine Center for Advanced Surgery, San Juan, Philippines

Department of Surgery, Cardinal Santos Medical Center, San Juan, Philippines

Department of Surgery, Quirino Memorial Center, Quezon City, Philippines

A. A. Buenafe
Philippine Center for Advanced Surgery, San Juan, Philippines

Department of Surgery, Cardinal Santos Medical Center, San Juan, Philippines

Department of Surgery, Rizal Medical Center, Pasig, Philippines

Department of Surgery, Batangas Medical Center, Batangas, Philippines

Department of Surgery, Asian Hospital and Medical Center, Alabang, Muntinlupa, Philippines

Indocyanine Green-Enhanced Imaging

History of Indocyanine Green (ICG). ICG-enhanced imaging is based on the properties of the cyanine dye. The Kodak research laboratories developed the ICG dye in 1955 for near-infrared photography [1, 2]. Its FDA-approved medical application began in 1956, initially used for quantitative measurement of hepatic and cardiac function; subsequently extended to use in ophthalmology with the investigation into its fluorescent properties in the 1970s [1]. Its use was hindered by technological limitations until recently with the development of improved digital imaging, allowing the broad application of ICG imaging.

Rationale for Using ICG. Use of ICG has several advantages: good signal-to-noise ratio where the target can be seen clearly due to the absence of background tissue auto fluorescence, rapid clearance of the dye allows repeated applications, the near-infrared light used to excite and

D. Lomanto et al. (eds.), *Mastering Endo-Laparoscopic and Thoracoscopic Surgery*,
https://doi.org/10.1007/978-981-19-3755-2_8

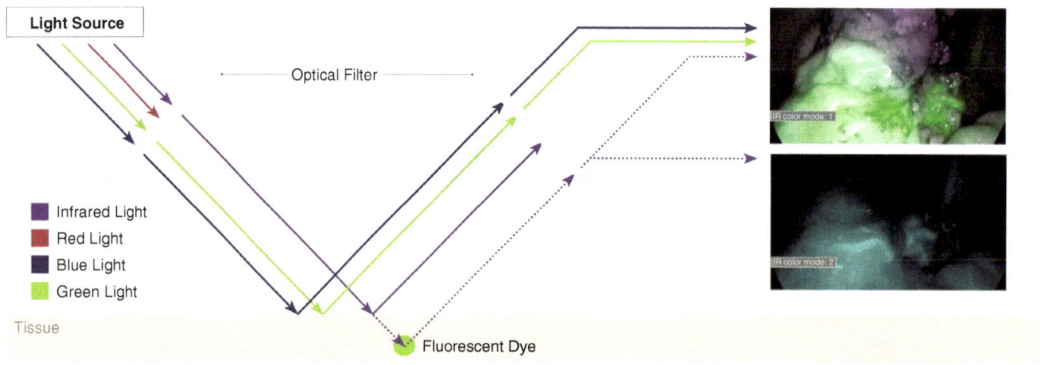

Fig. 1 How ICG-enhanced imaging works. (Source: Olympus)

fluorescence being viewed functions within the tissue optical window allowing visualization to about 5–10 mm deep, and the system itself merely requires simple affordable imaging devices [3]. The wavelengths below 700 nm are absorbed by hemoglobin and myoglobin, while that above 900 nm are limited by lipid and water absorption [4] (Fig. 1).

Properties of ICG. ICG is an amphiphilic, tricarbocyanine iodide dye with a molecular mass of 751.4 Da [1]. It is distributed as a powder and reconstituted with distilled water with good solubility, attaining an aqueous solution of 6.5 pH for intravenous injection. The solution has limited stability to light and must be used within 6–10 h on dilution; once injected, it attains spectral stabilization within seconds. The dye is excited with either filtered (near-infrared) light or laser between 750–800 nm [2]. The fluorescence is detected or viewed around the maximum peak of 832 nm with specifically designated scopes and cameras [1, 2]. It produces a nonlinear fluorescence quantum yield in relation to the concentration.

Injected intravascularly, around 98% binds to plasma proteins (serum albumin, α-, and β-lipoproteins) without altering the protein structure at the same time preventing dye extravasation and decreasing its tendency to aggregate. The concentration of the dye within the body should be kept below 15 mg/L, as it starts to aggregate at higher concentrations, which will result in "quenching" or a decrease in the fluorescence yield. The other 2% is free in the serum; eventually, both are taken up by the liver and

excreted unchanged into the bile. Hepatic clearance is at the rate of 18–24% per minute, with exponential clearance observed in the first 10–20 min. After the initial period, the clearance rate slows down, allowing trace amounts to remain for more than an hour; the half-life is around 3–4 min [5]. Multiple or repeated application is possible due to the rapid clearance of the dye [4, 6].

Injected interstitially, the dye similarly binds to proteins and is usually detected in the closest draining lymph nodes within 15 min and to the regional lymph nodes after 1–2 h [2].

The lethal dose (LD50) is 50–80 mg/Kg in animal studies and is practically nontoxic at the standard dosage of <2 mg/Kg (0.1–0.5 mg/ml/Kg) provided the patient has no iodide allergy [1, 2, 6].

Some Applications of ICG Imaging in MIS

Cholecystectomy. Bile duct injury (BDI) is the most dreaded complication of cholecystectomy; the incidence ranges from 0.3% to 1.5% for the laparoscopic technique. Even with the introduction of the Critical View of Safety (CVS) concept by Strasberg, the incidence of bile duct injury remains around 0.42% [7]. Often cited reasons were aberrant anatomy and the distortion or misinterpretation of the biliary tract anatomy due to inflammatory changes. While intraoperative cholangiography (IOC) is accepted to provide a

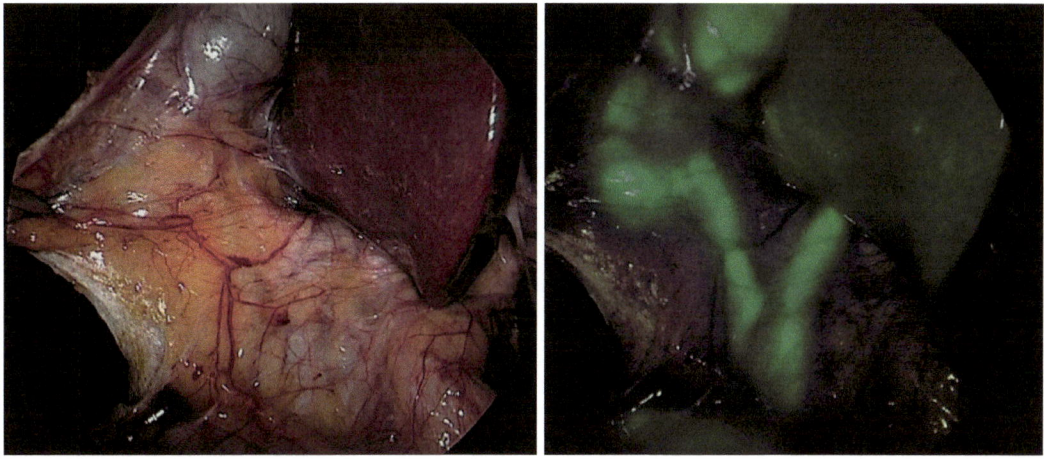

White (visible) Light   **Near Infrared (invisible) Light with ICG**

Photos courtesy of Prof Luigi Boni, MD, Fondazione IRCCS - Ca' Granda - Policlinico Hospital University of Milan

Fig. 2 Gallbladder and extrahepatic biliary ducts under white light (left) and the same area under ICG-enhanced imaging (right) show target outline beneath overlying tissues. (Source: Pfiedler Education, Fluorescence Guided Surgery: A Nurse's Guide to ICG. 2020)

roadmap during surgery, it has several shortcomings such as increased operative time, the need for dedicated radiologic instrumentation and trained staff, requiring partial dissection of the Calot's triangle and the cannulation of the cystic duct before IOC can be employed, and additional patient exposure to contrast and radiation. ICG allows real-time visualization of the biliary ducts and vessels before and during the dissection of the Calot's triangle [7] (Fig. 2).

There is a wide variation in the dosage and timing of the ICG solution infusion for cholecystectomy. The dosage ranges from a single fixed bolus of 2.5 mg to weight-based dosing (0.05–0.5 mg/Kg). The timing varies widely, from just after induction of anesthesia to as long as 48 h before surgery. Tsutsui et al. [3] suggested the optimal timing of infusion to be around 15 h before surgery to attain optimum contrast between the biliary tract against the background liver and surrounding soft tissue. Report by Graves et al. [8] of successful visualization of the cystic duct and common bile duct with direct injection of 0.025 mg/mL ICG-bile solution into the gallbladder of 11 patients for cholecystectomy; the drawback to this technique is obstruction of the cystic duct or gallbladder neck by

impacted stone, remedied by milking the stone into the gallbladder and allowing the gallbladder content to flow into the biliary duct. Intraoperative intravenous ICG injection (2–3 mL, 0.4 mg/Kg) may be done to clarify the cystic artery anatomy; it is usually visualized after 60 s and lasting about 32 s, repeat dosing may be done after 15 min to avoid quenching. In a comparative study against IOC by Osayi et al. [9], the biliary anatomy was visualized with ICG in 80% of cases where IOC could not. Similarly, Daskalaki et al. [10] noted a high visualization rate ranging 95.1–99% visualization of the biliary anatomy with ICG.

Bowel Anastomoses. Reconstruction after bowel resection in a gastrointestinal surgery has a wide rate for dehiscence (1–30%), with experienced hands, it is around 3–6%. One of the recognized risk factors for an anastomotic leak is the presence of poor local tissue oxygenation secondary to inadequate anastomotic vascular perfusion. Traditional blood flow assessment is subjective and based on surgical evaluation of bowel color, bowel peristalsis, pulsation of vessels, temperature, and bleeding from the marginal arteries [11]. Usually, more than 10 min are necessary for ischemia demarcation to become visible after vessel division [2]. More objective

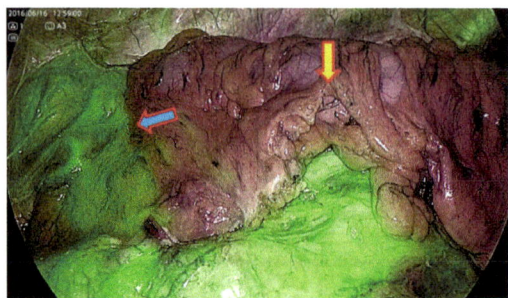

Fig. 3 Assessment of bowel perfusion for anastomosis: ICG lighting-up perfused bowel segment (blue arrow) distant from the planned bowel resection site (yellow arrow). (Source: Olympus)

means have been suggested, such as Doppler measurement; however, this is cumbersome and requires additional training. The injection of ICG would allow real-time evaluation of bowel perfusion before resection and completion of the anastomosis. To evaluate the perfusion of the bowel, intravenous ICG injection is given using two boluses of 5 ml each at a concentration of 0.4 mg/Kg; the first, after the division of the vascular pedicle to help choose the best-perfused site for resection and the second, just before performing the anastomosis to ensure adequate vascularization (Fig. 3). A systematic review on the use of ICG to assess perfusion in colorectal anastomosis concluded that the surgical plan was changed in 10.8% of cases after application of ICG, and the leak rate was reduced from 7.4% to 3.4% [11]. A meta-analysis reported by Shen et al. [12] also suggested that ICG was associated with a lower leak rate OR 0.27 (95% CI 0.13–0.53). The RCT looking into the use of ICG in colorectal anastomoses by Alekseev et al. [11] noted a decrease in the leak rate among low rectal anastomoses (14.4% from 25.7%, $p = 0.04$).

Summary

Currently, ICG imaging application in cholecystectomy for extrahepatic biliary tract visualization and the assessment of bowel perfusion for anastomoses have shown promising outcomes. Studies on its usage in other fields (gynecology, hepatobiliary surgery, neurosurgery, pediatric surgery, transplant, urology, etc.) are ongoing. In gynecology, oncology and endometrioses are the focus; detection of sentinel lymph nodes (SLN) with ICG may reduce the operative time and improve SLN detection, while endometrioses encounter a lack of robust evidence to conclude. In hepatobiliary surgery, investigations are directed towards liver mapping, cholangiography, tumor visualization, and liver graft evaluation; preliminary concerns exist regarding limited tissue penetration and instances of false positive or negative results. In general, there is a broad interest in applying ICG imaging to currently available diagnostic and therapeutic interventions, and there is a need for more robust studies to provide clear-cut conclusions and recommendations.

References

1. Reinhart MB, Huntington CR, Blair LJ, et al. Indocyanine green: historical context, current applications, and future considerations. Surg Innov. 2016;23(2):166–75.
2. Boni L, David G, Mangano A, et al. Clinical applications of indocyanine green (ICG) enhanced fluorescence in laparoscopic surgery. Surg Endosc. 2015;29(7):2046–55.
3. Tsutsui N, Yoshida M, Nakagawa H, et al. Optimal timing of preoperative indocyanine green administration for fluorescent cholangiography during laparoscopic cholecystectomy using the PINPOINT(R) endoscopic fluorescence imaging system. Asian J Endosc Surg. 2018;11(3):199–205.
4. Kaplan-Marans E, Fulla J, Tomer N, et al. Indocyanine green (ICG) in urologic surgery. Urology. 2019;132:10–7.
5. Desmettre T, Devoisselle JM, Mordon S. Fluorescence properties and metabolic features of indocyanine green (ICG) as related to angiography. Surv Ophthalmol. 2000;45(1):15–27.
6. Alander JT, Kaartinen I, Laakso A, et al. A review of Indocyanine green fluorescent imaging in surgery. Int J Biom Imaging. 2012;2012:940585.
7. Vlek SL, van Dam DA, Rubinstein SM, et al. Biliary tract visualization using near-infrared imaging with indocyanine green during laparoscopic cholecystectomy: results of a systematic review. Surg Endosc. 2017;31(7):2731–42.
8. Graves C, Ely S, Idowu O, et al. Direct gallbladder Indocyanine green injection fluorescence cholangiography during laparoscopic cholecystectomy. J Laparoendosc Adv Surg Tech A. 2017;27(10):1069–73.

9. Osayi SN, Wendling MR, Drosdeck JM, Narula VK, et al. Near-infrared fluorescent cholangiography facilitates identification of biliary anatomy during laparoscopic cholecystectomy. Surg Endosc. 2015;29(2):368–75.

10. Daskalaki D, Fernandes E, Wang X, et al. Indocyanine green (ICG) fluorescent cholangiography during robotic cholecystectomy: results of 184 consecutive cases in a single institution. Surg Innov. 2014 Dec;21(6):615–21.

11. Alekseev M, Rybakov EA-O, Shelygin Y, et al. A study investigating the perfusion of colorectal anastomoses using fluorescence angiography: results of the FLAG randomized trial. Colorectal Dis. 2020;22(9):1147–53. https://doi.org/10.1111/codi.15037.

12. Shen R, Zhang Y, Wang T. Indocyanine green fluorescence angiography and the incidence of anastomotic leak after colorectal resection for colorectal cancer: a meta-analysis. Dis Colon Rectum. 2018;61:1228–34.

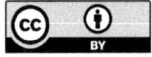

Instrumentations and Access Devices

Alembert Lee-Ong and Alfred Allen Buenafe

Introduction

Minimally Invasive Surgery (MIS) instruments are patterned after conventional hand instruments to perform similar specific functions; they are designed to pass and perform through small diameter ports and at a distance to the target tissues. The development of instruments has evolved since the early period of MIS, starting from the use of rudimentary gynecologic instruments; at that time. Gynecology was the only specialty widely performing laparoscopic procedures. The evolution in design, ergonomics, and variety has been pivotal for advancing endo-laparoscopic surgery to perform more complex surgical procedures with safety and better outcome. Various evolving concepts of MIS like Single-site or reduced Surgery, Natural Orifice Transluminal Endoscopic Surgery (NOTES), Needlescopic Surgery, and Robotic-assisted Surgery have also pushed the development of features such as articulation control, pre-bent configuration, smaller diameter, and robotic instruments to meet specific needs.

A better understanding of the features, ergonomics, characteristics, and different instrumentations is crucial for any surgeon before embarking on basic or advanced laparoscopic surgery.

We can divide the instrumentations into three categories: access the cavity or workspace, maintain the working space, and perform the surgical procedures. Let us analyze the role of these groups.

The development of these devices has also evolved to respond to the requirements of new MIS concepts.

In the first two groups: access devices are meant to gain entry into the workspace (i.e., abdominal cavity, chest, pre-peritoneal space, etc.) while other devices are needed to maintain the space by the insufflated CO_2 while allowing insertion of instruments necessary in the performance of surgery.

A. Lee-Ong (✉)
Department of Surgery, Manila Doctors Hospital, Manila, Philippines

Philippine Center for Advanced Surgery, San Juan, Philippines

Department of Surgery, Cardinal Santos Medical Center, San Juan, Philippines

Department of Surgery, Quirino Memorial Medical Center, Quezon City, Philippines

A. A. Buenafe
Philippine Center for Advanced Surgery, San Juan, Philippines

Department of Surgery, Cardinal Santos Medical Center, San Juan, Philippines

Department of Surgery, Rizal Medical Center, Pasig, Philippines

Department of Surgery, Batangas Medical Center, Batangas, Philippines

Department of Surgery, Asian Hospital and Medical Center, Alabang, Muntinlupa, Philippines

© The Author(s) 2023   51
D. Lomanto et al. (eds.), *Mastering Endo-Laparoscopic and Thoracoscopic Surgery*,
https://doi.org/10.1007/978-981-19-3755-2_9

Access Devices: Role and Characteristic

Access devices' primary purpose is to gain entry to the workspace, the insufflation of CO_2, maintain a pressurized workspace, and serve as a conduit for instruments to pass through.

1. Veress needle. A specially designed instrument to enter the abdominal or thoracic cavity using the closed technique (Fig. 1). It consists of an outer sharp cutting needle and an inner blunt spring-loaded stylet. During insertion, the needle encounters resistance; the blunt stylet retracts, exposing the sharp outer sheath which facilitates penetration of the structure; when it enters a cavity, the blunt stylet springs forward beyond the outer sheath to protect the viscera within. Once proper intraperitoneal placement has been ascertained using accepted maneuvers, insufflation of the peritoneal cavity may be initiated and followed by the insertion of working ports.
2. Hasson trocar. Composed of a cannula with an adjustable sliding cone and a blunt-tip trocar (Fig. 2). Intended to be inserted into the abdominal cavity after access is achieved with the open technique; the cone serves as a stopper preventing air leaks while the blunt trocar prevents visceral injury as it is inserted.
3. Optical trocar. It is a specially designed trocar that is utilized to access the abdominal cavity (Fig. 3). It is beneficial in certain situations like obesity or when the access with Veress or open technique is at risk of injury. The trocar has a transparent tip that allows a view through. The trocar accommodates an endo-laparoscope (0° scope preferred), allowing visualization of each layer of the abdominal wall as it is inserted into the abdominal cavity. The trocar may have either a cutting or a dilating tip, with the latter preferred.
4. Hand-assist port. Ports are designed to accommodate the passage of a hand (for assisting) while maintaining intraperitoneal pressure (Fig. 4).
5. Single or Reduced Ports. These ports are specifically designed for the single or reduced port technique. They are introduced through a single access point and allow multiple instruments and camera endoscope to be inserted. There are reusable and disposable devices, with different diameters and sizes. Also, the type and number of instrumentations that can

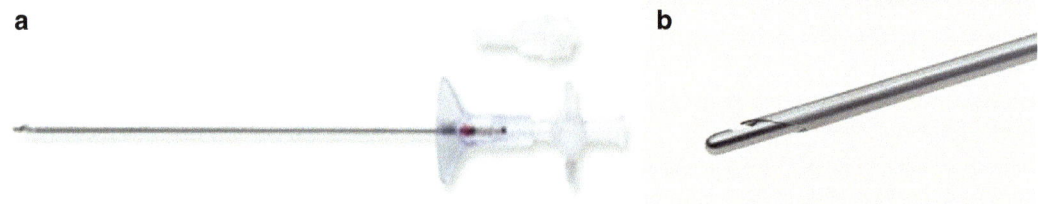

Fig. 1 (**a**) Veress needle. (**b**) Needle tip magnified showing inner blunt spring-loaded tip

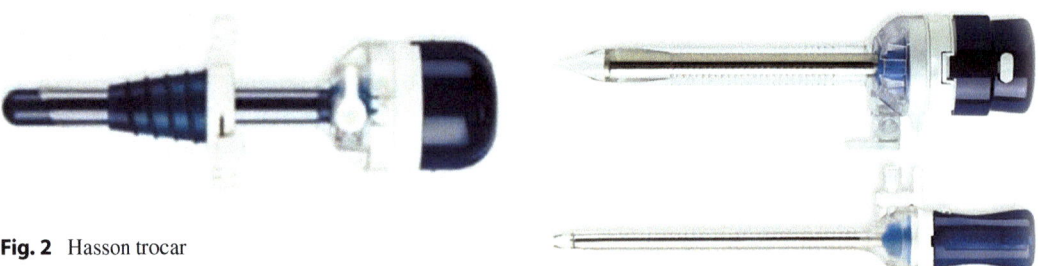

Fig. 2 Hasson trocar

Fig. 3 Optical trocars

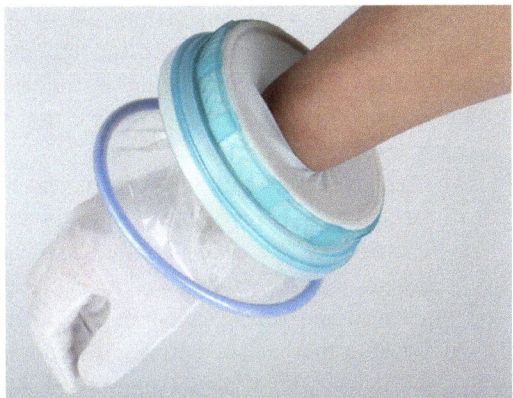

Fig. 4 Hand-assist port

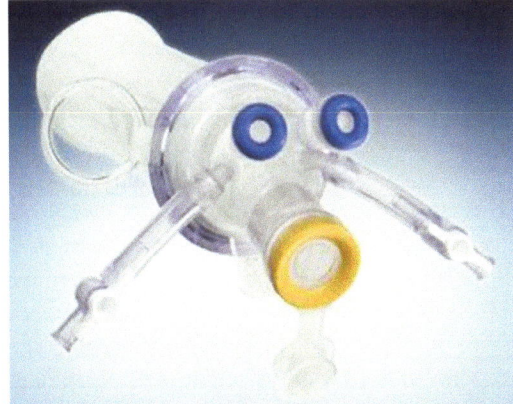

Fig. 5 Olympus Tri-port

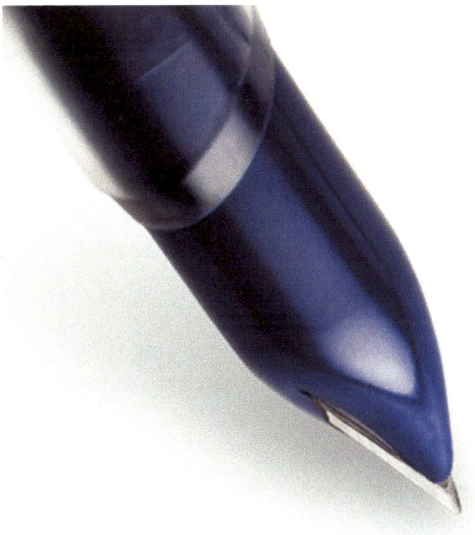

Fig. 6 Showing the extended cutting blade of a trocar

be inserted may vary. Fig. 5 shows Olympus Tri-port, a form of Single/Reduced port.

Device to Maintain the Working Space

Trocars or Conventional ports. The trocar or port is generally composed of two parts: the outer cannula and the inner trocar. The outer cannula usually has a valve that allows entry of hand instruments while maintaining the workspace, and a stopcock allows the insufflation and evacuation of the workspace. Like hand instruments, these can be reusable or single-use, have specific features to the outer sheath (flexible, ridges, or fixation balloon), and have varying trocar tip designs with different penetrating capabilities

(cutting or non-cutting). Maneuver during insertion through the abdominal wall: with long axis 90° to the wall, back and forth clockwise-counterclockwise rotation while slowly pushing in. Port can be held either two-handed (one hand on the head applying pushing and rotational force, while the second hand holds the cannula to prevent sudden slippage when the tip enters a cavity), or one-handed (the head in the palm with a finger or two along the cannula to act as a stopper when the tip enters a cavity)

(a) Bladed/Cutting—facilitated by a blade under a spring-loaded cover (Fig. 6) that springs forward, covering the cutting blade and locking in place once the device enters the abdominal cavity protecting the viscera within.

(b) Pyramidal—pyramidal tip is meant to expedite passage through tough tissue easier than the cone-tip, but with less trauma than a cutting-tip (Fig. 7).

(c) Dilating /non-cutting Tip—are usually pointed conical tip trocars intended to push aside the tissue fibers without cutting (Fig. 8).

We will now analyze the variety and characteristics of the instrumentations most frequently utilized to perform procedures. Instrumentations have different ergonomics, and they are mainly designed to accomplish a task or a determined action. Any surgeon must make proper and correct use of each one.

Endo-Laparoscopic Instruments: The Basic

The laparoscopic hand instruments (Fig. 9) are generally composed of three parts/sections:

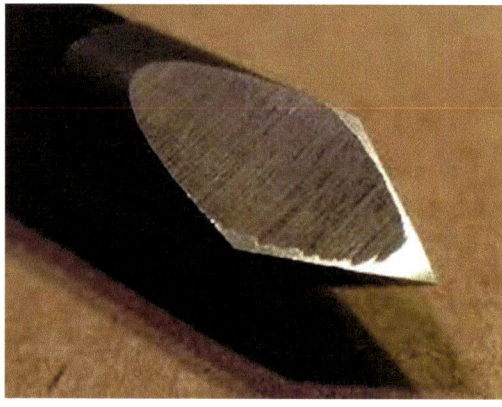

Fig. 7 Trocar with a pyramidal tip

Fig. 8 Trocar with a conical tip

1. Handle—this part controls the instrument tip and its function; it has features that contribute to the additional functions of the instrument and configuration that allows for the user's ergonomic preference.
   (a) Configuration/Design—the primary interface with the user provides control of the instrument's jaw action and has varying designs that allow for user preference that enhance comfort and ease of use (Fig. 10).
   (b) Locking mechanism—provides securing mechanism for the jaws to minimize hand strain when grasping tissues for extended periods.
   (c) Rotation knob—provides the means to rotate the instrument tip 360° around its long axis.
   (d) Electro-surgical post connects either monopolar or bipolar cable from the electro-surgical device to provide tissue coagulation or cutting capability.
2. Shaft—is a metal sheath through which the insert runs and connects to the instrument handle. Together with the insert, determine the instrument's length, based on the distance to the target tissue (dependent on varying factors: adult (33 cm) vs pediatric (23 cm), non-obese vs obese (43 cm), or preferred point of access). This part is usually covered by a non-conductive material (silicone or plastic) to isolate the current passing from the electro-surgical post to the instrument tip and prevent collateral injuries.
3. Instrument Insert/Tip—the main part that determines the function with specifically designed jaws.

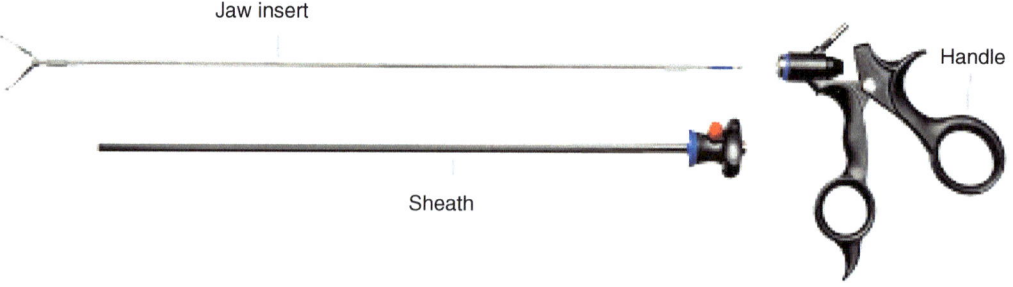

Fig. 9 Expanded view of the parts of a laparoscopic instrument

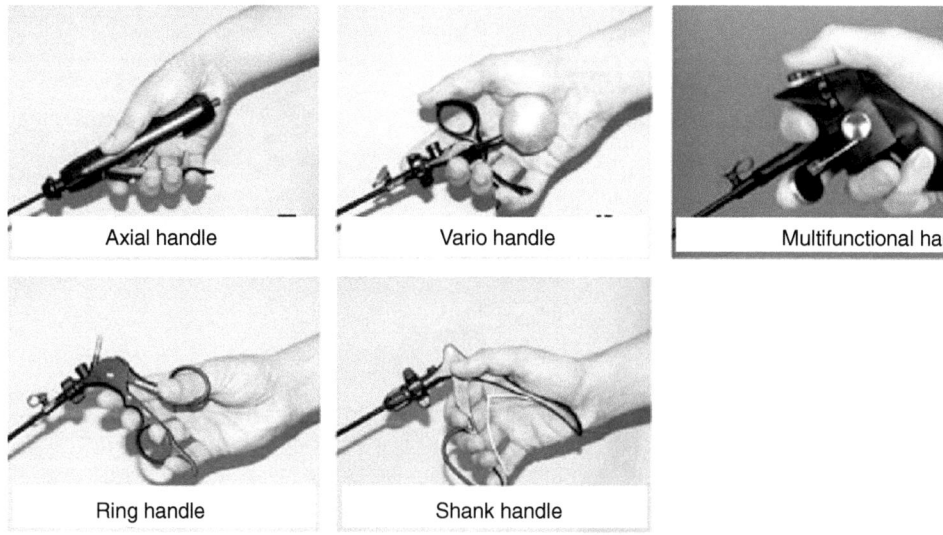

Fig. 10 Various handle designs in laparoscopic instruments

Fig. 11 Jaw action of laparoscopic instruments

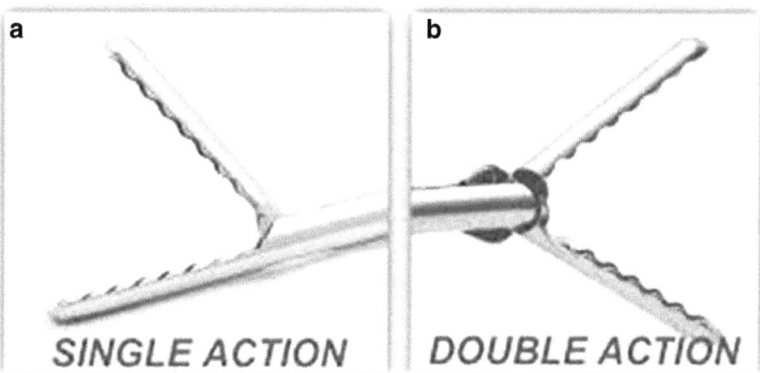

Concepts of Hand Instrument Variations

1. Jaw Action
   (a) Double-action—both jaws of the tip move; it is the preferred action for dissectors as it allows for greater tissue separation and access to varying tissue planes (Fig. 11b).
   (b) Single-action—one jaw moves while the other remains fixed; the mechanism allows for the force applied via the handle to be concentrated on the mobile jaw providing a firm grip. In instruments intended for delicate functions, this allows the user to focus on the mobile jaw (Fig. 11a).

2. Tip Function
   (a) Dissectors—are meant to expose, isolate, or separate tissue structures. The jaws are usually of the double-action type, fine-tipped, and with the curved jaws preferred by most users to allow better tip visualization. The most popular of which is the Maryland dissector (Fig. 12).
   (b) Graspers—are meant to hold on to structures to allow exposure, manipulation, or retraction. The jaws may be of atraumatic design for delicate tissues (Fig. 13), dou-

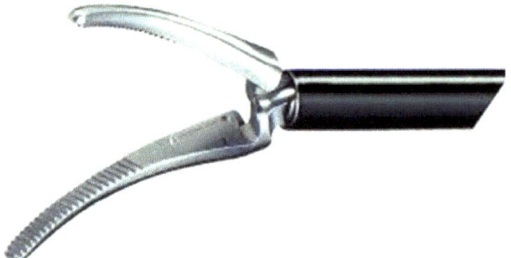

Fig. 12 Maryland dissector tip

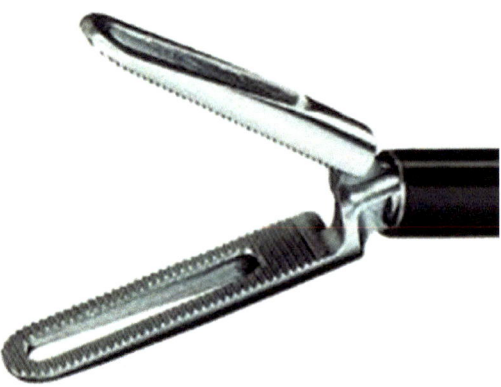

Fig. 13 Fenestrated atraumatic grasper tip

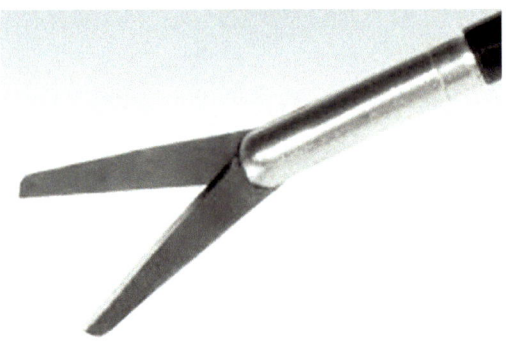

Fig. 14 Straight scissors

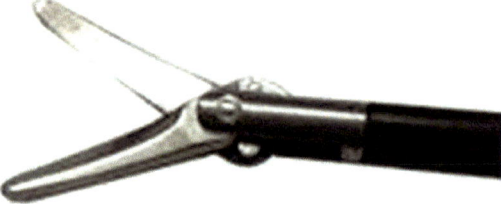

Fig. 15 Curved scissors

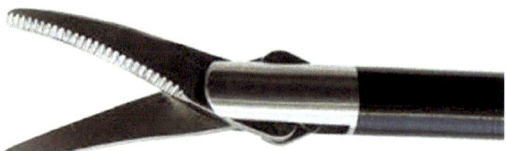

Fig. 16 Curved scissors with serrated blades

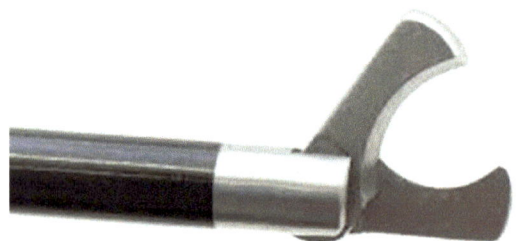

Fig. 17 Hook scissors

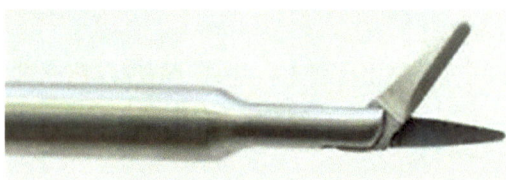

Fig. 18 Micro scissors

ble- or single-action, with or without fenestration (for a more secure grip, by
allowing the tissue to mold into the gaps),
with or without teeth (affords secure grip
on tougher tissues).

(c) Scissors/Shears—primarily meant for
cutting or sharp dissection, has varying
designs for specific functions.

   i. Straight scissors—mainly for cutting
      and dissection (Fig. 14).

ii. Curved scissors—preferred by most
    users, the curvature of the blade
    allows a better view of the tip
    (Fig. 15).

iii. Serrated scissors—ridges on the
     blade minimizes tissue or suture slip-
     page (Fig. 16).

iv. Hook scissors—encircles the struc-
    ture before cutting, assuring firm and
    solid grip (Fig. 17).

v. Micro scissors—facilitates partial
   cutting of structures (Fig. 18).

3. Insulation—In MIS, electro-surgical energy use plays a crucial part in dissection and hemostasis. The nonconducting material (usually plastic or silicone) covering the instrument shaft prevents the conduction of electrical current to surrounding tissues and isolates the flow toward the instrument's tip, allowing use even when the instrument shaft is in contact with other structures.

4. Reusability
   (a) "Reusable" instruments are meant to be used multiple times. They are constructed of durable materials, usually more rigid, and are expected to withstand repeated use and cleaning and sterilization processing cycles. They are also designed to be readily dismantled to allow thorough cleaning and have replaceable parts for easy maintenance.
   (b) "Disposable" instruments are also termed "single-use," they came about in response to the perceived high acquisition and maintenance cost of reusable instruments. They are usually manufactured from less costly materials, generally less robust, relatively flexible, cannot be dismantled for cleaning, and quickly wears down.
   (c) "Reposable" instruments arose from the combination of terms "reusable" and "disposable"; meant to describe the category of instruments having the beneficial characteristic of both. Reusable part (usually the handle) and disposable part (the insert and shaft, commonly scissors) components; supposed to integrate features: a sturdy instrument with low acquisition cost and eliminate the need for maintenance.

Specialized Endo-Laparoscopic Instruments

1. Irrigation and Suction instruments—meant to evacuate fluid by suction and dislodge adherent debris using pressurized water. The suc-

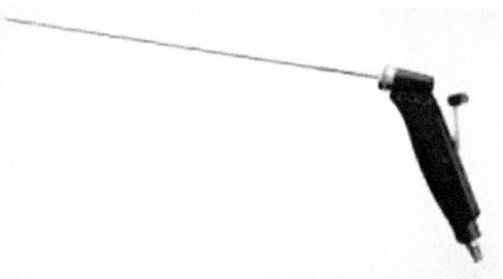

Fig. 19 Irrigation-suction instrument

tion tip usually has multiple fenestrations that not only facilitate suctioning but decrease the chance of obstruction by surrounding tissue (Fig. 19). Some are designed with an electro-surgical attachment that allows for simultaneous suctioning of fluids and coagulation of tissue, advantageous when the target area is constantly flooded.

2. Knot pushers—are usually long rods with specially designed tips used to perform extra-corporeal knot tying (Fig. 20a, b). The knots are thrown outside, utilizing this instrument to push the knot through the cannula and secure it inside.

3. Needle drivers/holders—are intended solely for executing intra-corporeal suturing and knot tying. These instruments have single-action, tough and robust jaws and, on occasion, may have tungsten inserts or diamond coating to ensure surface hardness and secure grip on the needle and suture, a rigid and sturdy shaft that can withstand applied rotational forces, and a ratchet mechanism. Various jaw configurations are available: straight, curved, and self-aligning (designed to orient the needle perpendicular to the jaws); the most versatile being the straight jaws which allow needle positioning in variable orientation (Fig. 21).

4. Retractors—similar to those used in open surgery, provide exposure by moving aside mobile structures such as small intestines, solid organs, or stomach. They may be hand-held or fixed to a bracket attached to the operating table.

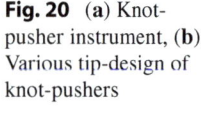

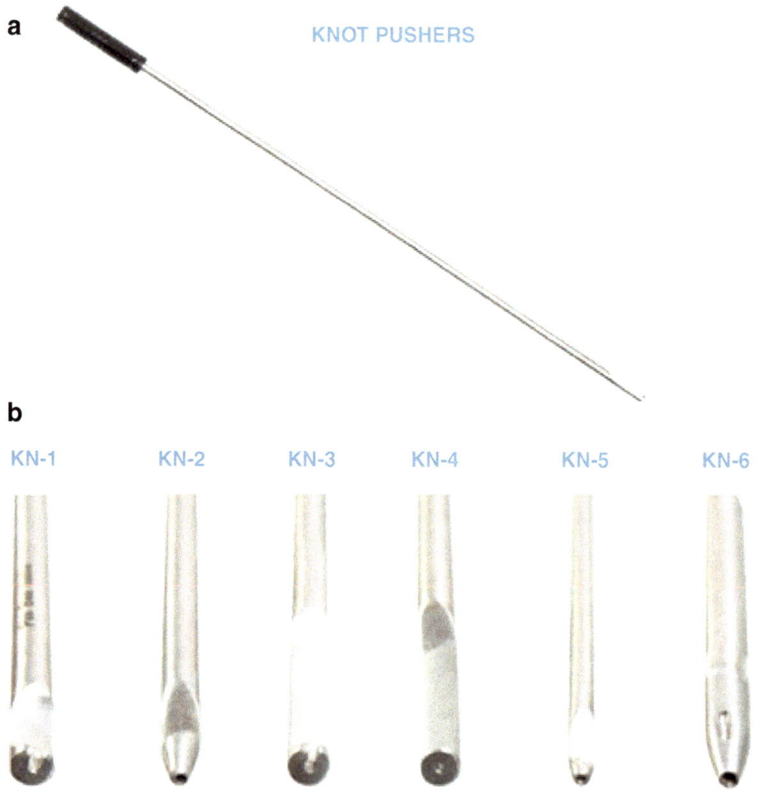

Fig. 20 (**a**) Knot-pusher instrument, (**b**) Various tip-design of knot-pushers

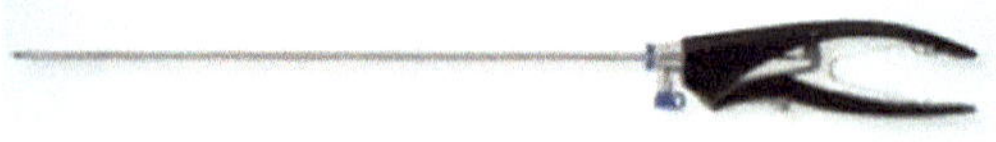

a

KNOT PUSHERS

b

| KN-1 | KN-2 | KN-3 | KN-4 | KN-5 | KN-6 |

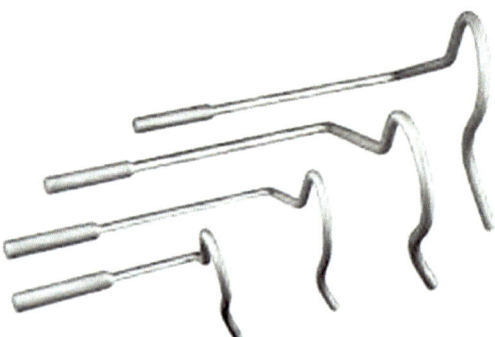

Fig. 21 Needle handler

Fig. 22 Nathanson retractor

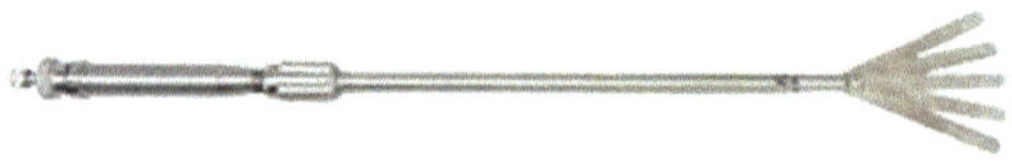

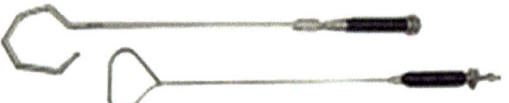

Fig. 23 Fan-retractor

Fig. 24 Snake-retractor

through an epigastric puncture site, maneuvered into position under the liver, and fixed to a bracket.

(b) The Hand-held retractors—meant to be operated by an assistant, allows for repositioning as the procedure progresses, a dynamic retractor. Once the desired retraction is achieved, it may also be fixed to a table-attached bracket and becomes a static retractor.

(a) The Nathanson retractor is designed to retract the liver (Fig. 22); it is inserted

i. Fan-retractor—has a folding head that spreads open like a hand-held fan when deployed (Fig. 23).

ii. Snake-retractor—is a floppy metallic tube that assumes a specified configuration and stiffens up when the tension knob is activated (Fig. 24).

Further Reading

Ahmed HO. Color atlas of laparoscopy. Suleimani: University of Suleimani; 2008. p. 31–140.

Adrales G, Park A. Technological and instrumentation aspects of laparoscopic hernia surgery. In: LeBlanc K, editor. Laparoscopic hernia surgery: an operative guide. Oxford University Press, Inc; 2003. p. 7–15.

Carol EH, Scott-Conner. The SAGES manual. New York: Springer-Verlag; 1998.

Goel A. Laparoscopic hand instruments, accessories and ergonomics. In: Kriplani A, Bhatia P, Prasad A, Govil D, Garg HP, editors. Comprehensive laparoscopic surgery. New Delhi: Sagar Printers; 2007. p. 9–19.

Palanivelu C. CIGES atlas of laparoscopic surgery. New Delhi: Jaypee Brothers Medical Publishers, Ltd.; 2000.

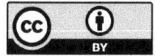

Operating Room Setup and Patient Positioning in MIS

Alembert Lee-Ong and Alfred Allen Buenafe

Crucial in any surgery, the performance and the outcome depend not only on the surgeon's skills and patient preparation but also on the setup of the operating room (OR) and positioning of the patients. In endo-laparoscopic surgery, we work with technology like cameras, monitors, insufflators, energy devices, and more. They are connected and interconnected by several cables and tubings. It is vital for patient's and OR Staff's safety that they be easily accessible in a fast and timely manner in case of any emergency or unexpected event. Avoid entangling of cables, or inter-

action between tubing and cables will make your surgery safer, elegant, and less stressful.

Moreover, the correct position of the patient to the endo-laparoscopic devices, monitor, and procedures is fundamental. The position depends on the procedure we intend to perform and where the surgical team will position in relation to the patient and the video monitor. Also, to surmount challenges like visceral retraction, we may need to tilt the patient, requiring preparation to avoid patient falling or sliding from the OR table.

Operating Room Setup

It depends on the size of your operating theater and the provision for the support of additional equipment. In general, the endo-laparoscopic camera system is on a cart and can be easily rolled and placed around the operating table accordingly. In other cases, the endo-laparoscopic camera system can be mounted on a boom arm and can be readily shifted around; in this so-called Integrated Operating Theater, additional monitors are placed on a swing arm that can be moved and adjusted to best fit the surgeon's needs. In general, the monitor stands along the axis: surgeon—target organ, the rest of the devices like insufflator, energy device, camera controller, recording, etc., can be placed nearby the operating table and are easy to access for monitoring and setup.

A. Lee-Ong (✉)
Department of Surgery, Manila Doctors Hospital, Manila, Philippines

Philippine Center for Advanced Surgery, San Juan, Philippines

Department of Surgery, Cardinal Santos Medical Center, San Juan, Philippines

Department of Surgery, Quirino Memorial Center, Quezon City, Philippines

A. A. Buenafe
Philippine Center for Advanced Surgery, San Juan, Philippines

Department of Surgery, Cardinal Santos Medical Center, San Juan, Philippines

Department of Surgery, Rizal Medical Center, Pasig, Philippines

Department of Surgery, Batangas Medical Center, Batangas, Philippines

Department of Surgery, Asian Hospital and Medical Center, Alabang, Muntinlupa, Philippines

© The Author(s) 2023

D. Lomanto et al. (eds.), *Mastering Endo-Laparoscopic and Thoracoscopic Surgery*, https://doi.org/10.1007/978-981-19-3755-2_10

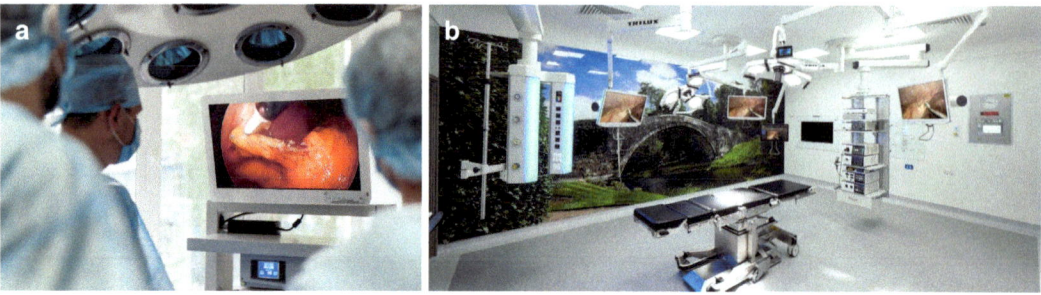

Fig. 1 Endo-laparoscopic system: (**a**) Endo-laparoscopic-cart mounted, (**b**) Boom-arm mounted

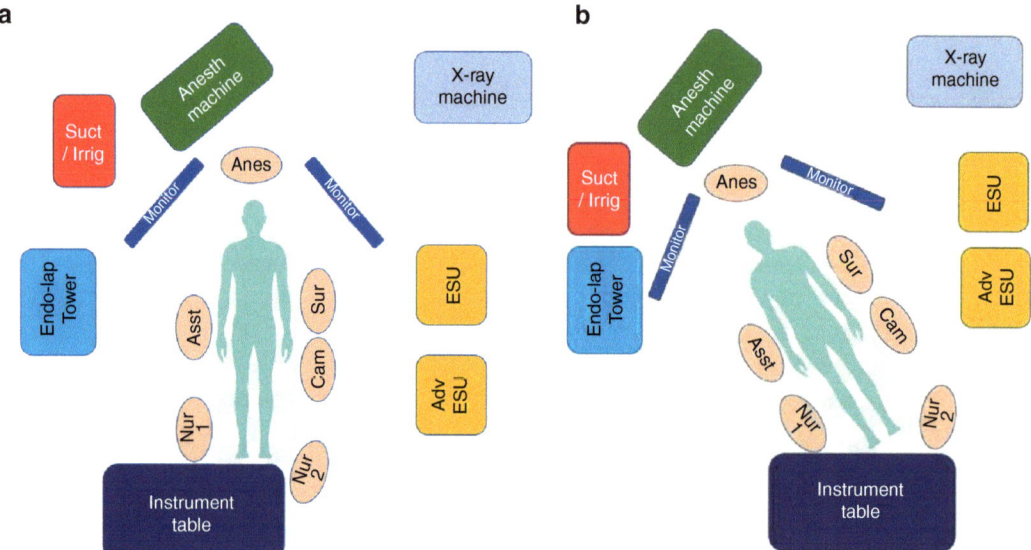

Fig. 2 Suggested OR setup in (**a**) large room, (**b**) small room

It is essential to plan everything ahead and before the patient is positioned on the table. Once the patient is draped, it will be cumbersome to reposition any devices. Allow enough space for the anesthesia team to move around and monitor the patient; if you need additional equipment like ultrasound, C-arm, various energy devices, laser, etc., plan and simulate the position. It is also essential to check that all the devices are correctly plugged in, powered, and working perfectly. For the OR Staff and the surgical team, allow good interaction and spacing. Usually, the operating surgeon and the camera assistant stand together on the same side of the patient and the opposite side of the targeted organ, allowing space for triangulation and the assistant on the contralateral side to help.

Figures 1a, b, 2a, b, and 3 are typical operating room setups for different surgical procedures.

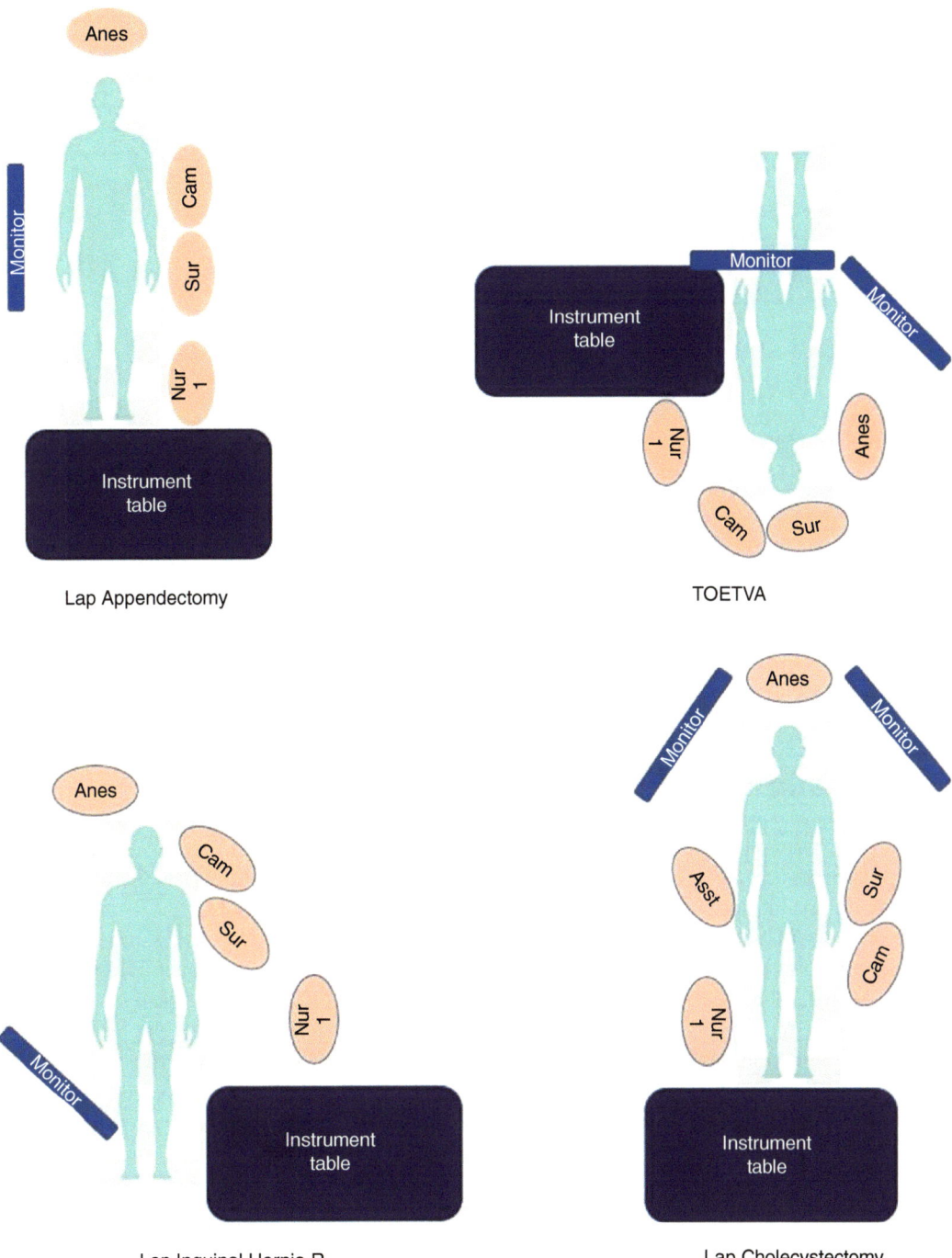

Fig. 3 Varying positions of the surgical team depending on the procedure

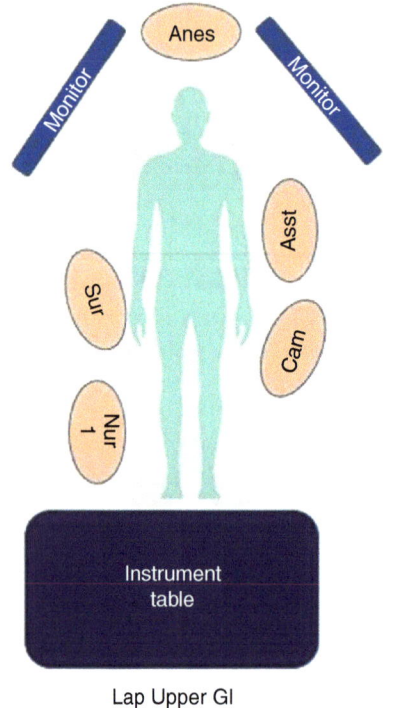

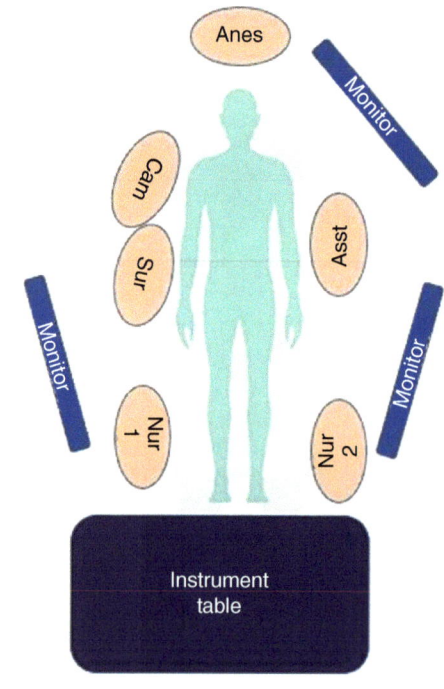

Lap Upper GI   Lap Lower GI Left

Fig. 3 (continued)

Introduction to Patient Positioning

Similar to exposure in open surgery, patient positioning is a necessary preparation in MIS; knowledge of the conduct of the operation provides comprehension of appropriate port placements and potential movement of the surgical team around the patient. Optimal patient positioning prevents inadvertent patient movement, protects the patient from injuries, ensures unhindered access to the port insertion area, and unencumbered instruments over and surgical team traffic around the patient.

The positioning augmented by intervals of unnatural positions (head down or up, or lateral tilt) allows gravity to retract the viscera away from the workspace. The prolonged operative time and maneuvering may generate compression, ischemia, shear, or stretch events that can cause positioning injuries like skin and tissue breakdown, transient neuropathies, compartment syndrome, and rhabdomyolysis [1]. The 2017 review by Zilloux and Krupski revealed the belief

these are rare events and comprehensive data on the general incidence is lacking; however, they gauged that postoperative neuropathies range 0.10–3.2% for MIS, 0.8–6.6% for robotic-assisted surgeries and suggests the overall incidence to be 2–5% [2, 3].

Factors such as operative time, body mass index (BMI), and the American Society of Anesthesiologists (ASA) physical status classification contributed to the development of positioning injuries. According to the study by Gelpi-Hammerschmidt et al. on renal surgeries, lengthy procedures (>5 h) have an increased chance of developing rhabdomyolysis. Correspondingly, other studies confirmed a decrease in positioning injuries and postoperative creatinine kinase as operative time decreases. BMI in both extremes is associated with an increased risk for injuries. High BMI presumably aggravates the underlying forces that produce damage, while the rationale for low BMI is the lack of subcutaneous soft tissue padding to protect the neurovascular structures. The poor ASA classification is linked to factors (malnutrition, diabetes, and peripheral vascular disease) that make a patient prone to neuromuscular insults [2].

General Guidelines for Patient Positioning

Pressure Redistribution. The use of pressure dispersing devices and surfaces is critical to reducing pressure-induced skin and tissue breakdown. The bony prominences of the body are areas where weight-bearing points come in contact with surfaces for prolonged periods and are prone to developing these injuries. Dispersal of focal pressure may be achieved using various types of padding material (blanket, foam, pillow, silicone, towel, or visco-elastic).

Deep Venous Thrombosis (DVT) Prevention. MIS procedures have inherent factors (long operative time, extremes of positioning, and pneumoperitoneum) that contribute to the risk of developing DVT. The application of anti-thromboembolic stockings and/or sequential compression devices has been shown to minimize DVT incidence in MIS [4].

Upper Extremities Positioning [1, 3]. The most effective means of avoiding brachial plexus injuries is to secure the arms carefully at the patient's sides, the palms resting against the patient with the elbows padded, and the draw sheet extends about the elbow and secured under the patient making sure it is not too tight to interfere with blood pressure cuff and intravenous lines. Avoid pronation of the arm, as this can expose the ulnar nerve to possible pressure. When arms are to be abducted, they should be placed level with the bed and not more than 90° from the patient's side. Avoiding shoulder braces and wrist straps is advised; however, the shoulder braces should be positioned at the acromioclavicular joints when needed.

Lower Extremities Positioning [1, 3]. For the lower extremities, especially for the lithotomy position, four elements of positioning should be kept in mind: (1) angle of hip flexion—60–170°, should never be >180° as it places strain on the lumbar spine, (2) angle of knee flexion—between 90–120°, greater flexion can put a strain on the sciatic nerve, lesser flexion can promote venous stasis that may lead to DVT, (3) angle of hip abduction—90° or less, a greater angle can put a strain on the obturator nerve, and (4) degree of external hip rotation—should be kept to the minimal, any degree of external rotation can increase strain on the femoral, obturator, and sciatic nerve leading to nerve injury; the use of boot stirrup can provide improved positioning of the lower extremity.

Standard Surgical Positions in MIS

Supine (Fig. 4). The supine position is the most common surgical position, also called the "dorsal recumbent" position. MIS procedures in this position include those requiring access to the neck area, the abdominal cavity through anterior access, or for inguinal hernias. The patient is positioned with the head and spine in a horizontal line with the hips parallel to each other with the legs positioned straight and uncrossed. The arms are positioned at the patient's sides or abducted. The table straps are applied loosely above the knees.

Modified Lithotomy (Fig. 5). In this position, the hips are flexed, with legs abducted, the knees bent, and the buttocks at the edge of the table; the arms may be secured at the sides or abducted. Procedures using this positioning may require concurrent or sequential access to several quadrants of the abdominopelvic cavity and the perineal area.

Prone (Fig. 6). Generally used for cases requiring access to the esophagus, the back, and the retroperitoneal area using dorsal access. After

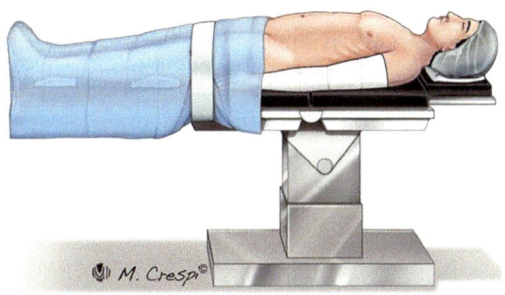

Fig. 4 Supine

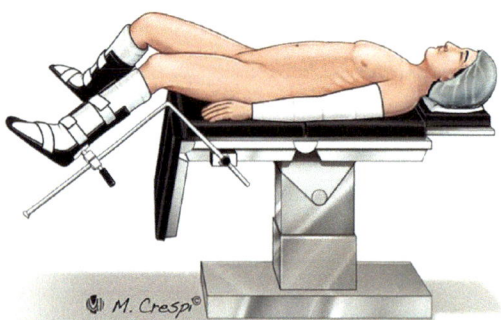

Fig. 5 Modified lithotomy

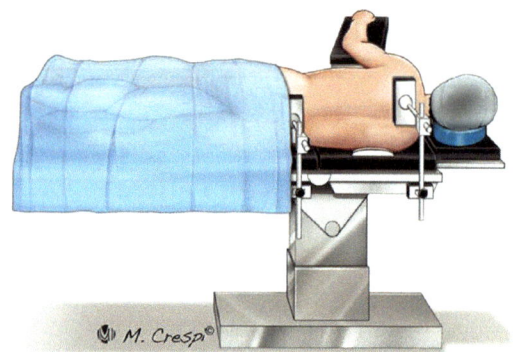

Fig. 7 Lateral decubitus

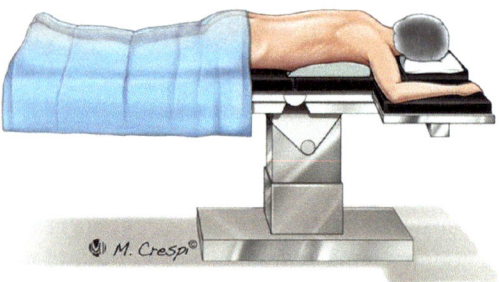

Fig. 6 Prone

induction of anesthesia, the patient is positioned face down with pads placed under the chest, hip, and thighs while verifying lung expansion is not restricted. The arms are brought down and forward next to the head, the elbows flexed, hands pronated, and padding at the elbows. The head may be turned to one side or placed on headrests designed to protect the airway.

Lateral/Lateral Decubitus (Fig. 7). The patient lies down on the side contralateral to the intended workspace side. The lateral positioning is used for access to the thorax, kidneys, and retroperitoneal space. Paddings are situated at the head, thorax, and legs; the arms are placed on supports, and bracing supports may be positioned at the back or anterior at the hip area.

Common Modifications

Trendelenburg and Reverse Trendelenburg (Fig. 8a, b). This modification may be added to any of the basic positions by placing the body on an incline. The Trendelenburg position elevates the feet above the head at an inclination of about 15–30°; the reverse Trendelenburg does the opposite—head elevated above the feet. The former allows gravity to pull the intra-abdominal organs away from the pelvis; the latter, the viscera to fall away from the upper abdomen.

Split Leg (Fig. 9). This variation applied to the standard supine position allows the surgeon to stand between the legs when the patient is in reverse Trendelenburg and be nearer to the upper abdomen access, which is frequently employed in bariatric and other upper gastrointestinal procedures.

Head extension (Fig. 10). The neck extension modification in the supine position is specific for access to the thyroid and parathyroid. The patient is initially positioned supine and anesthesia induced via nasotracheal intubation. The shoulders are raised with padding or sandbag, and the neck is slightly extended with the head secured over a donut ring.

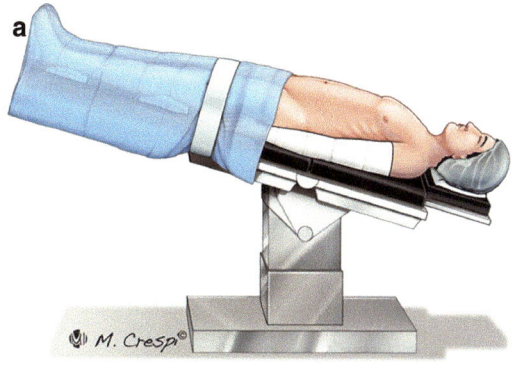

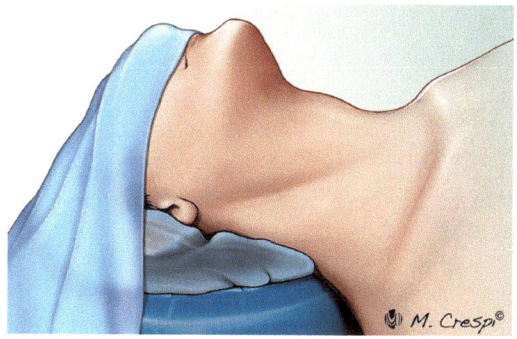

Fig. 10 Head extension

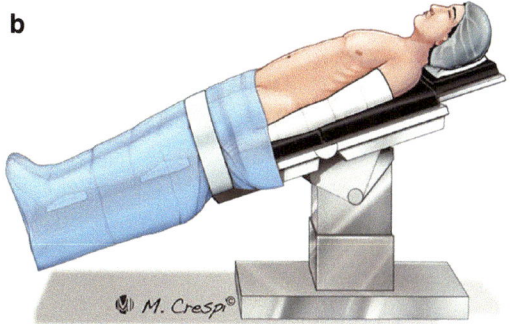

Fig. 8 (**a**) Trendelenburg and (**b**) Reverse Trendelenburg

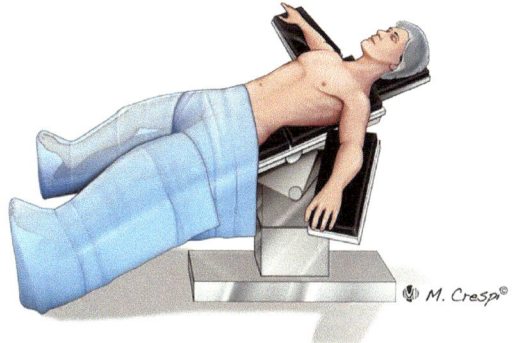

Fig. 9 Split Leg

References

1. Agostini J, Goasguen N, Mosnier H. Patient positioning in laparoscopic surgery: tricks and tips. J Visc Surg. 2010;147(4):e227–32.
2. Zillioux JM, Krupski TL. Patient positioning during minimally invasive surgery: what is current best practice? Robot Surg. 2017;4:69–76.
3. Barnett JC, Hurd WW, Rogers RM Jr, et al. Laparoscopic positioning and nerve injuries. J Minim Invasive Gynecol. 2007;14(5):664–72.
4. Millard JA, Hill BB, Cook PS, et al. Intermittent sequential pneumatic compression in prevention of venous stasis associated with pneumoperitoneum during laparoscopic cholecystectomy. Arch Surg. 1993;128(8):914–8. discussion 8–9

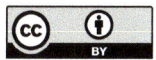

Surgical Smoke: Risks and Mitigation Strategies

Sajid Malik, Farah Khairi, and Sujith Wijerathne

Introduction

As the usage of electrocautery, ultrasonic scalpels, and lasers have become commonplace, operative staff and patients alike are at increased risk of exposure to dangerous surgical smoke emanating from these devices. Terms like "smoke," "plume," and less commonly "aerosol" are used to refer to by-products of laser tissue ablation and electrocautery, whereas "plume," "aerosol," and "vapor" are associated with ultrasonic dissection. "Smoke," although not formally accurate in all cases, is a widely accepted term used to describe surgically generated gaseous by-product [1].

Surgical smoke contains particulates like carbon monoxide, polyaromatic carbons, benzene, hydrogen cyanide, formaldehyde, viable and nonviable cellular material, viruses, and bacteria [2]. These particulates pose a risk to surgeons, operating theater personnel, and patients because they harbor these chemicals and biological components, and have shown to carry mutagenic and carcinogenic potential.

Factors affecting the amount and content of smoke produced does include type of procedure, surgeon's technique, pathology of target tissue (e.g., presence of bacteria or virus), type of energy device, power levels used, and the amount of cutting, coagulation, or ablation performed [3]. The smoke produced by each energy device has its own unique properties, comprising of aerodynamic particle size, chemical makeup, and biological constituents. For instance, electrocautery produces the smallest aerodynamic particle size, followed by laser tissue ablation creating larger ones while harmonic scalpels produce the largest particle size. The smaller the size, the further the distance these particles travel, and they pose a higher chemical concern. Larger particles, on the other hand, raise more concerns from a biological aspect [1].

Studies have compared the deposition of particulate matter in ten different tissues, and have shown that the liver produced the highest number of particles, skeletal muscle and renal tissues produced medium mass of particulate matter, while other tissues produced significantly less particulate mass [4].

Particles that are greater than 5μm can deposit on walls of the nose, pharynx, trachea, and bronchus whereas particles smaller than 2 μm are deposited in the bronchioles and alveoli. Considering that 77% of plume is in the inspirable range, it is concerning that smoke can cause

S. Malik (✉)
Department of General Surgery, Allama Iqbal Medical College, Lahore, Pakistan

F. Khairi
General Surgery Services, Alexandra Hospital, Queenstown, Singapore

S. Wijerathne
General Surgery Services, Alexandra Hospital, Queenstown, Singapore

Minimally Invasive Surgery Centre, National University Hospital Singapore, Singapore, Singapore

© The Author(s) 2023
D. Lomanto et al. (eds.), *Mastering Endo-Laparoscopic and Thoracoscopic Surgery*,
https://doi.org/10.1007/978-981-19-3755-2_11

acute and chronic inflammatory changes, including alveolar congestion, interstitial pneumonia, bronchiolitis, and emphysematous changes in the respiratory tract [5].

Multiple carcinogens have been identified in surgical smoke, with butadiene and benzene showing 17- and 10-fold higher concentrations than second-hand smoking. Several laboratory and animal studies have demonstrated smoke from laser and electrocautery surgery causing acute and delayed carcinogenic effects on humans. Although there is no direct evidence at present to show that surgical smoke is carcinogenic to humans, there are persistent concerns [5].

Besides chemical components, mutagenicity and cytotoxicity also pose great concerns to users of lasers, electrocautery, and powered surgical instruments. Tomita et al. quantified the mutagenic effect created by thermal destruction of just 1g of tissue to be equivalent to three to six cigarettes [6]. Additionally, studies have shown smoke produced from breast tissue has the mutagenicity of a TA98 strain of Salmonella, and another study demonstrated that it induced cytotoxicity in human small airway epithelial cells and mouse macrophages [7].

Surgical smoke, produced with or without a heating process, contains bio-aerosols with viable and nonviable cellular material that consequentially poses a risk of infection such as HIV, hepatitis B virus, and human papillomavirus (HPV) [8]. Although the possibility of disease transmission via surgical smoke exists, actual documented cases of pathogen transmission are rare. Only one such case has essentially been proven, whereby a surgeon contracted laryngeal papillomatosis after treating anogenital condyloma with a laser. HPV types 6 and 11, the same types in anogenital papillomatosis, were found in this individual's larynx, a very uncommon area of infection, which would suggest direct contact as a route of transmission [9].

Patients are also at risk from surgical smoke, particularly during laparoscopic procedures whereby smoke gets trapped in the peritoneal cavity. Potential complications include carbon monoxide toxicity, port-site metastases via chimney effect, and toxicity to peritoneal compartment and its contents [1]. The chimney effect, first described in 1995, stipulates that cancer cells are aerosolized during laparoscopic surgery and can leak from around the cannula during the procedure. The localized inflammation from the trauma caused by cannula and trocar insertion increases the potential for cancer cells to implant. It was also suggested that pneumoperitoneum creates a pressure gradient with resulting outflow of gas and floating tumor cells through port wounds, creating a chimney effect that does not occur in a standard wound [10]. Smoke also limits surgical field visibility, which poses direct harm to patients.

Mitigating the Risks

Once we recognize that surgical smoke is essentially an occupational hazard, it is important to minimize its production and have proper evacuation systems or protocols in place. It is also vital to raise awareness among surgeons and operating theater personnel regarding the dangers of surgical smoke.

Surgeons can minimize the production of surgical smoke by avoiding unnecessary tissue ablation and using shorter, precise bursts. Assistants may also aid in capturing smoke with a suction wand. A recently unpublished study had shown that a suction wand can effectively capture 95–99% of smoke if the tube's orifice is within 2 inches of the smoke source [11].

Small particles less than 1.1 μm constitute 77% of particulate matter found in surgical smoke [12]. Because of this, most conventional surgical masks do not have sufficient filtering or snug-fitting attributes to provide respiratory protection. A study by Gao et al. had shown that wearing at least N95 respirator and N100 filtering face piece respirator could offer more protection to wearers [13].

Evacuation Systems

The National Institute for Occupational Safety and Health (NIOSH) of the United States recommends a combination of general room and local exhaust ventilation (LEV) to remove airborne contaminants generated by surgical devices. They

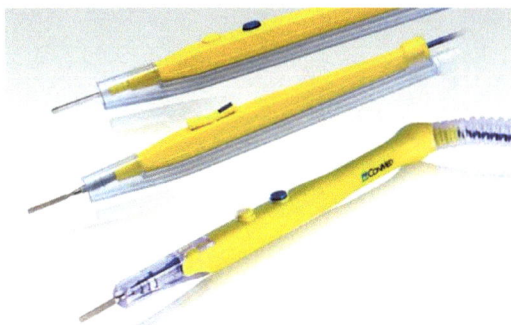

Fig 1 Smoke evacuation pencils and tubing

advocate suction devices with a capture velocity of 100–150 feet per minute [13]. Three such suction devices utilizing LEV include smoke evacuation wands, electrosurgical unit (ESU) pencils (Fig. 1), and cell foam technology.

ESU pencils are attached to tubing, which in turn connects to smoke evacuation filters. The latest device based on cell foam technology operates by having an open cell foam core sandwiched between layers of nonporous plastic to keep smoke within the device and prevent loss of suction power. The LEV machines used are in turn connected to ultra-low particulate (penetration) air (ULPA) filters that include activated charcoal which absorbs and deodorizes chemicals and odors present in smoke [13]. Filters should also be used in the exhaust port of the collection device to prevent contents of smoke from leaking [14].

Alternatively, high-efficiency particulate air (HEPA) filters that are placed on top entry ports of suction canisters can trap particulates effectively. Combination of HEPA filters with activated carbon called "high efficiency gas absorption" (HEGA) filters successfully prevent surgeons from volatile organic compounds and chemical vapors. Additionally, using activated carbon fiber filter during laparoscopic operations can dramatically reduce carcinogens by more than 85% [15].

Special Considerations

The COVID-19 pandemic had drastic ramifications towards society and many had to adapt to the "new normal" and change work practices.

The same applies to surgeons as there were raised concerns of the risk of coronavirus transmission in the operating room. Specifically, the elevated risk during intubation and extubation from the anesthetic standpoint, as well as the risk of release of potential infectious particulates in laparoscopic smoke.

Past research had shown that laparoscopy can lead to aerosolization of blood-borne viruses but there has been no evidence to support that this effect is seen with COVID-19, nor that it is isolated to laparoscopic procedures. However, to err on the side of caution, it is prudent to treat the coronavirus as exhibiting similar aerosolization properties. The UK and Ireland Intercollegiate Board have advised to consider laparoscopy only in selected cases whereby the clinical benefit of the patient outweighs the risk of viral transmission [16].

Assigning designated operating theaters for confirmed and suspect cases of COVID-19 can aid to streamline patient movements, limit the number of staff and equipment needed, as well as limiting contamination to specific areas. Negative pressure ventilation can curb contamination of surgical smoke via doors and vents. There had been recommendations to stop positive pressure ventilation during the procedure and for at least 20 min after the patient has left the theater; however, the risks associated with positive pressure ventilation have not been quantified [17].

Smoke extraction is crucial and can be achieved with a general ventilation system, local extraction at the site of surgery, and use of personal filtration masks, as discussed before. The smoke evacuator can be of two types one without the triple filter and the other one with a triple filtering tube (Figs. 2 and 3a, b). At present, the most effective smoke evacuation system is the triple filter, which includes a prefilter that traps large particles, an ULPA filter, and a special charcoal that captures toxic chemicals.

There are however nonfiltration devices available in the market that can evacuate smoke as well. The Ultravision™ system removes smoke particulates during electrosurgical procedures, as an aid to maintain clear visual field. This system is not restricted by particle size, and it has been

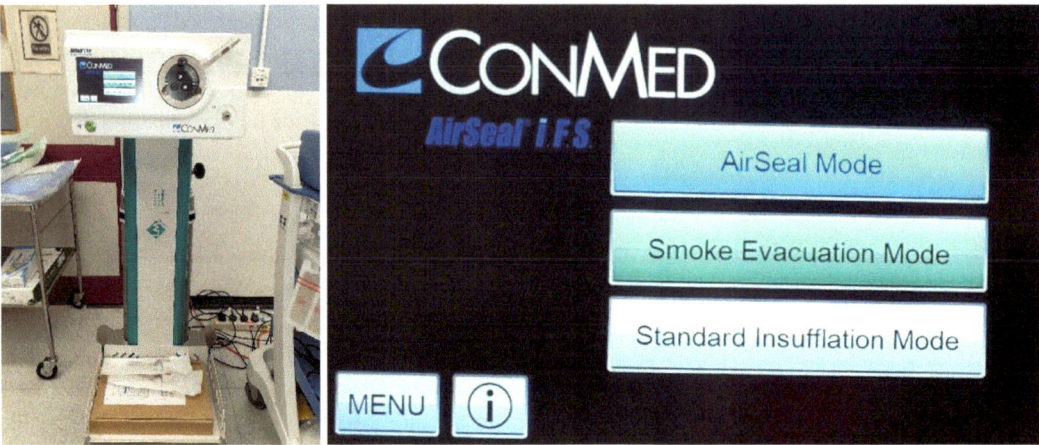

Fig 2 AirSeal intelligence unit

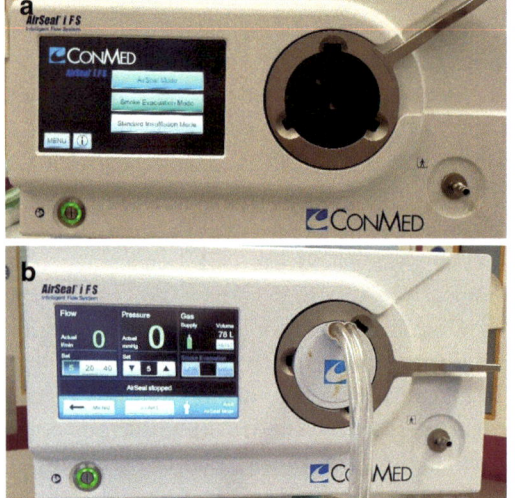

Fig 3 (**a**) Airseal iFS *without* Triple lumen filtered tube, (**b**) Airseal iFS *with* Triple lumen filtered tube

demonstrated to remove more than 99% of all smoke particulates [16].

Methods recommended for laparoscopic surgery include the use of balloon ports to reduce the risk of inadvertent displacement of trocars thus reducing the risk of loss of pneumoperitoneum to the operating theater environment. These trocars also have valves preventing gas leakage whenever an instrument is passed through into the peritoneal cavity. Pneumoperitoneum should be maintained throughout the procedure at the lowest possible pressure and decompressed

slowly at the end if an incision is required for specimen extraction [16].

Conclusion

Surgical smoke contains harmful particulates and although more research is required to determine its direct effect on health, we must be wary of its long-term effects. There are many mitigation strategies that can be applied, ranging from filtration masks to sophisticated smoke evacuation systems. The most important step however is to first and foremost educate healthcare workers that surgical smoke is an occupational hazard, and should be treated seriously as such.

References

1. Barrett W, Garber S. Surgical smoke: a review of the literature. Surg Endosc. 2003;17(6):979–87. https://doi.org/10.1007/s00464-002-8584-5.
2. Steege AL, Boiano JM, Sweeney MH. Secondhand smoke in the operating room? Precautionary practices lacking for surgical smoke. Am J Ind Med. 2016;59(11):1020–31. https://doi.org/10.1002/ajim.22614.
3. Gatti JE, Bryant CJ, Noone RB, Murphy JB. The mutagenicity of electrocautery smoke. Plastic Reconstr Surg. 1992;89(5):785–6. https://doi.org/10.1097/00006534-199205000-00002.
4. Karjalainen M, Kontunen A, Saari S, et al. The characterisation of surgical smoke from various tissues and its implications for occupational safety. PLoS

One. 2018;13(4):e0195274. https://doi.org/10.1371/journal.pone.0195274.

5. Liu Y, Song Y, Hu X, Yan L, Zhu X. Awareness of surgical smoke hazards and enhancement of surgical smoke prevention among the gynaecologists. J Cancer. 2019;10(2):2788–99. https://doi.org/10.7150/jca.31464.

6. Yoshifumi T, Shigenobu M, Kazuto N, et al. Mutagenicity of smoke condensates induced by CO2-laser irradiation and electrocauterization. Mutat Res. 1981;89(2):145–9. https://doi.org/10.1016/0165-1218(81)90120-8.

7. Sisler JD, Shaffer J, Soo J-C, et al. In vitro toxicological evaluation of surgical smoke from human tissue. J Occup Med Toxicol. 2018;13(1):12. https://doi.org/10.1186/s12995-018-0193-x.

8. Alp E, Bijl D, Bleichrodt R, Hansson B, Voss A. Surgical smoke and infection control. J Hosp Infect. 2006;62(1):1–5. https://doi.org/10.1016/j.jhin.2005.01.014.

9. Lobraico RV, Schifano MJ, Brader KR. A retrospective study on the hazards of the carbon dioxide laser plume. J Laser Applic. 1998;1(1):6–8. https://doi.org/10.2351/1.4745215.

10. Hubens G, Pauwels M, Hubens A, Vermeulen P, Marck EV, Eyskens E. The influence of a pneumoperitoneum on the peritoneal implantation of free intraperitoneal colon cancer cells. Surg Endosc. 1996;10(8):809–12. https://doi.org/10.1007/s004649900166.

11. Schultz L. An analysis of surgical smoke plume components, capture and evacuation. AORN J. 2014;99(2):289–98. https://doi.org/10.1016/j.aorn.2013.07.020.

12. Benson SM, Novak DA, Ogg MJ. Proper use of surgical N95 respirators and surgical masks in the OR. AORN J. 2013;97(4):457–70. https://doi.org/10.1016/j.aorn.2013.01.015.

13. Fan JK-M, Chan FS-Y, Chu K-M. Surgical smoke. Asian J Surg. 2009;32(4):253–7. https://doi.org/10.1016/s1015-9584(09)60403-6.

14. Gao S, Koehler RH, Yermakov M, Grinshpun SA. Performance of facepiece respirators and surgical masks against surgical smoke: simulated workplace protection factor study. Ann Occup Hyg. 2016;60:608–18. https://doi.org/10.1093/annhyg/mew006.

15. Choi SH, Choi DH, Kang DH, et al. Activated carbon fibre filters could reduce the risk of surgical smoke exposure during laparoscopic surgery: application of volatile organic compounds. Surg Endosc. 2018;32(10):4290–8. https://doi.org/10.1007/s00464-018-6222-0.

16. Mowbray NG, Ansell J, Horwood J, et al. Safe management of surgical smoke in the age of COVID-19. Br J Surg. 2020;107(11):1406–13. https://doi.org/10.1002/bjs.11679.

17. Team RCSEC. Intercollegiate General Surgery Guidance on COVID-19 UPDATE. The Royal College of Surgeons of Edinburgh. Published March 30, 2020. https://www.rsced.ac.uk/news-public-affairs/news/2020/march/intercollegiate-general-surgery-guidance-on-covid-19-update. Accessed 11 July 2020.

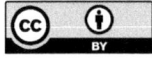

Part II

Anesthesia in Laparoscopic Surgery

Principles of Anesthesia

Emily Rose Nery

Introduction

The evolution of minimally invasive surgery in the last three decades led to better surgical experience, improvements in instrumentation, and application in a wide range of surgical procedures [1]. It has quickly emerged as the new gold standard versus traditional open surgical approaches. The advantages of laparoscopic surgery include reduced tissue trauma, reduced postoperative opioid analgesic requirement, improved postoperative pulmonary function, early recovery, and cost-effectiveness [2].

In laparoscopic surgery, the principles of anesthetic management centers around the interaction of the following elements: (1) intraperitoneal insufflation of carbon dioxide to create a pneumoperitoneum, (2) the systemic effects of carbon dioxide absorption, (3) the extreme changes in patient positioning, and (4) patient-related factors.

The advent of enhanced recovery programs with their goal of accelerating postoperative recovery, reducing the length of stay, and early return to preoperative status by reducing surgical stress response is seen as a complementary approach to minimally invasive surgery [3]. Established ERAS programs integrate several items among which short fasting time, perioperative fluid optimization, multimodal pain management, early mobilization, PONV prophylaxis, and treatment [4] as elements that overlap with the laparoscopic technique.

Physiologic Changes

The greatest impact on cardiovascular, pulmonary, and renal physiology stems from the pneumoperitoneum, the choice of carbon dioxide (CO_2) as insufflating gas, and the effects of patient positioning. Carbon dioxide is the preferred gas because it is highly soluble in blood, clears more rapidly, and is not combustible. The increase in intra-abdominal pressure (IAP) from CO_2 insufflation exerts mechanical and physiologic effects, while the systemic absorption of CO_2 produces hypercarbia and acidosis.

The determinants of cardiac output are systemic venous return and preload. Majority of the venous blood that enters the right atrium comes from the inferior vena cava (IVC). At IAP = 7.5 mm Hg, compression of the splanchnic circulation diverts the blood centrally and an early rise in cardiac output is observed [5].

E. R. Nery (✉)
Department of Anesthesiology, The Medical City, Pasig, Philippines

Acute and Critical Care Institute, The Medical City, Pasig, Philippines

Department of Anesthesiology and Perioperative Medicine, Rizal Medical Center, Pasig, Philippines
e-mail: ecnery@themedicalcity.com

© The Author(s) 2023
D. Lomanto et al. (eds.), *Mastering Endo-Laparoscopic and Thoracoscopic Surgery*,
https://doi.org/10.1007/978-981-19-3755-2_12

But as IAP continues to rise beyond 15 mm Hg, mechanical compression of the IVC and blood pooling in the lower extremities results in decreased venous return and a decrease in cardiac output [5].

Neuroendocrine responses and aortic compression results in increases in mean arterial pressure (MAP) and systemic vascular resistance (SVR). Reduction in cardiac output activates the renin-angiotensin system and release of vasopressin resulting in an increase in MAP. Stimulation of the sympathetic nervous system and release of catecholamines mediates the increase in SVR [6]. While vagal stimulation from abdominal distention and insertion of Veress needle may result in bradyarrhythmias and cardiac arrest [7]. Measures to attenuate the vagal response include slower insufflation time, lower IAP, and pharmacologic.

Cephalad displacement of the diaphragm secondary to pneumoperitoneum may impact pulmonary mechanics. Diaphragmatic displacement reduce lung volumes, reduce lung compliance, and increase airway pressures. The resulting decrease in functional residual capacity (FRC) and atelectasis may lead to V/Q mismatch [8].

Hypercarbia and acidosis as the result of CO2 absorption lead to cardiovascular and hemodynamic consequences [9]. Hypercarbia is addressed by increasing minute ventilation to maintain normal end-tidal CO_2.

Extreme changes in patient positioning in either a head-up (reverse Trendelenburg) or head-down (Trendelenburg) orientation affect cardiovascular and pulmonary functions. The head-up position leads to venous pooling affecting venous return to the heart. Catecholamines are also elevated in a head-up position, increasing SVR further reducing CO. The head-down position, on the other hand, moves the diaphragm and abdominal contents cephalad, reducing pulmonary compliance and increasing airway pressures. The reverse Trendelenburg favors pulmonary function, while the Trendelenburg favors venous return.

Anesthetic Management

Preoperative Evaluation

Preoperative evaluation and preparation of patients for laparoscopic surgery follow the same guideline equivalent to any surgery. A medical history and physical examination should be performed for all patients. The American Society of Anesthesiologists (ASA) classification aids in stratifying patients based on their physiologic reserves. Keeping in mind the physiologic derangements inherent with laparoscopy, further assessment of the patient's medical condition may be warranted.

Generally, laparoscopic surgery has a lower cardiovascular risk compared with open techniques. However, an understanding of the physiologic effects of the surgical technique that may increase the perioperative risk in specific patient population is essential. Adequate patient preparation, identification of risks, and anticipation of the hemodynamic and ventilatory effects together with a comprehensive anesthetic plan can mitigate the risk of adverse events and improve postoperative recovery.

Patients with cardiovascular diseases may not tolerate the increases in preload (↑ RAP, PCWP) and afterload (↑ SVR) and a decrease in cardiac output (CO). Those with decreased myocardial reserves may suffer decompensation brought about by further reductions in cardiac output. While the risk of myocardial ischemia in laparoscopic surgery is low, it may be precipitated by increases in myocardial oxygen demand brought about by increases in heart rate (HR), mean arterial pressure (MAP), and systemic vascular resistance (SVR). Mitigating measures include optimization of fluid status preoperatively, appropriate medications including continuing beta-blockers and heart failure medicine, close hemodynamic monitoring intraoperatively, avoidance of hypothermia, keeping the IAP < 15 mm Hg, and adequate pain management [10]. Morbid obesity is associated with comorbidities including diabetes mellitus, hypertension, obstructive sleep apnea, and restrictive lung disease. Pneumoperitoneum during laparoscopy alters the respiratory mechanics more in morbidly obese patients compared with patients of normal weight. Pulmonary compliance is reduced whereas inspiratory resistance is elevated requiring higher minute ventilation to maintain normocarbia [11]. Perioperative management includes avoiding steep head-down position, avoiding early extubation, and in some cases, extubation to CPAP/BIPAP.

Intraoperative Management

General anesthesia with endotracheal intubation and controlled mechanical ventilation is the most common choice of anesthesia technique. Balanced anesthesia employing either inhaled or intravenous anesthetics is chosen based on anesthesiologist's preference, the pharmacologic profile of the drugs, and the physiologic status of the patient. A total intravenous anesthesia (TIVA) using a propofol-based hypnotic has the added benefit of reducing postoperative nausea and vomiting.

Airway management with a cuffed endotracheal tube prevents aspiration pneumonitis and is still the airway of choice for most laparoscopic surgeries. Carbon dioxide insufflation shifts the diaphragm cephalad which increases airway pressure. This in turn increases the chance of air leaks, inadequate ventilation, and gastric insufflation that potentiates the risk of regurgitation and aspiration.

Several studies have compared the safety, efficacy, and complication risks of supraglottic airway devices (SGA) with endotracheal tubes (ETT). SGAs were found to be clinically useful in laparoscopy [12]. Second-generation SGAs with ventilation tube and gastric access provide higher oropharyngeal leak pressure than first-generation SGAs and reduce the risk of aspiration. These factors make a SGA device a viable option for airway management with the added benefits of attenuated hemodynamic changes compared with laryngoscopy and ETT as well as being well tolerated by patients with fewer incidences of coughing, laryngospasm, sore throat, and hoarseness.

Pneumoperitoneum in laparoscopy may cause derangements of the cardiopulmonary function and a lung-protective ventilation strategy using a combination of tidal volume of 6–8 ml/kg ideal body weight, a fraction of inspired oxygen (FiO2) of 0.5 ml, application of PEEP and recruitment maneuvers help improve lung mechanics and improve hypoxemia [13]. Controlled mechanical ventilation with pressure or volume modes is used to reduce peak inspiratory pressure and manage hypercarbia during laparoscopy.

Neuromuscular blocking agents (NMBA) help facilitate endotracheal intubation, improve surgical conditions by increasing the compliance of the abdomen and allow control of ventilation. The choice is guided by the drug's pharmacologic profile and anticipated length of surgery. Reversal of NMBAs is by metabolism or pharmacologic (neostigmine and sugammadex). Quantitative evidence of adequate reversal must be confirmed with train-of-four monitor.

Perioperative fluid management is very complex and clinically challenging. Hypervolemia increases the incidence of edema, impairs gut motility, and impairs wound healing. At the other end of the spectrum, hypovolemia may worsen hypotension, lead to oxygen mismatch, organ dysfunction, and lactic acidosis [14]. Static indicators of fluid balance like heart rate, central venous pressure, and urine output are unreliable. However, employing monitors for goal-directed fluid therapy remains controversial in laparoscopic surgery. The decision to use invasive and noninvasive monitors to guide fluid management must be based on the patient's condition and the extent of surgery.

Monitoring

Placement of routine monitoring equipment follows the basic standards of the ASA and includes pulse oximetry, noninvasive blood pressure monitoring, electrocardiography, temperature, and end-tidal carbon dioxide monitor. Additional monitors are warranted based on the duration of surgery, patient condition, and expected blood loss.

Positioning

Care must be taken to ensure that bony prominences and pressure points are well padded as in any surgery to prevent injury and peripheral nerve damage. Extremes in patient position necessitate the application of non-slip padding and body restraints to secure the patient to the operating table safely. Foot supports are employed in surgeries that require reverse Trendelenburg positions, while shoulder supports placed laterally at the acromioclavicular joint are used for steep Trendelenburg positions. The head is rested on a foam pillow with the neck in a neutral position. Arms are either tucked at the side or abducted to less than 90 on padded arm boards depending on the type of surgery and must be kept in a neutral thumbs-up or supinated position.

Postoperative Management

Pain expectations should be discussed preoperatively. The sources of pain from laparoscopic surgery are both somatic and visceral and the degree of pain depends on the specific surgery but is usually low to moderate. Evidence-based pain management recommends a combination of paracetamol, NSAID or cyclooxygenase-2-specific inhibitor, surgical site local infiltration, and dexamethasone [15]. A procedure-specific, multimodal approach capitalizing on preemptive analgesia and opioid-sparing techniques improve outcomes by providing adequate analgesia and reducing patient discomfort and adverse effects compared with a single opioid technique.

The advent of ultrasound-guided nerve blocks expanded the possibilities for pain management in laparoscopic surgeries. Currently, several techniques (i.e., transversus abdominis plane, paravertebral, and quadratus lumborum blocks) are being explored with promising results.

Postoperative Nausea and Vomiting (PONV)

PONV is one of the most distressing experience for patients after surgery. Although laparoscopy is identified as one risk factor for PONV, the literature is far from robust. Several predictors of risk of PONV in adults have been identified including (1) female gender, (2) history of motion sickness or PONV, (3) non-smoker, and (4) postoperative opioid use [16]. The risk increases with the number of factors present. Current recommendation is a multimodal antiemetic therapy based on the patient's level of risk using a combination of dexamethasone and 5-HT3 receptor antagonists. Additional antiemetic therapy may be used for very high-risk patients or as a rescue for intractable PONV [17].

References

1. Leonard IE, Cunningham AJ. Anaesthetic considerations for laparoscopic cholecystectomy. Best Pract Res Clin Anaesthesiol. 2002;16(1):1–20.
2. Keller DS, Delaney CP, et al. A national evaluation of clinical and economic outcomes in open versus laparoscopic colorectal surgery. Surg Endosc. 2016;30(10):4220–8.
3. Ni X, Jia D, et al. Is the enhanced recovery after surgery (ERAS) program effective and safe in laparoscopic colorectal cancer surgery? a meta-analysis of randomized controlled trials. J Gastrointest Surg. 2019;23(7):1502–12.
4. Gustafsson UO, Scott MJ, et al. Guidelines for perioperative care in elective colorectal surgery: Enhanced Recovery After Surgery (ERAS) Society Recommendations: 2018. World J Surg. 2019;43(3):659–95.
5. Kitano Y, Takata M, et al. Influence of increased abdominal pressure on steady-state cardiac performance. J Appl Physiol. 1999;86(5):1651–6.
6. Myre K, Rostrup M, et al. Plasma catecholamines and haemodynamic changes during pneumoperitoneum. Acta Anaesthesiol Scand. 1998;42(3):343–7.
7. Yong J, Hibbert P, et al. Bradycardia as an early warning sign for cardiac arrest during routine laparoscopic surgery. Int J Qual Health Care. 2015;27(6):473–8.
8. Atkinson. Cardiovascular and ventilatory consequences. 703.
9. Cunningham AJ. Laparoscopic surgery—anesthetic implications. Surg Endosc. 1994;8:1272–84.
10. Atkinson. Cardiovascular and ventilatory consequences. 701–702.

11. Sprung J, Whalley DG, et al. The impact of morbid obesity, pneumoperitoneum, and posture on respiratory system mechanics and oxygenation during laparoscopy. Anesth Analg. 2002;94:1345–50.

12. Park SK, Ko G, et al. Comparison between supraglottic airway devices and endotracheal tubes in patients undergoing laparoscopic surgery: a systemic review and meta-analysis. Medicine. 2016;95(33):e4598.

13. Valenza F, Chevallard G, et al. Management of mechanical ventilation during laparoscopic surgery. Best Pract Res Clin Anaesthesiol. 2010;24:227–41.

14. Rehm M, Hulde N, et al. State of the art in fluid and volume therapy. Anaesthesist. 2019;68(Suppl):S1–14.

15. Barazanchi AWH, MacFater WS, et al. Evidence-based management of pain after laparoscopic cholecystectomy: a PROSPECT review update. Br J Anaesth. 2018;121(4):787–803.

16. Horn CC, Wallisch WJ, et al. Pathophysiological and neurochemical mechanisms of postoperative nausea and vomiting. Eur J Pharmacol. 2014;722:55–66.

17. Gan TJ, Belani KG. Fourth consensus guidelines for the management of postoperative nausea and vomiting. Anesth Analg. 2020;131(2):411–48.

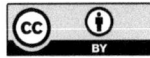

Physiologic Considerations in Laparoscopic Surgery

Alembert Lee-Ong

Introduction

MIS technique compared to the open technique is associated with substantial benefits for the patients, attributable to less surgical trauma; however, this does not imply the absence of physiologic changes when not anticipated may be deleterious. These physiologic alterations are triggered by a combination of the following: the insufflation gas used, the increase in intra-abdominal pressure (IAP), the extreme patient positioning during surgery, and the effect of the surgery itself [1].

Carbon Dioxide (CO_2) Effect

Carbon dioxide is the gas of choice used for insufflation in MIS, as it is nontoxic, nonflammable, rapidly soluble in blood, easily eliminated by the lungs, and relatively inexpensive [1]. Since CO_2 is a normal product of cellular metabolism, at physiological levels is nontoxic and an efficient means for its elimination is inherent in humans.

A. Lee-Ong (✉)
Department of Surgery, Manila Doctors Hospital, Manila, Philippines

Philippine Center for Advanced Surgery, San Juan, Philippines

Department of Surgery, Cardinal Santos Medical Center, San Juan, Philippines

Department of Surgery, Quirino Memorial Center, Quezon City, Philippines

The absorption rate of CO_2 is influenced by its partial pressure gradient between the cavity and the blood, its diffusion coefficient, the surface area of the cavity, and the perfusion of the walls of the cavity [2]. The CO_2 absorbed is dissolved in the blood and delivered to the lungs for excretion by ventilation, while the majority combines with water to form carbonic acid, which dissociates into hydrogen and bicarbonate. The hydrogen ions complex with hemoglobin and the bicarbonate diffuses into the plasma. These result in an increase in arterial pCO_2 and a fall in arterial pH.

The space insufflated with CO_2 influences the physiologic changes exerted by CO_2 absorption. Intraperitoneal insufflation with CO_2 is associated with an initial rapid rise in pCO_2 during the first 15 min and followed by plateau or second phase of slower change [2]. Extraperitoneal insufflation shows a significantly faster rise in pCO_2 and tends to persist into the postoperative period [3]. The magnitude of the rise in pCO_2 was not significantly different between extra- and intraperitoneal insufflation [2]. The faster rate seen in extraperitoneal insufflation may be due to concentrated absorption, vascularity of the extraperitoneal space, a faster diffusion in the extraperitoneal cavity, or a combination of these factors.

Mild hypercarbia (pCO_2 of 45–50 mm Hg) has minimal effect on hemodynamics; however, moderate to severe hypercarbia have both direct and indirect effects on the cardiovascular system: direct effects include myocardial depression and vasodilatation, while indirect effects are brought

D. Lomanto et al. (eds.), *Mastering Endo-Laparoscopic and Thoracoscopic Surgery*,
https://doi.org/10.1007/978-981-19-3755-2_13

83

about by catecholamine release eventually causing increase myocardial oxygen consumption [2]. While most healthy individuals will not be significantly affected by CO_2 elevation and can be corrected with moderate hyperventilation; those with cardiorespiratory compromise may not respond similarly and will need careful perioperative monitoring.

Insufflation with CO_2 results in a blunted immune response compared to open procedures. Acute-phase reactant (C-reactive protein) and cytokines (interleukin-6 and tumor necrosis factor-alpha) produced in response to tissue injury are likewise reduced in the presence of CO_2 [4].

Pneumoperitoneum/Increase Intra-abdominal Pressure Effect

Insufflation of the abdominal cavity results in shifting the abdominal wall outwards and the diaphragm upwards, resulting in an increase in intra-abdominal pressure (IAP) and reduction of thoracic volume, respectively. Respiratory compliance is reduced by 50% when the peritoneal cavity is insufflated to a pressure of 15 mm Hg [1, 5]. Pulmonary functions reduced with the decrease in lung compliance include forced expiratory volume in the first second (FEV1), functional residual capacity (FRC), total lung capacity, and vital capacity (VC) [1]; these changes can predispose to the development of ventilation-perfusion mismatch, leading to hypoxemia. Increasing the ventilatory rate is necessary to promote ventilation and maintain pCO_2 at or near-normal levels (Fig. 1).

Hemodynamic changes seen with pneumoperitoneum are the result of mechanical and neurohormonal responses. The increased IAP caused by pneumoperitoneum produces vascular compression of the inferior vena cava (IVC), aorta, splanchnic vasculature, and renal vasculature; this shifts the peripheral vascular volume to the central venous compartment, causing an initial increase in venous return [5]. A biphasic response is seen with an increase in the right atrial pressure (RAP), left atrial pressure (LAP), and cardiac output (CO) at 7.5 mm Hg IAP; as the IAP increases beyond 15 mm Hg, both the RAP and LAP remain

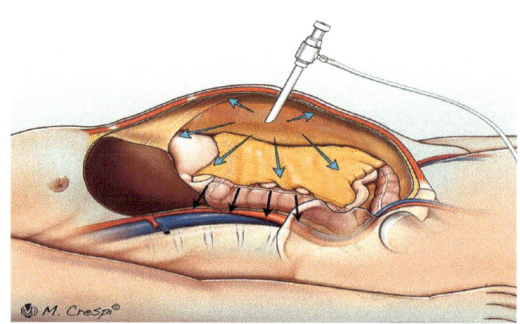

Fig. 1 Effects of increased intra-abdominal pressure on organs

elevated however the CO starts to decrease below the baseline [6]. The drop in CO is attributed to the decreased venous return caused by IVC compression and the pooling of the venous blood in the lower extremities. There is also an increase in afterload with an increase in IAP, seen as an increase in mean arterial pressure (MAP) and systemic vascular resistance (SVR) that contribute to the decrease in CO. The compression of the renal vasculature reduces renal blood flow stimulating the release of aldosterone and renin that contribute to the increase in MAP, and the release of atrial natriuretic peptide cortisol, epinephrine, norepinephrine, and vasopressin.

The hemodynamic changes will immediately return to baseline levels after desufflation among healthy individuals, in those with cardiovascular disease these can persist for at least 65 min. Those with cardiovascular compromise may experience an elevation in cardiac index, ejection fraction, heart rate, left ventricular stroke work index, and decrease in SVR; with 20% of these patients developing heart failure within 3 h after the MIS procedure [7]. Though laparoscopy appears to be safe in patients with cardiac disease, it will require special attention and additional intraoperative monitoring.

Patient Positioning Effects

Placing the patient in Trendelenburg or reverse Trendelenburg position facilitates optimal visualization of the surgical field in the lower abdomen or pelvis and the upper abdomen, respectively. Shifting from supine to Trendelenburg position displaces the diaphragm and abdominal contents cephalad. This enhances the pulmonary compromise associated with CO_2 insufflation, reduction of pulmonary compliance, and increase peak airway pressure. It however mitigates the effect on the hemodynamic changes with increased venous return and pulmonary capillary wedge pressure which minimize the decline in CO with an increase in IAP [5]. The reverse Trendelenburg position will generate positive ventilatory effects and negative hemodynamic effects.

Summary

The MIS technique imposes physiologic changes outside of that caused by anesthesia and the nature of surgery; these factors include CO_2 use, increase IAP, and patient positioning. These pulmonary and cardiovascular changes are generally well tolerated by the healthy patient during the procedure and recover immediately afterward. Cognizance of intraoperative and sustained effects afterward among patients with cardiopulmonary impairment would emphasize the need for thorough preoperative preparation and vigilant perioperative monitoring to mitigate the adverse effects.

References

1. Hasukic S. CO_2-pneumoperitoneum in laparoscopic surgery: pathophysiologic effects and clinical significance. World J Laparosc Surg. 2014;7(1):33–40.
2. Wright DM, Serpell MG, Baxter JN, et al. Effect of extraperitoneal carbon dioxide insufflation on intraoperative blood gas and hemodynamic changes. Surg Endosc. 1995;9(11):1169–72.
3. Demiroluk S, Salihoglu Z, Bakan M, et al. Effects of intraperitoneal and extraperitoneal carbon dioxide insufflation on blood gases during the perioperative period. J Laparoendosc Adv Surg Tech A. 2004;14(4):219–22.
4. Grabowski JE, Talamini MA. Physiological effects of pneumoperitoneum. J Gastrointest Surg. 2009;13(5):1009–16.
5. Sharma KC, Brandstetter RD, Brensilver JM, et al. Cardiopulmonary physiology and pathophysiology as a consequence of laparoscopic surgery. Chest. 1996;110(3):810–5.
6. Atkinson TM, Giraud GD, Togioka BM, et al. Cardiovascular and ventilatory consequences of laparoscopic surgery. Circulation. 2017;135(7):700–10.
7. Odeberg-Wernerman S. Laparoscopic surgery--effects on circulatory and respiratory physiology: an overview. Eur J Surg Suppl. 2000;585:4–11.

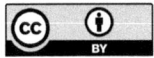

Part III

Diagnostic Laparoscopy

Staging Laparoscopy for Intra-Abdominal Carcinoma

Michael M. Lawenko

Introduction

Diagnostic laparoscopy is used for the diagnosis of intra-abdominal pathologies due to its capability to directly visualize intra-abdominal organs with the opportunity for gathering tissue biopsy, fluid aspiration, and tissue cultures [1] Its application for the staging of intra-abdominal cancers is known as staging laparoscopy.

Instruments

- 12 mm trocar
- 5 mm trocar × 2
- 30° laparoscope Atraumatic bowel graspers × 2
- Maryland forceps.
- Laparoscopic shears.
- Suction-Irrigation cannula.
- Punch biopsy forceps.
- Laparoscopic aspiration cannula.

General Indications [2]

1. Identification of occult metastatic disease or unsuspected locally advanced disease in patients with resectable disease based on preoperative imaging.
2. Assessment prior to administration of neoadjuvant chemoradiation.
3. Selection of palliative treatments in patients with locally advanced disease without evidence of metastatic disease on preoperative imaging.

General Contraindications

1. Verified metastatic disease.
2. Inability to tolerate pneumoperitoneum or general anesthesia.
3. Multiple adhesions/prior operations.
4. Intra-abdominal carcinoma complicated by obstruction, hemorrhage, or perforation in need of palliative surgery.

Surgical Technique

Under general anesthesia, a 10 mm umbilical incision is made for insertion of the Hasson's trocar with stay sutures to secure that trocar. A pneumoperitoneum at 12 mm Hg on medium flow (10–15 L/min) is created. The 30° telescope is then inserted through the 12 mm trocar and an

M. M. Lawenko (✉)
De La Salle Medical and Health Sciences Institute, Dasmarinas City, Philippines
e-mail: mmlawenko@dlshi.edu.ph

© The Author(s) 2023
D. Lomanto et al. (eds.), *Mastering Endo-Laparoscopic and Thoracoscopic Surgery*,
https://doi.org/10.1007/978-981-19-3755-2_14

initial exploration of the abdominal cavity is performed to evaluate for peritoneal as well as liver metastases. Port placement of the working trocars will now depend on the location of the pathology. The general rule is to apply the technique of triangulating the working ports in relation to the camera and the suspected pathology. A minimum of two trocars is advised, but additional trocars are deemed appropriate if needed. The size of the working trocars is variable depending on the instruments that you will use. Two 5 mm trocars would be sufficient to fit most instruments, being liberal to changing to a 10 mm working trocar as the need arises.

If no intra-abdominal metastasis is noted, definitive treatment can commence as planned.

In peritoneal carcinomatosis, biopsies can be performed by using Maryland forceps to pull down on the peritoneum where an area of metastasis is located and using the laparoscopic shears to cut that peritoneum together with the pathology. Minimal bleeding is usually encountered here which will eventually stop. For continuous bleeding, monopolar or bipolar hemostasis can be used. Aspiration of ascitic fluid can be achieved by letting the fluid gravitate using proper patient positioning and retraction of the bowels away from the field. An aspiration cannula with a 10 mm syringe attached at its end is inserted for getting a sample of fluid for cell cytology.

Depending on the type of carcinoma, different maneuvers can be done to visualize the pathology. These will be discussed in the succeeding chapters in more detail.

References

1. Ramshaw BJ, Esartia P, Mason EM, et al. Laparoscopy for diagnosis and staging of malignancy. Semin Surg Oncol. 1999;16:279–83.
2. SAGES guidelines for diagnostic laparoscopy. https://www.sages.org/publications/guidelines/guidelines-for-diagnostic-laparoscopy/

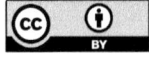

Diagnostic Laparoscopy

Michael M. Lawenko

Introduction

Diagnostic laparoscopy is used in endoscopic surgery for the diagnosis of intra-abdominal pathologies. This technique has the capability for directly visualizing intra-abdominal organs with the opportunity for gathering tissue biopsy, fluid aspiration, and tissue cultures. This procedure has the capability to aid other possible interventional alternatives.

There are several situations in which the role of diagnostic laparoscopy (DL) is useful in reducing the number of unnecessary laparotomies. Staging laparoscopy can be done for intra-abdominal cancer. Its application in the acute abdominal condition is also common. There is also DL for chronic conditions, such as infection, pelvic pain, cirrhosis, and cryptorchidism.

Instruments

- 12 mm trocar
- 5 mm trocar × 2.
- 30° laparoscope
- Atraumatic bowel graspers × 2.

M. M. Lawenko (✉)
De La Salle Medical and Health Sciences Institute, Dasmarinas City, Philippines
e-mail: mmlawenko@dlshsi.edu.ph

General Technique for Diagnostic Laparoscopy

Under general anesthesia, a 10 mm umbilical incision is made for insertion of the Hasson's trocar with stay sutures to secure that trocar. A pneumoperitoneum at 12 mm Hg on medium flow (10–15 L/min) is created. The 30° telescope is then inserted through the 12 mm trocar and an initial exploration of the abdominal cavity is performed. Port placement of the working trocars will now depend on the location of the pathology. The general rule is to apply the technique of triangulating the working ports in relation to the camera and the suspected pathology. A minimum of two trocars is advised, but additional trocars are deemed appropriate if needed. The size of the working trocars is variable depending on the instruments that you will use. Two 5 mm trocars would be sufficient to fit most instruments, being liberal to changing to a 10 mm working trocar as the need arises.

If a known pathology is suspected, for example, acute appendicitis. Upon insertion of the camera, a limited diagnostic laparoscopy is done around the abdominal cavity before focusing on the right lower quadrant. One working trocar is placed initially at the left lower quadrant for a bowel grasper to assist in exposing the appendix. Upon confirmation of acute appendicitis, the next working trocar can be placed on area of your preference as long as proper triangulation of the instruments in relation to the pathology is

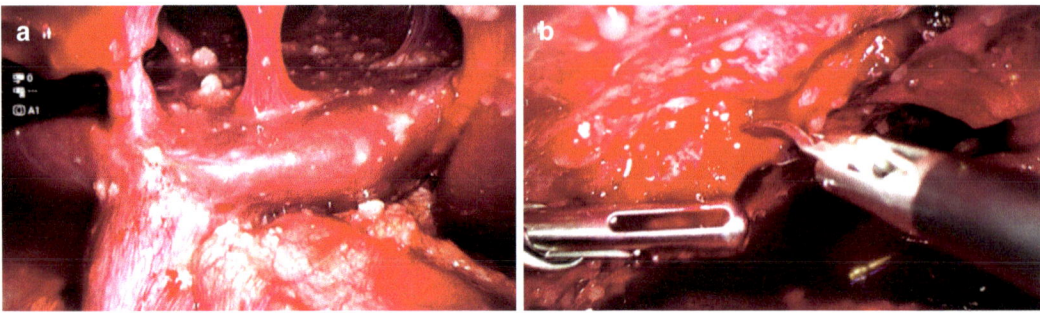

Fig. 1 (**a**) Intra-abdominal milliary tuberculosis during diagnostic laparoscopy with (**b**) biopsy

observed. If another pathology is to be suspected (and not appendicitis), then a formal diagnostic laparoscopy can commence.

For the above example, in performing a formal diagnostic laparoscopy, a second working trocar is placed at the right lower quadrant and the patient is placed in a reverse Trendelenburg position. Inspection of the right upper quadrant by visualizing the liver and the subdiaphragmatic area is done, going down to the subhepatic area to where the gallbladder and the extrahepatic biliary tree are located. The left upper quadrant is visualized by inspecting the anterior wall of the stomach, gastroesophageal junction, and splenic area. The patient is then placed in the Trendelenburg position to examine the pelvic area. Bowels are moved cephalad in order to visualize the posterior wall of the urinary bladder, sigmoid, and rectum, in addition to the uterus, ovaries, and fallopian tubes in females. Once the patient is returned to the supine position, the bowels are now inspected from the duo-

denum down to the sigmoid using both bowel graspers to run the bowels. If needed, the greater sac of the stomach is opened to visualize the pancreas retroperitoneally.

Specimen collection can be accomplished in various ways. For pedunculated nodules on the peritoneum or abdominal organs, a sharp dissection of the nodules can be achieved, followed by appropriate hemostasis (Fig. 1). For evacuation and examination of fluids like ascites and puss, needle aspiration instruments connected to syringes can be done.

Further Reading

Ramshaw BJ, Esartia P, Mason EM, et al. Laparoscopy for diagnosis and staging of malignancy. Semin Surg Oncol. 1999;16:279–83.
SAGES guidelines for diagnostic laparoscopy. https://www.sages.org/publications/guidelines/guidelines-for-diagnostic-laparoscopy/

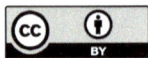

Part IV

Emergency Laparoscopy

Perforated Ulcer Treatment

Mika Yamamoto and Kiyotaka Imamura

The perforated ulcers were treated by open gastrectomy or simple suture until 1937 then Graham introduced the method using a free omental graft, which is called the "Graham patch procedure" [1]. This procedure has long been a golden standard of surgical treatment for perforated peptic ulcers. The idea of laparoscopic treatment had arisen in the 1990s, and the comparison of superiority between laparoscopy and open surgery has long been discussed [2].

Recently reported meta-analysis had shown the significance of laparoscopic repair over the open repair for postoperative pain in the first 24 h and postoperative wound infection, and equivalence of multiple clinical outcomes [3]. In addition, explorative laparoscopy will be useful to gain more information about the perforation site and decide to move on to laparoscopic repair or switch to open repair. Therefore, in a facility where there is a surgeon that is well trained in the laparoscopic procedure, laparoscopic repair is a better choice for the patient.

Indications for Operation

- Perforated ulcer with no evidence of spontaneous seal.

Indications for Nonoperative Management

- Clinically stable, without signs and symptoms of sepsis, and with good radiologic evidence that the perforation has sealed.
- Low risk (Boey score* of 0,1).

*Boey score: shock on admission, ASA grade III–IV, symptom duration(>24 h) [4]. The maximum score is 3, which is indicated high surgical risk.

Contraindications for Laparoscopic Repair

- High-risk patient (Boey score of 3).
- Clinical evidence of concomitant bleeding ulcer.
- Previous abdominal surgery (relative).

Preoperative Assessment

- Fluid resuscitation.
- Preoperative antibiotics (cover gram-negatives, anaerobes, mouth flora, and fungi).

M. Yamamoto
Department of Surgery, Teine Keijinkai Hospital, Sapporo, Japan

K. Imamura (✉)
Minimally Invasive Surgery Center, Yotsuya Medical Cube, Tokyo, Japan
e-mail: k-imamura@mcube.jp

D. Lomanto et al. (eds.), *Mastering Endo-Laparoscopic and Thoracoscopic Surgery*,
https://doi.org/10.1007/978-981-19-3755-2_16

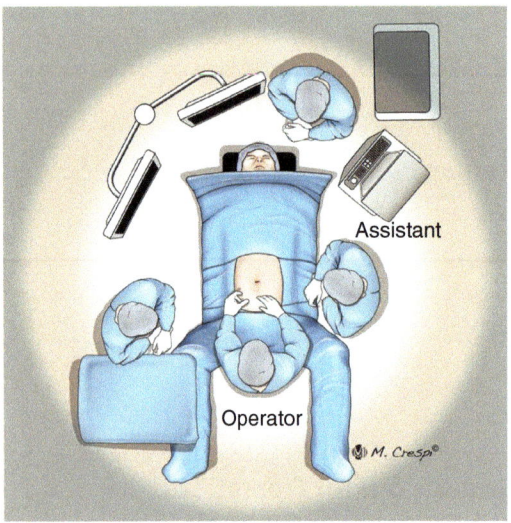

Fig. 1 OT setup and patient position

- Intravenous PPI.
- Kept NPO and insertion of nasogastric (NG) tube.
- Adequate analgesics.
- Prophylactic anticoagulation.

OT Setup and Patient's Position

- Patient is placed in the modified lithotomy position (Lloyd-Davies).
- Surgeon stands between the legs of the patient.
- Assistant stands on the left side of the patient.
- Monitor is positioned above the patient's right shoulder (Fig. 1).

Instrumentations Required

- 10 mm 30° laparoscope
- Scissors.
- Grasper.
- Needle holder.
- Suction device.
- 3–0 absorbable suture needle
- 10 mm periumbilical trocar
- Two 5 mm trocars are positioned on either side along the midclavicular line at the level of the umbilicus.
- One 5 mm trocar at the subxiphoid region is placed for retraction of liver or gallbladder.

Surgical Technique

Identification of the Site of Perforation

- Insert camera and the rest of the trocars in place. Pneumoperitoneum is established and maintained 10–12 mm Hg. Change the patient's position to reverse Trendelenburg position and retract the liver to the cranial side to expose the stomach and duodenum.
- Gently investigate the organs and look for the perforation site. Bacteriologic and fungal cultures are taken. A biopsy is recommended to perform for gastric ulcer perforation since malignancy can be occasionally seen.
- Even in the case of perforated gastric cancer, a two-stage procedure should be performed in most cases, consisting of suture closure of the perforation followed by a second-stage gastrectomy [5].

Peritoneal Washing

- Start with exploring the entire abdomen and removing purulent collections and gastric/bowel contents using suction to gain proper field of view. Change the patient's position to Trendelenburg position when exploring the pelvic cavity. If the patient has suffered more than 24 h after the onset, some fibrin formation may be seen throughout the entire abdomen.
- Be sure to conduct lavage enough so that the omentum is clean without any pleural collections, gastric/bowel contents, or fibrin before moving on to coverage of the perforation with omentum.

Closure of the Perforation

Method of closure depends on the size of the perforation;

<1 cm: closure by interrupted sutures covered with a pedicled omentum on top of the repair (Cellan-Jones repair [6]).

Applicate standard stitches with 3–0 absorbable sutures to close the perforation. When pull-

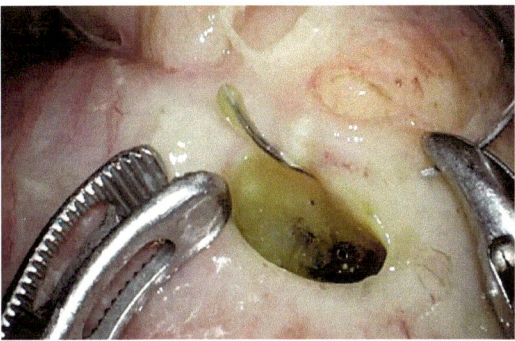 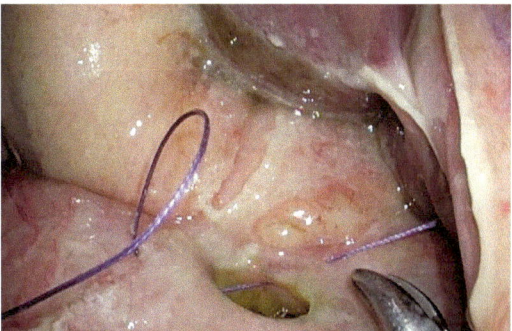

Fig. 2 Perforated ulcer with full-thickness wall suturing

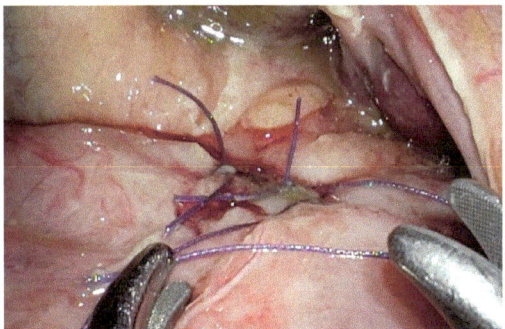 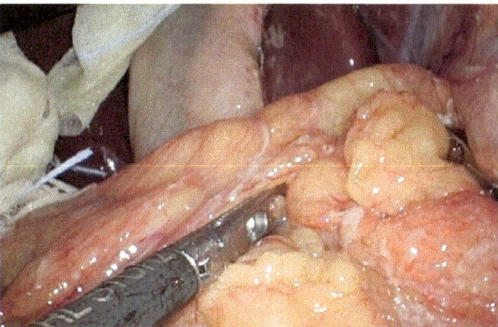

Fig. 3 The sutures are tied using the intracorporeal technique

Fig. 4 Omentum is brought up to the site of perforation to ensure adequate length without tension. The omentum was fixed with the falciform ligament to prevent dislodging

ing the omentum to cover the suture line, be sure to avoid any tension. Do 3–4 additional stitches to fix the omentum to the suture line. The last procedure may be omitted; some studies which compared the sutureless onlay omental patch method with sutured omental patch method showed that either group never had postoperative leaks, and the former method had significantly shorter operative time and length of stay [7].

Perforated duodenal ulcer repair is done by placing sutures through the full thickness of the bowel wall with 3–0 absorbable suture (Figs. 2 and 3).

1–2 cm: plugging the perforation with a free omental plug (Graham patch [1]).

If the perforation is 1 ~ 2 cm, the standard stitch may give too much tension to the suture line. Therefore, the operator should skip the standard suture process and directly move on to covering and fixing the omentum to the perforation. If the perforation is too big or damaged too much

to suture, stuffing the omentum into the perforation would be enough (Fig. 4).

>2 cm: If the perforation size is more than 2 cm, it may be difficult to proceed graham patch closure. The operator should consider converting to laparotomy.

After Closure

After the perforation is properly covered, irrigate the peritoneal cavity with at least 5 l of warm saline to wash off the impurities. To confirm the closure is watertight, instillation of intragastric air or methylene blue via the NG tube is useful. Drains are optional; however, there is no evidence to support their routine use. Remove trocars one after another and be sure that there is no active hemorrhage of trocar sites. Close the skin with sutures.

Complications and Management

- Leakage: repeat laparoscopy and rerepair laparoscopically or convert to an open procedure.
- Intra-abdominal abscess: percutaneous drainage.
- Intestinal obstruction.

Postoperative Care

- NG tube is removed after 24 h when the residual gastric aspirates are minimal.
- Oral intake is commenced once there is a return of bowel function.
- PPI.
- Antibiotics.
- Upper endoscopy is performed 6–8 weeks later to check H.pylori status and to assess for healing in gastric ulcer perforation.

References

1. Graham RR. The treatment of perforated duodenal ulcers. Surg Gyecol Obstet. 1937;64:235–8.
2. Lau H. Laparoscopic repair of perforated peptic ulcer: a meta-analysis. Surg Endosc. 2004;18:1013–21.
3. Cirocchi R, et al. Meta-analysis of perioperative outcomes of acute laparoscopic versus open repair of perforated gastroduodenal ulcers. J Trauma Acute Care Surg. 2018;85:417–25.
4. Boey J, et al. Risk stratification in perforated duodenal ulcers. A prospective validation of predictive factors. Ann Surg. 1987;205:22–6.
5. Mouly C, et al. Therapeutic management of perforated gastro-duodenal ulcer: literature review. J Visc Surg. 2013;150:333–40.
6. Cellan-Jones CJ. A rapid method of treatment in perforated duodenal ulcer. Br Med J. 1929;1:1076–7.
7. Wang YC, et al. Sutureless onlay omental patch for the laparoscopic repair of perforated peptic ulcers. World J Surg. 2014;38:1917–21.

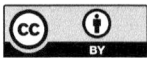

Laparoscopic Appendectomy

Michael M. Lawenko and Eva Lourdes Sta Clara

Introduction

Appendicitis is one of the most common causes of a surgical abdomen. In 1894, McBurney performed a new technique in treating appendicitis, which eventually became the gold standard for acute appendicitis [1]. However, in 1980, Kurt Semm, a gynecologist from Switzerland performed the first laparoscopic appendectomy [2]. The laparoscopic approach has several advantages over the open appendectomy like lesser postoperative pain, faster recovery, fewer wound infections, and lesser incidence of adhesions. In addition, the complication rates were comparable in laparoscopic and open appendectomy. Laparoscopic appendectomy is also safe to perform in patients with perforated appendicitis, but it is dependent on the surgeon's expertise. It offers lesser wound contamination during operation and direct visualization during peritoneal washing.

Another advantage of laparoscopy is the visualization of the abdominal cavity to rule out other pathologies and address them simultaneously. It is also preferable in women for cosmetic reasons.

M. M. Lawenko
De La Salle Medical and Health Sciences Institute, Dasmarinas City, Philippines

E. L. Sta Clara (✉)
Training Officer (UMIST) and Training Committee, Department of Surgery, Cardinal Santos Medical Center, Manila, Philippines

Department of Surgery, Rizal Medical Center, Manila, Philippines

Department of Surgery, Asian Hospital Medical Center, Manila, Philippines

Department of Surgery, University of Perpetual Help Dalta Medical Center, Manila, Philippines

Indications

- Any patient with signs and symptoms of acute appendicitis.
- Patient who are fit for general anesthesia.

Contraindications

- Severely septic with generalized peritonitis.
- Severe pulmonary disease in whom carbon dioxide pneumoperitoneum may exacerbate their condition.
- Hemodynamic instability.
- Patient not fit for general anesthesia.
- Advanced stage of pregnancy wherein the intra-abdominal working space would be suboptimal.

© The Author(s) 2023
D. Lomanto et al. (eds.), *Mastering Endo-Laparoscopic and Thoracoscopic Surgery*,
https://doi.org/10.1007/978-981-19-3755-2_17

Preoperative Preparation

- In female patients, an adequate menstrual history and a pregnancy test.
- The minimum ancillary diagnostic test would be a complete blood count and urinalysis.
- CT scan may be warranted if the physical examination and laboratories are equivocal.
- Adequate intravenous hydration.
- Prophylactic intravenous antibiotics with coverage for gram-negative and anaerobes.
- Insertion of a urinary catheter to decompress the urinary bladder and minimize injury to it and allow for a bigger working space.
- Informed consent with the potential to convert to an open procedure.

OT Setup

The patient is in supine position in a Trendelenburg position with the right side up to expose the right lower quadrant. The anesthesiologist and the anesthesia machine are at the patient's head (Fig. 1). The surgeon stands on the left side of the patient opposite the appendix and the assistant stands at the right side of the surgeon. The video monitor is positioned directly across the surgeon at the right side of the patient.

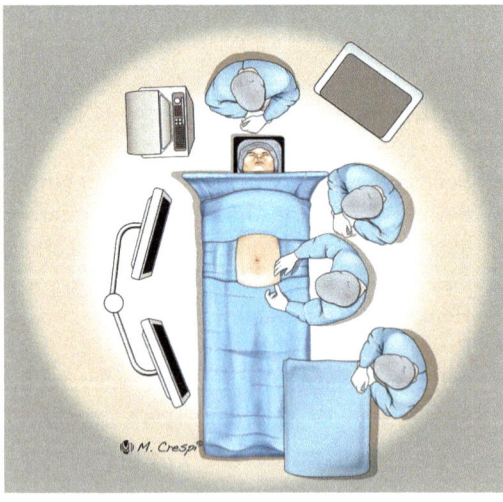

Fig. 1 OT setup

Surgical Technique

The patient is under general anesthesia. The 10 mm port is inserted at the umbilicus using Hasson's technique and pneumoperitoneum is created with CO_2 pressure at 12 mmHg and flow rate at medium or 20 L/min. A 5 mm port is then placed at the left lower quadrant and another 5 mm trocar is inserted at the suprapubic area under direct vision to avoid any injury to any intrabdominal organs and vessels. A limited diagnostic laparoscopy is then done to exclude other pathologies.

The appendix is identified by locating the cecum and tracing the taenia coli to the base of the appendix. Careful dissection is done if there are adhesions between the appendix and the surrounding organs to avoid iatrogenic injury to the bowels. Once the appendix is freed, this is then grasped then the mesoappendix is isolated by using either one of the following:

1. Monopolar hook with diathermy dissection to isolate the artery.
2. Maryland dissector to bluntly isolate the artery.

Then the appendiceal artery is isolated and ligated using the following techniques:

1. Clip application using either small polymer or titanium clips.
2. Bipolar vessel sealing (Fig. 2).

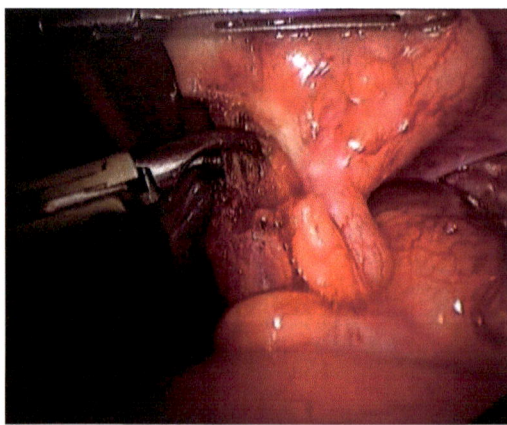

Fig. 2 Vessel sealing

3. Ultrasonic vessel sealing for a small artery less than 8 mm in size.

The sealed artery can be cut using laparoscopic shears or the included cutter in the advanced bipolar instruments. As with open appendectomy, the base of the appendix must be exposed completely and should be devoid of fat in preparation for its ligation via the following techniques:

1. Simple suture ligation via intracorporeal suturing with a 2–0 braided suture on a round half circle needle with two sutures on the patient side and one on the specimen side [3].
2. Simple suture ligation via extracorporeal knot tying of a 2–0 braided suture in creating a loop ligation around the base of the appendix. Applying 2 sutures on the patient side and one on the specimen side.
3. Commercially available preformed suture loops (i.e., Endoloop™, Johnson & Johnson, USA) of a 2–0 braided suture in creating a loop ligation around the base of the appendix. Applying two sutures on the patient side and one on the specimen side (Fig. 3).
4. Plastic clips (i.e., hem-o-lok™, Teleflex Medical, USA) with two clips at the patient side and one at the specimen side [4].

The ligated appendiceal base can now be cut using the laparoscopic shears (Fig. 4). The appen-diceal mucosa on the stump is suctioned to make sure that no fecalith remains and is burned with bipolar energy to prevent the rare incidence of mucocele formation [5].

Inspection of the stump and nearby surrounding area for fecal soilage, bleeding and bowel perforation is done. Suction is used for pooled clotted blood and a few purulent materials. Copious use of lavage is optional depending on the presence of fecal soilage.

A sterile 10 × 5 cm plastic bag with a 35 cm nonabsorbable suture with a Roeder's knot attached is placed in the umbilical port. The appendix is placed in the bag, closed and extracted together at the umbilical port. This is done to decrease the incidence of infection at the umbilical incision [6].

Alternative options can be the following:

1. The appendix is extracted from the abdomen with the use of a condom, which is inserted at the umbilical port. The appendix is placed inside the condom and then telescoped into the 10 mm port as the camera is pulled out.
2. Use of a commercially available specimen bag which is inserted through the umbilical port. A 5 mm scope is placed in the left lower quadrant trocar while a bowel grasper is in the suprapubic port to assist in placing the specimen in the bag. The bag is closed and retracted under direct vision together with the trocar.

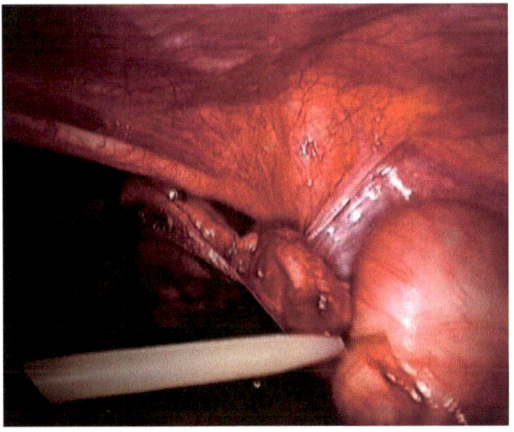

Fig. 3 Endoloop for ligation at the base of the appendix

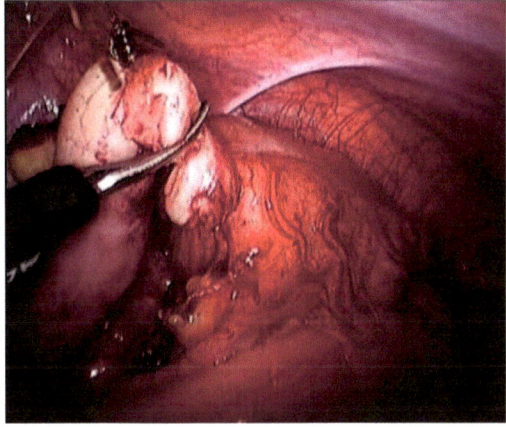

Fig. 4 Cutting the appendiceal base with shears

3. If the appendix is thin (<1 cm) and not grossly purulent, a 5 mm scope is placed at the left lower quadrant while a bowel grasper at the suprapubic trocar feeds the specimen to the grasper in the umbilical port for direct withdrawal of the specimen.

Peritoneal lavage can be done if needed. A closed suction drain is inserted in cases of perforated appendix. After extracting the specimen, desufflation is done together with direct visualization through a scope in the umbilicus of the working trocars to check for port site bleeding. Appropriate hemostasis is achieved prior to a figure of eight sutures with a 2–0 braided, absorbable suture at the fascial level of the umbilical incision. Subdermal interrupted skin closure with 4–0, monofilament, absorbable sutures are done to close the skin incisions. Film dressings are applied to the incision sites.

Complications and Management

The most common postoperative complication in laparoscopic appendectomy is wound infection, which can be treated by antibiotics and/or drainage. However, compared to open appendectomy, this is markedly lower with a rate of less than 2%.

Other complications which might occur is intra-abdominal abscess, which can be managed by percutaneous drainage.

Late complications include the following: incisional hernia, stump appendicitis, and small bowel obstruction due to postoperative adhesions.

Post-op Care

Patient is advised to ambulate once fully awake and with adequate pain control. Diet is progressed as tolerated and the patient is expected to be discharged on the first postoperative day for uncomplicated appendicitis.

Patient is then seen 1 week after for follow up.

References

1. Mcburney. The incision made in the abdominal wall in cases of appendicitis, with a description of a new method of operating. Ann Surg. 1894;20(1):38.
2. Semm K. Endoscopic appendectomy. Endoscopy. 1983;15(02):59–64.
3. Sayyadinia M, Hamadiyan H, Mokaripoor S, et al. Comparing the complications of purse-string and simple ligation of appendix stump in appendectomy: a randomized clinical trial. Int J Med Res Health Sci. 2016;5(10):55–60.
4. Abou-Sheishaa MS, Negm A, Abdelhalim M, et al. Ligation versus clipping of the appendicular stump in laparoscopic appendectomy: a randomized controlled trial. Ann Emerg Surg. 2018;3(1):1029.
5. El Ajmi M, Rebai W, Safta ZB. Mucocele of appendiceal stump—an atypical presentation and a diagnostic dilemma. Acta Chirurgica Belgica. 2009;109(3):414–5.
6. Fields A, Lu P, et al. Does retrieval bag use during laparoscopic appendectomy reduce postoperative infection? Surgery. 2019;165(5):953–7.

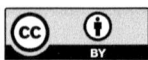

Meckel's Diverticula

Eva Lourdes Sta Clara

Introduction

Meckel's diverticulum is one of the most common congenital anomalies of the small intestine, which resulted from the incomplete obliteration of the vitelline duct during embryogenesis. It is usually located at the terminal ileum 45–90 cm proximal to the ileocecal valve on its antimesenteric border. Almost half of the patients with this anomaly have ectopic gastric or pancreatic mucosa, which might cause some complications [1].

Patients with Meckel's diverticulum are usually asymptomatic and are commonly diagnosed as an incidental finding. However, life threatening complications might occur like bleeding, inflammation, intestinal obstruction, and perforation.

Treatment of symptomatic Meckel's diverticulum is definitive surgery either via diverticulectomy, wedge or segmental resection. Laparoscopically, it can be managed by diverticulectomy with endostaplers, wedge or segmental resection with extracorporeal or intracorporeal anastomosis. Simple diverticulectomy is not advised if the base is broad and/or the diverticulum is noticeably short because of a risk of leaving behind heterotropic tissue [2]. Thus, segmental resection followed by anastomosis is preferable to diverticulectomy and wedge resection or tangential mechanical stapling because of the risk of leaving behind abnormal heterotropic mucosa [3]. Laparoscopic surgery compared to open laparotomy has equivalent outcomes [4]. However, the choice of surgical approach still depends on the patient's condition, surgeon's expertise, and the availability of laparoscopic instruments.

Indications

- Symptomatic patients with Meckel's diverticulum.
- Patient fit for general anesthesia.

Contraindications

- Severe pulmonary disease in whom carbon dioxide pneumoperitoneum may exacerbate their condition.
- Hemodynamic instability.
- Patient not fit for general anesthesia.

E. L. Sta Clara (✉)
Training officer (UMIST) and Training Committee, Department of Surgery, Cardinal Santos Medical Center, Manila, Philippines

Department of Surgery, Rizal Medical Center, Manila, Philippines

Department of Surgery, Asian Hospital Medical Center, Manila, Philippines

Department of Surgery, University of Perpetual Help Dalta Medical Center, Manila, Philippines

© The Author(s) 2023
D. Lomanto et al. (eds.), *Mastering Endo-Laparoscopic and Thoracoscopic Surgery*,
https://doi.org/10.1007/978-981-19-3755-2_18

Preoperative Preparation

- Fluid resuscitation.
- Blood transfusion (if needed for bleeding Meckel's diverticulum).
- Correction of electrolyte imbalances simultaneously with hydration especially for Meckel's diverticulum which initially presented as an obstruction.
- Prophylactic intravenous antibiotics with coverage for gram negative and anaerobes.

Meckel's diverticulum is difficult to diagnose. It usually mimics other abdominal pathologies like appendicitis and is usually confirmed only during laparotomy. Some imaging studies might help in its diagnosis like technetium pertechnetate/Meckel's scan, CT scan, colonoscopy, or wireless capsule endoscopy but they yield a high false-negative result [5]. Therefore, its diagnosis requires a high degree of suspicion as the preoperative clinical and investigational diagnosis is difficult to be made with accuracy [6].

Operating Theater Setup

Instruments

- 10 mm 30° angled laparoscope
- Trocars.
- 10 mm optical or Hasson's trocar
- 12 mm trocar
- (2) 5 mm trocar.
- Graspers and atraumatic graspers.
- Hook.
- Scissors.
- Suction.
- Endostaplers/Laparoscopic linear cutter staplers.
- Needle holder.
- Ultrasonic energy devices (e.g., Harmonic™, Ethicon, Mexico).
- Specimen bag.

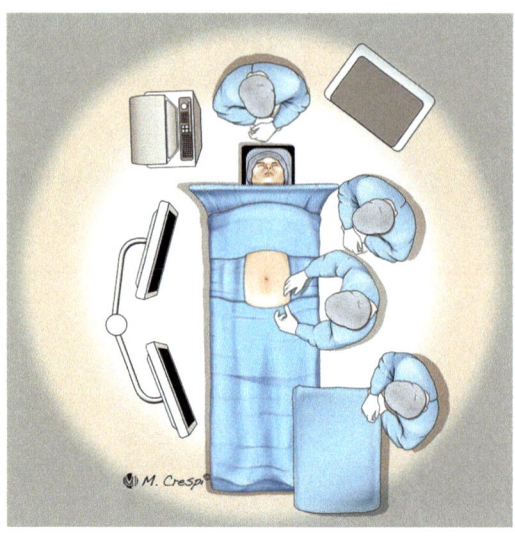

Fig. 1 OT setup

Patient and Surgical Team Positioning

Patient is in supine position in a Trendelenburg position with the right side slightly up to expose the right lower quadrant. The anesthesiologist and the anesthesia machine are at the patient's head. The surgeon stands on the left side of the patient and the assistant stands on the right side of the surgeon. The video monitor is positioned directly across the surgeon on the right side of the patient (Fig. 1)

Surgical Technique

The patient is under general anesthesia with arms tucked in. Then a 10 mm port, which will serve as the camera port, is inserted at the left midclavicular line midpoint between the left costal margin level and anterior superior iliac spine (ASIS) level. This can be done using an optical view trocar or via Hasson's technique. Avoid going too lateral to avoid injuring the descending colon. Pneumoperitoneum is created with CO_2 pressure at 12 mmHg and flow rate at medium or 20 L/min. A 5 mm port is then inserted in between the 10 mm port and ASIS and a 12 mm port, which will serve as the working port, in between the 10 mm port and costal margin. The 5 mm and 12 mm ports can be interchanged depending on the preference of the surgeon. Avoid putting it too near the costal margin and the ASIS as the bones might limit your movements. All of this is done under direct vision to avoid injuring any vessels or intestines. A diagnostic laparoscopy is done.

A bowel run from the ileocecal area is done using atraumatic graspers until the Meckel's diverticulum is located. Dissect free the Meckel's diverticulum if there are any adhesions using a hook or an ultrasonic energy device.

If a simple diverticulectomy is planned, this can be done using an endostapler/linear cutter stapler. The diverticulum is transected at the base. Making sure not to compromise the lumen of the intestine and not to leave behind a stump of the diverticulum.

On the other hand, if segmental resection is to be done, mesenteric openings are made around 5 cm from the base of the diverticulum proximally and distally. The mesentery connecting to the diverticulum is then serially ligated and transected using an ultrasonic energy device.

The Meckel's diverticulum is then transected segmentally using linear cutter staplers. The proximal and distal small intestines are then aligned in preparation for a side-to-side anastomosis, and a stay suture is placed at the proximal and distal small intestines to stabilize it. Always make sure that the intestines are not twisted. Another 5 mm port can be inserted so that another grasper can be used to hold the stay suture and lift the intestines to be anastomosed.

A small enterotomy is done at the proximal and distal intestine. Inspect the lumen if there is any bleeding. After which anastomose the proximal and distal intestine using the endostaplers/linear cutter staplers. The common channel is then closed via intracorporeal suturing with 2–0

sutures in a running single layer fashion. Check for any bleeding. The mesenteric defect is closed with figure of 8 sutures to prevent herniation of the intestines. Copious irrigation is done if there is spillage of intestinal contents or if dealing with a perforated Meckel's diverticulum.

The Meckel's diverticulum is then placed inside a specimen/collection bag and extracted. Remove the trocars under direct vision to observe for any port side bleeding. Desufflation is then done. The fascia at the 10 mm and 12 mm ports is closed with figure of 8 sutures to minimize the formation of a hernia in the future. Subdermal interrupted skin closure with 4–0, monofilament, absorbable sutures is done to close the skin incisions.

Postoperative Care

Antibiotics is continued to complete for 7 days with adequate pain control. Patient is advised to ambulate as soon as possible. Oral intake is started once return of bowel functions is observed. Patient is discharged once vital signs are stable with complete return of bowel function and able to tolerate oral intake. Patient is then seen after 7–10 days for follow-up.

Complications and Management

One of the possible complications of resecting a Meckel's diverticulum is anastomosis leakage. If this is suspected immediate repair is warranted either via laparoscopy or open laparotomy. Intra-abdominal abscess might also occur, which can be managed by intravenous antibiotics and percutaneous drainage. Wound infection might also be encountered. This can be treated by antibiotics and drainage. Another possible complication as with other abdominal operations is intestinal obstruction secondary to postoperative adhesions.

References

1. Ajaz AM, Bari SU, et al. Meckel's diverticulum–revisited. The Saudi Journal of Gastroenterology. 2010;16(1):3–7.
2. Palanivelu C, Rangarajan M, Senthilkumar R, Madankumar MV, Kavalakat AJ. Laparoscopic management of symptomatic Meckel's diverticula: a simple tangential stapler excision. JSLS. 2008;12:66–70.
3. Lequet J, Menahem B, Alves A, et al. Meckel's diverticulum in the adult. Journal of visceral sugery. 2017;152(4):253–9.
4. Hosn MA, Lakis M, Faraj W, Khoury G, Diba S. Laparoscopic approach to symptomatic meckel diverticulum in adults. JSLS. 2014;18:e2014.00349. https://doi.org/10.4293/JSLS.2014.00349.
5. Rho JH, Kim JS, Kim SY, Kim SK, Choi YM, Kim SM, Tchah H, Jeon IS, Son DW, Ryoo E, et al. Clinical features of symptomatic meckel's diverticulum in children: comparison of scintigraphic and non-scintigraphic diagnosis. Pediatr Gastroenterol Hepatol Nutr. 2013;16:41–8.
6. Sharma RJ, Jain VK. Emergency surgery for Meckel's diverticulum. World Journal of Emergency Surgery. 2008;3:27.

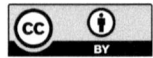

Emergency Groin Hernia Repair

George Pei Cheung Yang

Introduction

Laparoscopic groin hernia repair (inguinal, femoral, and obturator hernias) has become one of the gold standard for elective groin hernia treatment since its introduction in 1990 [1]. For almost 30 years onward, the techniques of laparoscopic groin hernia repair are divided into two mainstreams, namely the transabdominal preperitoneal (TAPP) [2, 3] and totally extraperitoneal (TEP) [4] approaches. These two surgical techniques have withstood the test of time, with high success and low morbidity rate [5–7].

As the techniques become more mature, also deeper understanding of the preperitoneal anatomy, and with more structural surgical training, naturally surgeons have broadened its applications into more complex scenarios. Now it has expanded from elective noncomplicated groin hernia to complex and emergency groin hernia situations [8, 9], similar to laparoscopic cholecystectomy for acute cholecystitis.

Many expert centers have applied laparoscopic approach in the management of acute emergency groin hernia situations with a favorable outcome. The difference in outcome between laparoscopic and open surgery is believed to be due to the switch in surgical steps sequence in the management of emergency groin hernia situations. In open approach, once the strangulated bowel is isolated, then time is spent for the bowel to show any sign of recovery. If the extent of strangulation is unclear, or viability is in doubt, then laparotomy or bowel resection will be performed. In the laparoscopic approach, after diagnostic laparoscopy and reduction of the strangulated bowel is carried out, instead of purely waiting for the recovery of the bowel viability, surgeons will proceed to groin hernia repair first, either laparoscopically or open repair. Once the hernia repair is completed, the surgeon then comes back to recheck the viability of the bowel. That in turn gives ample time for the strangulated bowel to recover hence reducing the bowel resection rate. The clear advantages of laparoscopy in accessing the strangulated content, and the extended time allowed for the strangulated bowel to recover in a warm intra-peritoneal environment, all of these are the key factors in reducing the rate of unnecessary laparotomy and bowel resection in emergency laparoscopic of groin hernia [10–12]. It is well known that the moment when laparotomy is decided, that is the major cause for subsequent morbidity and mortality.

In this chapter, we will be mainly discussing the technical aspect of Laparoscopic approach in the management of acute emergency groin hernia situations.

G. P. C. Yang (✉)
Hong Kong Hernia Society, Hong Kong, China

Hong Kong Adventist Hospital, Hong Kong, China
e-mail: george.yang@hkah.org.hk

© The Author(s) 2023   107
D. Lomanto et al. (eds.), *Mastering Endo-Laparoscopic and Thoracoscopic Surgery*,
https://doi.org/10.1007/978-981-19-3755-2_19

Indications

Any adult patient who is hemodynamically stable with acute strangulated or incarcerated groin hernia can benefit from laparoscopic approach.

Those with previous appendicectomy through grid iron incision; and those with previous upper midline laparotomy for upper gastrointestinal or hepatobiliary surgery can also benefit from laparoscopic approach.

Contraindications

As with all laparoscopic approaches for emergency surgical pathologies, there are some common contraindications:

1. For clinically and hemodynamically unstable patients, open surgery should be a lifesaving choice.
2. In cases where there is markedly distended abdomen, open surgery should be the choice of approach. The limited space in the peritoneal cavity will substantially increase the difficulty of the surgery, prolong the time of surgery, and increase the chance of injury to peritoneal viscera;
3. In patients who have a limited cardiopulmonary reserve, pneumo-peritoneal will run the risk of destabilizing their cardiopulmonary system function;
4. Those groups of patients which post a higher risk of mesh infection and postoperative complications, including those with ascites from liver cirrhosis and renal failure patients with peritoneal dialysis. In these conditions, open tissue repair should be considered.
5. Those patients who have gone through multiple laparotomies previously, an open approach should be the choice of surgery.
6. If there is a lack of supporting equipment to perform laparoscopic approach, then an open approach should be the considered;
7. If the surgeon has inadequate training in laparoscopic management of emergency surgical condition, open surgery should be performed;

There are specific contraindications for particular steps in the laparoscopic approach for emergency groin hernia situations, such that alternative techniques should be considered:

1. In a patient who is on anticoagulant because of cardiovascular or cerebrovascular reasons, laparoscopic hernia repair should probably not be the choice. It is because the area of dissection is far greater than open hernia repair. Any bleeding after TAPP or TEP can accumulate into a substantial amount before the tamponade effect takes place to slow down the bleeding.

   However, the rest of the steps including diagnostic laparoscopy, laparoscopic-assisted reduction of strangulated hernia, and bowel resection to be performed through smaller extended sub-umbilical port wounds can be carried out to reduce postoperative morbidity and mortality.
2. If the operating surgeons or theater assisting staffs are not familiar with laparoscopic surgery, open approach should be considered;
3. If the surgeon has inadequate training on laparoscopic hernia repair, the hernia repair part should be performed as open repair;
4. If there is no progress after prolonged period of time, most likely in the reduction of strangulated hernia, hybrid approach—which means making an incision over the strangulated mass to openly assist in releasing the strangulation and reduction of the herniated content should be carried out.

Preoperative Assessment

Anesthetic assessment, routine blood test like complete blood count, renal function, clotting profile, ECG, and CXR should be done preoperatively because this is a surgical emergency with operation requiring pneumo-peritoneum under general anesthesia.

Preoperative CT scan of the abdomen and pelvis:

The fundamental disadvantage of laparoscopic surgery for any surgical emergency is the limited working space to perform the surgery. This limited working space will

1. Obscure the visual fields such that sometime other pathology might be missed;
2. It also increases the risk of visceral injury during surgery.

To minimize these disadvantages, a preoperative CT scan of the abdomen and pelvis should be done so that the surgeon can get as much information as possible on the site of hernia pathology, any concurrent pathology within the abdomen, any free gas and bowel vascularity on contrast phase scan, and the extend of bowel dilatation as well.

This preoperative CT scan helps to direct the surgeon on where to look for once they enter the peritoneal cavity laparoscopically, and thereby reducing the operative time. It also helps to reduce the chance of any unexpected surprise, such as strangulated urinary bladder herniation through direct inguinal hernia, in such case the surgeon should be prepared for a hybrid approach to reduce the strangulated bladder.

Operating Theater Setup

The operative theater setup should be one that is equipped for laparoscopic surgery including carbon dioxide insufflator, laparoscopic imaging and light source unit, and monitors.

Instruments

1. A 10 mm 30° laparoscope.
2. A 10 mm and two to four 5 mm laparoscopic trocar, should all be Blunt tip ports to avoid inadvertent injury to the bowel.
3. Standard 5 mm a-traumatic laparoscopic bowel grasper.
4. Laparoscopic 5 mm Diathermy scissor (optional).
5. Mesh (either laparoscopic groin hernia mesh or open groin hernia mesh depends on surgeon preference).

6. Absorbable Tacker (optional).
7. Cyanoacrylate glue for mesh fixation (optional).
8. Laparoscopic needle holder and sutures (optional).
9. Ultrasonic dissector (optional).

Patient Position

This is similar to routine laparoscopic groin hernia repair;

- The patient is positioned supine with both arms tucked by the side and patient strapped securely as titling of the patient is often required;
- Foley catheter should be inserted to reduce bladder distension and also monitor urine output intra- and postoperatively for any surgical emergency;
- The surgeon stands on the opposite side of the pathology;
- The assistant if available should stand beside the surgeon near the cephalad part of the patient;
- The video monitor should be placed at the patient legs side caudally;

The working trocars port should be as follow:

- A 10 mm sub-umbilical port for laparoscope;
- (The surgeon has to decide whether TAPP or TEP will be used before placing the working intraperitoneal 5 mm trocars for reduction of strangulated hernia. It is because if the surgeon prefers TEP approach, then the peritoneal laparoscopic working ports should be placed well away from the TEP working fields to avoid a gas leak.)
- Usually, for peritoneal laparoscopic bowel reduction, two 5 mm ports should be placed, one on each flank of the patient (Fig. 1).
- For TEP hernia repair, additional two 5 mm working ports should be placed at the lower midline position, or as the surgeon's usual preference.

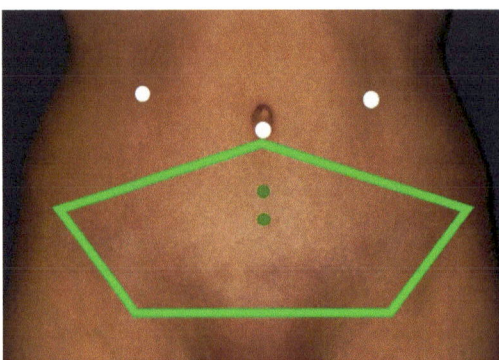

Fig. 1 Port placement

Surgical Technique

Acute surgical emergency for groin hernia refers to strangulated groin hernia (inguinal/femoral/obturator) with the involved viscera having a variable degree of ischemia. This is a disease with a wide spectrum of presentation. Fortunately, in the majority of the cases, the ischemic viscera are reversible after reduction. Only with the extreme spectrum where gangrenous changes occur or even more extreme situations when perforation occurs.

1. Diagnostic laparoscopy via sub-umbilical wound
   (a) The creation of sub-umbilical wound should take extra care because of the possibility of injuring the underlying bowel loops. Before making the incision on the fascia, the surgeon should pull the umbilicus as far up as possible to lift the umbilicus away from the underlying bowel loop. The surgeon should carefully incise the fascia without piercing through the peritoneum. The peritoneum should be punctured using blunt grasping forceps. And most importantly only use blunt tip trocars.
   (b) Two additional 5 mm ports are usually required to manipulate the bowel for clear assessment. These two 5 mm trocars should be inserted under direct vision and blunt tip trocars should always be used to avoid inadvertent injury to the dilated bowel.

2. Identify the site of hernia and the strangulated viscera
   (a) The patient should be tilted to aid the exposure of the pelvis, at least 45 head down or more. Therefore, preoperatively the surgeon should make sure the patient is securely strapped.
3. Laparoscopic reduction of the strangulated viscera
   (a) The reduction of strangulation is probably the most difficult part and determining steps in the whole surgery. It is vital to avoid any injury to the strangulated bowel. So external compression in the correct axis directed by laparoscopy should be carried out, assisted by gentle pulling from inside using a traumatic bowel grasper.
   (b) Tips and tricks in reduction of strangulated contents including.
      i. Grasping on and reducing the nonessential part, including omentum, mesentery but need to avoid injuring the mesenteric vessels;
      ii. Compression of the strangulated content to reduce edema;
      iii. Manual compression externally to reduce the strangulated content;
      iv. In extreme cases where the strangulated content could not be reduced, a hybrid approach should be employed. This means open reduction, with an additional incision over the herniated mass, release of the strangulation ring or adhesion in order to aid the complete reduction of the strangulated content;
4. Groin hernia repair
   (a) After reduction of the strangulated viscera, the surgeon should now decide on the mode of hernia repair. In most cases of strangulation, it is either the small bowel or omentum involvement. As long as there is no perforation, mesh repair for groin hernia should be feasible. The surgeon can decide if laparoscopic or open groin hernia repair should be carried out.

(b) Contralateral groin hernia if found should be repaired at the same time as well. It is quite often to encounter bilateral femoral or obturator hernia. And also concurrent femoral/obturator hernia can be found in patients with inguinal hernia. These pelvic floor hernias should all be repaired in the same session.

(c) For pelvic floor hernia, laparoscopic repair should be employed;

(d) Laparoscopic groin hernia repair—which method of repair, namely TAPP or TEP, is rather based on the surgeon's preference and his surgical training. The surgeon should use his/her best-trained technique.

   i. For TAPP there is the advantage of using the same laparoscopic ports and operating within the same peritoneal space.

   ii. For TEP, there are advantages in working in a completely different plane so as to reduce the chance of bowel injury, avoid the need for cutting instruments to create the peritoneal flap, and also have the mesh without ever touching the peritoneal cavity.

(e) TAPP—using the same 5 mm working port, peritoneal flap is created and hernia repair is carried out. However, with TAPP technique the surgeon should take extra care when the instruments are moving in and out of the working ports. It is because, with dilated bowel and patient position tilted, the instruments can cause direct puncture injury to the bowel loops during insertion through the trocars; therefore, iatrogenically cause fecal contamination to the peritoneum.

(f) TEP—the surgeon enters the preperitoneal space through the same sub-umbilical port skin wound, incised on the anterior fascia, enters the retromuscular plane and then the preperitoneal plane. Additional two 5 mm working ports are inserted at the lower midline. Usual TEP groin hernia repair is carried out. Since the surgeon is working at a different plane to the dilated bowel loops in the peritoneal cavity, it is much safer and also the mesh has less chance to come into contact with the peritoneal fluid and bowel loops thus theoretically less chance of contamination.

(g) Open groin hernia repair. The surgeon can carry out groin incision and open groin hernia repair for inguinal hernia, and open repair for femoral hernia.

5. Re-laparoscopy for the reassessment of the strangulated viscera viability.

   (a) During this part of surgery, the strangulated bowel should be assessed by several factors:

   (b) If there is any pulsation along the mesenteric artery supplying the involved segment of the bowel.

   (c) If the serosa surface of the involved bowel is intact.

   (d) If there is peristalsis of the involved bowel.

   (e) If there is any improvement in the vascularity of the involved bowel (picture should be taken before and during this time for comparison).

6. Decision if bowel resection is required.

   (a) If small bowel resection is required, it should be performed through an extended sub-umbilical port wound. Usually, a 3–4 cm length wound is all that requires to bring out the small bowel for section.

   (b) In an extremely rare situation, if large bowel resection is required, an expert colorectal laparoscopic surgeon should be called in for assistance to perform a laparoscopic large bowel resection. If none is available, then a conversion to an open approach should be carried out.

7. Conclusion of the surgery

   (a) During recheck peritoneal laparoscopy, most importantly the surgeon must make sure there is no inadvertent injury to the bowel loops. If occult injury goes unnotice, major morbidity or even mortality will arise postoperatively. The occult injury can be caused by instruments going in and out of the trocar during surgery while the patient is titled with bowel loops sitting right in front of the trocars, especially with cutting instruments. This is why some surgeons prefer TEP rather than TAPP in order to minimize this possibility.

(b) Recheck the strangulated segment of the bowel loop together with its mesenteric vessels.

(c) Recheck if there is any peritoneal defect which might expose the mesh.

Complications and Management

The major complication one needs to avoid during laparoscopic surgery for emergency hernia condition is an inadvertent injury to the dilated bowel loop leading to fecal peritoneum.

That is why the surgeon has to take extra care when the laparoscopic instruments go in and out of the trocars, especially when sharp cutting instruments and energy device is being used and when the patient is tilted to gain additional working space.

It is also important to prevent any occult injury to the bowel which the surgeon might miss during the operation. This is usually iatrogenic caused by instrumentation. That is why TEP repair is the preferred choice of repair by some surgeons. Since working in a completely different plane, it minimized the chance of iatrogenic bowel injury.

In case there is a bowel injury, the surgeon must quickly control the injured site and consider conversion to open surgery. Because the bowel loops are usually distended, and therefore leaking of fecal fluid might be very extensive once the injury occurs. Plan B should always be in the surgeon's mind to handle a situation like this during the surgery.

Mesh infection is not common in emergency hernia surgery, even in open approach with Lichtenstein's repair.

It depends on the degree of bowel ischemia and contamination of the operative field. Mesh should be avoided in the extreme end of the spectrum where bowel ischemia with perforation is encountered.

Postoperative Care

Because this is a disease with a spectrum of presentation ranging from (1) omentum strangulation; (2) strangulation of bowel with different levels of ischemia which recovered after reduction; and (3) strangulation with gangrenous bowel required bowel resection. The speed of recovery directly depends on their disease status.

For group 1, the patient can effectively resume oral feeding once they are fully awake after the surgery, and consider discharge home within the next 24 h.

For group 2, the patient can resume on clear water to soft diet depending on the level and time of bowel ischemia. They can usually be discharged within 24–48 h.

For group 3, because of bowel resection and anastomosis, they should be kept nil by mouth for several days until the anastomosis heal.

Antibiotics should be given, intraoperatively and continue for a course postoperatively to lower the risk of wound infection and mesh infection rate.

During the postoperative recovery period over the next 24–48 h, patient abdominal condition and vital signs should be monitored. This is to detect if there is any occult bowel injury that might be missed during surgery. So if there is any deterioration, or rapid recovery does not occur, the surgeon should be cautious and investigate the causes and subsequent salvage surgery should be performed as soon as possible if occult bowel injury is the case. In this respect, TEP approach after laparoscopic reduction of the strangulated bowel should be considered.

References

1. Ger R, Monroe K, Duvivier R, et al. Management of indirect inguinal hernias by laparoscopic closure of the neck of the sac. Am J Surg. 1990;159:370–3.
2. Arregui ME, Davis CJ, Yucel O, Nagan RF. Laparoscopic mesh repair of inguinal hernia using a preperitoneal approach: a preliminary report. Surg Laparosc Endosc. 1992;2:53–8.
3. Dion JM, Morin J. Laparoscopic inguinal herniorrhaphy. Can J Surg. 1992;35:209–12.

4. Barry McKernan J, Laws HL. Laparoscopic repair of inguinal hernias using a totally extraperitoneal prosthetic approach. Surg Endosc. 1993;7:26–8.

5. Memon MA, Cooper NJ, Memon B, Memon MI, Abrams KR. Meta-analysis of randomized clinical trials comparing open and laparoscopic inguinal hernia repair. Br J Surg. 1900;12:1479–92.

6. Hernia Trialists Collaboration EU. Laparoscopic versus open groin hernia repair: meta-analysis of randomized trials based on individual patient data. Hernia. 2002;6(1):2–10.

7. Neumayer L, Giobbie-Hurder A, Jonasson O, Fitgibbons R Jr, Dunlop D, Gibbs J, Reda D, Henderson W. Open mesh versus laparoscopic mesh repair of inguinal hernia. N Engl J Med. 2004;350:1819–27.

8. Legnani GL, Rasini M, Pastori S, Sarli D. Laparoscopic trans-peritoneal hernioplasty (TAPP) for the acute management of strangulated inguino-crural hernias: a report of nine cases. Hernia. 2008;12:185–8.

9. Miki Y, Sumimura J, Hasegawa T, et al. A new techniques of laparoscopic obturator hernia repair: report of a case. Jpn J Surg. 1998;28:652–6.

10. Yang GPC, Chan CTY, Lai ECH, Chan OCY, Tang CN, Li MKW. Laparoscopic versus open repair for strangulated groin hernias:188 cases over 4 years. Asian J Endosc Surg. 2012;5(3):131–7.

11. Lavonius MI, Ovaska J. Laparoscopy in the evaluation of the incarcerated mass in groin hernia. Surg Endosc. 2000;14:488–9.

12. Hayama S, Ohtaka K, Takahashi Y. Laparosopic reduction and repair for incarcerated obturator hernia: comparison with open surgery. Hernia. 2015;19:809–14.

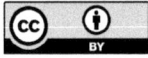

Laparoscopic Subtotal Cholecystectomy

Michael M. Lawenko

Introduction

Severely inflamed gallbladders due to acute or chronic infections are challenging to operate on laparoscopically. This is due to the difficulty of adequate ductal identification using the critical view of safety (CVS), which increases the risk of bile duct injury. The safer method would be to avoid dissection in the hepatocystic triangle and perform a subtotal laparoscopic cholecystectomy. The two types of subtotal cholecystectomy, based on the remaining remnant gallbladder would be fenestrating (no remnant) and reconstituting (remnant present) [1].

Indications [2]

- Severe cholecystitis.
- Cholelithiasis in liver cirrhosis and portal hypertension.
- Empyema or perforated gallbladder.

Contraindications

- Severe adhesions make it hard to access the gallbladder.
- Hemodynamic instability (systolic pressure < 90 mmHg).
- Bleeding and clotting problems.

Instruments

- Laparoscopic hook.
- Laparoscopic blunt graspers.
- Laparoscopic toothed graspers.
- Maryland forceps.
- Laparoscopic needle holders.
- Suction-Irrigation cannula.
- Advanced bipolar forceps (if available).

Conduct of the Operation

A 10 mm umbilical incision for a 10 mm Hasson Trocar. Three 5 mm incisions at the right subcostal area for 5 mm working trocars. Pressure is set initially at 8 mmHg with a flow rate of low flow (5 L/min). Once an ideal pneumoperitoneum is established, pressure is increased to 12 mmHg and high flow is established (20 L/min). The patient is set wherein the head is elevated (reverse Trendelenburg position) and the right side of the patient is also elevated just enough to let the bowels fall for exposure of the gallbladder.

M. M. Lawenko (✉)
De La Salle Medical and Health Sciences Institute, Dasmarinas City, Philippines
e-mail: mmlawenko@dlshsi.edu.ph

© The Author(s) 2023

D. Lomanto et al. (eds.), *Mastering Endo-Laparoscopic and Thoracoscopic Surgery*,
https://doi.org/10.1007/978-981-19-3755-2_20

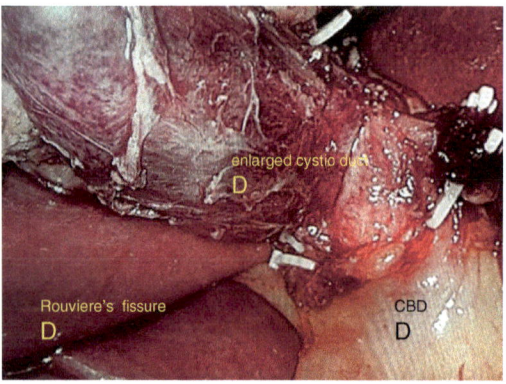

Fig. 1 Cystic duct is greatly enlarged making it unsafe to continue dissecting into the cystohepatic triangle

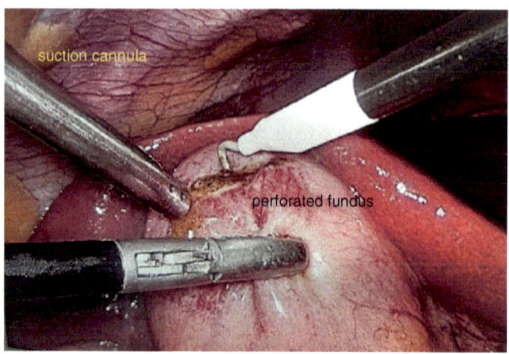

Fig. 2 Decompression of a distended gallbladder

A limited diagnostic laparoscopy is conducted by sweeping the scope around the abdomen to check for concomitant abdominal pathologies, active bleeding at port site insertions, and/or bowel injuries that might have occurred during trocar insertions. The area of the gallbladder (GB) is assessed for accessibility. In the presence of dense and hard omental adhesions or significant bowel adhesions to the GB, a decision to convert to an open procedure is executed due to difficulty to access. If the GB is readily visualized, dissection proceeds to isolate the cytic duct and artery. Additional maneuvers like the fundus down approach can be done at this point. If the cystohepatic triangle is fused with the cystic artery and/or the cystic duct cannot be safely dissected, a decision will be made to abort dissection into the cystohepatic triangle and initiate a laparoscopic subtotal cholecystectomy, so as to avoid a bile duct injury (Fig. 1).

Fenestrating Subtotal Cholecystectomy

Decompression of the GB is started with an open laparoscopic bowel grasper, on the lateral most trocar, which is used to push the GB cephalad. A suction cannula on the surgeon's left hand is situated at the fundus while a monopolar hook is on the surgeon's right hand to puncture the fundus of the GB just large enough to fit the suction can-

nula tip. Decompression of the GB is continued by suctioning the liquid contents present in the GB [3] (Fig. 2).

The bowel grasper is replaced with a toothed grasper, situated inside the newly created puncture in the fundus to grasp the GB and push it upwards with just enough space to carry out dissection around the GB. Dissection to remove the anterior wall of the GB is started at the fundus and carried down either medially or laterally towards the neck of the GB. A monopolar hook can be used, being mindful to address small arterial bleeding with bipolar forceps. An alternative is to carry out dissection with advanced bipolar forceps to minimize bleeding, as this has both cutting and vessel sealing capability (Fig. 3). The posterior wall of the GB is left attached to the liver with the mucosa exposed. Monopolar energy is applied to the exposed mucosa so as to limit the production of mucin.

During dissection of the GB, a specimen bag is placed inside beside the GB so that the stones extracted can be safely set aside by placement in a specimen bag. Smaller stones can be suctioned off. This prevents stones from being scattered around the abdomen, which can be challenging for multiple small stones. The removed anterior wall of the GB can also be placed inside the specimen bag at this point.

It must be noted that there must be no more stones inside the GB stump and bile flow is visualized in the orifice of the cystic duct. This is the time that intracorporeal suturing of the orifice of the cystic duct with a 2–0, braided, nonabsorbable suture via purse string closure is done.

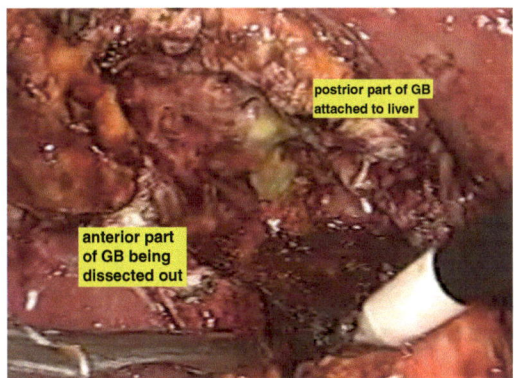

Fig. 3 Fenestrating subtotal cholecystectomy wherein part of the GB is attached to the liver

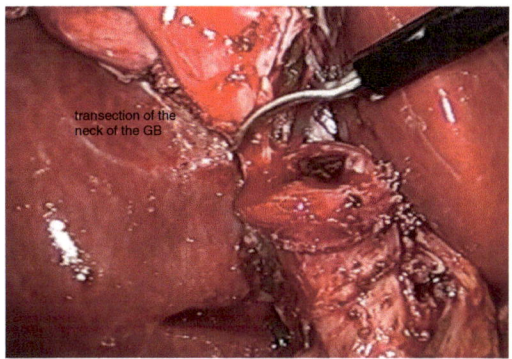

Fig. 4 Reconstituting subtotal cholecystectomy by transecting the neck of the GB

Using the suction irrigation cannula, copious lavage with plain saline solution for irrigation is done at the operative field, around the inferior and lateral borders of the liver to clean out small stones and spilled bile. A closed suction drain is placed at the inferior margin of the liver close to the GB stump with the proximal end exiting the most lateral 5 mm trocar. A last look to assess the integrity of the anatomy of the extrahepatic biliary tree is done by taking note that there are no signs of bleeding and bile leak. The remaining working trocars are removed under direct vision making sure that there are no signs of active port site bleeding. Dessuflation is done and the specimen bag is extracted through the umbilical incision. Proper closure of incision sites is done.

Reconstituting Subtotal Cholecystectomy

With the same indications for doing a subtotal cholecystectomy, since it is very difficult to approach the hepatocystic triangle, the fundus of the GB is perforated with the same technique discussed above. A dome-down technique is commenced wherein the GB is separated from the liver by a monopolar hook from the posterior part of the fundus up to the posterior part of the neck of the GB [4] (Fig. 2). Bleeding is common in this step, wherein control can be done with advanced bipolar forceps from time to time. If the

GB has a thickened wall, a 5 mm advanced bipolar forceps can be used throughout the dissection, being cautious when reaching the neck of the GB as the common hepatic duct can be adherent to the inflamed neck of the GB. It is of importance that dissection has proceeded to a point that the GB is freed from the liver up to the area of the neck. This is the point wherein transection of the neck of the GB is done, either with a monopolar hook or an advanced bipolar forceps (Fig. 4). Proper hemostasis must be done once arterioles are transected. The stones are removed and placed into a specimen bag, together with the transected part of the GB. Visualization of the orifice of the cystic duct is done with minimal probing with the Maryland forceps just to make sure that there are no stones lodged inside the cystic duct and that flow of bile is noted. Burning of the stump mucosa is commenced with a monopolar hook. Intracorporeal suturing with a 2–0 absorbable barbed suture is needed to close off the stump (Fig. 5).

Copious suction and irrigation are done around the operative field so as to clean away small stones and bile. A closed suction drain is placed lateral and inferior to the gallbladder stump with the distal end coming out of the lateral trocar insertion site. A last look to assess the integrity of the anatomy of the extrahepatic biliary tree is done by taking note that there are no signs of bleeding and bile leak. Remaining working trocars are removed under direct vision mak-

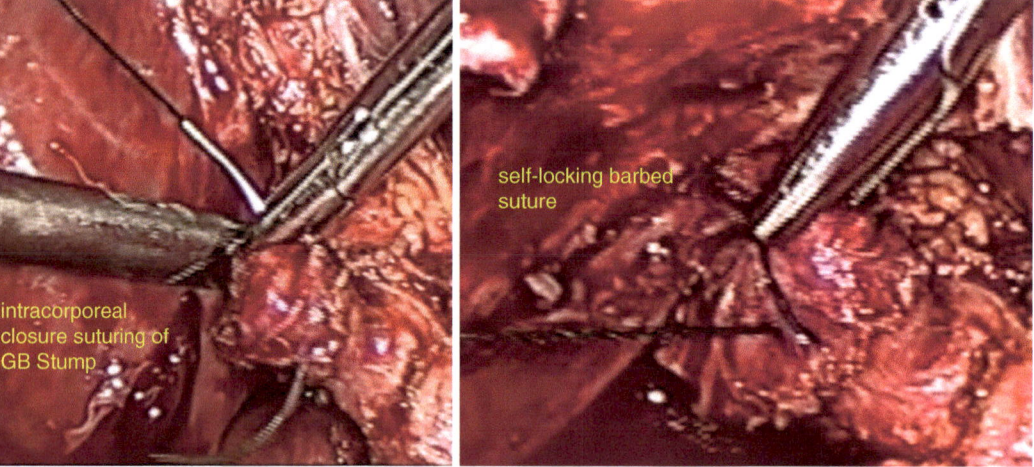

Fig. 5 Closure of the GB stump with a barbed suture

ing sure that there are no signs of active port site bleeding. Dessuflation is done and the specimen bag is extracted through the umbilical incision. Proper closure of incision sites is done.

References

1. Strasberg SM, Pucci MJ, Brunt ML, et al. Subtotal cholecystectomy-"Fenestrating" vs "reconstituting" subtypes and the prevention of bile duct injury: definition of the optimal procedure in difficult operative conditions. J Am Coll Surg. 2016;222(1):89–6.

2. Elshaer M, Gravante G, Thomas K, et al. Subtotal cholecystectomy for "difficult gallbladders" systematic review and meta-analysis. JAMA Surg. 2015;150(2):159–68.

3. Shin M, Choi N, Yoo Y, et al. Clinical outcomes of subtotal cholecystectomy performed for difficult cholecystectomy. Ann Surg Treat Res. 2016;91(5):226–32.

4. Purzner RH, Ho KB, Al-Sukhni E, et al. Safe laparoscopic subtotal cholecystectomy in the face of severe inflammation in the cystohepatic triangle: a retrospective review and proposed management strategy for the difficult gallbladder. J Can Chir. 2019;62(6):402–41.

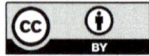

Adhesiolysis for Bowel Obstruction

Raquel Maia

Introduction

Abdominal surgery is the major cause of peritoneal adhesion formation. Although being part of the body's healing process, it is estimated that intra-abdominal adhesions are developed in 90–95% of patients. Other causes of intra-abdominal adhesions include pelvic inflammatory disease, spontaneous bacterial peritonitis, and complicated diverticulitis [1].

Consequences of adhesions may range from chronic pain, infertility to partial or total intestine obstruction, bowel necrosis, and death if not addressed adequately.

Laparoscopy for adhesiolysis has some advantages when compared to the open approach: (1) earlier recovery of gastrointestinal function; (2) decrease in incidences of ventral hernias; and (3) shorter length of hospitalization. However, Yao et al., in a study with 156 patients submitted to either open or laparoscopic approach for adhesiolysis concluded that the incidence of reoperations for obstruction was higher in the laparoscopic group (7.7 vs. 0%) [2].

In another study, Kelly et al., evaluate more than 9.000 patients from a database, comparing the 30 days outcome in both laparoscopic and open groups. As expected, the rate of major incision complications was less frequent in the laparoscopic group, but also the mortality at 30 days was higher in the open group (4.7 vs. 1.3%) [3].

Indications

Patients with small bowel obstruction (SBO) should be carefully selected for laparoscopic adhesiolysis. Moreover, all attempts must be taken to treat stable patients conservatively. Some bowel obstructions can be successfully resolved with no oral intake, nasogastric tube for decompression, intravenous fluid resuscitation, bladder catheter to closely follow the urine output, and antibiotics if fever or leukocytosis is present. The ultimate goal is to avoid a scenario where small bowel necrosis is installed. Physical examination, radiologic study of the abdomen with water-soluble contrast, and tomography are valuable tools to follow up on the evolution of SBO cases. If it all fails in 24–48 h, the surgical approach must be considered without further delay.

Patients with (1) partial obstruction; (2) SBO that fails with conservative management in a stable patient; (3) Chronic pain and (4) recurrent obstruction are the best indications for laparoscopic adhesiolysis [4].

Contraindications

- Diffuse peritonitis.
- Vascular compromise or perforation.

R. Maia (✉)
Brazilian College of Gastric Surgeons,
Sao Paolo, Brazil

© The Author(s) 2023
D. Lomanto et al. (eds.), *Mastering Endo-Laparoscopic and Thoracoscopic Surgery*,
https://doi.org/10.1007/978-981-19-3755-2_21

- Hemodynamic instability.
- Patient who is unable to tolerate pneumoperitoneum or refuse the procedure.
- "Frozen" abdomen due to carcinomatosis or matted adhesions.

Preoperative Assessment and Patient Preparation

- Abdominal radiography especially if a complete obstruction is suspected (Fig. 1).
- Tomography (CT) to identify major complications such as necrosis, presence of pneumatosis of the bowel, transition point of obstruction, and cause of SBO.
- Fluid and electrolytes replacement and acidosis correction.
- Preoperative antibiotics.
- Nasogastric tube in low continuous suction.
- DVT prophylaxis.
- Bladder catheterization.
- General anesthesia.
- Laparotomy tray available.
- Bipolar or harmonic scalpel.

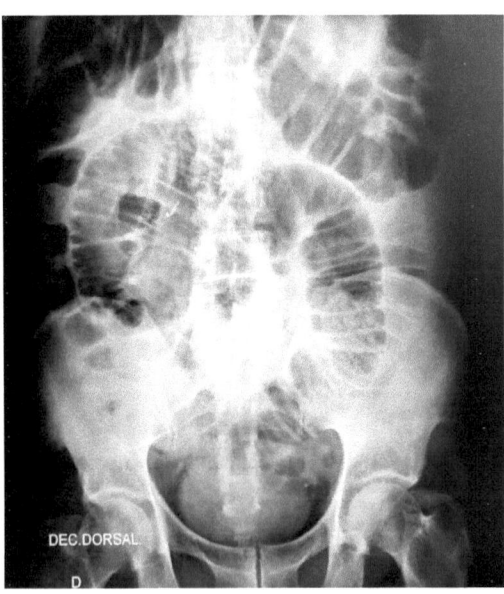

Fig. 1 Rx of small bowel obstruction (personal file)

OT Setup

The patient should be placed in supine position with arms tucked at the sides and both arms and legs are safely secured in a flat position. Keep in mind that a steep Trendelenburg or reverse Trendelenburg position might be needed during the procedure.

Two monitors should be placed either on each side of the patient's head or one in the head and the other one near the opposite hip, depending on the surgeon's discretion.

The surgeon must be placed on the opposite side of the first trocar placement site [5].

The instruments needed must include:

- 3–5 trocars;
- Angled scopes.
- Laparoscopic atraumatic graspers.
- Blunt-tipped scissors.
- Handport device in case of a hybrid approach for bowel suturing or resection (optional).
- Laparoscopic staple if bowel anastomosis is needed.
- Suction-irrigators for aqua dissection (optional).

Surgical Technique

- The first trocar should be placed in virgin territory, at least 5 cm away from any previous scar, and using Hasson's technique. Both RUQ and LUQ are good options for entering the abdomen.
- The second trocar is placed in an area away from adhesions. Keep in mind the triangulation when positioning the trocars.
- Start the procedure by releasing the adhesions to the anterior abdominal wall that looks filmy and avascular.
- Use gravity, CO_2 pneumoperitoneum, and work above the adhesions to delineate a plane.
- Scissor is the best tool to release the adhesions. Insert a blunt—tip scissor in an avascular plane between the peritoneum or omentum and the adhesion, open and withdraw it

opened. Repeat this step as many times as needed to clear the adhesions. Use gentle atraumatic traction to expose the plane.

- Always start from a plane where is easier to identify the anatomy, rather than an unknown territory.
- When facing a thick, dense, and vascular adhesion, use electrosurgical energy to cauterize and then divide the plane. A harmonic scalpel is a better option, but consider that the jaws are hot when in use. Avoid thermal injury.
- Any incidental enterotomies must be repaired as soon as they are detected to avoid cavity contamination.
- Any nonviable ischemic bowel segment should be resected and an end-to-end or side-to-side anastomosis is performed. Surgical staples can be used and in more complex cases a hybrid approach, e.g., hand-assisted laparoscopy is of use.
- Move into the pelvis to release adhesion with the omentum. Keep in view both ureters' trajectories to avoid damage.
- When the obstruction stopping point is freed from adhesions, run the bowel with gentle atraumatic graspers to search for any unnoticed bowel injury.
- Carefully review the hemostasis and wash the cavity copiously.

Tips

- Start from a clear anatomical site, then move to the more complex areas of adhesions.
- Avoid thermal injuries. Late thermal bowel injury might not be noted until hours or days after the surgery. Scissors are the best tool.
- All mesenteric defects should be closed.
- Establish a realistic timeline for the laparoscopic procedure. If not successful DO NOT hesitate to convert.

- At any time, do not hesitate to convert if adhesions are too dense, if pneumoperitoneum cannot be achieved due to bowel distention, and especially if bowel resection is needed.
- If the integrity of an anastomosis is uncertain, a diverting ostomy should be considered.
- Be patient!

Postoperative Care

- Analgesia with non-opioid medication.
- A liquid diet can be initiated on the first day.
- The patient can be discharged once bowel movements have returned and flatus are present.

References

1. Eillis H. The clinical significance of adhesions: focus on intestinal obstruction. Eur J Surg Suppl. 1997;(577):5–9.
2. Yao S, Tanaka E, Matsui Y, Ikeda A, Murakami T, Okumoto T, et al. Does laparoscopic adhesiolysis decrease the risk of recurrent symptoms in small bowel obstruction? A propensity score-matched analysis. Surg Endosc [internet]. 2017;31(12):5348–55. https://doi.org/10.1007/s00464-017-5615-9.
3. Kelly KN, Iannuzzi JC, Rickles AS, Garimella V, Monson JRFF. Laparotomy for small-bowel obstruction: first choice or last resort for adhesiolysis? A laparoscopic approach for small-bowel obstruction reduces 30-day complications. Surg Endosc. 2014;(1):65–73.
4. Di Saverio S, Birindelli A, Ten BR, Davies JR, Mandrioli M, Sallinen V. Laparoscopic adhesiolysis: not for all patients, not for all surgeons, not in all centres. Updates Surg [Internet]. 2018;70(4):557–61. https://pubmed.ncbi.nlm.nih.gov/29767333
5. Villanueva MSS, Roberts KEM. Laparoscopic Adhesiolysis [Internet]. Medscape. 2019 [cited 2020 Sep 10]. https://emedicine.medscape.com/article/1829759-overview#a2

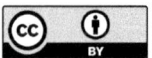

Emergency Laparoscopic Small Bowel Resection

Abdul Gafoor Mubarak

The small bowel forms the majority of "real estate" particularly in the lower abdomen and remains to this day one of the most formidable challenges that a laparoscopic surgeon faces when he is performing surgery [1]. The common conditions that will require the laparoscopist attention includes.

1. Blockages either due to adhesions or are congenital.
2. Bleeding, infection, and ulcers due to disease process, i.e., Chron's disease.
3. Cancer and carcinoids.
4. Small bowel injury.
5. Meckel's Diverticulum.
6. Precancerous polyps.
7. Non-cancerous benign tumors.

Inadvertently the most common reason for a small bowel resection would be adhesions [2]. For simplification purposes, this part will focus on acquired and not congenital issues which need small bowel resections.

Almost all small bowel resections can be done by laparoscopy [1]. If the patient is fit for general anesthesia, they should be fit for a laparoscopic resection option as well. Absolute contraindication for resection would include

- Poor blood supply to bowel ends (i.e., radiation-injured bowel).
- Unclear bowel viability after a revascularization procedure.
  - Both ends of the small bowel may be brought up to skin level as temporary ostomies if the distal small bowel is involved. A proximal small bowel ostomy will create a high-output fistula that is difficult to manage.
  - Alternatively, both ends can be stapled closed and a plan made for a second-look laparotomy in 24–48 h.
  - In extreme situations (e.g., acute mesenteric ischemia with gangrene extending from the ligament of Treitz to mid colon), the likelihood of survival is very small. This is an absolute contraindication to attempted resection and anastomosis [3].
- Inadequate tumor margins.
  - If a tumor is unresectable, and small bowel obstruction is likely to occur, a side-to-side anastomosis in the uninvolved bowel proximal and distal to the obstruction may be performed as a bypass procedure, leaving the tumor in situ.

A. G. Mubarak (✉)
Island Hospital, Penang, Malaysia

Relative Contraindications Would Include

- Peritoneal sepsis.
- Hemodynamically precarious patient.
- Extensive Crohn's disease.
  - Stricturoplasty should be considered to minimize the need for extensive resection and the risk of short gut syndrome; 90 cm is the approximate shortest length of small bowel that might still support a viable oral nutrition program.

The limiting factor is however the operator. The resection requires an experienced surgeon whereby some suggest the experience should be at least someone who is able to perform intracorporeal knotting and suturing comfortably. The other requirement is the knowledge of patient orientation and usage of the operating table including the functions of rotations and various positions. The small bowel is a precarious organ that flops around and good control over the mobility of the organ is essential.

Preoperative assessment is a vital step in performing small bowel resections [3]. The availability of information regarding the location of pathology, nature of pathology, and the extent of contamination would affect the positioning of the patient and also placement of trocars. A contrast CT scan would be able to show the nature of the pathology and also avail information regarding contamination if present. This would then be translated into planning the operation itself. In laparoscopic small bowel resection, the consideration should be if the operator is required to stand in

between the patient's legs in either a Trendelenburg or reverse Trendelenburg position (Fig. 1).

It is my contention that if the pathology is located in the upper small bowel, i.e., the duodenum or the jejunum it would be better to position the patient in a head-down position with the operator standing between the patient's legs. However, if the pathology is located in the lower small bowel, i.e., a Meckel's diverticulum, the operator should be standing on either side of the patient with a slight tilt up on the opposite side (Fig. 2).

The patient should be catheterized if the operation is expected to take some time, i.e., more than 90 min and there should be considerations for DVT prophylaxis according to local norms and practices. Prophylactic and empirical antibiotics are also as per local norms and practices. Other imaging modalities that can be used to aid are as follows:

- Small bowel follow-through and small bowel enteroclysis.
- As indicated for bleeding:
  - Esophagogastroduodenoscopy, push enteroscopy, or double balloon enteroscopy.
  - Capsule endoscopy.
  - Nuclear scan.
  - Angiography.

The three positioning for port placement for patients for small bowel surgery is illustrated in the diagram below (Fig. 3). The placement of ports and selection of port placement should be dictated by the pathology itself. As mentioned before a CT scan is essential in this regard. The aim is to not only triangulate the pathology and working space

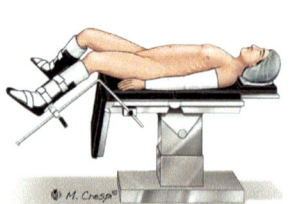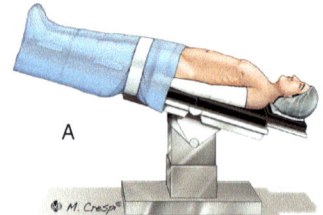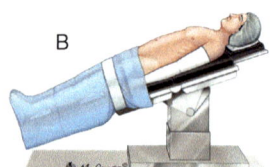

Fig. 1 Split leg, trendelenburg, and reverse trendelenburg position

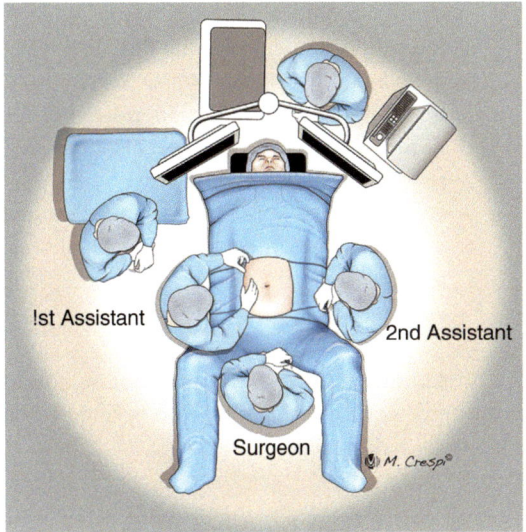
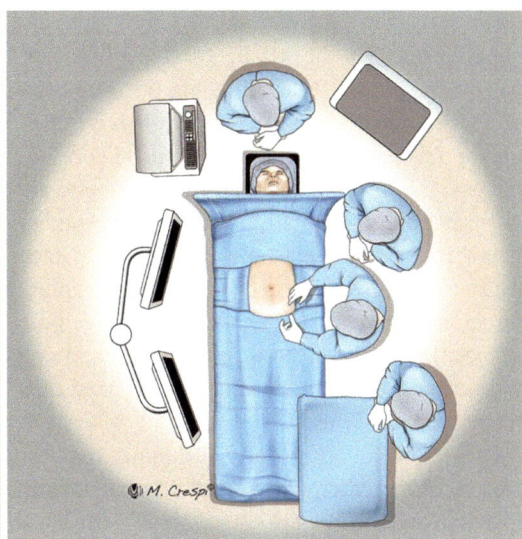

!st Assistant 2nd Assistant

Surgeon

Fig. 2 Surgeon standing in between legs or on either side of the patient

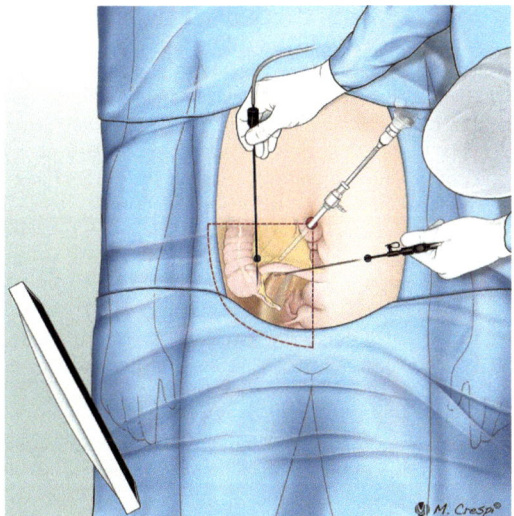

Fig. 3 Triangulate pathology during port placement

ergonomically but also to ensure that adequate room is available for not only resection but also to accommodate stapler devices and aid in closure using intracorporeal sutures. The likely positions for port placement are illustrated below. The most general consideration would be for adhesions. The pathology does not allow very much planning but in general I prefer to place a supraumbilical port by an open technique followed by diagnostic laparoscopy before inserting the other ports. Once the

adhesiolysis is undertaken, the working port can be enlarged to accommodate the stapler device and aid in resection and closure.

Surgical Technique and Synthesis

Small bowel resections laparoscopically are always a balance of finesse and precision [2]. The operator has to determine the viability of the segment that remains and how much of the small bowel is actually going to be resected. The consideration is further confounded by the general condition of the patient, i.e., is the patient septic or bleeding due to an injury. Once the affected segment is identified, the surgeon has to perform a detachment procedure whereby the small bowel is denuded of the blood supply. Often an energy device is used for this purpose and the author's preference is the Ligature device from Medtronic or the Harmonic Ace by Johnson and Johnson. The addition of separating the function of sealing and cutting allows more control when performing this step. Often however the operator can get carried away by the ease of the instrument and fail to dissect clear and large vessels before sealing them and this will lead to obscurity of vision and unexpected bleeding.

Once the segment of the bowel is denuded from the blood supply the resection is undertaken. It is often done with staplers and the height required depends on the thickness of the tissue however in general a stapler device using a height of 2.6–3.6 mm is sufficient for the job. It is essential for the operator to place the segment of resection away from the trocar site for this step to aid in resection and then anastomoses. Another important tip is to use an anchoring stitch to keep the two bowel segments together before stapling for the anastomoses. In general, we can use three staples, i.e., two for the resection ends and one for the anastomosis or anastomose first and then resect which will usually always end with three staples as well. The former technique requires closure of the enterotomy created by the stapler insertion and the latter does not.

The closure of the omental defect after performing small bowel resection is debatable however it is the author's opinion that all defects should be closed and the closure of this defect is relatively easy to perform. Drains are not routinely recommended.

Postoperative Management and Complication

Post surgery the patient can be started on clear fluids almost immediately in ward and following bowel movement, up-scaled to a nourishing and normal diet. There is a lot of evidence to support the fact that bowel movements are faster after laparoscopic bowel resections as opposed to open surgery however the overall postoperative stay may not be affected. There is no need for the continuation of antibiotics unless there has been evidence of contamination or infection during the surgery and patients are encouraged to ambulate and mobilize as soon as possible.

Common Complications Include

- Surgical site infection (either deep or superficial).
- Bleeding.

- Systemic complications of major surgery, including pneumonia, venous thromboembolism, and cardiovascular events.
  - Small bowel obstruction, stricture, and the need for further surgery are also potential risks of small bowel resection.
  - Patients with extensive intra-abdominal sepsis or who are in a malnourished state are at increased risk for anastomotic leak and enteric fistula.

In summary, small bowel resection is a delicate and precise procedure that can be undertaken safely by laparoscopy.

References

1. Gerson LB, Fidler JL, Cave DR, et al. ACG clinical guideline: diagnosis and management of small bowel bleeding. Am J Gastroenterol. 2015;110:1265–87. https://doi.org/10.1038/ajg.2015.246.
2. Pennazio M, Spada C, Eliakim R, et al. Small-bowel capsule endoscopy and device-assisted enteroscopy for diagnosis and treatment of small-bowel disorders: European Society of Gastrointestinal Endoscopy (ESGE) clinical guideline. Endoscopy. 2015;47:352–76. https://doi.org/10.1055/s-0034-1391855.
3. Schottenfeld D, Beebe-Dimmer JL, Vigneau FD. The epidemiology and pathogenesis of neoplasia in the small intestine. Ann Epidemiol. 2009;19:58–69. https://doi.org/10.1016/j.annepidem.2008.10.004.
4. Cloyd JM, George E, Visser BC. Duodenal adenocarcinoma: advances in diagnosis and surgical management. World J Gastrointest Surg. 2016;8:212–21. https://doi.org/10.4240/wjgs.v8.i3.212.
5. Achille A, Baron A, Zamboni G, et al. Molecular pathogenesis of sporadic duodenal cancer. Br J Cancer. 1998;77:760–5.
6. Markogiannakis H, Theodorou D, Toutouzas KG, et al. Adenocarcinoma of the third and fourth portion of the duodenum: a case report and review of the literature. Cases J. 2008;1:98. https://doi.org/10.1186/1757-1626-1-98.
7. Edge SB, Byrd DR, Compton CC. American joint committee on cancerstaging manual. 7th ed. New York: Springer; 2010. p. 127.

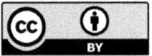

Laparoscopic Hartmann's Procedure

Yen-Chen Shao, Ming-Yin Shen, and William Tzu-Liang Chen

Introduction

Hartmann's procedure, Hartmann's resection, or Hartmann's operation is the surgical resection consisting of sigmoidectomy without intestinal restoration. It contains an end-colostomy and closure of a rectal stump. It was first described by Henri Albert Hartmann (1860–1952) for resection of rectal or sigmoid cancer [1]. Nowadays, Hartmann procedure is usually used in treating malignant obstruction of left-sided colon or in emergent conditions, such as sigmoid colon perforation [2], mostly because of diverticulum disease. The advantage of Hartmann's procedure is reduction in morbidity and mortality in emergent settings because it avoids the possibility of complications from a colorectal anastomosis. For patients with unstable hemodynamic status, or multiple comorbidity or inflammatory condition of the intestinal tissue, which would make performing a colorectal anastomosis difficult or have a higher risk of anastomotic leakage, this procedure is simple and fast, and meanwhile preserve the chance of restoration of intestine continuity after patients' general condition got improvement. However, the Hartmann reversal rate is variable in different studies, ranging from 0 to 50% [3, 4]. The morbidity rate of Hartmann reversal is up to 55%, and the mortality rate is ranging from 0 to 14% [5–7]. A study showed reversal of Hartmann between 3 and 9 months associated with increased risk of postoperative complications [8]. The mean interval from Hartmann procedure to its reversal is ranging from 7.5 to 9.1 months [3, 5]. We usually delay the reversal of Hartmann's operation at least 6 months later in our daily practice. Hartmann's procedure and/or reversal of Hartmann's procedure could be conventional or laparoscopic. Laparoscopic reversal of Hartmann's procedure is associated with less complications compared to the conventional method, especially in wound infection, anastomotic leakage, and cardiopulmonary complications [3].

Indications

This procedure is used for left-sided colonic disease, usually in emergent situations, either preoperatively or peri-operatively noted. Generally speaking, when a patient is mandated to a sigmoidectomy, who also has unstable vital signs (shock status) or multiple comorbidities (ASA IV patients), which increase the risks of postoperative complications, especially in anastomotic condition, Hartmann's procedure is an alternative method. Besides, when the intestine tissue condition is not healthy, such as distention and edematous change resulting from obstruction, ischemic

Y.-C. Shao · M.-Y. Shen · W. T.-L. Chen (✉)
Division of Colorectal Surgery, Department of Surgery, China Medical University Hsinchu Hospital, Zhubei City, Hsinchu County, Taiwan
e-mail: wtchen@mail.cmuh.org.tw

© The Author(s) 2023
D. Lomanto et al. (eds.), *Mastering Endo-Laparoscopic and Thoracoscopic Surgery*,
https://doi.org/10.1007/978-981-19-3755-2_23

change, and inflammatory fibrosis, or any condition would make a colorectal anastomosis difficult to perform, Hartmann's procedure provides a damage control method and avoid any complications followed by an anastomosis.

These indications include [9].

1. Colorectal cancer obstruction,
2. Perforated diverticulitis with peritonitis,
3. Ischemic colitis.
4. Sigmoid volvulus.
5. Anastomotic complications, such as leakage or stricture.
6. Abdomen trauma.

Other less common indications

1. Severe low anterior syndrome, mostly when a patient received an ultra-low anterior resection complicated with a poor rectal reservoir function.
2. Surgery in patients with preexisting anal incontinence.

Contraindications

Patient with unstable hemodynamic status who could not tolerate general anesthesia is contraindicated. Patient who could not tolerate prolonged pneumoperitoneum is contraindicated for laparoscopic Hartmann's procedure. In an oncological setting, any condition that would compromise the result is a relative contraindication, such as low rectal cancer invading the pelvic floor, in such situation, abdominal-perineal combined resection should be performed.

Preoperative Assessment

Preoperative Preparation

First, an informed consent should be obtained. The indication and risks should be explained to the patient. Most of Hartmann's procedure is performed under emergent condition, and these patients were initially scheduled to receive an anterior resection or sigmoidectomy with anastomosis, the possibility of stoma creation (either end stoma or loop stoma) should be informed. In fact, we suggest informing the possibility of stoma creation in all colonic procedures before doing a surgery, not only for left-sided colonic lesion. According to many retrospective studies, only half of the patients could receive a reversal of Hartmann's procedure in the seeing future therefore possible permanent stoma placement should be explained.

Preoperative Testing

Before surgery, one should receive preoperative studies to evaluate the surgical plan and potential life-threatening condition.

Laboratory Studies

Complete blood counts and differential count (CBC/DC), renal function tests (serum BUN and creatinine), electrolytes (Serum sodium and potassium), liver function tests (serum AST and ALT, direct/total bilirubin), pre-transfusion study (ABO and Rh typing), prothrombin time and activated partial thromboplastin time (PT and aPTT), are routinely checked preoperatively in patients who will receive major surgery in our institute.

Chest X-Ray (CxR)

CxR is routinely checked in our institute, it provides information on some major comorbidities, such as pleural effusion, cardiomegaly, or pulmonary tuberculosis (especially in South-East Asia). It is not the gold standard for the diagnosis of lung metastasis in colorectal cancer.

Electrocardiogram (ECG)

Electrocardiograms are noninvasive, quick, and effective in detecting potential heart disease. It is routinely checked in major surgery in our hospital.

Abdominal Computed Tomography (CT)

Abdominal CT scan with intravenous contrast is useful to assess the disease severity in diverticulitis disease or tumor obstruction/perforation. In perforated diverticulitis disease, it provides information to evaluate whether the surgery would be a sigmoidectomy with/without diverting stoma, or Hartmann's procedure. In a patient who has malignant obstruction or perforation, it provides not only the surgical choices but also the possibility of combined resection of adjuvant organ which invaded by the tumor. Oral or rectal contrast is usually not recommended in emergent condition.

Magnetic Resonance Imaging (MRI)

Pelvic MRI is now widely accepted as the gold standard for rectal malignancy; however, it is usually not available in patients under emergent condition.

OT Setup

Patient's Position

It is better to put the patient in a modified Trendelenburg lithotomy position (Fig. 1) than in a supine position. However, in many cases, colorectal surgeons are consulted in the operation theater by general surgeons for patients with colonic disease, and these patients are receiving the surgery under the indication of hollow organ perforation initially. In such cases, these patients are usually put in the supine position.

The operator should be positioned to patient's left and the cameraman positioned next to the

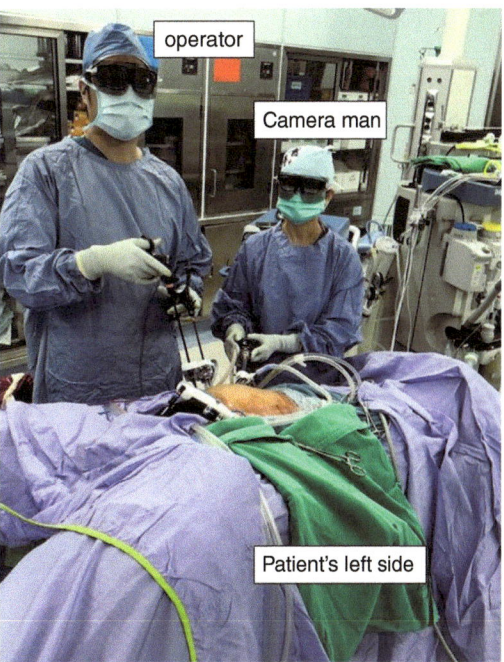

Fig. 2 Operator and camera man

operator (Fig. 2). If there is an assistant, he or she should be positioned on the patient's left side.

Instrumentations

- Trocars:
- 12 mm trocars ×2: One for camera, another as working port
- 5 mm trocars ×2–4.
- Laparoscopic instruments:
  - Bowel grasping forceps ×2–3.
  - Metzenbaum scissor ×1.
  - Hook electrode or spoon electrode ×1.
  - Right angle dissection forceps ×1.
  - Energy devises ×1 (alternative: bipolar forceps).
  - Suction and irrigation system.

Surgical technique

1. Under general anesthesia, the patient should be put in modified Trendlenburg lithotomy position.

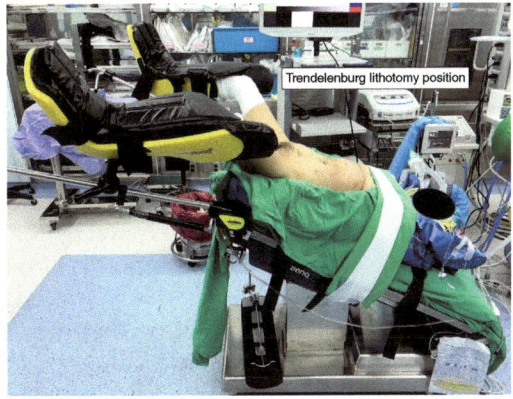

Fig. 1 Trendelenburg lithotomy position

2. A 12 mm camera trocar is inserted near umbilicus. A 12 mm trocar should be inserted via right lower quadrant of abdomen; another 5 mm trocar should be inserted via right abdomen, 8–10 cm away from the 12 mm trocar (Fig. 3a). You can insert an additional 5 mm trocar via left lower quadrant of abdomen for assistant (Fig. 3b).

3. Identified the lesion in diseased sigmoid colon or rectum, if there is a perforated hole, do damage control first. Close the perforated hole with sutures and irrigate the peritoneal cavity copiously with warm saline.

4. Gently separate the inflamed tissue surrounding the lesion. Use hand instruments to grab a piece of wet gauze and wipe out the adhesive tissue. Avoid direct dissection between severely inflamed tissue unless there is a clear surgical plane.

5. Use electrode to free the sigmoid colon from its peritoneal attachment along the line of Toldt proximally from the descending colon and distally to the pelvic inlet (Fig. 4).

6. If the lesion is malignant, such as tumor obstruction or tumor perforation, adequate

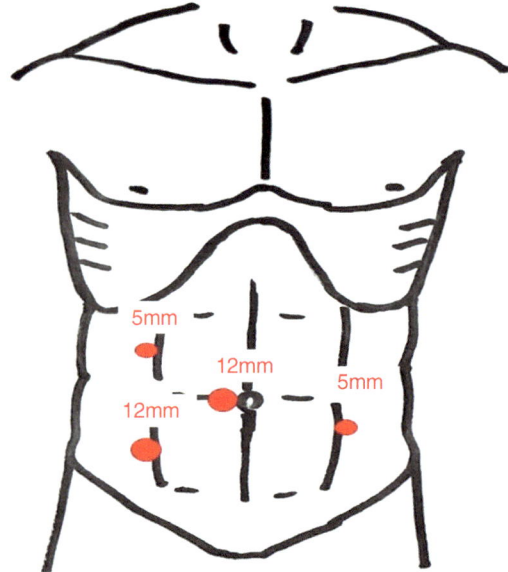

Fig. 3b Port placements

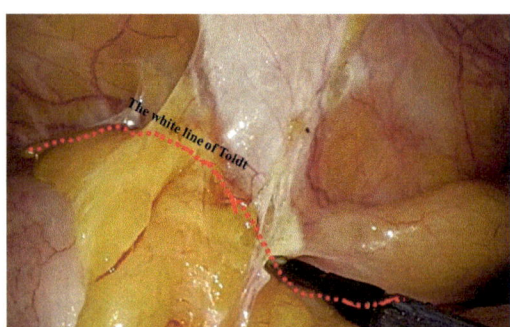

Fig. 4 Dissection along the white line of Toldt

lymph nodes sampling is recommended. Ligate inferior mesentery artery at its root just above abdominal aorta (Fig. 5). Perform complete mesocolon excision as standard colon cancer surgery. If the lesion is benign, such as diverticulitis perforation, stercoral ulcer perforation, or other nonmalignant diseases, dissect mesocolon at the level of marginal vessels to preserve a better blood supply to colon is feasible.

7. Select the transection point proximally and distally. If inferior mesentery artery was ligated at its root, bowel transection point at upper rectum would be better. Use endocut-

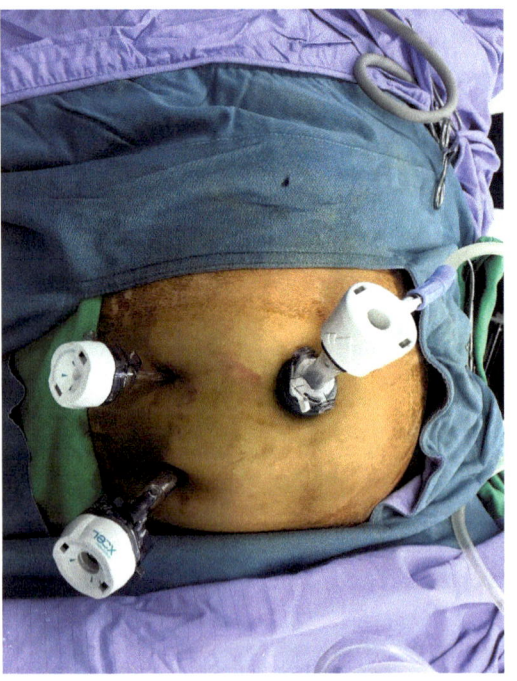

Fig. 3a Trocar insertion

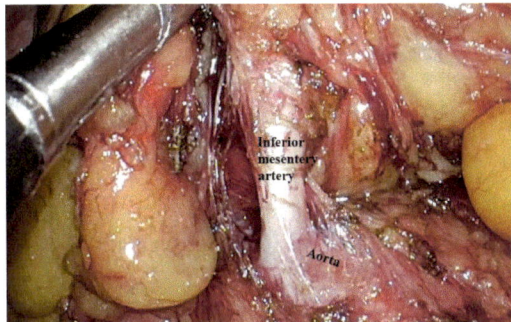

Fig. 5 Ligate root of inferior mesentery artery

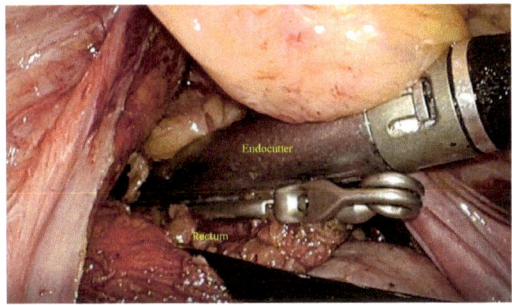

Fig. 6 Divide rectum by endocutter

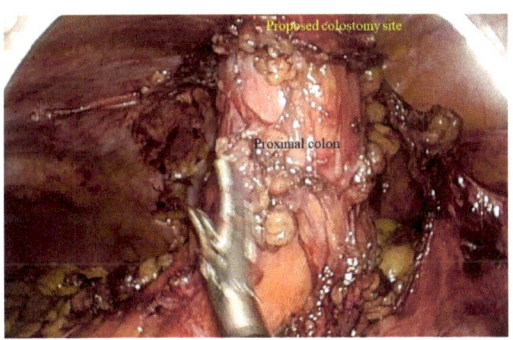

Fig. 7 Proposed end-colostomy without tension

ter to divide the bowel proximally and distally (Fig. 6).

8. Make sure the proximal colon could reach the proposed colostomy site without tension. Make a circular incision at the proposed colostomy site. Split rectus abdominis and pull out the proximal colon through the incision (Fig. 7).

9. Enlarge the 12 mm camera port, set a wound protector, and remove the specimen through the incision. Reestablish pneumoperitoneum, check hemostasis, and place a drainage tube if indicated.

10. Close the trocar wounds layer by layer. Mature the end-colostomy.

Complications and Management

Wound Infection

Hartmann's procedure is usually associated with emergent settings, and therefore has a higher risk of wound infection than elective surgery. Laparoscopic Hartmann's procedure has less infection rate than conventional Hartmann's procedure [10] however it still has 5–10% wound infection rate. Adequate fluid drainage with antibiotic treatment for 7–10 days should be given for patients with wound infection. Parastomal infection needs specialized nursing care, treated with adequate abscess drainage and antibiotic therapy.

Ureteral Injury

In the medial-to-lateral approach for sigmoid colon mobilization during the surgery, a surgical plane is made below inferior mesentery artery. The left ureter and gonadal vessels should be swept away and injury to these structures could be avoided if the plane is accurate. Under ideal conditions, a ureter can be identified by Kelly's sign, a visible vermiculation by direct press. A precise dissection along the surgical plane avoids ureteral injury. However, in the emergent setting, severe inflammatory change and adhesions result in difficulty identifying ureter. Latrogenic ureteral injury has been documented at 0.3–1.5% incidence rate. Despite preventing ureteral injury by inserting a ureteral double-J stent before colon resection remains controversial, it provides immediate identification of ureteral injury. Once the ureter is injured, immediate repair with ureteral stenting placement for 2 weeks avoids reoperation [11]. Usually, the ureteral stent is removed after the ureter was tested and healed.

Urinary Bladder Injury

Bladder injury is a rare complication during colon surgery, the incidence is less than 5% [11]. It is associated with an infectious or inflammatory process. A Foley catheter insertion before surgery avoids potential trocar injury during surgery. Urinary bladder injury is usually identified by urine leakage during surgery, the most reliable confirmation is a visible Foley catheter balloon in the bladder. Immediate repair with a Foley catheter left for 2 weeks is indicated. The Foley catheter will be removed after cystogram is performed.

Vessel Injury

It is more common to see vessel injuries in laparoscopic Hartmann's procedure than in other laparoscopic surgeries. Severe inflammation, infectious process, and adhesion are risk factors that contribute to vessel injuries. Compare to traditional D3 dissection with vessel ligation at the root of inferior mesentery artery, it occurs more often in vessel ligation along intermittent vessels or marginal vessels. Immediately control the bleeding vessels by laparoscopic energic device or end clips would be helpful.

Bowel Injury

In diverticulitis or tumor perforation diseases, small intestine or right-sided colon may adhere to the inflamed colon. Irrigate the peritoneal cavity with warm saline copiously and gently separate adhesion between bowel loops by grabbing a wet gauze to mimic incidentally bowel injuries. Seromuscular tear of the bowel wall can be repaired by suturing.

Intra-abdominal abscess formation:

A few days after surgery, if persisted fever or positive peritoneal sign was noted, intra-abdominal abscess formation should be considered. It can be diagnosed by abdominal echogram or computed tomography (CT). Superficial abscess just beneath the wound can be drained by opening the wound. Deep abscess in the perito-

neal cavity should be treated by percutaneous drainage, either by echogram-guided or CT-guided. Obtain bacterial culture and blood culture sampling and then give empiric antibiotics until the pathogen was yielded in the laboratory, usually 7–10 days of antibiotic treatment is adequate.

Post-OP Care

Adequate fluid maintenance to keep hemodynamic status stable. Vasopressor therapy initially targets a mean artery pressure of 65 mmHg. Intravenous fluid can be tapered after the patient tolerates oral intake. Postoperative ileus is common after emergent colorectal surgery, it ranges from days to weeks. A nasogastric tube indwelling is helpful in poor gastric emptying. Remove nasogastric tube when the drainage gastric juice decreased, and on diet as soon as patients can tolerate. Normalized bowel movement could be observed by feces or gas retention in the colostomy bag.

Education on colostomy nursing care is important for patients and their caregiver, usually their spouse or children. An enterostomal therapist is essential for postoperative care in Hartmann's procedure. A comprehensive health education avoids most of the complications of colostomy, such as poor appliance, parastomal dermatitis, or dehydration. A patient could be discharged after he/she is well-educated in colostomy care.

References

1. Hartmann H. New procedure for the removal of cancers of the terminal part of the pelvic colon. 1921
2. DeMaio EF, Naranjo C, Johnson P. Hartmann's pouch, the Hartmann operation, the Hartmann procedure: an enigma of terminology. Surg Endosc. 1996;10(1):81–2.
3. van de Wall BJM, Draaisma WA, Schouten ES, Broeders IAMJ, Consten ECJ. Conventional and laparoscopic reversal of the Hartmann procedure: a review of literature. J Gastrointest Surg. 2010;14(4):743–52.
4. Guerra F, Coletta D, Del Basso C, Giuliani G, Patriti A. Conventional versus minimally invasive Hartmann

takedown: a meta-analysis of the literature. World J Surg. 2019;43(7):1820–8.

5. Vermeulen J, Mannaerts GHH, Weidema WF, Lange JF. Restoration of bowel continuity after surgery for acute perforated diverticulitis: should Hartmann's procedure be considered a one-stage procedure? Colorectal Disease. 2009;11(6):619–24.

6. Bell C, Fleming J, Anthony T. A comparison of complications associated with colostomy reversal versus ileostomy reversal. Am J Surg. 2005;4

7. Salem L, et al. Primary anastomosis or Hartmann's procedure for patients with diverticular peritonitis? A systematic review. Colon Rectum. 2004;47(11):12.

8. Fleming FJ, Gillen P. Reversal of Hartmann's procedure following acute diverticulitis: is timing everything? Int J Color Dis. 2009;7

9. Barbieux J, Plumereau F, Hamy A. Current indications for the Hartmann procedure. J Visc Surg. 2016;153(1):31–8.

10. Celentano V, Giglio MC, Bucci L. Laparoscopic versus open Hartmann's reversal: a systematic review and meta-analysis. Int J Color Dis. 2015;30(12):1603–15.

11. Ferrara M, Kann B. Urological injuries during colorectal surgery. Clin Colon Rectal Surg. 2019;32(03):196–203.

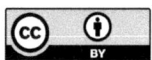

Remote Access Endoscopic Thyroidectomy

Marilou B. Fuentes and Rainier Lutanco

Introduction

This technique makes use of incisions that is outside the exposed neck requiring advanced laparoscopic skills. Because its scar is hidden, the technique became attractive especially for females, but with issues with extensive dissection from the remote access to reach the target organ. Remote access is divided into two: Extracervical (Transaxillary, retro auricular, breast and chest wall approach) and Cervical Approach (Video-assisted central approach, lateral endoscopic, and anterior endoscopic approach) [1].

Indications

- Patient factor—thin habitus because the absence of fat on flap trajectory makes it easier to do dissection [2].
- Thyroid factor—well circumscribed nodule ≤3 cm, thyroid lobe <5–6 cm largest dimension, no evidence of thyroiditis on UTZ [2].
- Approach—axilla and sternal notch distance should be <15–17 cm for axillary approach [2].

Contraindications

- Evidence of thyroid Cancer with nodal and extrathyroidal extension, Graves disease, substernal extension, and previous neck surgery [2].

Preoperative Assessment

- Ultrasound of Neck, Thyroid function test, Chest X-ray, 12 lead ECG, CBC, and Bleeding parameters.

Instruments

- Trocars.
- Retractor for flap elevation.
- 30° Endoscope.
- Tunneler.
- Electrocautery with long tip.
- Hemoclip.
- Suction-irrigator.
- Needle driver.
- Ultrasonic shears.
- Maryland forceps.
- Retrieval bag.
- Two 10 mL syringes.
- Spinal needle.
- Intraoperative nerve monitoring (IONM) probe.

M. B. Fuentes (✉) · R. Lutanco
Department of Surgery, The Medical City, Pasig, Manila, Philippines

© The Author(s) 2023
D. Lomanto et al. (eds.), *Mastering Endo-Laparoscopic and Thoracoscopic Surgery*,
https://doi.org/10.1007/978-981-19-3755-2_24

139

Cervical Approach

Video-Assisted Central Approach, Gases or *MIVAT* (Minimally Invasive Video-Assisted Thyroidectomy)

This technique widespread and well-studied endoscopic assisted thyroidectomy was developed by Miccoli et al. in 1998 and makes use of 1.5 cm incision at the sternal notch (Fig. 1). Although considered as the least invasive of minimally invasive thyroidectomy (MIT), still has the drawback of exposed scar [3]. Exposure of linea alba using retractors and inserting a 5 mm 30° endoscope as the endoscopic phase of the procedure. Thyroid lobe is pulled caudally to expose the upper pedicle and in cutting this pedicle, Sonicision is preferred because of its size and high power of coagulation. After the superior pole is freed, thyroid is pulled medially and using Tuberculum of Zuckerkandl as landmark, Recurrent Laryngeal Nerve (RLN) is identified and preserved. RLN should be followed and dissected until its insertion into the larynx, finishing the procedure with transection of the lobe at the Berry ligament and closure of strap muscles and hemostasis [4]. Below are the indications and contraindications for the procedure (Table 1).

Lateral Endoscopic Approach

This approach is for unilateral lesions since it uses the plane between Sternocleidomastoid muscle (SCM) and carotid sheath laterally and

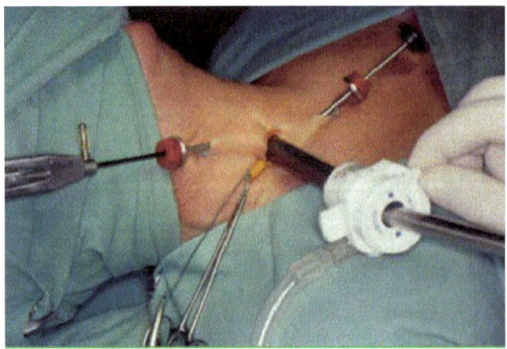

Fig. 1 Sternal notch incision

Table 1 Indications and contraindications for MIVAT [4]

Indications	Contraindications
Nodule not exceeding 35 mm (largest diameter)	Presence of metastatic/suspicious nodes in the lateral neck compartment
Volume not exceeding 25 cc via ultrasound	Thyroid cancers located very posteriorly
Fit for level 6 lymphadenectomy	Thyroiditis

strap muscles medially. 10 mm optic port is placed on the medial border of SCM which has direct access to posterior aspect of the gland. CO_2 insufflation at 8 mmHg to maintain working space. Same dissection steps for lobectomy are utilized [1].

Anterior Endoscopic Approach

Since the procedure uses midline access, bilateral dissection of the thyroid gland can be achieved. 5 mm Optical trocar is placed above the suprasternal notch, while two 2 mm trocars and one 5 mm trocar are placed at the superior medial border of SCM. Same steps for lobectomy/total thyroidectomy as mentioned in previous approach [1].

Extra-Cervical Approach

Trans-Axillary Approach

This approach was first accounted for by Ikeda et al. in 2000, having a remarkable cosmesis with a hidden scar at the axilla sparing the breast and having direct access to the gland. The lateral view with this approach has the advantage of easy identification of RLN and parathyroid glands; however, downside is clashing of instruments that is positioned close to each other [2, 5].

Indications [3]

- Adenomatous goiter or follicular nodule w max diameter < 6 cm.
- dx of benign nodule by FNAC.
- Tumors <15 mm and confined to thyroid gland, without LN mets and local invasion.

Position—patient supine, arm, and shoulder on vertical height with the neck slightly extended. The arm on the pathological side is positioned cephalad and flexed above the head (Modified Ikeda's position) or an alternative is positioning the ipsilateral arm to the lesion to 180° cephalad [1] and to avoid brachial plexus injury, it was suggested to have a limited extension across elbow and shoulder joints [2].

Incisions—place an imaginary line between sternal notch and axilla, an inferior limit of incision that is directed posteriorly to hide the scar. A 60° oblique line was drawn from thyrohyoid membrane to axilla, marking the superior border of the incision. After infiltration of 10 mL of 1% lidocaine with 1 in 200,000 adrenaline solution, a 5–6 cm vertical incision is made intersecting oblique and anterior axillary line defining the inferior limit (Fig. 2). Tissue handling in the incision area is important to avoid keloid.

Working space—defined by the clavicular head above the omohyoid that is parallel to the superior pole of the thyroid. A subcutaneous flap is created using monopolar electrocautery along the subplatysmal plane up to the clavicle. Retractors are used to maintain the plane; after clavicle identification, the SCM heads are dissected to create a wide midline neck access. Sternothyroid muscle has to be dissected from the superior pole using EBD and CO_2 insufflation maintained at 4–9 mmHg [1, 6].

Surgical Resection—Middle thyroid vein is divided using Harmonic scalpel. Superior pole is then pulled in inferomedial direction exposing superior thyroid vessels which are ligated, parathyroid identified and preserved. Traction at tracheoesophageal groove helps in RLN identification but it is recommended to use IONM to assure its integrity. Inferior pole is released by sealing the vessels and subsequent division of the isthmus and removal of the specimen using endobag. Closure once hemostasis is assured.

Retro-Auricular Approach

Compared to transaxillary approach, retroauricular has the advantage of easier positioning, shorter distance to the target gland, elimination of brachial plexus paralysis, and chest paraesthesia. However, issues with transient greater auricular nerve hyperaesthesia and the need for bilateral incisions for total thyroidectomy if needed [1, 3].

Indication—length and circumference of the neck is a major determinant of good exposure, short and slender being the best candidate. Thyroid required to be benign lesions, small and early-stage carcinoma, this with neck metastasis but no gross extracapsular spread.

Instruments—retractors and self-retaining retractors, suction, long tip electrocautery and hemo clip, 30° endoscope, and ultrasonic dissector.

Patient position—supine under GA (ET tube 6 to allow IONM) and head turned 30° away from the side dissection.

Incisions—postauricular crease incision extending to the occipital area below the hairline and it is important to avoid acute angle incisions to avoid flap necrosis.

Working space—a subcutaneous flap superficial to platysma is created with Metzenbaum scissors superficial to the greater auricular nerve. Dissection continues until the omohyoid is iden-

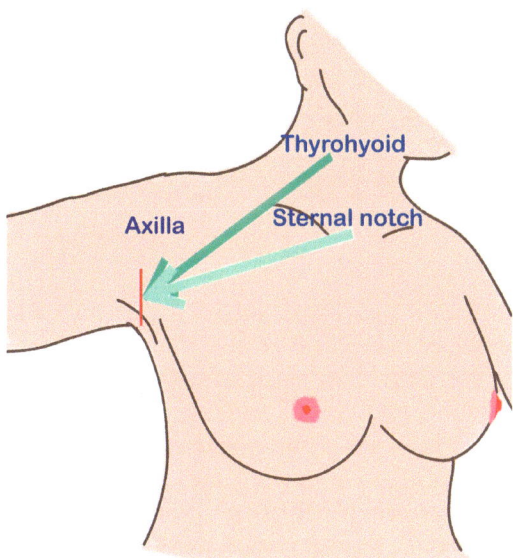

Fig. 2 Patient position and skin incision

tified, this serves as a landmark for strap muscles that will be a guide going to the central neck area [1, 6].

Plane of dissection for flap is above the SCM fascia, Great auricular nerve and external jugular vein are identified and preserved. Flap dissection is continued until the anterior border of SCM.

Borders of dissection are submandibular gland superiorly, midline of the neck anteriorly, and sternal notch inferiorly. Anterior border of SCM is retracted posteriorly to expose the carotid sheath, followed by identification and dissection of omohyoid and strap muscles which are both retracted superiorly to expose the superior pole of the thyroid (Fig. 3). The same procedure for conventional thyroidectomy, bear in mind that RLN is noted to be in a higher position than expected because of the medial reaction of the gland.

Complications—hypothyroidism, temporary corner of the mouth deviation (indirect injury to marginal mandibular nerve), and transient earlobe numbness (indirect injury to great auricular nerve) all managed conservatively. Minor complications such as hematoma or skin flap necrosis, hair loss along the incision line, wound infection and keloid are encountered.

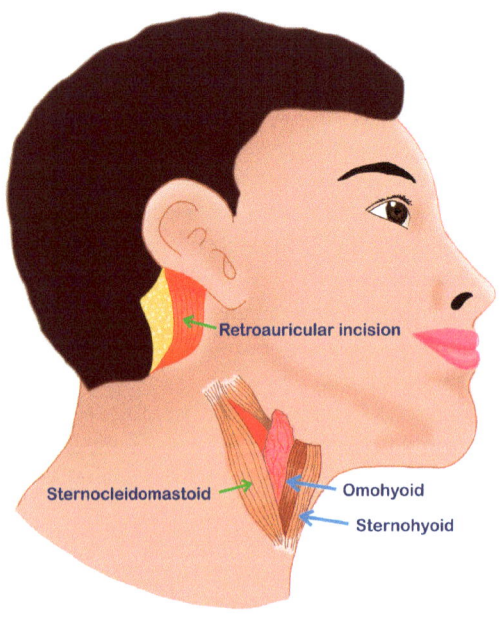

Fig. 3 To expose thyroid gland: SCM retracted posteriorly and omohyoid and strap muscles superiorly

Postoperative care—acoustic (perceptive scale, voice handicap index, fundamental frequency, and maximal vocal pitch) and functional evaluation (swallowing, pain/sensory, and cosmesis) are done postoperatively at 1 week, 1 month, 3, 6, and 12 months.

Breast Approach

A technique developed by Ohgami et al. in 2000, makes use of two 15 mm circumareolar incisions and another 5 mm at 3 cm below the ipsilateral clavicle. 12 mm trocar is inserted to create the working space. Then proceed with dissection like the open thyroidectomy but will begin at the inferior pole and then goes posterolaterally to expose the gland [2, 3].

This technique has two different approaches:

Axillo-Bilateral Breast Approach (ABBA)

Was first introduced by Shimazu et al. He modified incision to resolve the issues of narrow view and limited mobility using an axillary instead of the previous parasternal incision. This allowed better cosmesis, easy identification of structures from the lateral view, and provides freedom of movement accounting for shorter operative time [3, 5, 7].

Indication:

- Low risk thyroid carcinoma not large than 1 cm,
- Follicular neoplasm <3 cm,
- Benign thyroid nodules.

OT Setup:

Patient position: supine, ipsilateral arm extended to expose the axilla.

Incisions: Subcutaneous epinephrine-saline solution injection of anterior chest wall and working space in the subplatysmal area done (hydrodissection—makes the dissection easy and decreases bleeding). A 2.5 cm incision was made at the level of skin crease of the ipsilateral axilla. Using the tunneler, blunt dissection of skin from pectoralis muscle was done and a 12 mm trocar was inserted. Succeeding two

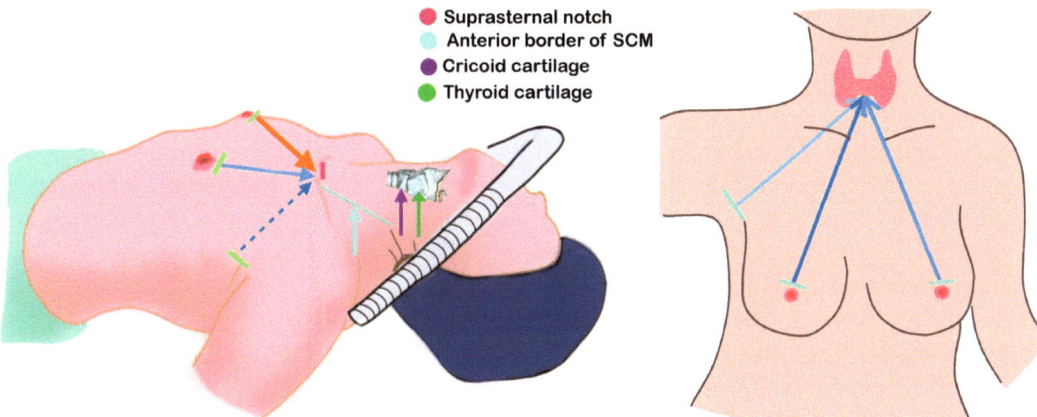

Fig. 4 Landmarks for dissection

5 mm trocars placed on the ipsilateral and contralateral upper circumareolar area and blunt dissection towards the sternal notch done. After the creation of working space, insufflation was done with CO_2 gas at 6 mmHg at the 12 mm port. Once the landmark for dissection such as anterior border of SMC is identified we then proceed with freeing the thyroid gland from sternohyoid and Sternothyroid muscles (Fig. 4). Control of superior, middle, and inferior thyroid vessels using Harmonic scalpel, staying as close to the glands possible to avoid injury to external branch of superior laryngeal nerve and RLN [3, 7].

Bilateral Axillo-Breast Approach (BABA)

Developed in 2007 by Choe et al. as a modification of Shimazu's ABBA technique with addition of contralateral axillary port. This technique has the advantage of having a symmetrical view of both lobes, is more ergonomic, and allows central node dissection. It also prevents the clashing of instruments with its large operative angles as compared to the other remote access approaches [2, 3, 6]. Although this is an appealing technique, patients who have breast implants will be an extra challenge for the surgeon. They have to deal with smaller space and the possibility of implant rupture. Other surgeons also considered this technique quite invasive due to extent of the dissection [5].

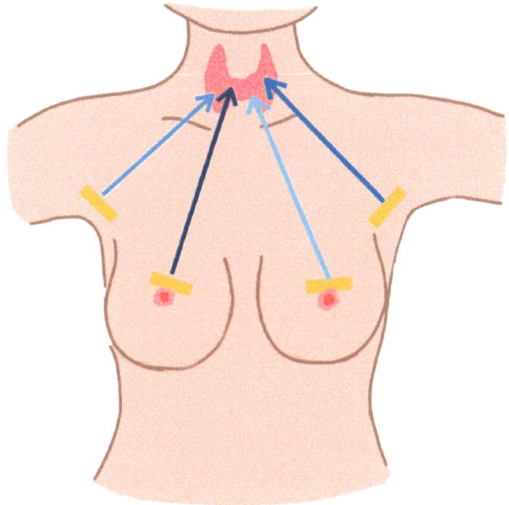

Fig. 5 Port placement

The 8–12 mm ports are placed on both superomedial circumareolar incisions while two axillary incisions for instruments were made as 5 mm port (Fig. 5). The same steps for subcutaneous dissection are carried out for endoscopic thyroidectomy breast approach [2].

Complications

1. Hematoma can be prevented by adequate hemostasis but if there are early signs of airway compromise, one can do reexploration and evacuation of blood clots.

2. Nerve injury (RLN, mandibular nerve, external branch of SLN, and brachial plexus) is avoided by mastery of anatomy and identification of structures during dissection. Permanent palsies lasting for 12 months is noted to be at .3–3% of cases. It is standard practice to use IONM in thyroidectomy to prevent this kind of complication [1]. Brachial plexus neuropraxia can be prevented by cautious positioning of ipsilateral arm.
3. Hypoparathyroidism can be transient and permanent (hypocalcemia >6 months) for total thyroidectomy patients. Patients are given oral Calcium supplement upon discharged and adjusted according to serum Calcium levels on follow-up [1].
4. Seroma.
5. Wound infection.

Postoperative Care

- Patient is seen after 1 week and 3 months postoperatively [2].

Tips [8]

Areolar Approach
- The short distance between optics and instruments interferes with the view: adjust the incisions (if areola is small, make incisions a few mm distant from the other incision).
- Ecchymosis: plane should be between deep and superficial fascia and between subplatysmal and deep cervical fascia.
- Subcutaneous emphysema: maintain CO_2 at 6 mmHg pressure.
- Smoke: clear operative field is affected by plume when electrocautery or ultrasonic device is used. Lens should be withdrawn and use aspirator for continuous smoke evacuation.
- RLN injury—good exposure to RLN is the key and is done by pulling strap muscles laterally. If available in your institution, you may use IONM. During dissection at the area of ligament of Berry, move a few mm away when using ultrasonic shears.

Transaxillary Approach
Brachial plexus injury: modification of arm positioning and use of brachial plexus monitoring.

References

1. Bhatia P, Mohamed HE, et al. Remote access thyroid surgery. Gland Surg. 2015; https://doi.org/10.3978/j.issn.2227-684X.2015.05.02.
2. Berber E, Bernet V, et al. American thyroid association statement on remote-access thyroid surgery. Thyroid. 2016; https://doi.org/10.1089/thy.2015.0407.
3. Sephton BM. Extracervical approaches to thyroid surgery: evolution and review. Minimally Invasive Surgery. 2019; https://doi.org/10.1155/2019/5961690.
4. Miccoli P, Fregoli L, et al. Minimally invasive video-assisted thyroidectomy (MIVAT). Gland Surg. 2019; https://doi.org/10.21037/gs.2019.12.05.
5. Aidan P, et al. Gasless trans-axillary robotic thyroidectomy: the introduction and principle. Gland Surg. 2017; https://doi.org/10.21037/gs.2017.03.19.
6. Russell J, Noureldine S, et al. Minimally invasive and remote access thyroid surgery in the era of the 2015 American Thyroid Association guidelines. Laryngoscope investigative Otolaryngology. 2016; https://doi.org/10.1002/lio2.36.
7. Hong HJ, Kim WS, et al. Endoscopic thyroidectomy via axillo-breast approach without gas insufflation for benign thyroid nodules and micropapillary carcinomas: preliminary results. Yonsei Med J. 2011; https://doi.org/10.3349/ymj.2011.52.4.643.
8. Jia G, Tian Z, et al. Comparison of the breast and areola approaches for endoscopic thyroidectomy in patients with microcarcinoma. Oncol Lett. 2017; https://doi.org/10.3892/ol.2016.5439.

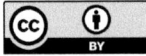

Transoral Endoscopic Thyroidectomy

Marilou B. Fuentes and Rainier Lutanco

Introduction

With the advancement in different MIS procedures across subspecialties, endocrine surgeons convene and embark on improving thyroidectomy techniques adhering to proper management of thyroid pathology while achieving optimal cosmetic result and safety [1, 2].

In 2007, New European Surgical Academy had an interdisciplinary assembly on NOTES on various procedures including the thyroid section. It emphasized on the criteria for minimally invasive endoscopic thyroidectomy which is respecting surgical planes, minimizing trauma, requiring access to be as close as possible to the gland, optimal cosmesis, and safety. Investigations on evolving techniques were done to evaluate its safety and clinical application. They observed that Totally Transoral Video-assisted thyroidectomy (TOVAT) has serious concerns on safety and application due to the important structures that are prone to injury at the submandibular triangle once trocars are inserted. Transoral vestibular approach comes into favor because it makes use of naturally predetermined cervical layers that can be bluntly separated rather than divided and leave no visible scars [3, 4]. Learning curve studies were conducted to investigate surgeon's proficiency in learning the new technique. It was noted to be 11 cases of endocrine surgeons who had no considerable training with laparoscopic procedures done by Razavi et al. [5] while Lee et al., believed that the learning curve should stabilize only after 20 procedures [6].

Evolution of Transoral Endoscopic Thyroidectomy

Sublingual Approach

The idea was started using cadavers and pigs by Witzel et al., using a single 10 mm sublingual incision with addition of two 3.5 mm located at external neck for triangulation of rigid instruments used [7].

Combined Sublingual and Oral Vestibular Approach

Another simulation done by Benhidjeb et al., introduced the transoral video-assisted thyroidectomy (TOVAT) on human cadavers and makes use of one 5 mm and two 3 mm trocars at the floor of the mouth and oral vestibule [7, 8].

M. B. Fuentes (✉) · R. Lutanco
Department of Surgery, The Medical City,
Pasig, Manila, Philippines

© The Author(s) 2023   147
D. Lomanto et al. (eds.), *Mastering Endo-Laparoscopic and Thoracoscopic Surgery*,
https://doi.org/10.1007/978-981-19-3755-2_25

Oral Vestibular Approach

Richmond et al. first described oral vestibular approach with assistance of the robot (Transoral robotic-assisted thyroidectomy-TRAT) and concluded that using oral vestibule for optics is better. Another modification of the technique was designed by Nakajo et al. (Transoral video-assisted neck surgery—TOVANS) a single 25 mm incision at the center of oral vestibule combined with the gasless technique by using Kirschner wire as an external retractor to maintain working space [9] while Wang et al., combined the three transoral incisions and make use of CO_2 insufflation in maintaining the working space [7]. With an increasing interest in this promising procedure, Dr. Angkoon who has the most number of cases, modified the incisions on the oral vestibule placing the two lateral ports in between the incisor and canine thus avoiding mental nerve injury—Transoral endoscopic thyroidectomy vestibular approach (TOETVA).

Indications

For beginners, it is suggested to start with female patients with uncomplicated right lobectomy since the majority of surgeons are right-handed and to avoid male patients for the main reason that the thyroid cartilage interferes with vision and dissection [10].To standardize the Criteria for the procedure as seen in Table 1, an International Transoral Neck Surgery (TONS) Study Group conference was held and consensus for modifications, preparation, techniques, and postoperative care for patients was reached [11].

Table 1 Inclusion criteria

Inclusion Criteria	Modifications for Robotic TOETVA
Ultrasound: Gland size– < 10 cm	
Volume– < 45 mL	
Nodule size– < 5 cm	
Histopathologic: Bethesda 3 or 4	

Table 1 (continued)

Inclusion Criteria	Modifications for Robotic TOETVA
1° papillary microcarcinoma without local/distant metastasis	Papillary Ca with minimum extra thyroidal extensions (T1, T2, and T3)—papillary CA with or without evidence of cervical lymph node metastasis (N0, N1a)
Patient request	Grave's disease with volume of ≤50 mL

Contraindications

TOETVA is suitable for most thyroid cancers but not for those with extensive extrathyroidal invasion and lateral neck metastasis, patients who cannot tolerate general anesthesia, previous radiation in head and neck and upper mediastinum, previous neck surgery, recurrent goiter, UTZ findings: volume ≥ 45 mL, nodule >5 cm, documented node/distant metastasis, tracheal and esophageal infiltration, preoperative laryngeal palsy, hyperthyroidism, mediastinal goiter, oral abscess and poorly differentiated cancer, dorsal extra thyroidal radius and lateral neck metastasis [12].

Preassessment

All patients need to have routine thyroid function tests, neck ultrasound, and fine needle aspiration biopsy. Direct laryngoscopy is done a day before surgery to document palsy. Oral cavity preparation is done using 0.05% Hibitane H_2O 5 min and IV antibiotic 1.2 g Amoxicillin+Clavulanic acid given 30 min prior to incision [11].

Operative Setup

Instruments

- 30° scope 10 mm/5 mm
- Tissue grasper
- Needle holder
- Vascular clips

- Veress needle
- Maryland dissector
- Energy-based device (EBD)
- Trocars: 1 (10 mm) and 2 (5 mm)
- Kelly clamp
- Endobag
- Straight vascular tunneler (Fig. 1)
- Ball-tip stimulator Intraop Neuromonitoring probe (IONM) 230 mm long

Patient Position

Patient is placed on supine,15° Trendelenburg position, neck slightly extended using shoulder pad and feet toward the monitor [1, 13]. Nasotracheal intubation fixed at the corner of the

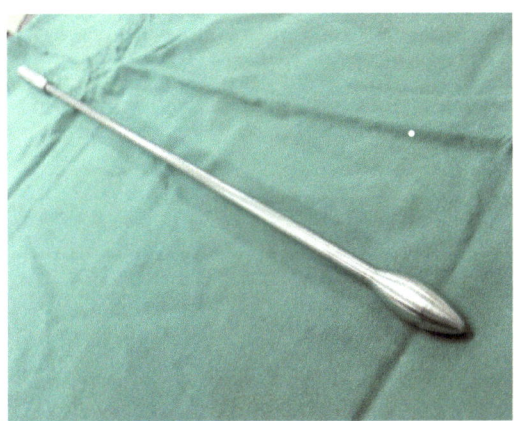

Fig. 1 Straight vascular tunneler

mouth, neck, and lower face prepped and draped. (Fig. 2)

The surgeon at the head area of the patient with full view of the oral cavity and monitor and assistants on the side of the patient.

Surgical Technique

1. *Working space creation*: first 10 mm incision is made at the center of the oral vestibule just above the inferior labial frenulum, Kelly clamp is tunneled through the chin until submandibular area is reached. Long Veress needle is used for hydrodissection (30 mL solution of 1 mg of adrenaline diluted with 500 mL normal saline) to expose the subplatysmal flap, the oral vestibular area of lower lip down to anterior neck and laterally to the central working space (Fig. 3) [1, 11, 13].

2. *Port placements*: Blunt-tip tissue dissector is inserted at the central incision, advancing about 2 cm distally to the chin in a fan-shaped manner to widen the working space followed by introduction of 10 mm trocar (Fig. 4) [11]. Insufflation was maintained at 6 mmHg and CO_2 with 15–20 mL/min flow rate to avoid subcutaneous emphysema. The two lateral 5 mm trocars are placed at the junction between incisor and canine on both sides and just in the inner aspect of inferior lip to avoid mental nerve injury.

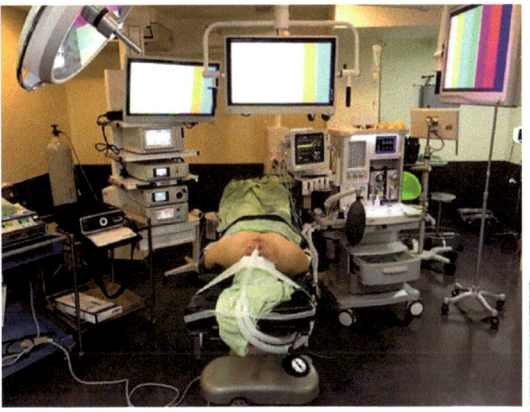

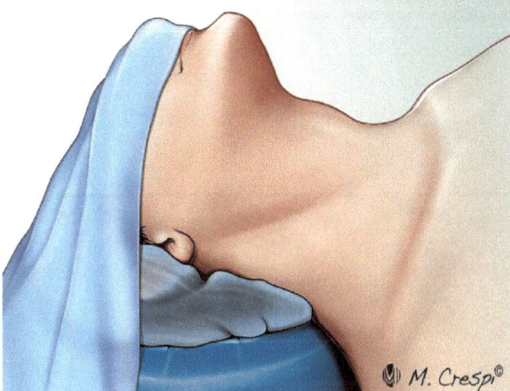

Fig. 2 Extended neck position

3. *Borders*: Superior border is the larynx, inferiorly by suprasternal notch and both sternocleidomastoid muscles laterally (Fig. 5).

4. A 30°, 10 mm endoscope inserted, on a craniocaudal view, strap muscles are divided and retracted laterally. Isthmus is divided exposing the trachea while the strap muscles are dissected from thyroid lobes. External hanging sutures can be laid at this time for additional mechanical retraction (optional).

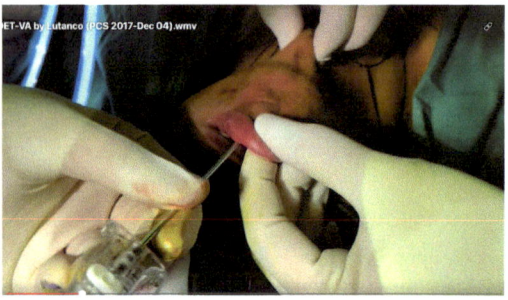

Fig. 3 Hydrodissection with veress needle to expose the flap

Thyroid vessels are ligated and divided in sequence starting with the middle thyroid vein followed by the superior thyroid vessels. During dissection, upper pole is lifted up to improve the identification of recurrent laryngeal nerve (RLN) especially in dissection near the ligament of Berry. IONM is performed using stimulation level 3 mA, location of RLN is evaluated while doing blunt dissection to explore the RLN at its entry point and traced inferiorly using IONM forceps [1, 7, 8, 11, 14] Different IONM stimulators were chosen according to purpose; if RLN location is to be evaluated, a high level (3 mA or more) is appropriate while a low level (1 mA) may be used for identification and confirmation of its integrity. After dissecting the thyroid capsule away from RLN, ligament of Berry's was identified and divided using harmonic scalpel while preserving the parathyroid glands. The thyroid lobe was lifted medially and lower pole was identified and divided from perithy-

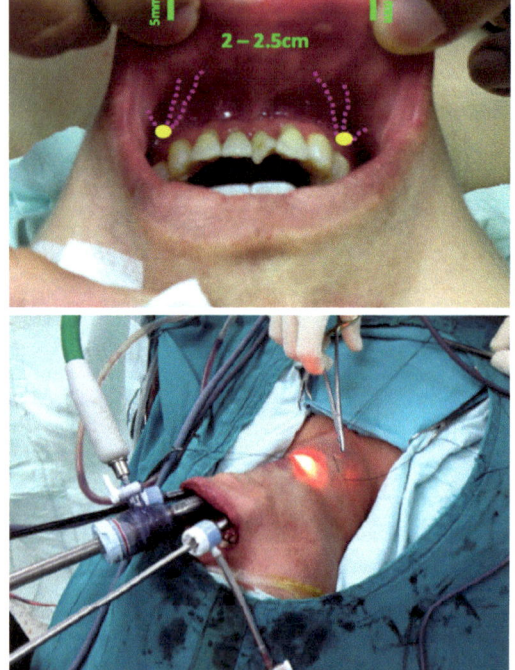

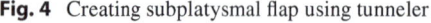

Fig. 4 Creating subplatysmal flap using tunneler

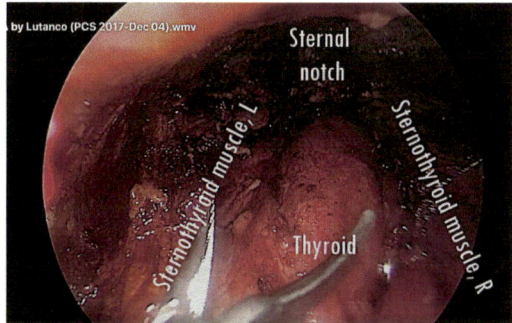

Fig. 5 Borders of dissection

roidal tissues. The specimen was placed in the endocatch bag and removed through 10 mm incision. Meticulous hemostasis was done prior to strap muscle approximation with 3–0 absorbable sutures. The same technique was applied to contralateral side for total thyroidectomy [1, 6, 9, 13, 14].

Complications and Management

1. Hypoparathyroidism—seen in 5.6% of cases which could be prevented by parathyroid gland angiography with indocyanine green (ICG). The transient hypoparathyroidism can be managed by giving calcium and vitamin D supplementation [6].
2. RLN injury—seen in 3.1% of cases hence IONM is required during dissection especially if total thyroidectomy is contemplated [3].
3. Mental nerve injury—is seen in 1.5% which lead to modification of incision at the vestibular area.
4. Subcutaneous emphysema was observed when the CO_2 pressure was increased to more than 6 mmHg. With conservative management, subcutaneous emphysema has gradual reabsorption in 6–12 h although 48 h is needed to achieve complete resolution [6, 9].
5. Minor complications like seroma (2.5%), hematoma, and infection which were conservatively managed.

Postoperative Care

No dressing is required but oral antibiotic and mouthwash are prescribed three times a day for 5–7 days. Patient is allowed to have a soft diet in the same evening of surgery. Hospital discharge depends on the result of postoperative direct laryngoscopy and serum Ca (if total thyroidectomy is done).

Tips and Tricks

- Identification subplatysmal plane—each patient has a varied thickness, decussations, shape, and size, when not identified will go through the strap muscles or even deeper causing subcutaneous emphysema worst pneumomediastinum [9].
- Subcutaneous emphysema/Pneumomediastinum—CO_2 insufflation should be strictly maintained at 6 mmHg pressure with 15–20 mL/min flow rate.

References

1. Fernandez-Ranvier G, Meknat A, et al. Transoral endoscopic thyroidectomy vestibular approach. J Soc Laparoendosc Surg. 2019; https://doi.org/10.4293/JSLS.2019.00036.
2. Witzel K, Hellinger A, et al. Endoscopic thyroidectomy: the transoral approach. Gland Surg. 2015; https://doi.org/10.4293/JSLS.2018.00026.
3. Chen S, Zhao M, et al. Transoral vestibule approach for thyroid disease: a systematic review. Eur Arch Otorhinolaryngol. 2018; https://doi.org/10.1007/s00405-018-5206-y.
4. Benhidjeb T, Stark M, et al. Transoral thyroidectomy–from experiment to clinical implementation. Transl. Cancer Res. 2017; https://doi.org/10.21037/gs.2017.03.16.
5. Razavi C, Vasiliou E, et al. Learning curve for transoral endoscopic thyroid lobectomy. Otolaryngol Head Neck Surg. 2018; https://doi.org/10.1177/0194599818795881.
6. Wang Y, Yu X, et al. Implementation of intraoperative neuromonitoring for transoral endoscopic thyroid surgery: a preliminary report. J Laparoendosc

Adv Surg Techn. 2016; https://doi.org/10.1089/lap.2016.0291.

7. Anuwong A, Kim HY, et al. Transoral endoscopic thyroidectomy using vestibular approach: updates and evidences. Gland Surg. 2017; https://doi.org/10.21037/gs.2017.03.16.

8. Nakajo A, Arima H, et al. Trans-oral video-assisted neck surgery (TOVANS). A new transoral technique of endoscopic thyroidectomy with gasless pre-mandible approach. Surg Endosc. 2013; https://doi.org/10.1007/s00464-012-2588-6.

9. Zhang D, Che-Wei W, et al. Lessons learned from a faulty transoral endoscopic thyroidectomy vestibular approach. Surg Laparosc Endosc Percutan Tech. 2018;28:e94–9.

10. Zhang D, Sun H, Anuwong A, et al. Indications, benefits and risks of transoral thyroidectomy. Best Pract Res Clin Endocrinol Metab. 2019; https://doi.org/10.1016/j.beem.2019.05.004.

11. Anuwong A, Sasanakietkul T, et al. Transoral endoscopic thyroidectomy vestibular approach (TOETVA): indications, techniques and results. Surge Endosc. 2017; https://doi.org/10.1007/s00464-017-5705-8.

12. Dionigi G, Chai YJ, et al. Transoral endoscopic thyroidectomy via vestibular approach: why and how? Endocrine. 2017; https://doi.org/10.1016/j.ijscr.2018.07.018.

13. Dionigi G, Bacuzzi A, et al. Transoral endoscopic thyroidectomy: preliminary experience in Italy. Updat Surg. 2017; https://doi.org/10.1007/s13304-017-0436-x.

14. Erol V, Dionigi G, et al. Intraoperative neuromonitoring of the RLNs during TOETVA procedures. Gland Surg. 2020; https://doi.org/10.21037/gs.2019.11.21.

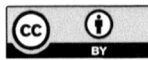

Laparoscopic Adrenalectomy Abdominal Approach

Henry Chua and Vincent Matthew Roble II

Introduction

Since its first description by Gagner et al., in 1992, laparoscopic adrenalectomy has become the gold standard for the surgical treatment of most adrenal conditions [1]. It has generally replaced open adrenalectomy for small- and medium-sized adrenal lesions [2]. The advantages of LA include shorter hospital stays, less postoperative pain, and better cosmetic results [3].

The lateral transabdominal approach to the adrenals is currently one of the most widely used technique. It allows an optimal comprehensive view of the adrenal region and surrounding structures and provides adequate working space [4]. The magnification of the endoscope is particularly helpful in the course of dissection in this area. A detailed knowledge of retroperitoneal anatomy with gentle tissue manipulation and precise hemostatic technique are essential requirements for a successful laparoscopic adrenalectomy.

H. Chua (✉)
Section of Minimally Invasive Surgery, Cebu Doctors' University Hospital, Cebu, Philippines

Advanced Minimally Invasive Surgery Fellowship Program, Cebu Doctors' University Hospital, Cebu, Philippines

V. M. Roble II
Advanced Minimally Invasive Surgery Fellowship Program, Cebu Doctors' University Hospital, Cebu, Philippines

Indications

More than 75% of LA's are performed for endocrine causes of hypertension such as aldosteronoma, Cushing's syndrome and disease, and pheochromocytoma. Other indications adrenal cyst, metastases, myelipoma, primary adrenocortical neoplasm, androgen-secreting tumors, adrenal hemorrhage, ganglioneuroma, and adrenal tuberculosis [5] (Table 1).

Adrenalectomy is generally indicated in the following:

- Biochemically functioning tumors.
- Suspected primary adrenal malignancies.

Careful consideration of the imaging characteristics of the lesion (CT/MRI/PET-CT) should be done to assist in decision-making.

Contraindications

Absolute contraindication to LA are patients who are unable to tolerate laparoscopy.

Relative contraindications to laparoscopy include presence of locally invasive tumors that require contiguous resection of other structures, persistent coagulopathy, and inability to perform the procedure safely with minimally invasive techniques.

The size limit to consider LA has been increased progressively from 6 cm, to 8 cm, and

© The Author(s) 2023

D. Lomanto et al. (eds.), *Mastering Endo-Laparoscopic and Thoracoscopic Surgery*,
https://doi.org/10.1007/978-981-19-3755-2_26

Table 1 Indications and contraindications for laparoscopic adrenalectomy [6]

Indications	Relative contraindications	Absolute contraindications
• Functional unilateral benign adrenal mass (<6–10 cm) • Nonfunctional unilateral benign adrenal mass (>4 cm, lesion growth, or concern for malignancy) • Primary unilateral adrenal hyperplasia • Unilateral adrenal metastasis	• Functional or nonfunctional unilateral benign adrenal mass (10–15 cm) • Malignant adrenal mass (small, encapsulated, noninvasive) • Previous nephrectomy, splenectomy, and/or hepatectomy. • Surgeon inexperience with laparoscopic adrenalectomy	• Functional or nonfunctional unilateral benign adrenal mass (>15 cm) • Invasive malignant adrenal mass

to 10–12 cm, depending on the experience of the surgical team [7]. Large adrenal tumors have a higher malignant rate. Sturgeon et al. discovered more malignant incident rate of large adrenal tumor (<4 cm = 5%, > or = 4 cm = 10%, and > or = 8 cm = 47%) [8]. Intraoperative findings, rather than strict reliance on tumor size, should determine whether a patient undergoes laparoscopic versus open adrenalectomy for adrenal cortical tumors [9].

Preop Preparation [6]

1. Blood pressure control and correction of electrolyte abnormalities are done preoperatively in patients with functional adrenal mass and hypertension.
2. All patients with hypercortisolism should receive intravenous stress-dose corticosteroids and are given immediately before and after adrenalectomy.
3. For patients with pheochromocytoma, alpha adrenergic receptor blockade is started 7–10 days prior to surgery. The goal is to achieve control of hypertension and achieve mild orthostasis. Beta adrenergic blockade should be initiated if tachycardia persists, or the tumor is epinephrine secreting.
4. Close discussion with the anesthetist team in the preparatory phase is important, particularly in the hemodynamic management of patients with pheochromocytoma.
5. Preoperative antibiotic prophylaxis is administered prior to the beginning of the procedure.

6. Anti-thrombotic stockings are placed prior to induction of anesthesia and a sequential compression device is utilized.
7. Foley catheters are placed in patients with larger tumors or more difficult cases.
8. Cross-matched blood should be prepared for vascular tumors or tumors with invasion.

Operating Theater Setup

Instrumentation [10]

- Veress needle.
- 10 mm 30 and 0 laparoscopes.
- 5 mm 30 and 0 laparoscopes.
- One 12 mm and three (left) or four (right) 5 mm non-bladed trocar.
- 5 mm Suction Aspirator (Stryker, Kalamazoo, MI).
- Ultrasonic curved shears—Harmonic scalpel (Ethicon Endosurgery, Cincinnati, OH).
- Laparoscopic scissors.
- 5-mm right angle forceps.
- Graspers-locking and non-locking [2].
- Bipolar forceps (Aesculap or Wolf).
- 5 mm polymer locking clip and applier (Hem-O-Lok-Weck, NC).
- 10 mm specimen retrieval bag (Ethicon or US Surgical).
- PEER retractor (Jarit, Hawthorne, NY).
- Diamond-Flex triangular retractor (Snowden-Pencer, Tucker, GA).
- Optional: 5 mm Ligasure laparoscopic forceps (Valleylab, Boulder, CO).
- Optional: Carter Thomasson Inlet Closure device (Inlet Medical, Eden Prairie, MN).

Patient Position [10]

Patient is placed in a lateral decubitus position with the affected side elevated around 60°. A bean bag is placed to help support the patient in the required position. Axillary pads are placed under the contralateral axilla and the arms are secured with padding. The patient is securely fastened with adequate padding to the operating room table using tape over the leg, thigh, pelvis, and chest. Flex the operating table to increase flank exposure (Fig. 1). Position the video monitors near the patient's head. The surgeon and first assistant stand on the abdominal side of the patient. The second assistant stands on the side of the patient's back (Fig. 2).

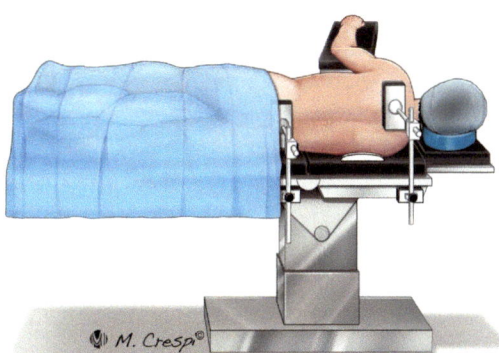

Fig. 1 Patient positioning

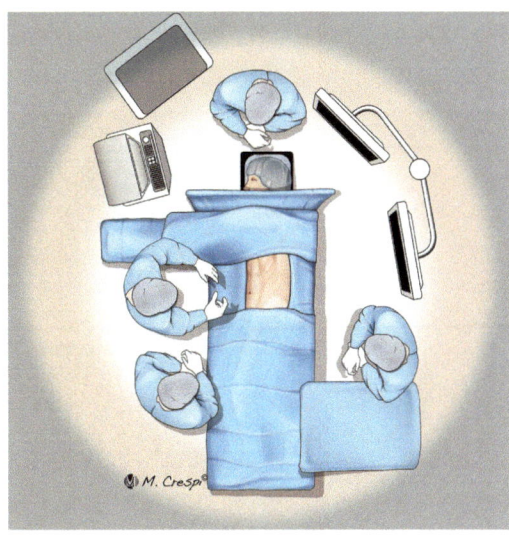

Fig. 2 Surgical team position [11]

Port Placement

Right Adrenalectomy [6]

1. Mark the anterior and posterior axillary lines before prepping the patient
2. Open technique is the preferred approach on entering the abdominal cavity using a blunt tipped cannula. Access to the peritoneal cavity may also be done using a closed technique with a Veress needle.
3. Insert first 10 mm trocar along anterior axillary line two fingers' breadths below the costal margin.
4. The endoscope is then inserted and a diagnostic laparoscopy is performed. Look for signs of local invasion.
5. Under direct vision, insert second 5 mm trocar in the subcostal area medial to the first trocar. This port is for the graspers, energy devices, and peanut swabs used for dissection.
6. Insert the third 5 mm trocar between the anterior axillary line and the epigastrium. This will be used to retract the liver.
7. Insert the fourth 5 mm trocar at the subcostal triangle.

Left Adrenalectomy [6]

1. Mark the anterior and posterior axillary lines before prepping the patient.
2. Access peritoneal cavity using closed technique with Veress needle. Open technique may also be used using a blunt tipped cannula.
3. Insert first 10 mm trocar along anterior axillary line two fingers' breadths below the costal margin.
4. The endoscope is then inserted and a diagnostic laparoscopy is performed. Look for signs of local invasion.
5. Two other 5 mm trocars are placed under direct vision about 7 cm on each side of the first trocar below the costal margin.
6. The fourth trocar, when necessary, is positioned below the first trocar at a distance of 4–5 cm.

Surgical Technique [6]

Right Adrenalectomy

Right Adrenalectomy is potentially more hazardous than left adrenalectomy due to the anatomy of the adrenal vein and its drainage to the inferior vena cava. Dissection of the right adrenal gland involves meticulous dissection of the lateral border to the inferior vena cava.

1. After pneumoperitoneum has been established, a 5 mm retractor is inserted through the most medial subcostal port to elevate the right lobe of the liver.
2. The right triangular ligament is dissected to achieve partial mobilization of the liver. Incise the posterior peritoneum along the inferior margin of the liver to expose the adrenal gland. The liver is then retracted upwards and medially to expose the adrenal gland and the inferior vena cava. The plane between the medial edge of the adrenal gland and the inferior vena cava is dissected (Fig. 3).
3. Dissection of the lateral edge of the vena cava should start from the right renal vein and head superiorly.
4. Identify the right adrenal vein. Dissect with right angle forceps and is doubly clipped and divided (Fig. 4).
5. Proceed to dissection of the inferior aspect of the adrenal en bloc with the periadrenal fat (Fig. 5).

6. The adrenal is then lifted up and the posterior, lateral, superior aspect of the gland is dissected (Fig. 6).
7. Identify and divide the three main adrenal arteries and accessory veins with energy

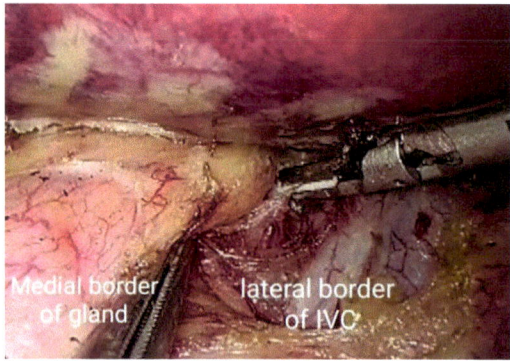

Fig. 4 Dissection of medial border of the gland

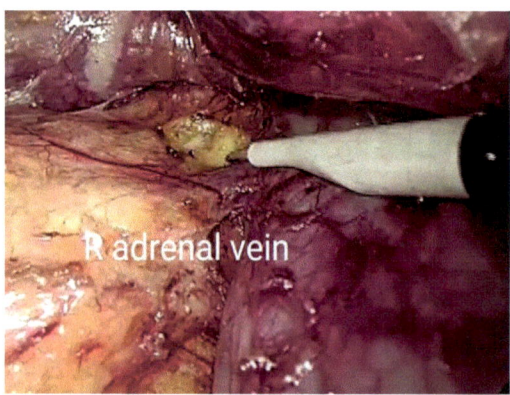

Fig. 5 Isolation of R adrenal vein

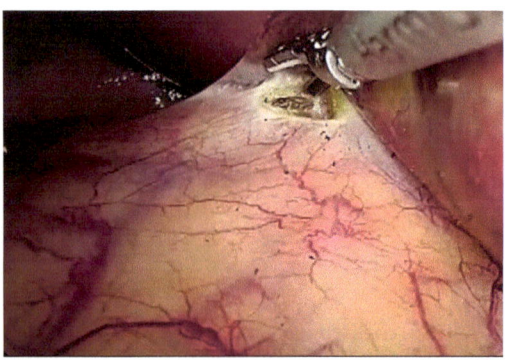

Fig. 3 Division of right triangular ligament

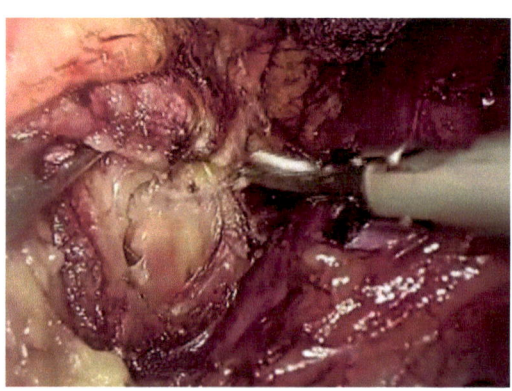

Fig. 6 Dissection of the posterior aspect of the adrenal

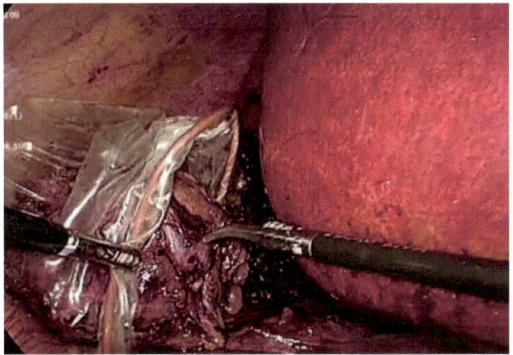

Fig. 7 Placement of adrenal within a retrieval bag

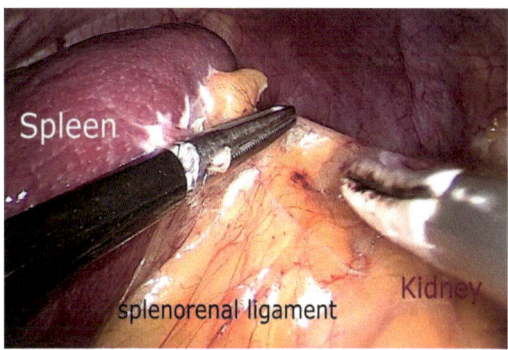

Fig. 8 Dissection of the splenorenal ligament

devices. Typically, the adrenal arteries are not prominent and may not be intentionally identified.

8. Place the adrenal within a retrieval bag and remove it through the 10 mm trocar (Fig. 7).
9. Drain placement is optional. Port site closure is done.

Left Adrenalectomy

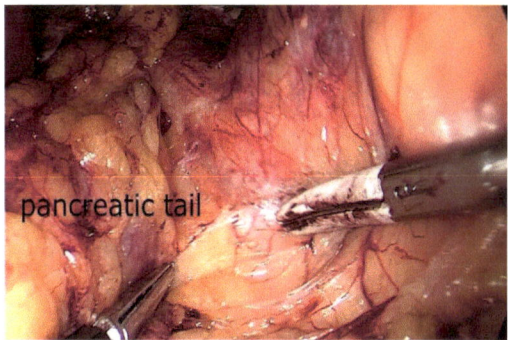

Fig. 9 Medial rotation of the pancreatic tail

Several factors such as the lack of a major anatomic landmark, relatively small size of the left adrenal gland, main vein within the retroperitoneal fat, and close proximity to the pancreatic tail may render left adrenalectomy a challenging procedure. Careful dissection and mobilization of adjacent organs such as the spleen and pancreatic tail are needed to avoid injury.

1. Mobilization to the splenic flexure.
2. Division of the splenorenal ligament and rotate the spleen medially (Fig. 8).
3. Dissect the plane between the kidney and the tail of the pancreas and medially rotate the pancreas (Fig. 9).
4. Identify the adrenal gland near the superior and medial aspect of the kidney (Fig. 10).
5. Identify the medial and lateral borders of the gland and follow these borders caudally to the inferior margin of the gland where the adrenal vein lies.

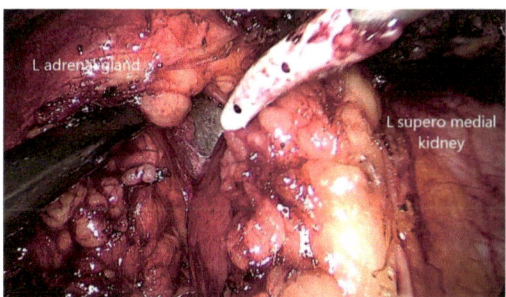

Fig. 10 Identification of the adrenal gland

6. Visualize the left renal vein during medial dissection and elevate the adrenal gland from this vessel.
7. Identify the left adrenal vein running obliquely from the inferomedial aspect of the adrenal gland to its junction with the left renal vein. Isolate and doubly clip and divide (Fig. 11).
8. Completely dissect the adrenal gland from the surrounding tissue.

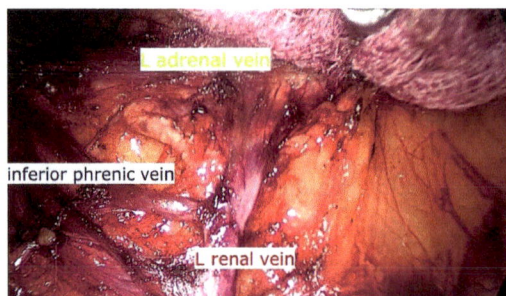

Fig. 11 Identification of the L adrenal vein

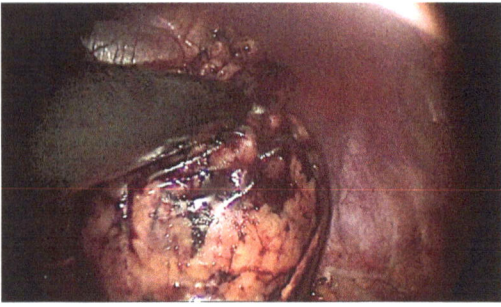

Fig. 12 Placement of specimen in a retrieval bag

9. Visualize and ligate with clips or with energy device arterial branches of the renal artery. The small adrenal arteries may not be easily identified but these are divided with the energy devices during the dissection of the adrenal gland.
10. Place the adrenal within a retrieval bag and remove it through the 10 mm trocar (Fig. 12).
11. Drain placement is optional. Port site closure is done.

Post-op Management [6]

Most patients can be admitted to a regular surgical nursing unit. Patients with hemodynamically significant pheochromocytoma or major underlying cardiopulmonary disease should be admitted to an intensive care unit.

Diet may be advanced as tolerated. Oral analgesics may be taken 24 h postoperatively. A complete blood count and metabolic panel may be drawn as clinically indicated.

Most patients are discharged after 24–48 h without restrictions to physical activities. Patients may return to work within 7–14 days. A follow-up exam at the office should be performed 2–3 weeks after discharge. Patients are generally advised to avoid strenuous activities for 2–4 weeks.

For patients with hypercortisolism and those who undergo bilateral adrenalectomy, intravenous stress-dose corticosteroids are given in the immediate perioperative period. Once the patient resumes diet, intravenous doses may be stopped and replaced with oral corticosteroid therapy.

Patients with Cushing syndrome may require replacement therapy for 6–12 months while the contralateral gland recovers. This may be gradually tapered off as tolerated.

Complications

Complication rate for laparoscopic adrenalectomy ranges from 2.9% to 15.5% [7].

Hemorrhage [12]
Bleeding is the most prevalent intra-op and post-op complication considering the gland is highly vascularized and adjacent to major blood vessels. Intraoperative hemorrhage can be easily identified and may require conversion to an open procedure if hemostasis cannot be achieved. Postoperative bleeding is best detected by monitoring vital signs, urine output, and physical diagnosis of the abdomen.

Organ Injury [11]
The key to the prevention of inadvertent organ injury is familiarity with the anatomy and gentle dissection. Damage to the liver and spleen will present as intraoperative bleeding.

Care should be taken while dissecting the superior aspect of the left adrenal gland to prevent injury to the pancreatic tail. Damage to the pancreas can present early as pancreatitis or late as pancreatic pseudocyst. These can be self-limited but may require medical or surgical management.

High dissection in the abdomen may cause diaphragmatic injury, potentially leading to a tension pneumothorax. Closure with chest drainage would be the appropriate solution.

Others [11]

Appropriate pharmacologic blockade is mandatory before surgery of pheochromocytoma to prevent hypertensive crisis intraoperatively. Hemodynamic instability particularly hypertensive and hypotensive episodes (post-excision of tumor) may occur after laparoscopic adrenalectomy for pheochromocytoma. Sufficient hormonal replacement is mandatory after bilateral adrenalectomy in Cushing's disease.

References

1. Tsuru N, Suzuki K. Laparoscopic adrenalectomy. J Minim Access Surg. 2005:165–72.
2. Gagner M, Lacroix A, Bolte E. Laparoscopic adrenalectomy in Cushing's syndrome and pheochromocytoma. N Engl J. 1992;327:1033.
3. Gill I. The case for laparoscopic adrenalectomy. J Urol. 2001;166:429–36.
4. Raffaelli M, De Crea C, Bellatone R. Laparoscopic Adrenalectomy. Gland Surg. 2019:S41–52.
5. Mckinlay R, Mastrangelo M, Park A. Laparoscopic adrenalectomy: indications and technique. Curr Surg. 2003;60:145–9.
6. Bittner JG, Brunt L. Laparoscopic adrenalectomy. New York: Lippincott Williams & Wilkins; 2013.
7. Gumbs A, Gagner M. Laparoscopic adrenalectomy. Best Pract Clin Endocrinol Metab. 2006;20:483–99.
8. Duh QY. Laparoscopic adrenalectomy for isolated adrenal metastasis: the right thing to do and the right way to it. Ann Surg Oncol. 2007:3288–9.
9. Sturgeon C, Kebebew E. Laparoscopic adrenalectomy for malignancy. Surg Clin North Am. 2004;83(4):755–74.
10. Mellon MJ, Sethi A, Sundaram CP. Laparoscopic adrenalectomy: surgical techniques. Indian J Urol. 2008:583–9.
11. Assalia A, Gagner M. Laparoscopic adrenalectomy. In: Scott-Conner CE, editor. The SAGES manual, fundamentals of laparoscopy, thoracoscopy, and gi endoscopy. New York: Springer; 2006. p. 252–464.
12. Brunt L. The positive impact of laparoscopic adrenalectomy on complications of adrenal surgery. Surg Endosc. 2002;16:252–7.

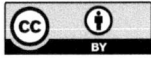

Laparoscopic Adrenalectomy: Retroperitoneal Approach

Marilou B. Fuentes and Cheah Wei Keat

Introduction

With the advent of advances in radiologic imaging, there is an increase in the number of diagnosed cases of Adrenal Incidentaloma (adrenal mass ≥ 1 cm diameter, discovered on imagining done for other organs). Prevalence of which is around 2% and noted to increase with age, affecting 4% of middle-aged and increases to 10% in elderly patients. Tumor of the adrenal gland more than 4 cm in diameter or if the mass enlarges by 1 cm during observation period is recommended to be surgically removed after thorough endocrine clearance. The concept of minimally invasive surgery changed the approach to adrenal tumors but did not changed the indications and goals of treatment [1–4]. Posterior retroperitoneal adrenalectomy has the advantage of direct approach without mobilizing adjacent structures justifying the shorter operative time and lower blood loss. The only drawback of this technique is the unfamiliar anatomic view of retroperitoneal space [5]. A study on learning curve for retroperitoneoscopic approach done by Barczynski and Walz showed that 20–25 cases should be done by an apprentice under the supervision of an experienced surgeon before being able to have a mean operative time of 90 min [6].

Anatomy

Right adrenal gland is mostly suprarenal and located in front of 12th rib, while the left is prerenally located in front of 11th and 12th ribs both lateral edges of vertebral column.

Posteriorly, it is in close proximity to diaphragmatic crus and lateral arcuate ligament. Anteriorly the right adrenal is lateral to inferior vena cava and the left adrenal is with adjacent organs such as spleen and the pancreatic tail.

Arterial supply: Superior adrenal artery from inferior phrenic artery.

- Middle adrenal artery from aorta
- Inferior adrenal artery from renal artery

Venous: each adrenal is usually drained by a single adrenal vein, the importance of handling this in tumors that secrete excess hormones.

M. B. Fuentes (✉)
Department of Surgery, The Medical City, Pasig, Philippines

Ateneo School of Medicine and Public Health, Quezon City, Philippines

C. W. Keat
General Surgery, Ng Teng Fong General Hospital, Singapore, Singapore

Division of General Surgery (Thyroid and Endocrine Surgery), Department of Surgery, University Surgical Cluster, National University Hospital, Kent Ridge, Singapore

D. Lomanto et al. (eds.), *Mastering Endo-Laparoscopic and Thoracoscopic Surgery*,
https://doi.org/10.1007/978-981-19-3755-2_27

- Right vein is usually short (5–10 mm length) and drains to IVC (Fig. 1).
- Left vein is longer (about 30 mm in length) empties to left renal vein.
- Accessory veins in 5–10%.

Retroperitoneal Endoscopic Adrenalectomy

Retroperitoneoscopic approach was introduced by Martin Walz in mid-1990s as the more favorable technique for adrenal tumors. The advantage of less extensive dissection, and with bilateral adrenalectomy done in same position, is gaining popularity since its introduction [7].

Advantages—does not need extensive mobilization, is not affected by previous abdominal surgeries, same position for bilateral adrenalectomy, short surgery time. Tumors that are close to vena cava, this approach offers a direct access therefore less manipulation of vena cava avoiding injury [8].

Disadvantages—difficult to learn because there is a need for retroperitoneal view familiarity. This technique is not suitable for obese patients and large tumor because of limited working space.

Indications

Oncological Recommendations
- Over 30 HU by enhanced CT with tumor size diameter of >4–5 cm and fast tumor growth without local invasion [1].

Endocrinological Indications
- All cases of biochemically confirmed pheochromocytoma; Cushing's syndrome, primary hyperaldosteronism, and hyperandrogenic syndrome [1].

Contraindications

1. Large adrenal lesions (>8–10 cm).
2. Unstable comorbidities.
3. Contraindications to anesthesia and pneumoperitoneum.
4. Previous retroperitoneal surgery.

Preoperative Preparations

1. Control of hypertension, correction of electrolyte abnormalities.

Fig. 1 Venous drainage of the adrenal gland

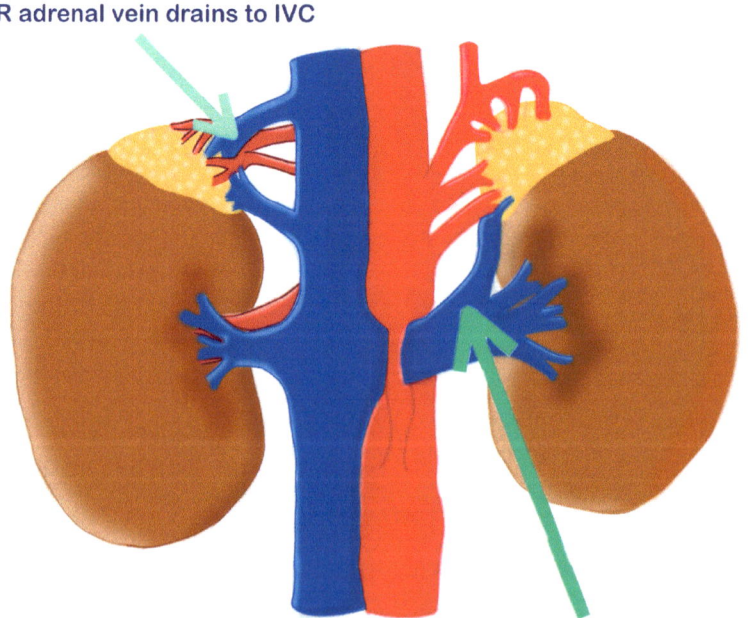

R adrenal vein drains to IVC

L adrenal vein drains to L renal vein

(a) For pheochromocytoma, alpha blocker administration for 2–3 weeks preoperatively for heart rate normalization [1]. For potassium preparation, low sodium and high potassium diet with Spironolactone 100–400 mg/daily for few weeks [4].

(b) If 1°aldosteronism is suspected, adrenal venous sampling is routinely performed for lateralization and patient started on spironolactone for at least 1 month preoperative. BP should be maintained below 150/100 mm Hg [2].

2. Evaluation and optimization.

3. Diagnostic criteria: Adrenal protocol CT, biochem marker screening for 1° aldosteronism, Cushing syndrome, and Phaeochromocytoma. Screening laboratory tests: like ECG, chest x-ray, electrolytes, clotting parameters, and blood type.

Instruments

- Two 12 mm port.
- Maryland dissector.
- Harmonic scalpel.
- One 5 mm port.
- Clip applicator.
- Suction/irrigation device.
- 30° scope.
- Curved scissors.
- Specimen retrieval bag.
- Atraumatic graspers   .
- Hook diathermy.

Prone or semi-jackknife position with the hips flexed (Fig. 2).

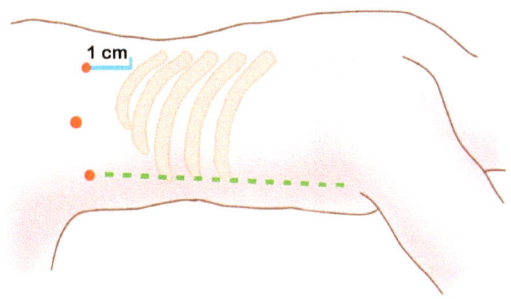

1 cm

Fig. 2 Patient and port positions

Surgical Technique

Walz's technique—patient on prone jackknife position with bent hip joints at 90° angle to maximally open the space between 12th rib and iliac crest. Surgeon stands on the adrenal side to be removed and the assistant on the opposite side. The first 1.5 cm incision is placed approximately 1 cm inferior to the tip of 12th rib, followed by creation of retroperitoneal space by finger dissection. Two additional incisions were made at the posterior axillary line and between the first trocar site and mid-axillary line at the lower tip of 11th rib [2].These two 5 mm ports are placed about a palm breadth apart from the first port to avoid being too close that may interfere with instrument handling. CO_2 insufflation can be set from 12 mm Hg to a maximum of 25 mm Hg, depending on how to achieve the best exposure for the adrenal gland [6, 9].

Exposure: The first step is visualization and mobilization of the upper pole of the kidney. Dissection is from superior pole from lateral to medial and inferior aspect of the adrenal.

For Right Adrenalectomy

Investing fascia is opened transversely at the upper pole until the IVC is identified and continues along the lateral edge to the right adrenal vein which is usually located posterolateral to IVC. Once identified can be clipped and may proceed to complete mobilization of the gland. Early transection of feeding arteries between Gerota's fascia and psoas muscle results in tumor shrinkage and good bleeding control [4, 9].

For Left Adrenalectomy

The Gerota's fascia is opened at the superior aspect of the kidney and dissection continued medially along the renal vein until the adrenal vein is identified, clipped with Hem-o-lock clips, and divided. There is identifiable feeding arteries which are often seen around renal pedicle and just above posts muscle can be ligated with a vessel sealing system [4, 9].

Importance of early ligation of adrenal central vein in Pheochromocytoma patients cannot be over-emphasized. This maneuver reduces the excessive catecholamine secretion thereby preventing intraoperative fluctuation of blood pressure [10].

Indications for Conversion

- Uncontrolled hemorrhage.
- Cardiac arrhythmias.

Conversion rate was noted to be 2–14% [11], Shen et al. reported that the significant independent predictive factors for conversion to open were tumor size >5 cm, BMI of ≥24 kg/m^2, and Pheochromocytoma [12].

Complications

The most common intraoperative complications are bleeding from adrenal and renal vein and vena caval injuries while the postoperative complications are retroperitoneal hematoma and hyponatremia [11].

1. Neuromuscular pain—noted in 9% in one of the largest series done by Walz et al. This is secondary to subcostal injury during trocar insertion but is only temporary [13].
2. Wound infection especially in patient's with Cushing's syndrome.

Postoperative Care

Hypotension is a possible problem postoperatively because of catecholamine decrease leading to vasodilatation reducing the cardiac output. Cortisol, ACTH concentration, and serum electrolyte are requested to assess if the patient will require steroid coverage after surgery. Patients

requiring steroid replacement are observed for 72–96 h prior to discharge [4]. Steroid replacement is mandatory for patients post-surgery for Cushing's syndrome for several months until adequate functioning of the remaining adrenal gland. Patients are allowed to ambulate, start on diet, and require minimal analgesic [11]. Diagnostics such as full blood count and electrolytes may be done as clinically indicated. Periodic glucose monitoring for Pheochromocytoma patients.

Practical Tips and Tricks [14]

- Complication rate—0–15% for unilateral, rises to 23% for bilateral.
- Male sex and high BMI correlate significantly with duration of OR.

Position
- 90° angle between spine and legs should be obtained to optimize distance between rib and iliac crest.

Trocar Position
- Correct and planned angle and position to avoid clashing of instruments and hand fatigue. If 11th rib is noted to be long, the trocar should be adjusted to more cranial position to allow a better degree of freedom for movement.

CO_2 Insufflation Pressure
- Can be increased to max of 25 mm Hg and can be adjusted according to the anatomy/working space of the patient. This helps to create good working space and in small vessel bleeding tamponade; air embolism is a possibility but none was reported even with the largest series of Walz et al. [8]

Dissection
- Early identification of landmarks is crucial [8] It is best to start at the upper pole of the kidney, conducted clockwise starting from 3 to 9 o'clock on the right and counterclockwise 9–3 o'clock on the left.

Choice of Patient

- for early part of surgical experience, do not go for tumors larger than 4 cm, should be smaller and avoid patients with BMI of >35 because these patients have dense retroperitoneal fat adherent to capsule of the kidney, making dissection difficult.

References

1. Bednarczuk T, Bolanoswki M, et al. Adrenal incidentaloma in adults- management recommendations by polish Society of Endocrinology. Endokrynol Pol. 2016; https://doi.org/10.5603/EP.a2016.0039.
2. Uludağ M, Aygün N, et al. Surgical indications and techniques for adrenalectomy. Med Bull Sisli Etfal Hospital. 2020; https://doi.org/10.14744/SEMB.2019.05578.
3. Gagner M, Pomp A, et al. Laparoscopic adrenalectomy: lessons learned from 100 consecutive procedures. Ann Surg. 226(3):238–47.
4. Arezzo A, Bullano A, et al. Transperitoneal versus retroperitoneal laparoscopic adrenalectomy for adrenal tumours in adults. Cochrane Database Syst Rev. 2018; https://doi.org/10.1002/14651858.CD011668.pub2.
5. Vrielink OM, Wevers KP, et al. Laparoscopic anterior versus endoscopic posterior approach for adrenalectomy:a shift to a new golden standard? Langenbeck's Arch Surg. 2017; https://doi.org/10.1007/s00423-016-1533-x.
6. Hisano M, Vicentini F, et al. Retroperitoneoscopic adrenalectomy in pheochromocytoma. Clinics. 2012;67(51):161–7.
7. Maccora D, Walls GV, et al. Bilateral adrenalectomy: a review of 10 years' experience. Ann R Coll Surg Engl. 2017;99(2) https://doi.org/10.1308/rcsann.2016.0266.
8. Ma J, Wang Y, et al. Outcome and safety of retroperitoneoscopic and transperitoneal laparoscopic adrenalectomy: a comparative study of 178 adrenal tumor patients. Int J Clin Exp Med. 2018;11(9):9701–7.
9. Shiraishi K, Kitahara S, et al. Transperitoneal versus retroperitoneal laparoscopic adrenalectomy for large pheochromocytoma: comparative outcomes. Int J Urol. 2018;26(2) https://doi.org/10.1111/iju.13838.
10. Ban EJ, Yap Z, et al. Hemodynamic stability during adrenalectomy for pheochromocytoma: a case control study of posterior retroperitoneal vs lateral transperitoneal approaches. Medicine. 2020;99(7):e19104. https://doi.org/10.1097/MD.0000000000019104.
11. Conzo G, Tartaglia E, et al. Minimally invasive approach for adrenal lesions: systematic review of laparoscopic versus retroperitoneoscopic adrenalectomy and assessment of risk factors for complications. Int J Surg. 2016;28:S118–23. https://doi.org/10.1016/j.ijsu.2015.12.042.
12. Hirano D, Hasegawa R, et al. Laparoscopic adrenalectomy for adrenal tumors: a 21-year single-institution experience. Asian J Surg. 2014;38:79–84. https://doi.org/10.1016/j.asjsur.2014.09.003.
13. Walz A, et al. Posterior retroperitoneoscopic adrenalectomy- 560 procedures in 520 patients. Surgery. 2006; https://doi.org/10.1016/j.surg.2006.07.039.
14. Alesina P. Retroperitoneal adrenalectomy - learning curve, practical tips and tricks, what limits its wider uptake. Gland Surg. 2019;8 Suppl (1) S36-S40. https://doi.org/10.21037/gs.2019.03.11

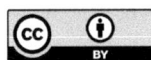

Endoscopy-Assisted Breast Surgery for Breast Cancer

Tang Siau Wei

Introduction

Modified radical mastectomy was traditionally the preferred method for treating operable breast cancer. With advances in surgical techniques over the past few decades, breast-conserving surgery (BCS) and sentinel lymph node biopsy are now acceptable treatments for early breast cancer. Over the last two decades, endoscopic techniques had initially been adapted to facilitate cosmetic breast augmentation surgery but are now increasingly adopted in the surgical management of breast cancer [1–3]. It is often done to optimize the cosmetic outcome by performing surgery through small wounds hidden in the axilla or periareolar areas. If endoscopic mastectomy is performed, it is often followed by immediate reconstruction.

Indications [1, 3, 4]

- Early stage breast cancer (ductal carcinoma in situ (DCIS), stage I or II).
- A tumor size less than 3 cm for endoscopic breast conserving surgery (EBCS) or no larger than 5 cm for endoscopic-assisted total mastectomy (EATM).
- No evidence of multiple lymph node metastasis.
- No evidence of skin or chest wall invasion.

Contraindications [1, 3, 4]

- Multifocal/multicentric lesions (for EBCS).
- Inflammatory breast cancer.
- Paget's disease of the nipple/nipple discharge.
- Breast cancer with nipple, pectoralis major/chest wall, or skin invasion.
- Locally advanced breast cancer.
- Breast cancer with extensive axillary lymph node metastasis (stage IIIB or later).
- Patients with severe comorbid conditions, such as heart disease, renal failure, liver dysfunction, and poor performance status as assessed by the primary physicians.

Pre-op Assessment

- Thorough history and physical examination.
- Histopathologic confirmation of breast cancer.
- Routine investigations as to hospital protocol for fitness to undergo general anesthesia.
- Breast imaging—Mammogram/Ultrasound/MRI (for EBCS) to delineate the extent of disease.

T. S. Wei (✉)
Division of General (Breast) Surgery, Department of Surgery, National University Hospital, Singapore, Singapore

Division of Surgical Oncology, National University Cancer Institute, Singapore, Singapore
e-mail: siau_wei_tang@nuhs.edu.sg

D. Lomanto et al. (eds.), *Mastering Endo-Laparoscopic and Thoracoscopic Surgery*,
https://doi.org/10.1007/978-981-19-3755-2_28

Preoperative Preparation

- Preoperative marking of inframammary fold, extension of breast tissue at the lateral and superior aspects performed with the patient in an upright position.
- For nonpalpable lesions undergoing EBCS—hookwire placement.
- EBCS—preoperative marking of resection margins under ultrasound guidance with either methylene blue or indocyanine green dye with at least a 1 cm margin.
- Preoperative radiocolloid (^{99m}Tc) is injected to aid in identification of the sentinel lymph node.

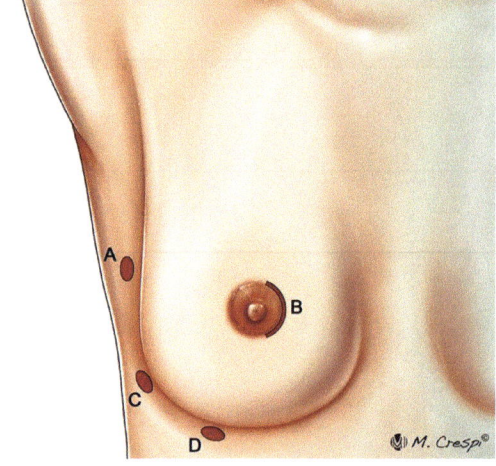

Fig. 1 Skin incisions

OT Setup

Instruments Required
- Lighted retractor (Vein harvest, Ultra Retractor, Vein Retractor).
- 30 straight rigid 5 mm endoscope.
- Bipolar scissors/electrocautery or Energy device (e.g., Harmonic scalpel).
- Wound protector.
- OptiView port.
- Endocatch retrieval bag.

Patient Position
- The patient is in supine position.
- Both arms are abducted to 90°.
- Endoscopic video monitors are positioned on the opposite side of the patient.
- 5 ml of diluted 0.5% Patent blue dye is injected into the upper outer quadrant of the periareolar after induction of anesthesia for sentinel lymph node biopsy.

Surgical Technique [1, 4–8]

Incisions
- 2 cm axillary incision (A).
- Semicircular Periareolar incision (less than half of circumference of areolar) (B).
- If required, additional 5 mm incisions are placed at the lateral breast and/or at inframammary fold for trocars to assist in dissection (C/D) (Fig. 1).

Sentinel Lymph Node Biopsy (SLNB)
- 2 cm transverse axillary incision is made close to the site of the hottest nodes that are detected using a hand-held gamma probe.
- The axillary tissue is dissected to identify any blue ducts, which is traced to identify the sentinel lymph node.
- SLNB is then confirmed with the hand-held gamma probe and sent for intraoperative frozen section.
- If the frozen section results show malignancy in the sentinel lymph node, axillary dissection is performed through the same incision after completion of the breast surgery.

Posterior Dissection
- After completing the SLNB, the dissection is carried out to the lateral border of the pectoralis major muscle.
- Dissection in the retromammary space, between the pectoralis muscle fascia and posterior breast parenchyma is carried out using a retractor with an optical system (endoscopic vein harvest, Ultra retractor, Vein Retractor) with blunt dissection (Fig. 2).
- The surrounding tissue is pulled up using the endoscopic retractor and a suction tube to create sufficient working space and to evacuate mist and smoke.
- The penetrating vessels are coagulated and cut with bipolar scissors, harmonic scalpel, or

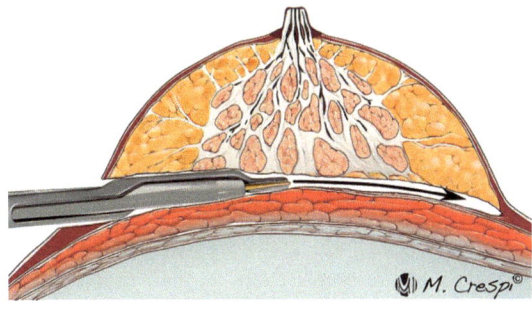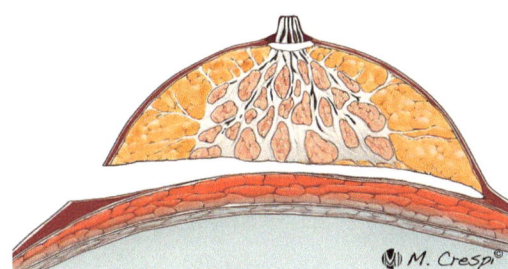

Fig. 2 Retromammary space dissection

electrocautery to ensure a clear visual field and uncomplicated hemostasis.

- Alternatively, the retromammary space could be dissected using a pre-peritoneal dissection balloon or carbon dioxide insufflation.
- For mastectomy, the dissection is carried out throughout the whole retromammary space to the anatomic margins of the breast.
- For EBCS, dissection is performed to cover an area further beyond the tumor margins (marked preoperatively) to facilitate tissue mobilization for closure of the defect [9].

Subcutaneous Skin Flap Development

- A semicircular periareolar incision is made. An appropriately sized wound protector is placed into the incision to protect the periareolar wound and ensure adequate visualization.
- The retroareolar tissue is dissected and the nipple base tissue is sampled and examined by intraoperative frozen section.
- If the frozen section is positive for malignancy, the whole nipple areolar complex is removed.
- A combination of normal saline, lignocaine 0.05%, and epinephrine 1:1000000 as a tumescent solution is infiltrated subcutaneously into the breast to facilitate dissection and minimize bleeding (Fig. 3).
- A 5 mm thick skin flap is created using the optical bladeless trocar (Xcel port) using the "subcutaneous tunnelling method," whereby the trocar is used to separate the breast parenchyma from the overlying skin and subcutaneous tissue under direct endoscopic visualization (Fig. 4).
- The "septa" created between the tunnels are then dissected using bipolar scissors, electro-

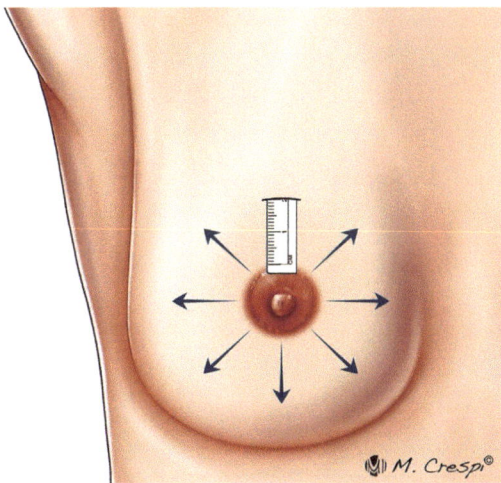

Fig. 3 Saline injection

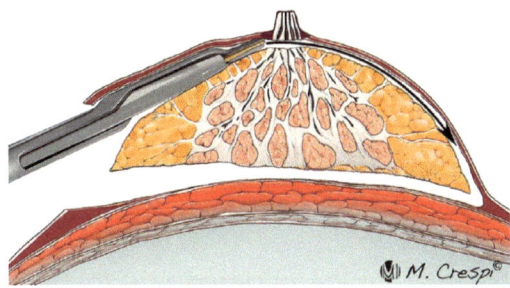

Fig. 4 Subcutaneous tunneling method

cautery, and/or energy devices (e.g., harmonic scalpel).

- For mastectomy, the dissection is carried out throughout the whole anterior surface of the breast to the anatomic margins of the breast (Fig. 5).
- For EBCS, dissection is performed to cover an area further beyond the tumor margins

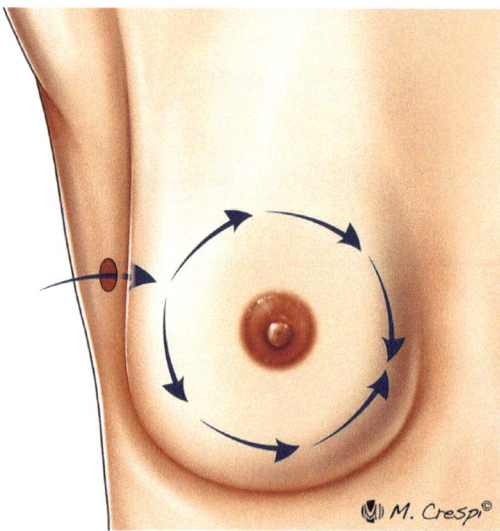

Fig. 5 Dissection along the anterior surface of the breast

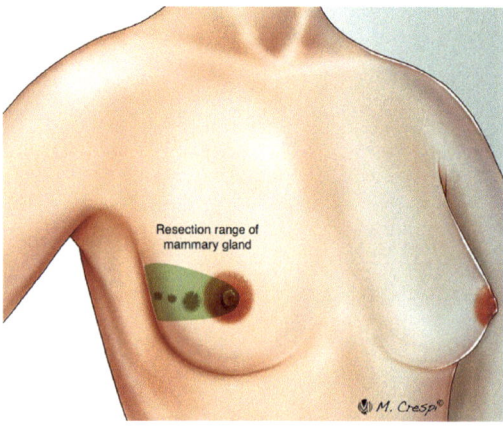

Fig. 6 Dissection beyond tumor margins

(marked preoperatively) to facilitate tissue mobilization for closure of the defect [9] (Fig. 6).

Specimen Excision and Reconstruction

- For mastectomy, the anterior subcutaneous dissection will meet the posterior retromammary space dissection at the anatomic margins of the breast to complete the mastectomy.
- For EBCS, the breast tissue is then divided according to the preoperative markings using bipolar scissors, energy devices, or electrocautery with the help of the endoscopic light retractor completing the lumpectomy [9].

- The surgical specimen can then be removed through the axillary incision or periareolar incision (with or without an endocatch).
- For mastectomy, immediate reconstruction can then be performed using implants or autologous tissue, and a drain may be placed in the surgical cavity [10].
- For EBCS, surgical clips are placed in the cavity and the breast tissue is then mobilized to close the defect, with or without oncoplastic techniques [9].

Postoperative Care

- Similar to open surgery, would depend on reconstructive technique (if any).
- Standard analgesia as required.
- Regular diet as tolerated.
- Discharge the patients when comfortable and able to drink, eat, and walk.

Complications and Management [1, 8]

- The complications reported with endoscopic breast surgery are generally similar to that of open surgery—e.g., Seroma, superficial or deep skin burns, ecchymoses, infection; and can be managed in a similar manner.
- If insufflation is used to develop the surgical planes, the patient may have subcutaneous emphysema in the breast and surrounding tissues postoperatively. This is usually self-limiting and will resolve spontaneously.
- For EBCS, the patient may develop fat necrosis if there are wide areas of tissue mobilization for resection and reconstruction.

References

1. Mok CW, Lai HW. Endoscopic-assisted surgery in the management of breast cancer: 20 years review of trend, techniques and outcomes. Breast. 2019;46:144–56.
2. Sakamoto N, Fukuma E, Higa K, Ozaki S, Sakamoto M, Abe S, Kurihara T, Tozaki M. Early results of an endoscopic nipple-sparing mastectomy for breast cancer. Ann Surg Oncol. 2009;16:3406–13.

3. Tamaki Y, Nakano Y, Sekimoto M. Transaxillary endoscopic partial mastectomy for comparatively early-stage breast cancer: an early experience. Surg Laparosc Endosc. 1998;8:308–12.

4. Lai H-W, Chen S-T, Chen D-R, Chen S-L, Chang T-W, Kuo S-J, et al. Current trends in and indications for endoscopy-assisted breast surgery for breast cancer: results from a six-year study conducted by the Taiwan endoscopic breast surgery cooperative group. PLoS One. 2016;11(3):e0150310.

5. Du J, Liang Q, Qi X, Ming J, Liu J, Zhong L, Fan L, Jiang J. Endoscopic nipple sparing mastectomy with immediate implant-based reconstruction versus breast conserving surgery: a long-term study. Sci Rep. 2015;7:45636.

6. Ho WS, Ying SY, Chan ACW. Endoscopic-assisted subcutaneous mastectomy and axillary dissection with immediate mammary prosthesis reconstruction for early breast cancer. Surg Endosc. 2002;16:302–6.

7. Kitamura K, Ishida M, Inoue H, Kinoshita J, Hashizume M, Sugimachi K. Early results of an endoscope assisted subcutaneous mastectomy and reconstruction for breast cancer. Surgery. 2002;131(1):S324–9.

8. Soybir G, Fukuma E. Endoscopy assisted oncoplastic breast surgery (EAOBS). J Breast Health. 2015;11:52–8.

9. Lee E-K, Kook S-H, Park Y-L. Endoscopy-assisted breast-conserving surgery for early breast cancer. World J Surg. 2006;30:957–64.

10. Lai HW, Wu HS, Chuang KL, Chen DR, Chang TW, Kuo SJ, Chen ST, Kuo YL. Endoscopy-assisted total mastectomy followed by immediate pedicled transverse rectus abdominis musculocutaneous (TRAM) flap reconstruction: preliminary results of 48 patients. Surg Innov. 2015;2(4):382–9.

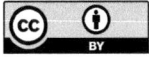

Laparoscopic Omental Flap Partial Breast Reconstruction

Siau Wei Tang

Introduction

Oncoplastic breast surgery combines oncological resection of a breast malignancy with plastic surgical techniques for immediate reconstruction of the defect using volume replacement or volume displacement techniques. As breast-conserving surgery increases in popularity, partial breast reconstruction using volume replacement techniques has evolved to allow excision of larger tumors while minimizing cosmetic deformity. Lateral chest wall perforator flaps (thoracodorsal artery perforator (TDAP) flap and the lateral intercostal artery perforator (LICAP) flap) are commonly used for tumors in the outer half of the breast; superior epigastric artery perforator (SEAP) flaps are commonly used for lower inner quadrant tumors. Upper inner quadrant defects present a challenge for volume replacement in partial breast reconstruction as there are limited options for local flaps and would require adequate mobilization for a longer pedicle if perforator flaps are utilized.

Historically, the omental flap has been used to reconstruct chest and upper abdominal wounds from oncologic resections or trauma [1]. However, the morbidity associated with a laparotomy to harvest the flap has limited its use. With advances in endoscopic surgery, laparoscopic harvesting of the omental flap has made it a viable option in breast reconstruction surgery [2–4], particularly for defects in the upper and lower inner quadrant of the breast, with minimal donor site morbidity.

Indications

- Breast conserving surgery where 20–50% of the breast volume is resected.
- Tumor location in the upper inner quadrant, lower inner quadrant, or lower outer quadrant of the breast.

Contraindications

- If a large amount of skin over the tumor is resected, omental flap is not a suitable reconstructive option.
- Extensive disease involving more than 50% of the breast (as it is difficult to estimate the omental volume preoperatively and may have inadequate volume for replacement).
- Tumor location in the upper outer quadrant.
- Patients with previous upper midline laparotomy/peritonitis/intra-abdominal malignancy.
- Morbid obesity (BMI >35).

S. W. Tang (✉)
Division of General (Breast) Surgery, Department of Surgery, National University Hospital, Singapore, Singapore

Division of Surgical Oncology, National University Cancer Institute, Singapore, Singapore
e-mail: siau_wei_tang@nuhs.edu.sg

© The Author(s) 2023
D. Lomanto et al. (eds.), *Mastering Endo-Laparoscopic and Thoracoscopic Surgery*,
https://doi.org/10.1007/978-981-19-3755-2_29

Pre-op Assessment

- Histopathologic confirmation of breast cancer.
- Routine investigations as to hospital protocol for fitness to undergo general anesthesia.
- Breast imaging—Mammogram/Ultrasound/ MRI (for EBCS) to delineate the extent of disease.
- The volume of omentum is often unpredictable and is difficult to estimate with current imaging modalities. Some surgeons may opt to do a separate diagnostic laparoscopy to estimate the omental volume (particularly if considering reconstruction of >50% of the breast) and to evaluate for any adhesions/intraabdominal pathology prior to the oncoplastic surgery.
- Pre-op marking of the inframammary fold and midline on the sternum is performed in the standing position.
- The distance between the IMF and the costal margin is assessed in the supine position.
- The breast tumor and resection margins are outlined on the skin of the breast.
- Preoperative placement of hook wire is required if the tumor is nonpalpable.
- Prophylactic antibiotics are given at induction of anesthesia.

OT Setup

- Two separate teams can operate on the breast and abdomen concurrently

Instruments Required

- Veress needle (Optional).
- 30° telescope 10 mm and 5 mm
- Atraumatic graspers 5 mm.
- Energy device (e.g., Harmonic scalpel).
- Curved Maryland dissector 5 mm.
- Suction/irrigation device.
- Wound protector.

Patient Position

- The patient is in supine position or split legs (French) position.
- Both arms are abducted to 90°.
- Endoscopic video monitors are positioned next to the patient's head on the patient's left.
- Surgeon to stand on the right of the patient or between the patient's legs (French position).
- The assistant is standing on the patient's left.

Surgical Technique [4–7]

- Wide local excision of the tumor is performed by the breast surgeon, ideally through an incision at the medial end of the inframammary fold (IMF).

Incisions

- 12 mm camera port is inserted at the umbilicus using the open technique.
- Two 5 mm working ports are inserted at the right midclavicular line, at the right upper quadrant and right lower quadrant.
- 5 mm assistant port is inserted at the left lower quadrant midclavicular line.
- Additional 5 mm assistant port may be inserted in the left upper quadrant midclavicular line (if required).

Laparoscopic Harvesting of the Omental Flap

- After a 30°laparoscope is inserted through the umbilical port, pneumoperitoneum is maintained at 10 mmHg and the three other 5 mm trocars are inserted under direct vision.
- Diagnostic laparoscopy is performed, where the omentum is evaluated for size and adhesion.
- The omentum is moved toward the upper abdomen and the lesser sac is entered.

- The omentum is dissected from the left side of the transverse colon toward the splenic flexure using an energy device (e.g., Harmonic scalpel). It is transected toward the lower pole of the spleen, and the left gastroepiploic vessels are divided (Fig. 1).
- The omentum is then dissected from the stomach toward the greater curvature, with care taken to preserve the right gastroepiploic vessels as the main pedicle.
- The dissection is then continued to dissect the omentum from the right transverse colon and the duodenum and pylorus, where the fusion between the posterior leaf of the gastrocolic ligament and the anterior leaf of the transverse mesocolon is carefully divided toward the anterior capsule of the pancreas head.
- Fatty tissue at the root of the right gastroepiploic artery and vein are resected to enable a long and narrow pedicle of the flap to minimize the risk of a subsequent ventral hernia, completing the dissection of the omental flap.

Partial Breast Reconstruction

- The IMF incision used to perform the wide local excision is used to exteriorize the omental flap.
- A subcutaneous tunnel is created from the medial side of the IMF incision toward the xiphoid process, over the anterior sheath of the rectus muscle. Subcutaneous fat around the tunnel is resected to avoid a bulge from the pedicle (after it has been exteriorized).
- A 3 cm longitudinal incision is made in the linea alba (just below the xiphoid process) to enter the abdominal cavity.
- The pedicled omental flap is carefully exteriorized through this tunnel, with care taken to avoid torsion or kinking of the pedicle.
- The linea alba incision may need to be widened to allow the omental flap to be exteriorized. If so, it must be partially closed again after, to minimize the risk of ventral hernia in the future.
- When exteriorized, hemostasis of the omental flap is performed, and vascularity of the flap is reassessed (Fig. 2).
- The size of the omental flap is then assessed in relation to the size of the defect in the breast.

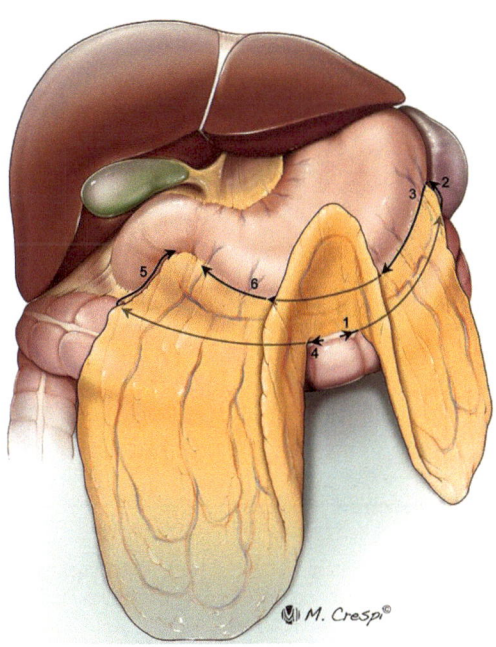

Fig. 1 Steps for laparoscopic dissection of the omentum

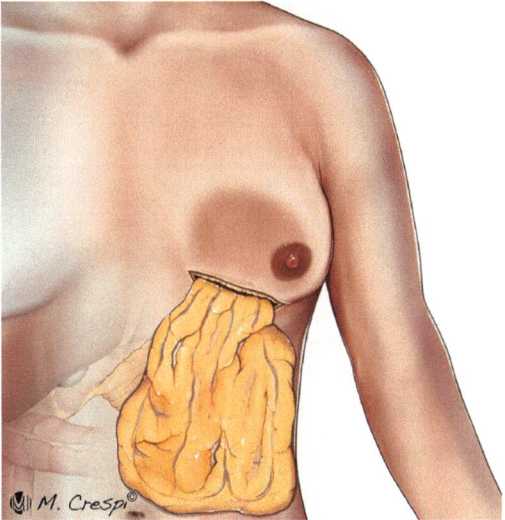

Fig. 2 Assessment of vascularity of omental flap

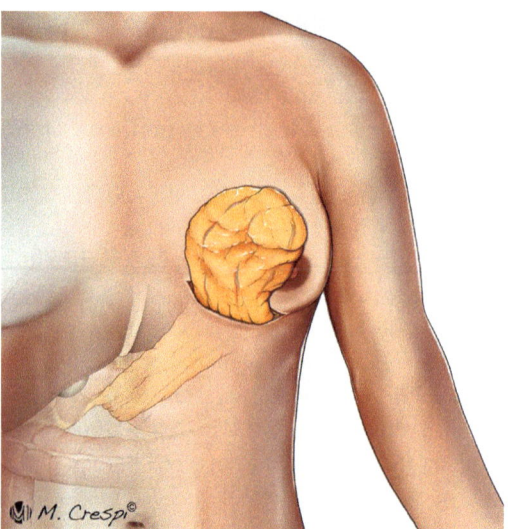

Fig. 3 Assessment of omental flap in relation to breast size defect

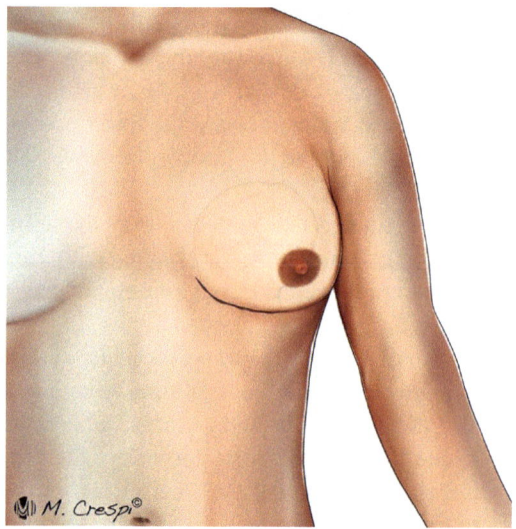

Fig. 4 Skin closure by layers

If it is too large, the periphery of the omentum is trimmed (Fig. 3).

- Pneumoperitoneum should then be reinstated, and laparoscopy performed to check for any tension in the pedicle. High tension in the pedicle will cause traction on the distal stomach, which may lead to gastric outlet obstruction.
- The appropriately sized omental flap is then tucked into the breast defect to fill the cavity. If there was an extensive subcutaneous or prepectoral dissection of the breast tissue around the defect, the edges of the residual breast tissue should first be fixed onto the pectoralis major muscle in its original position, to avoid movement of the omental flap.
- Fixation of the omental flap to the chest wall is usually not necessary. A closed suction drain may be placed in the breast cavity.
- The skin wound is then closed in layers, recreating the IMF (Fig. 4).

Postoperative Care

- Standard analgesia as required.
- Regular diet as tolerated.
- If close suction drain is used in the breast cavity, it can be removed when the average drainage over 24 h is <50mls.

- Discharge the patient when she is comfortable and able to drink, eat, and walk.

Complications

- Vascular injury—if inadvertent injury is made to the pedicle, the omentum may no longer be viable and alternative reconstructive methods should be considered (e.g., Latissimus dorsi flap).
- Bleeding/hematoma.
- Seroma.
- Infection.
- Bowel injury (small/large bowel injury).
- Skin flap necrosis.
- Graft fat necrosis.
- Late complication—ventral hernia, intra-abdominal adhesions.

References

1. Claro F Jr, Sarian LO, Pinto-Neto AM. Omentum for mammary disorders: a 30-year systematic review. Ann Surg Oncol. 2015;22:2540.
2. Cothier-Savey I, Tamtawi B, Dohnt F, Raulo Y, Baruch J. Immediate breast reconstruction using laparoscopically harvested omental flap. Plast Reconstr Surg. 2001;107:1156–63.

3. Góes JCS, Macedo ALV. Immediate reconstruction after skin-sparing mastectomy using the omental flap and synthetic mesh. In: Spear S, editor. Surgery of the breast: principles of the art. 2nd ed. Philadelphia, PA: Lippincott; 2006. p. 786–93.

4. Zaha H, Inamine S, Naito T, Nomura H. Laparoscopically harvested omental flap for immediate breast reconstruction. Am J Surg. 2006;192:556–8.

5. Zaha H. Omental flap reconstruction; in partial breast reconstruction. In: Losken A, Hamdi M, editors. Techniques in oncoplastic surgery. 2nd ed; 2017. p. 369–86.

6. Zaha H, Inamine S. Laparoscopically harvested omental flap: results for 96 patients. Surg Endosc. 2010;24(1):103–7.

7. Zaha H, Sunagawa H, Kawakami K, et al. Partial breast reconstruction for an inferomedial breast carcinoma using an omental flap. World J Surg. 2010;34(8):1782–7.

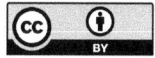

Part VII

Video Assisted Thoracic Surgery

Basic Principles and Advanced VATS Procedures

Narendra Agarwal and Bharti Kukreja

Introduction

In the era of growing enthusiasm for minimally invasive surgical approaches, many general and thoracic surgeons have fostered a resurgence of interest in thoracoscopy. Over the last two decades, surgeons have expanded the use of thoracoscopic or video-assisted thoracic surgery (VATS), procedures to address a variety of thoracic pathologies classically managed through open thoracotomy. The goal of this chapter is to guide minimal invasive surgeons who are trained in open thoracic procedures, and thoracic surgeons beginning their thoracoscopic experience with the basic operative setup for thoracoscopic (VATS) surgery.

Historical Background

The evolution of VATS can be traced back to the early nineteenth century when Bozzini used an endoscope to examine the urinary bladder (cystoscopy) [1]. Driving in the same direction, a couple of years later Carson induced artificial pneumothorax for the treatment of pulmonary Kochs [2]. Almost a decade later, in the early 1900s, Jacobaeus introduced thoracoscopic examination and use of thoracoscope for releasing pleural adhesions [3]. Further research and development of microcameras in the 1980s led to the arrival of Video-assisted thoracoscopic surgery in 1990s [4].

VATS has since been used and different modifications for the same are being done all over the world from VATS under GA, to awake VATS [5]; from three ports to single port surgery (uniportal) [6]; further developments are anticipated.

Basic Principles of VATS

The primary operative strategy is to orient the thoracoscopic instruments and the camera in triangulation, so that all are being used in the same general direction facing toward the target pathology [7] (Fig. 1).

To accomplish the basic maneuvers of thoracoscopy and to conduct effective VATS operations, several basic principles should be applied.

1. The trocar sites and thoracoscope should be placed keeping the target pathology and following in mind.

   - Ability to achieve a panoramic view and provide room to manipulate the tissue.
   - Strategic positioning of the thoracoscopic camera and the endoscopic instruments is vital to the success and efficiency of the procedure.

N. Agarwal (✉)
Department of Thoracic Surgery, Fortis Memorial Research Institute, Gurgaon, India

B. Kukreja
Medanta the Medicity, Gurgaon, India

© The Author(s) 2023
D. Lomanto et al. (eds.), *Mastering Endo-Laparoscopic and Thoracoscopic Surgery*,
https://doi.org/10.1007/978-981-19-3755-2_30

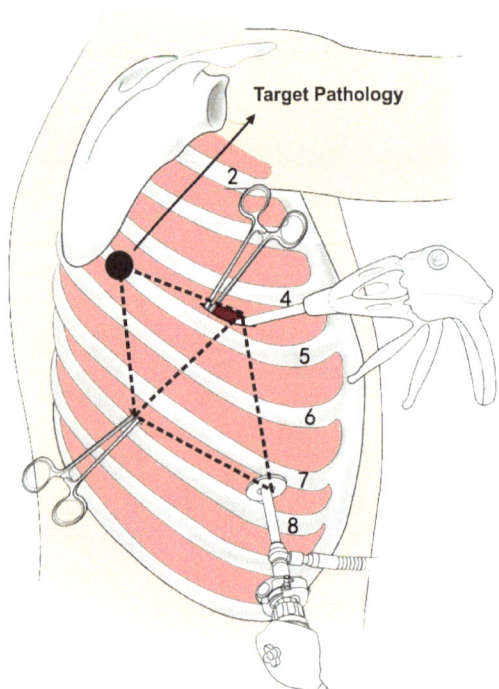

Fig. 1 Baseball diamond: Principle for port placement

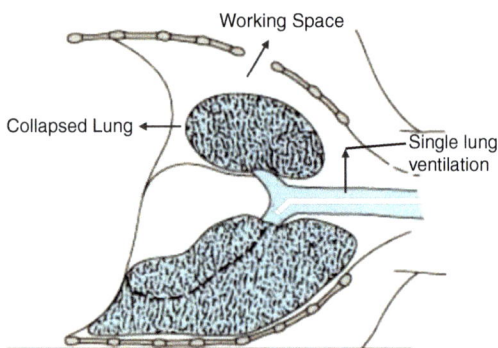

Fig. 2 Doube lumen single lung ventilation

- Avoid instrument crowding, which may otherwise result in "fencing" during instrument manipulation.
- Avoid mirror imaging by positioning instruments and thoracoscope (approach the lesion in the same general direction with instruments and camera).

2. To avoid operative chaos, move or manipulate instruments or the camera one by one, rather than randomly or synchronously.
3. Instruments should be manipulated only when seen directly through the thoracoscope.
4. All instruments should have a long working length to avoid operative struggle.

Anesthesia

Anesthesia used most commonly is General anesthesia along with single lung ventilation using Double lumen endotracheal tube or bronchial blocker (Fig. 2).

The indications for double lumen tube intubations mainly are:

- To prevent cross-contamination of a noninvolved lung from blood or pus.
- To control the distribution of ventilation in cases where there is a major air leak—such as Broncho pleural fistula, tracheobronchial trauma, or in major airway surgery.
- To perform Broncho pulmonary lavage.
- Pneumonectomy.
- Lobectomy.
- Thoracic aneurysm repair.

Use of a single lumen tube is done in procedures like esophagectomy or mobilization of esophagus, thymectomy, thoracic spine access, sympathectomy, and diagnostic procedures using insufflation of carbon dioxide into the thorax at the beginning of the procedure to facilitate a more complete and expeditious collapse of the lung. In such cases, the intrapleural pressure is measured and kept lower than 10 mm Hg to avoid mediastinal tension and hemodynamic compromise. It is necessary to use air-tight valves (reusable or disposable) trocars to seal the gas within the thorax when this carbon dioxide insufflation technique is used.

Preoperative Work Up

The role of the preoperative evaluation is to determine the risk and morbidity associated with the proposed procedure. The assessment should focus on pulmonary and cardiac conditions, as these represent the most common complications after thoracic surgery.

Cardiac Risk Assessment: The American Heart Association recommends noninvasive testing as a minimum for such patients, with additional invasive testing and intervention as indicated.

- History of a cardiac condition prior to myocardial infarction, congestive heart failure, diabetes, and cerebrovascular disease and cardiac medications.
- Unable to climb more than two flights of stairs.

Pulmonary function test: Adequate pulmonary reserve is assessed through the use of pulmonary function testing, with occasional use of perfusion scanning and exercise testing when appropriate.

This algorithm evaluates pulmonary function in three areas:

- Respiratory mechanics (forced expiratory volume in 1 s [FEV_1]).
- Parenchymal function (diffusing capacity for carbon monoxide [DLCO]).
- Cardiopulmonary interaction (Vo_2max).
- Laboratory studies: Standard blood work should include:
- Complete blood count.
- Electrolyte panel.
- Clotting parameters.
- Liver function tests.
- Preoperative imaging studies: they help to confirm the planned extent of resection and the suitability of a VATS approach.
- Contrast-enhanced computed tomography (CT).
- Positron emission tomography (PET) in suspicious malignancy or malignant cases.

Indications

Indications are as below according to organ/tissue involved:

Lung

- Lung cancer.
- Bronchiectasis.
- Aspergilloma and other fungal infections.
- Hydatid cyst in the lung.
- Emphysema.
- Destroyed lung: tuberculosis.
- Complications of Tuberculosis.
- Spontaneous pneumothorax.

Pleura

- Undiagnosed/complex/recurrent effusion.
- Empyema.
- Pericardial effusion.
- Diagnostic biopsy.
- Pleurodesis and pleurectomy.

Mediastinum

- Mediastinal mass.
- Disease of thymus.
- Parathyroid adenoma excision.

Esophagus

- Benign esophageal tumors.
- Esophageal cancer.
- Esophageal diverticula.

Diaphragm

- Eventeration.
- Hernia.

Thoracic duct ligation

Sympathectomy.

Positioning

The patient is positioned in lateral decubitus position (Fig. 3) with the thorax surgically prepared in case conversion to an open thoracotomy is necessary during the course of the operation. This is accompanied by flexion of the operating table at the level of the tip of the scapula to widen the intercostal space [8–11]. The flexion is achieved either by putting a bolster or flexing the operating table, with the operative lung facing up and nonoperative lung in the dependent position. The lateral decubitus posi-

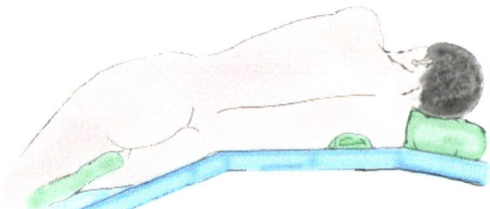

Fig. 3 Position of VATS: Lateral deubitus

tion provides adequate access to most thoracic structures which include the lungs, pleura, esophagus, and pericardium among other mediastinal structures. Care must be taken at all times to avoid nerve injury by adequately padding pressure points The patient's shoulder and arm are extended and secured to a side rest.

Port Placement

Using sterile techniques, the port site is created by making incisions in the intercostal space. The incisions are parallel to the long axis of the intercostal space. The surgeon must take care that these incisions are in the center of the space to avoid injury to the intercostal nerves that run in a groove at the lower border of the ribs. Then using a hemostat bluntly spread the fascia and muscle layers until the pleural cavity is entered.

The first port incision should be at the maximum distance from the target site of dissection or inspection to allow better visualization. Mostly the choice of incision is at the seventh or eighth intercostal space at the anterior to midaxillary line. This incision is best suited for the placement of chest tube at the end of the procedure. Surgical interventions are made over the rib to prevent any injury to the neurovascular bundle.

The second incision site is the anterior fourth and fifth intercostal space between the midclavicular and anterior axillary line.

The third incision is posterior, at the fifth and sixth intercostal space adjacent to the scapula (Fig. 4).

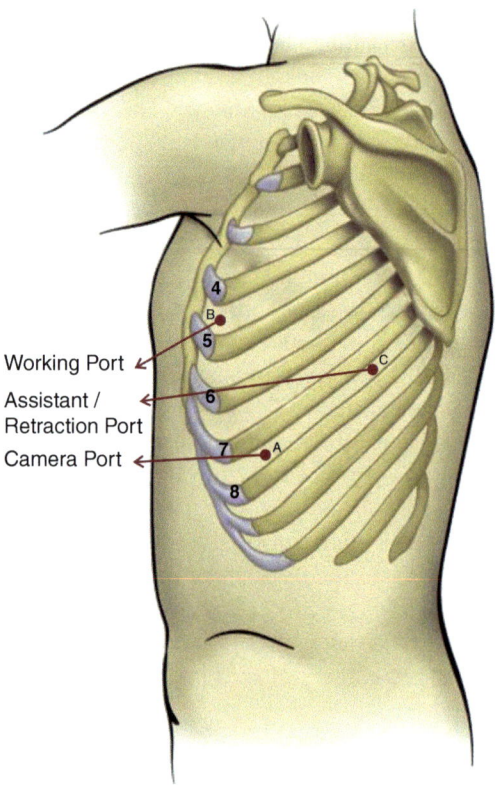

Working Port
Assistant /
Retraction Port
Camera Port

Fig. 4 VATS: Port placement

There are many different port placements in VATS being used throughout the world. The earliest established was referred to as "baseball diamond" which consist of 10–12 mm incisions with the placement varying from surgeon to surgeon according to their preferred approach for the particular patients. Multiple different variations of the above have been seen now including the two port and even single port technique. With two port technique using an anterior and an inferior port, and single port technique using the camera and multiple instruments through the same port.

Instruments

The instruments generally used in VATS have salient features like long working length which provides the familiarity of traditional handles for

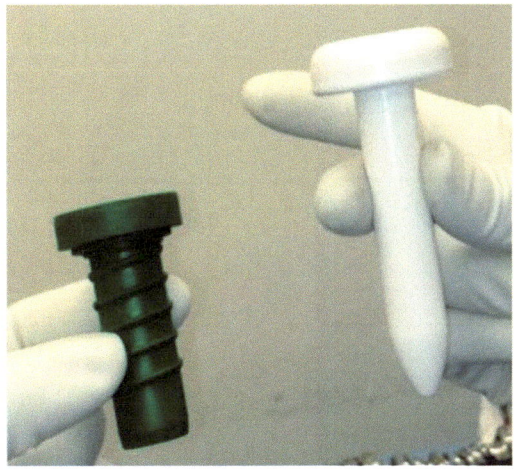

Fig. 5 VATS: Short trocars

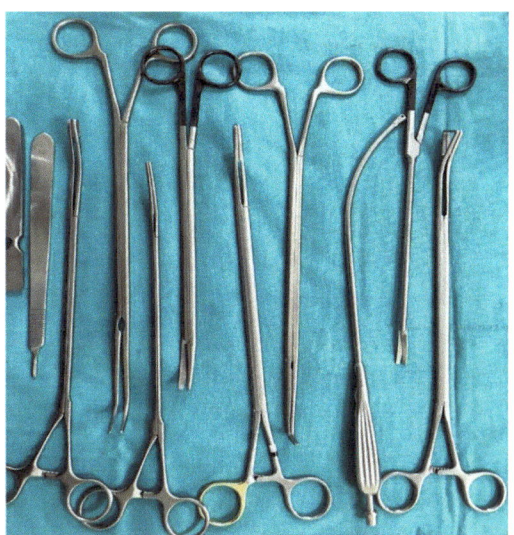

Fig. 6a VATS Instrument: Thin Shaft and Curved shape Instruments

secure manipulation and superior tactile response. The Sliding Shafts enable the instrument to be fully functional when placed through a port or very small incision and also minimize Patient Trauma. Continuous technical advancements in vats instrumentation have happened in the last decade.

Commonly used instruments during VATS procedure are:

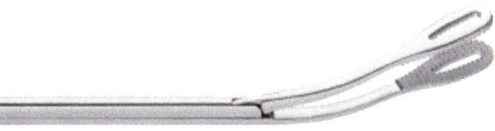

Fig. 6b Decortication Forcep

- Short trocars (Fig. 5).
- 30/45 telescope
- Usual range of 5 mm thoracic/endoscopic instruments (grasping forceps, decortication ring forceps (Fig. 6b), DeBakey forceps, small and large dissectors, scissors, suction) (Fig. 6a).
- 5 mm bipolar shears.
- 5 mm vessel sealing device.
- 5 mm endo peanuts.
- 10 mm clip applier.
- Endo-stapler, preferably with curved tip.
- Large retrieval bag.
- Conventional open thoracic instrumentation ready on a separate table.

The OR Setup

The operating room should be fully equipped that allows the surgeon at any immediate potential to convert to open thoracotomy. Video-assisted thoracic surgery (VATS) requires a high definition (HD) video monitor, together with VATS instruments allowing the surgeon to view a sharp, high-resolution image within the chest cavity. The organization of the operation room is done based on the surgeon's surgical approach.

There are two types of approaches:

- Anterior (Fig. 7a).
- Posterior (Fig. 7b).

Fig. 7a Anterior
appoach: Video-assisted
thoracic surgery

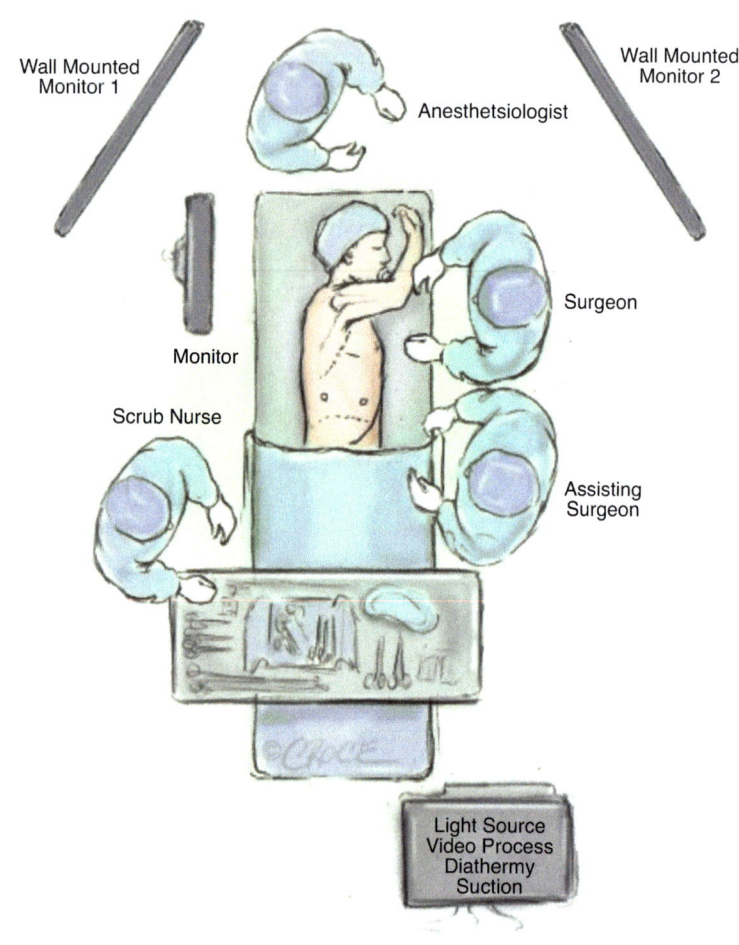

Fig. 7b Posterior
approcah: Video-assisted
thoracoscopic surgery

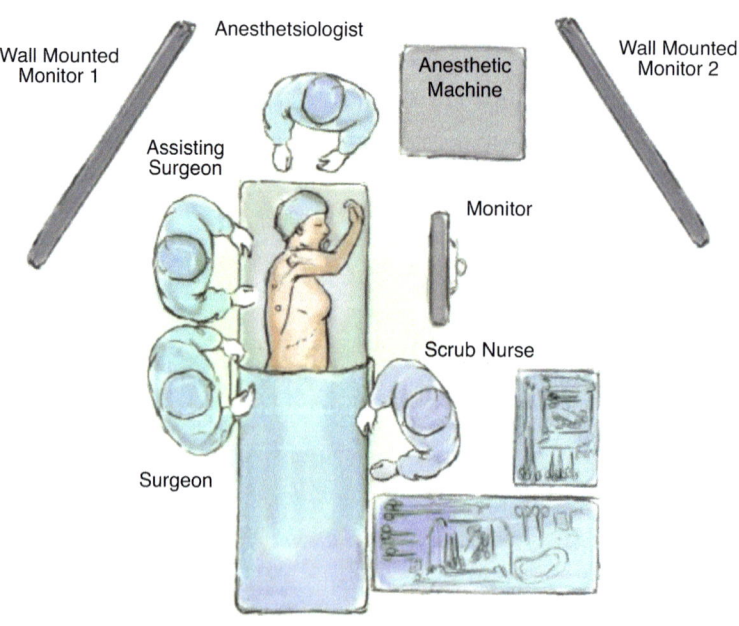

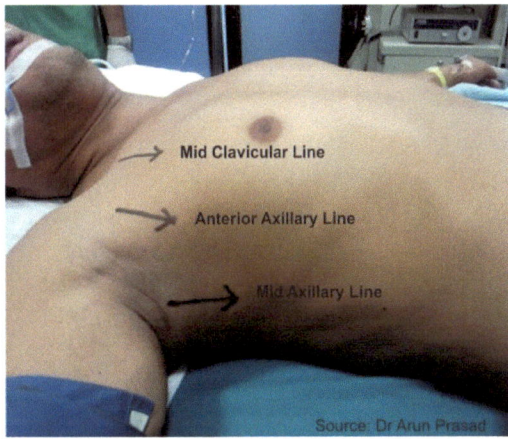

Fig. 8 Anatomical landmark for port placement in sympathectomy

VATS Sympathectomy

It is a surgical procedure in which a portion of the sympathetic nerve trunk in the thoracic region is destroyed [1, 2]. The most common area targeted in sympathectomy is the upper thoracic region, that part of the sympathetic chain lying between the first and fifth thoracic vertebra (Fig. 8).

Indications

- Hyperhidrosis [12].
- Splanchnic pain.
- Reflex sympathetic dystrophy (RSD).
- Upper extremity ischemia is also appropriate when nonsurgical treatment fails.
- Prolonged QT interval.

Position

The patient is positioned supine with both arms outstretched on arm boards and the trunk in a 30° Fowler position. The position helps the apex of the lung to fall apart.

Anesthesia

General anesthesia, along with single lung intubation [13], a bilateral two port VATS approach is performed.

Technique

- The sterile field includes the neck, both axillae and upper arms down to the costal margin bilaterally.
- At fourth or fifth intercostal space with an anterior axillary line, approximately 1 cm incisions are made for camera port (Fig. 8).
- Insufflation of carbon dioxide for active lung collapse using intra pleural Pressure up to 8 mmHg.
- The zero-degree thoracoscope is introduced through the port.
- The thoracic chain is readily identified and covered by the thin layer of the parietal pleura.
- A diathermy hook is inserted through the third midclavicular line intercostal space (Fig. 8).
- The sympathetic chain is visualized behind the parietal pleura, which is then scored on either side using the cautery to delineate the position of the chain and the extent of the planned cauterization which corresponds to the extent of the chain destroyed.
- Using the ribs as reference, the sympathetic chain is then cauterized and divided from T2 to T3 for patients with predominantly palmar hyperhidrosis and from T2 to T4 for patients with predominantly axillary hyperhidrosis [14]. Possible anatomical variations such as the Kuntz nerve, a transverse dissection along the rib is performed (Fig. 9).
- The thoracoscope is then removed and replaced with a small red rubber catheter. With positive pressure ventilation, the catheter is then removed under suction to allow expansion of the lung.

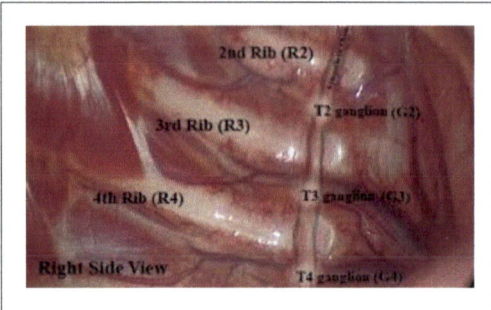

CAMERA IMAGE

ILLUSTRATION

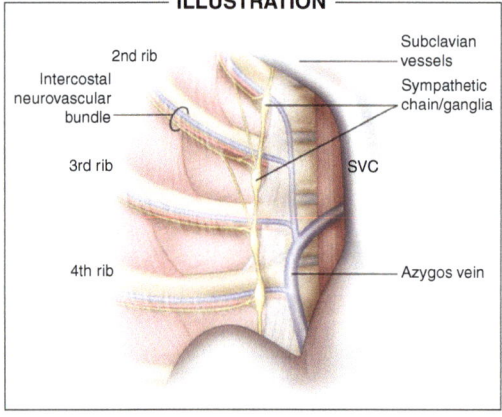

Fig. 9 Thoracic sympathetic chain

- The skin incision is closed with a single absorbable 3–0 suture followed by the placement of skin types.
- Contralateral sympathectomy is performed in a similar manner without changing the patient's position.

Postoperative

- No chest tubes are routinely placed at the end of the procedures.
- All resected sympathetic chain specimens are sent for histopathology.
- Patients are generally discharged the same day.

Complications

- Compensatory sweating.
- Horner's syndrome.
- Bleeding.

- Pneumothorax.
- Recurrence.

Vats Wedge Resection

It is a minimally invasive technique for nonanatomical limited resection of a lung. It is preferred over open as it is muscle sparing non-rib spreading and does not involve thoracotomy [15]. It is better suited for peripherally located lesions compared to deep-seated central pathology which is very arduous and difficult to secure sufficient surgical margin [16] (Fig. 10). To attempt such deep-seated resections can cause prolonged air leak and delayed recovery. Lesions at the periphery or outer one-third of the lung are considered the most suitable indications for wedge resections.

Indications

It has both diagnostic and therapeutic roles.

Therapeutic

- Early-stage (NSCLC; T1N0M0) and early-stage in patients with limited cardiopulmonary reserve (although lobectomy is preferred).

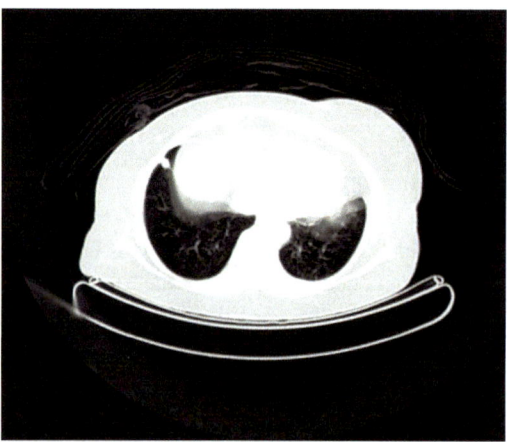

Fig. 10 High-resolution computed tomography of solitary lung lesion

- Metastasectomy for pulmonary metastases due to renal, breast, colon malignancy, melanoma, sarcoma.
- Ground-glass opacification lesions on chest CT scan in patients with past or present cancer [16].
- Localization and excisional biopsy of ill-defined or small pulmonary lesions [17]
- Resection of hamartoma.
- Resection of pulmonary sclerosing hemangioma.
- Resection of intralobar sequestrated lung.
- Resection of localized peripheral bronchiectasis.
- Lung volume reduction surgery in end-stage emphysema.
- Resection of pulmonary arteriovenous malformation (PAVMs) [18, 19].
- Infectious tubercular granulomas, aspergilloma, and focal organizing pneumonia.

Diagnostics

- Excision biopsy of solitary/pulmonary nodules.
- Excisional biopsy of ill-defined or small pulmonary lesions [17].
- Interstitial lung disease (ILD), wedge resections for diagnostic purposes, the lingula or the middle lobe are usually preferred, although alternative segments may be selected.
- Pulmonary fibrosis.
- Resection of ruptured/bullous lung.
- Resection of pulmonary sclerosing hemangioma.

Surgical Technique

- In lateral decubitus and ports, placement are done as described above.
- Localization of the pathologic site is done based on visceral pleural changes such as puckering, dimpling, raised lesions over a deflated lung, increased vascularity, or overlying pleural adhesions (Fig. 11).
- Gentle handling of the lung parenchyma to avoid unnecessary air leak or bleeding due to tear.

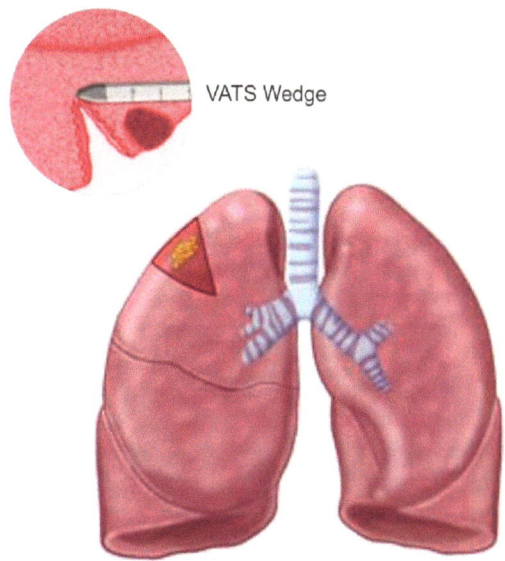

Fig. 11 Wedge resection

- Since there are limitations of finger palpation of the target site other techniques used to identify target site are preoperative CT-guided needle placement, hook-wire localization, or placement of radio-opaque dye (methylene blue). These can be used for guidance and lesion detection intraoperatively with fluoroscopy.
- After localization resection is done by using endostaplers, larger lesions require planning with numerous staple runs. The deflated lung tissue can be rotated from the apex or base to lie over hilum to allow alignment for straight staple cuts.
- Tissue is delivered using endo bag from the anterior working port.
- Before closing the ports lung is inspected for any air leaks.
- Chest tube with underwater seal is placed from inferior port and lung is allowed to expand completely.

Postoperative

- Postoperative pain management consists of narcotics and/or NSAIDS.
- Chest physiotherapy and early ambulation are recommended.

- Chest tube is removed when the pleural effusion is lower than 200 mL/day and air leak flow <40 mL/min for more than 8 h (and without spikes of airflow greater than this value) [20].

Complications

- Wound infection.
- Persistent air leak.
- Subcutaneous emphysema.
- Hemothorax.
- Pneumonia.
- Atelectasis.
- Broncho pleural fistula.
- Local and port-site recurrence of malignancy [8] (more common with wedge resection than with lobectomy).

VATS Bullectomy and Pleurodesis

VATS bullectomy is a minimally invasive surgery to remove bulla, i.e., dilated air space or air-filled pockets from the lung parenchyma (Fig. 10). Pleurodesis is the procedure of sticking together the coverings of the visceral and the parietal pleura of the lung together.

VATS bullectomy and pleurodesis together have been seen in various studies to improve the outcomes in patients with spontaneous/recurrent pneumothorax or emphysema [21, 22].

Indications

- In asymptomatic cases: Large bullae occupying more than 30% of lung volume (with underlying lung comparatively nonemphysematous).
- Symptomatic cases: after ruling out other causes of dyspnoea.
- When patient presents with complications due to ruptured bulla such as pneumothorax, infection, chest pain, or hemoptysis (refractory to treatment).
- The controversy arises in cases of giant bullas in which some surgeons prefer operating early

[23] in asymptomatic patients whereas some prefer to wait for the occurrence of symptoms before surgery to avoid the risk of complications in otherwise clinically asymptomatic patients [24].

Preoperative

CT should be done to record the progress, size of bulla or bullae, identify the proper anatomy of the bulla as well as its surrounding tissue, and therefore help the surgeon to plan the procedure (Fig. 12).

Anesthesia

Single lung ventilation by use of a double-lumen endotracheal tube or bronchial blocker. Placement of a thoracic epidural catheter for postoperative pain control.

Procedure

- The first step in the surgery is the placement of the ports in the lateral decubitus position described above. The first incision should be taken very carefully after accessing the computed tomography imaging as the lungs might be adhered to the chest wall. Adhesiolysis lead

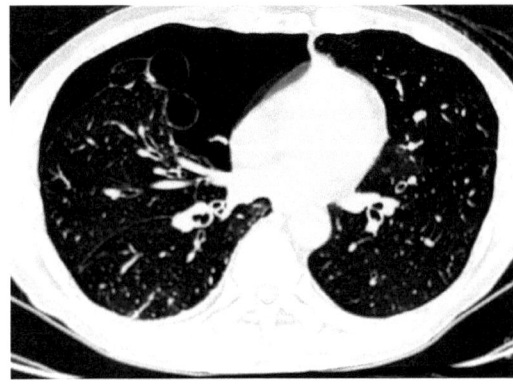

Fig. 12 High-resolution computed tomography of bullous lung

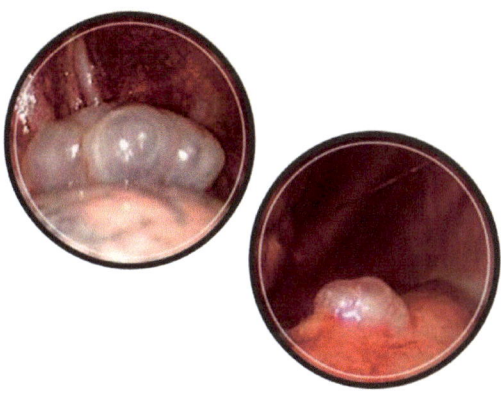

Fig. 13 Camera view: Bullous lung

to space for removing the bulla and increases the visibility of the lungs (Fig. 13).

- Next step is to locate and grasp the bulla and fire the stapler across the base. In case of large bullas which are difficult to manipulate, the bulla is punctured and deflated for effortless handling. The staple line should be put in normal lung tissue to avoid air leak.
- Sizing should be carefully planned, otherwise inadequate sealing due to small stapler or leakage in case of too large stapler, some surgeons prefer buttressing of the staple lines is also done to prevent air leakage.
- Chest cavity is reinstalled with normal saline and reinflation of the lungs to check for any visible leak.
- Pleurodesis is done with mechanical abrasion along with talc or with the help of other chemicals.
- Placement of pleural drains to avoid air or fluid collection in the operated area and to ensure complete expansion of lung.
- Pleurodesis works when the lung is completely expanded. Closure of the ports.

Post-op Management

- Drain placed can be attached to negative pressure suction as per the surgeon's choice. There have been controversies regarding the use of negative pressure suction as few authors believe it continues to have air leak and hence

delay in healing however the author has preferred using negative pressure suction as it helps pleurodesis by increasing lung volume and decreasing chances of atelectasis.
- NSAIDS or opioids.
- Chest physiotherapy and incentive spirometry.

Complications

- Air leak: Inside the lungs can lead to pneumothorax and collapse of healthy lung tissue. To avoid this we place the drain connected to negative suction, It should be checked routinely that the drain is patent.
- Atelectasis: Incomplete expansion of lungs can lead to atelectasis. Pre-op and post-op physiotherapy helps prevent the same.
- Pneumonia: Chances of infection due to an invasive process possible. Use of empirical antibiotics should be considered. Proper post-op care with vitals, i.e., temperature, pulse, and BP should be monitored hourly.
- Sputum retention: This can also be prevented with help of chest physiotherapy and nebulization if and when needed.

Vats Decortication

The ability to completely drain the thoracic cavity, break up pockets of pleural fluid, completely visualize all aspects of the pleural space, by thoracoscopy and avoid the morbidity of a thoracotomy. VATS drainage of empyema and decortication has become an attractive procedure in the management of empyema and hemothorax.

Indications

- An effusion which is loculated or occupying 50% of hemithorax [25].
- An infected pleural effusion.
- An empyema of less than approximately 3 weeks, in the exudative or fibro purulent stage 4 [25].
- Hemothorax.

- Descending mediastinitis.
- When the nature of the pleural process is undiagnosed, this allows for a directed pleural biopsy that is likely to make the diagnosis while avoiding the morbidity of a thoracotomy.

Contraindications

- Prior thoracotomy.
- Prior talc pleurodesis.
- The inability to tolerate single lung ventilation.
- Fibrothorax.

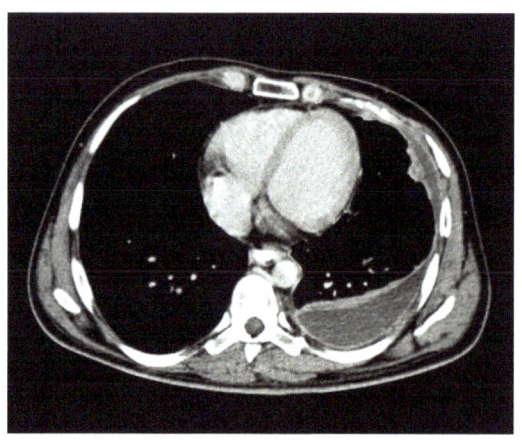

Fig. 14 High-resolution computed tomography of empyema

Surgical Technique

- The first incision should be taken very carefully after accessing the computed tomography imaging as the lungs might be adhered to the chest wall. The camera port is placed in the seventh or sixth intercostal space in the line of the anterior superior iliac spine or just anterior to this. Rest of the ports are placed as discussed above; generally, 2–3 ports are made for drainage of empyema and hemothorax [26]. However, in cases of dense adhesions at the primary camera port, different positions can be chosen for insertion of first port.
- After entering the chest wall, a Yank Auer suction is used to drain the chest of effusion or blood. The suction along with a finger is then used to break up simple loculations while continuing suction if necessary. The preoperative CT scan (Fig. 14) helps guide this "blind" initial drainage and creates a working pleural space for the thoracoscopic instruments. Gelatinous fibrinous deposits and blood clots are removed with a curved ring forceps/decortication forceps (Fig. 6a). The visceral pleural peel can be debrided if needed using ring forceps, a curette, and a peanut dissector as in an open decortication.
- Once a pleural space has been created the removal of fibrinous material is performed over the lateral part of the pleural cavity starting from the apex of the lung and proceeding to the diaphragm or vice versa.

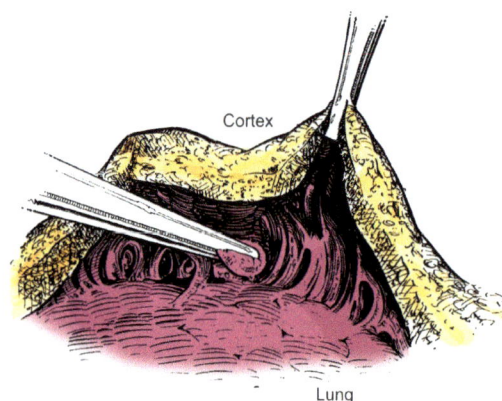

Fig. 15 Technique to peel of cortex

- The suction and ring clamp/decortication forceps are used together to remove the fibrinous material from the pleural cavity and the curette, peanut, and ring clamp are used to dissect the cortex on the lung (Fig. 15).
- At the inferior aspect of the pleural cavity, it is helpful to identify and separate the lower lobe of the lung from the diaphragm. This plane is developed posteriorly and anteriorly allowing for the lung to fill the cost diaphragmatic sulcus once the decortication is complete [27]. Next, the posterior aspect of the pleural space is debrided and the underlying lung is decorticated.
- Intermittent ventilation of the lung is used to assess the completeness of the decortication as the dissection proceeds [28] (Fig. 16).

- Particular care should be taken with hemostasis both on the parietal and visceral pleura [29].
- If adequate progress is not being made or there is inadequate expansion of the lung to fill the chest, then conversion to open decortication should be performed. Conversion to open is performed when necessary and should not be considered a failure of thoracoscopy [30].
- Once adequate debridement has been accomplished, irrigation is performed and the lung expansion is visualized to ensure the pleural cavity is filled by the lung [31].
- Chest tubes can be placed anteriorly and posteriorly for air and fluid drainage.

Postoperative

- Chest physiotherapy and incentive spirometry.
- The chest tubes are maintained on suction to make sure there is complete lung expansion and adequate drainage of the pleural space.
- Once the drainage is less than 200 cc/24 hrs and the air leak has been reduced to minimum, the tubes can be removed.
- For patients with empyema, intravenous antibiotics are continued during postoperative period and for 14 days of oral antibiotics once the patient is discharged [32].

Complications

- Inadequate lung expansion.
- Infection and recurrence [33].
- Prolonged air leak.

Basic Principles: Vats Anatomical Lung Resection

Types of Anatomical Lung Resection (Fig. 17)

- Pneumonectomy: complete removal of affected lung
- Lobectomy: resection of one of the lobes of either lung along with their respective blood supply.

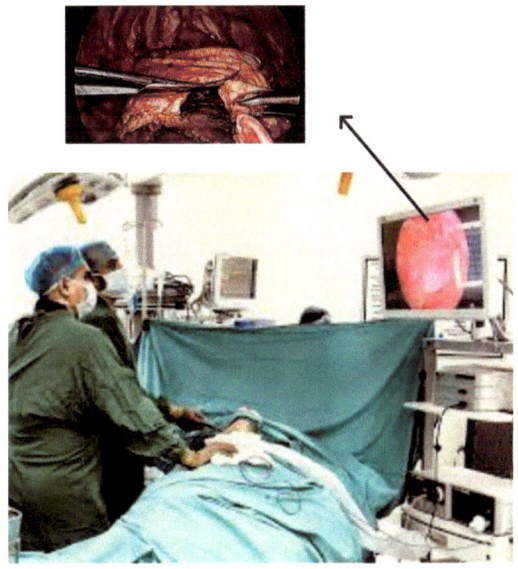

Fig. 16 VATS decortication

Fig. 17 Anatomical lung resection

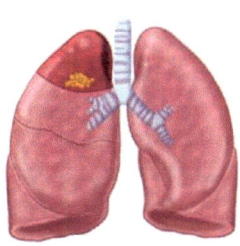

Segmentectomy

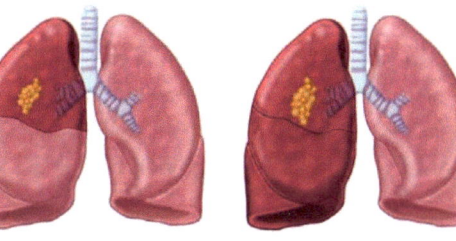

Lobectomy   Pneumonectomy

- Segmentectomy: lung segment has a separate group of bronchi, arteries, and segmental veins shared with the adjacent segments. A resection based on their anatomy will not damage other lung segments. Therefore, for certain lesions that are restricted to one lung segment, especially benign lesions, a segmentectomy may be considered [34].

Anesthesia

General Anesthesia with Single lung ventilation [13] by use of a double lumen endotracheal tube or bronchial blocker. Placement of a thoracic epidural catheter should be done for postoperative pain control.

Position: Lateral decubitus position.

Approach: depends upon where surgeon choice while operating.

- Anterior (Fig. 7a).
- Posterior (Fig. 7b).

Procedure

- The surgical procedure is facilitated by aligning the view of the camera with the general direction of the dissection. Use of angled, either at 30 or 45 from the long axis of the scope.
- Thorough knowledge of the hilar anatomy (Fig. 18) greatly enhances the safety of all of these techniques. Vital structures such as the phrenic nerve or recurrent laryngeal nerve should be identified early and preserved.
- Use of sharp, blunt, or cautery techniques is also at the discretion of the surgeon's comfort, as long as the individual dissection and ligation of the lobar and hilar structures are observed.
- Pulmonary vessels and bronchi within the hilum are ligated separately using endoscopic staplers.
- Bronchial arteries may be cauterized or clipped, or stapled in rare cases involving long-standing pulmonary infection.

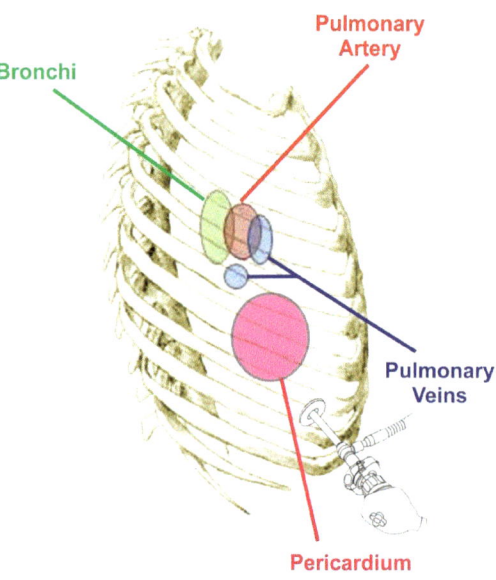

Fig. 18 Illustration of the hilar structure

- It is important to introduce the stapler into the chest such that, once around the vessel or bronchus, it exits freely on the other side and not encumbered by other structures. This will avoid injury to other tissues, and assure a secure closure of the target.
- Specimen removal is achieved with the use of a specimen bag, to minimize contact with the soft tissues at the access incision site which reduces recurrence at port sites.
- In malignant cases, nodal dissection may be performed either before or after completion of the pulmonary resection.

Conclusion

It is imperative that minimal access surgeries such as VATS be taught to a surgeon in the early training period to shorten the learning curve as multiple studies done on the same show the improvement in the prognosis of patients needing thoracic surgery. The morbidity and mortality have drastically decreased and hence it has been widely accepted all over the world. VATS has progressively replaced open thoracotomies in most thoracic surgery centers around the world because of its safety profile in elderly patients, better pain control, faster recovery times, and better access to apical structures. It has been shown to decrease the length of hospital stay compared to open thoracotomy.

More improvements in the same are bound to happen with time with help of young surgeons and creative minds like Bozzini's.

References

1. Ramai D, Zakhia K, Etienne D, Reddy M. Philipp Bozzini (1773-1809): the earliest description of endoscopy. J Med Biogr. 2018;26(2):137–41. https://doi.org/10.1177/0967772018755587.
2. Dubovsky H. Artificial pneumothorax in the treatment of lung tuberculosis. S Afr Med J. 1992;81(7):372–5.
3. Hatzinger M, Kwon ST, Langbein S, Kamp S, Häcker A, Alken P. Hans Christian Jacobaeus: inventor of human laparoscopy and thoracoscopy. J Endourol. 2006;20(11):848–50. https://doi.org/10.1089/end.2006.20.848.
4. Roviaro G, Rebuffat C, Varoli F, Vergani C, Mariani C, Maciocco M. Videoendoscopic pulmonary lobectomy for cancer. Surg Laparosc Endosc. 1992;2(3):244–47.
5. Gonzalez-Rivas D, Bonome C, Fieira E, et al. Non-intubated video-assisted thoracoscopic lung resections: the future of thoracic surgery? Eur J Cardio-thoracic Surg. 2016;49(3):721–31. https://doi.org/10.1093/ejcts/ezv136.
6. Ng CSH, Rocco G, Wong RHL, Lau RWH, Yu SCH, Yim APC. Uniportal and single-incision video-assisted thoracic surgery: the state of the art. Interact Cardiovasc Thorac Surg. 2014;19(4):661–6. https://doi.org/10.1093/icvts/ivu200.
7. Hansen HJ, Petersen RH. Video-assisted thoracoscopic lobectomy using a standardized three-port anterior approach - the Copenhagen experience. Ann Cardiothorac Surg. 2012;1(1):70–6. https://doi.org/10.3978/j.issn.2225-319X.2012.04.15.
8. Colice GL, Shafazand S, Griffin JP, Keenan R, Bolliger CT. Physiologic evaluation of the patient with lung cancer being considered for resectional surgery: ACCP evidenced-based clinical practice guidelines (2nd edition). Chest. 2007;132(3Suppl):161S–77S https://doi.org/10.1378/chest.07-1359.
9. Yim APC, Rendina EA, Hazelrigg SR, et al. A new technological approach to nonanatomical pulmonary resection: saline enhanced thermal sealing. Ann Thorac Surg. 2002;74(5):1671–76. https://doi.org/10.1016/S0003-4975(02)03901-2.
10. Dowling RD, Keenan RJ, Ferson PF, Landreneau RJ. Video-assisted thoracoscopic resection of pulmonary metastases. Ann Thorac Surg. 1993;56(3):772–5. https://doi.org/10.1016/0003-4975(93)90977-p.
11. Sakuma T, Sugita M, Sagawa M, Ishigaki M, Toga H. Video-assisted thoracoscopic wedge resection for pulmonary sequestration. Ann Thorac Surg.
2004;78(5):1844–5. https://doi.org/10.1016/j.athoracsur.2003.07.028.
12. Cerfolio RJ, De Campos JRM, Bryant AS, et al. The society of thoracic surgeons expert consensus for the surgical treatment of hyperhidrosis. Ann Thorac Surg. 2011;91(5):1642–8. https://doi.org/10.1016/j.athoracsur.2011.01.105.
13. Benumof JL. Physiology of the open chest and one-lung ventilation. In: Anesthesia T, editor. Churchill-Livingstone. New York: NY; 1983. p. 287–316.
14. Kux M. Thoracic endoscopic Sympathectomy in palmar and axillary hyperhidrosis. Arch Surg. 1978;113(3):264–6. https://doi.org/10.1001/archsurg.1978.01370150036005.
15. Landreneau RJ, Herlan DB, Johnson JA, Boley TM, Nawarawong W, Ferson PF. Thoracoscopic neodymium: yttrium-aluminum garnet laser-assisted pulmonary resection. Ann Thorac Surg. 1991;52(5):1176–8. https://doi.org/10.1016/0003-4975(91)91309-J.
16. Wang Y, SurgWang Y. Video-assisted thoracoscopic surgery for non-small-cell lung cancer is beneficial to elderly patients. International journal of clinical and experimental Medicinery for non-small-cell. Int J Clin Exp Med. 2015;8(8:13604–09.
17. Lin F, Xiao Z, Mei J, et al. Simultaneous thoracoscopic resection for coexisting pulmonary and thymic lesions. J Thorac Dis. 2015;7(9):1637–42. https://doi.org/10.3978/j.issn.2072-1439.2015.09.09.
18. Shiiya H, Suzuki Y, Yamazaki S, Kaga K. Polypoid pulmonary arteriovenous malformation causing hemothorax treated with thoracoscopic wedge resection. Surg Case Rep. 2018;12;4(1):21. https://doi.org/10.1186/s40792-018-0428-1.
19. Bakhos CT, Wang SC, Rosen JM. Contemporary role of minimally invasive thoracic surgery in the management of pulmonary arteriovenous malformations: report of two cases and review of the literature. J Thorac Dis. 2016;8(1):195–197. https://doi.org/10.3978/j.issn.2072-1439.2015.12.67.
20. Campisi A, Dell'Amore A, Giunta D, Congiu S, Daddi N, Dolci G. Micro-incision thoracoscopic treatment of primary spontaneous pneumothorax: the "loop" technique. J Vis Surg. 2018;10;4:35. https://doi.org/10.21037/jovs.2018.02.01.
21. Sano A, Fukami T, Murakawa T, Nakajima J. Recurrent pneumothorax related to Swyer-James syndrome. Ann Thorac Cardiovasc Surg Off J Assoc Thorac Cardiovasc Surg Asia. 2014;20 Suppl:539–41. https://doi.org/10.5761/atcs.cr.12.02102.
22. Panagopoulos N, Papavasileiou G, Koletsis E, Kastanaki M, Anastasiou N. VATS bullectomy and apical pleurectomy for spontaneous pneumothorax in a young patient with Swyer-James-mc Leod syndrome: case report presentation and literature review focusing on surgically treated cases. J Cardiothorac Surg. 2014;9–13. https://doi.org/10.1186/1749-8090-9-13.
23. Huang W, Han R, Li L, He Y. Surgery for giant emphysematous bullae: case report and a short literature review. J Thorac Dis. 2014;6(6):E104-7. https://doi.org/10.3978/j.issn.2072-1439.2014.04.39.

24. Tian Q, An Y, Bin XB, Chen LA. Treatment of giant emphysamous bulla with endobronchial valves in patients with chronic obstructive pulmonary disease: a case series. J Thorac Dis. 2014;6(12):1674–80. https://doi.org/10.3978/j.issn.2072-1439.2014.11.07.

25. Light RW. Parapneumonic effusions and empyema. Proc Am Thorac Soc. 2006;3(1):75–80. https://doi.org/10.1513/pats.200510-113JH.

26. Wurnig PN, Wittmer V, Pridun NS, Hollaus PH. Video-assisted thoracic surgery for pleural empyema. Ann Thorac Surg. 2006;81(1):309–13. https://doi.org/10.1016/j.athoracsur.2005.06.065.

27. Roberts JR, Weiman DS, Miller DL, Afifi AY, Kraeger RR. Minimally invasive surgery in the treatment of empyema: intraoperative decision making. Ann Thorac Surg. 2003;76(1):225–30. https://doi.org/10.1016/S0003-4975(03)00025-0.

28. Cassina PC, Hauser M, Hillejan L, Greschuchna D, Stamatis G, Deslauriers J. Video-assisted thoracoscopy in the treatment of pleural empyema: stage-based management and outcome. J Thorac Cardiovasc Surg. 1999;117(2):234–38. https://doi.org/10.1016/S0022-5223(99)70417-4.

29. Navsaria PH, Vogel RJ, Nicol AJ. Thoracoscopic evacuation of retained posttraumatic hemothorax. Ann Thorac Surg. 2004;78(1):282–5. https://doi.org/10.1016/j.athoracsur.2003.11.029.

30. Lardinois D, Gock M, Pezzetta E, et al. Delayed referral and gram-negative organisms increase the conversion thoracotomy rate in patients undergoing video-assisted thoracoscopic surgery for empyema. Ann Thorac Surg. 2005;79(6):1851–6. https://doi.org/10.1016/j.athoracsur.2004.12.031.

31. Shimizu K, Otani Y, Nakano T, Takayasu Y, Yasuoka Y, Morishita Y. Successful video-assisted Mediastinoscopic drainage of descending necrotizing Mediastinitis. Ann Thorac Surg. 2006;81(6):2279–81. https://doi.org/10.1016/j.athoracsur.2005.07.096.

32. Hope WW, Bolton WD, Stephenson JE. The utility and timing of surgical intervention for parapneumonic empyema in the era of video-assisted thoracoscopy. Am Surg. 2005;71(6):512–4.

33. Luh SP, Chou MC, Wang LS, Chen JY, Tsai TP. Video-assisted thoracoscopic surgery in the treatment of complicated parapneumonic effusions or empyemas: outcome of 234 patients. Chest. 2005;127(4):1427–32. https://doi.org/10.1378/chest.127.4.1427.

34. He J, Xu X. Thoracoscopic anatomic pulmonary resection. J Thorac Dis. 2012;4(5):520–47. https://doi.org/10.3978/j.issn.2072-1439.2012.09.04.

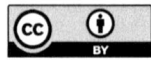

Part VIII

Upper Gastrointestinal Surgery: Esophageal Surgery

Achalasia

Javier Lopez-Gutierrez and B. Mario Cervantes

Introduction

Achalasia is the result of a progressive degeneration process of the ganglion cells of the myenteric plexus, located in the esophageal wall. The disorder motility that characterizes achalasia appears to result primarily from the loss of inhibitory neurons within the wall of the esophagus itself. This loss of the inhibitory innervation in the LOS causes the basal sphincter pressure to rise and renders the sphincter muscle incapable of normal relaxation. The loss of inhibitory neurons from the smooth muscle portion of the esophageal body results in aperistalais [1]. The manifestations of the disease depend on the degree and location of ganglion cell loss [2]. Loss of peristalsis in the distal esophagus and LOS failure to relax with swallowing, both impair esophageal emptying. Most of the signs and symptoms of achalasia are due to the defect in LES relaxation. Esophagogastric junction (OGJ) outflow obstruction. The risk of developing esophageal cancer increases up to 3.3% after a mean symptom duration of 13 years [3].

J. Lopez-Gutierrez (✉)
Minimally Invasive Surgery and Gastrointestinal Endoscopy CMN 20 de Noviembre, ISSSTE CDMX, Mexico City, Mexico

B. M. Cervantes
Minimally Invasive Surgery and Robotic Surgery CMN 20 de Noviembre, ISSSTE CDMX, Mexico city, Mexico

Clinical Features and Manifestations

- Usually has an insidious onset of mild symptoms, with gradual progression through the years.
- Mean duration of symptoms before proper diagnosis is 4.7 years [4].
- The most frequent manifestations are:
  - Dysphagia for solids 91%.
  - Dysphagia for liquids 85%.
  - Regurgitation of undigested food or saliva in up to 91%.
  - Aspiration of retained material in the esophagus.
  - Vomit induction.
  - Difficulty in belching in 85%.
  - Substernal chest pain.
  - Heartburn in 40–60%.
  - Hiccups.
  - In order to overcome the distal obstruction:
- Patients slow down when they eat.
- Adopt specific maneuvers (neck lifting and throwing the shoulders back) in order to enhance esophageal emptying.
  - Mild weight loss.
  - Significant weight loss may suggest malignancy (psuedoachalasia).

© The Author(s) 2023
D. Lomanto et al. (eds.), *Mastering Endo-Laparoscopic and Thoracoscopic Surgery*,
https://doi.org/10.1007/978-981-19-3755-2_31

Diagnostic Evaluation

- Clinical History.
- Chest X-Ray.
- Barium Swallow Study.
- OGD:
  - Dilated esophagus.
  - Food debris.
  - Mucosal ulcerations (esophagitis).
  - Mild resistance on passing the endoscope through the union.
- Esophageal manometry. Typical manometric findings are:
  - Aperistalsis in the distal two-thirds of the esophagus.
  - Incomplete LOS relaxation.
  - Elevated resting LOS pressure. The loss of inhibitory neurons may cause resting LOS pressures to rise above 45 mmHg.
  - High-resolution manometry. Achalasia is diagnosed by an elevated median integrated relaxation pressure (IRP), which indicates impaired OGJ relaxation, and absence of normal peristalsis.
- Endoscopic Ultrasound.

Findings Include

- Bird beak sign or rat-tail sign
- Esophageal dilatation.
- Pooling or stasis of barium in the esophagus when the esophagus has become atonic or noncontractile (a late feature in the disease).
- Failure of normal peristalsis to clear the esophagus of barium when the patient is in the recumbent position, with no primary waves identified.
- When the barium column is high enough (with the patient standing), the hydrostatic pressure can overcome the lower esophageal sphincter pressure, allowing passage of esophageal content [5].
- Endoscopic evaluation to exclude malignancy at the esophageal-gastric junction that can mimic achalasia. It may reveal a dilated esophagus with residual material. LOS appearance may range from normal to thick-ened muscular ring with a rosette configuration on retroflexed view. The contracted LOS may appear with an increase in the passage of the endoscope through the esophagogastric junction. However, endoscope can usually be traversed easily with a gentle pressure of the endoscope. The esophageal mucosa usually appears normal [6]. Some nonspecific changes may be seen. Stasis may predispose to esophageal candidiasis, which may be seen as adherent whitish plaques.

Differential Diagnosis

Achalasia may be misdiagnosed as gastroesophageal reflux disease, especially in patient with chest pain of a burning quality of heartburn. The differential diagnosis includes other motility disorders and pseudo achalasia due to malignancy or Chagas disease.

Treatment

1. **Pharmacological therapy.**
2. **Endoscopic Therapy.**
   (a) **Pneumatic Dilation** [7].
   (b) **Peroral endoscopic myotomy (POEM)** [8].
   (c) **Botulin Toxin (BT) injection** [9].
3. **Surgical Myotomy for Achalasia**.

Dr. Heller described in 1913 a surgical myotomy with a fundoplication as the optimal surgical treatment of achalasia [10]. The effectiveness of symptom control ranges from 90 to 97% of patients [11]. The muscle fibers of the lower esophageal sphincter are incised without disrupting the mucosal lining of the esophagus. The primary goal is to relieve the functional obstruction of the LOS while preventing reflux. Original Heller's technique was modified to anterior myotomy only, and nowadays, is the most common operative procedure to treat achalasia [12]. The esophagus can be approached through the abdomen or thorax.

Patient Selection Criteria The key component for selecting the appropriate patient for surgical management is to differentiate achalasia from other motility disorders, pseudoachalasia, malignancy, and mechanical obstruction.

POEM Vs Heller's Myotomy For patients not willing to have surgical treatment, or have relative surgical contraindications, POEM may be an option. It is an incisionless surgery, using flexible endoscopes. Submucosal tunneling is made, and the dysfunctional circular muscle of the LOS is divided leaving the longitudinal muscle layer intact, which differs from surgical myotomy, where both layers are incised. POEM has an additional margin of safety. However, the incidence of pneumoperitoneum or pneumothorax remains high (up to 40%). More long-term studies are needed in order to appreciate the real advantages and disadvantages compared with Heller's Myotomy, as well as to evaluate the long-term results [14].

Contraindications Patients who prefer to avoid surgery have undergone multiple prior abdominal surgeries or would be unable to tolerate the pneumoperitoneum required for the laparoscopic procedure.

Surgical Technique

Patient Position Patient can be placed in supine, split leg position for optimal ergonomics. Surgeon stands between the legs. The patient is positioned in a steep reverse Trendelenburg position, which allows the stomach and other organs to fall away from the esophageal hiatus.

Abdominal Access and Port Placement We can establish pneumoperitoneum by open Hasson technique, Veress needle, or optical trocar entry. After establishing the pneumoperitoneum, we insert the first port, preferably with an optical trocar. Then, four more ports (two for the surgeon, one for the scope, and the rest for the assistant) are placed under direct laparoscopic vision. Liver

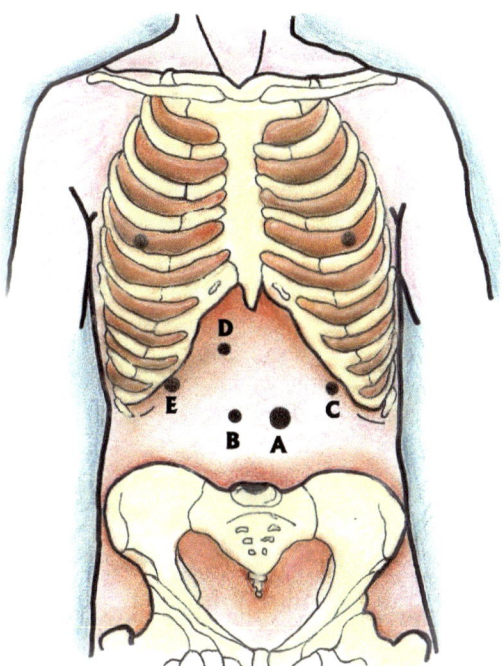

Fig. 1 Port placement

retraction should always be considered and can be achieved by one of many different devices available for that purpose (Fig. 1).

Mobilization of the Gastroesophageal Junction and Proximal Stomach

1. Incise the gastrohepatic ligament (Pars flaccida) in an avascular plane.
2. Preserve the nerve of Latarjet and avoid injury to an accessory or replaced hepatic artery.
3. Divide the anterior phrenoesophageal ligament and the peritoneum overlying the anterior abdominal esophagus.
4. Preserve the anterior vagus nerve, which lies immediately posterior to the right anterior phrenoesophageal ligament.
5. If a posterior partial or a total fundoplication is performed, a posterior esophageal window is created, then divide the left phrenogastric ligaments by dividing the short gastric arteries, starting at the inferior pole of the spleen to the exposed left crus of the diaphragm. In creating this window, the posterior vagus nerve is identi-

fied and protected. If an anterior fundoplication (Dor) technique is used, a posterior esophageal window is unnecessary unless a hiatal hernia and/or a relatively short esophagus is encountered and there is a need for further mobilization to allow more intra-abdominal length in order to construct a proper fundoplication.

Mobilization of the Mediastinal Oesophagus
The distal portion of the mediastinal esophagus is mobilized to achieve sufficient length to perform a myotomy incision that divides the entire length of the LOS and permits a tension-free fundoplication.

Myotomy When performing the myotomy, it is essential to have adequate visualization and exposure in order to prevent mucosa injuries.

1. The cardioesophageal fat pad and the anterior vagus must be cleared from the esophagus and the OGJ.
2. Once cleared, a myotomy is performed on the esophagus and the stomach. This is done using a grasper in the left hand and Maryland forceps in the right hand. The muscles are gently split layer by layer till the submucosa is clearly seen this would help avoid injury to the mucosa.
3. It is useful to have a stable platform and lighting. A lighted bougie may be used, or even better, an endoscope, in order to illuminate, stretch the muscle fibers by insufflation, and, therefore, facilitate their division.
4. The anterior surface of the esophagus is completely exposed, and slight tension is created by retracting caudally with a Babcock retractor.
5. The incision may be started on the stomach or the esophagus.
6. The myotomy is performed by individual dividing the esophageal and gastric muscle fibers. Longitudinal muscle fibers are divided first, which exposes the underlying circular muscles (Fig. 2).
7. Division of the circular layer reveals a bulging mucosa plane that should appear smooth and white. The esophageal portion of the myotomy should be approximately 6 cm in length.
8. The most critical and challenging factor is to create a 3 cm myotomy caudal to the OGJ,

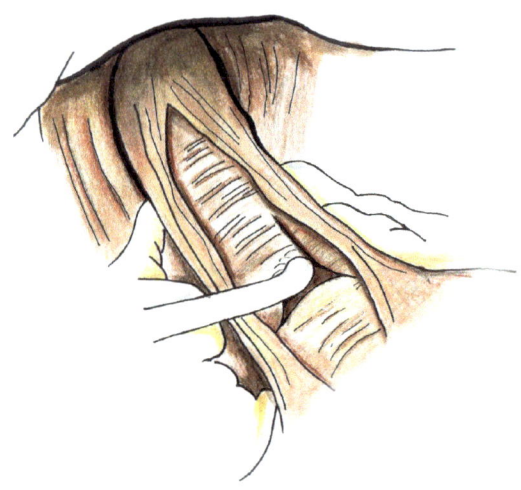

Fig. 2 Esophageal myotomy

where the tissue plane becomes less readily identifiable. A careful layer-by-layer dissection helps prevent injury.
9. The total length of the myotomy should be 9 cm.
10. It is highly advisable to perform an endoscopic inspection of the mucosa, before the next steps, in order to identify and repair any mucosal perforations.
11. Perform a hiatal closure and when possible, it is advisable to perform a fundoplication procedure, partial or total. Please refer to the fundoplication chapter for further details (Fig. 3).
12. During fundoplication take care to do the following: Place an inner row of interrupted sutures to secure the medial aspect of the fundus to the left side of the myotomy. A second row of interrupted sutures is placed to fix the leading edge to the right side of the myotomy.

Intraoperative Technical Risks

- Esophageal or gastric perforation—It ranges from 10 to 16%. The mucosal perforations, when adverted, should be repaired with 4–0 or 5–0 absorbable monofilament suture. The Dor fundoplication will buttress the repair.
- Division of vagus nerve—It is rare. If an injury to the anterior or posterior vagus nerve occurs, it is not repaired.
- Splenic injury—Ranges from 1 to 5%.
- Pneumothorax.

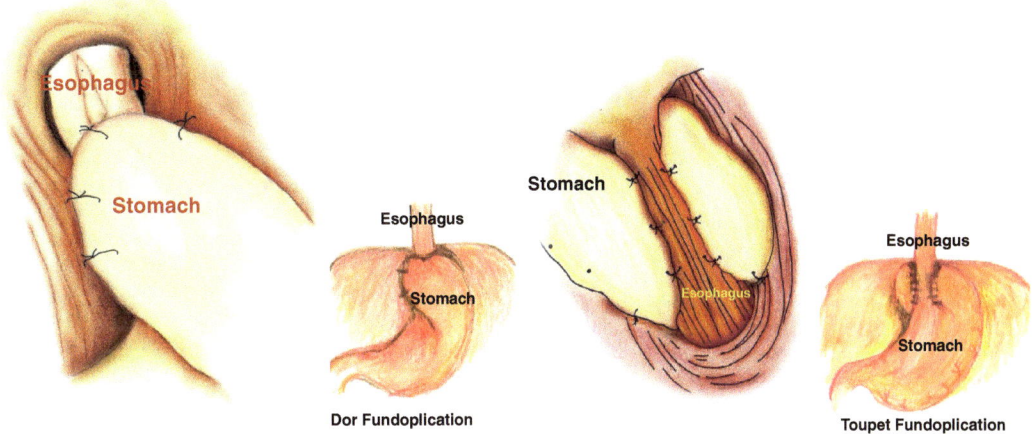

Fig. 3 Partial fundoplication

Postoperative Complications

The morbidity rate ranges between 1 and 10%. The mortality rate is <0.1% in the first 30 days after the procedure [15, 16].

Perforation It is the most common early postoperative complication and occurs in 1–7% of patients [17]. Late perforations usually result from either direct unrecognized mucosal injury or inadvertent thermal injury. Perforations may result in peritonitis or mediastinitis, or both, and may be life-threatening [16]. When a perforation is suspected, a water-soluble contrast radiograph should be obtained. Thoracic and abdominal CT scan with oral water-soluble contrast may show liquid extravasation and collections on abdomen and/or thorax. OGD is controversial. Once the perforation is confirmed, early reexploration is advisable with lavage and drainage placement. Primary repair may have acceptable results if performed in the first 24 hours after the perforation was produced [18].

Recurrent Dysphagia Is usually a late complication of a Heller myotomy + fundoplication. It presents in 3–10% of patients [19, 20]. The most common cause is incomplete myotomy. Is more common in patients that underwent thoracic approach [21]. Other reasons for dysphagia include herniated fundoplication, perihiatal scarring, peptic stricture, and tumors.

GORD If the patient underwent only a myotomy, the rate of GORD is higher [13]. If this happened despite a fundoplication, they should be treated medically.

Other Complications Bleeding is a rare complication and is reported in approximately 3% of patients.

Postoperative Care

- Analgesics.
- Antiemetics. Very important in order to avoid nausea and retching that may increase pressure on the myotomy, increasing the risk of complications.
- Clear liquids may be started the night of the day of the procedure, or when bowel function returns.
- If the patient does not present dysphagia after liquids, diet may be advanced to a soft diet the following day.
- If the patient develops early symptoms suggestive of perforation, a contrast X-ray should be considered. Symptoms include chest pain, epigastric pain, fever, tachycardia, emphysema (subcutaneous or mediastinal), and leukocytosis.

References

1. Sadowski DC, Ackah F, Jiang B, Svenson LW. Achalasia: incidence, prevalence and survival. A population-based study. Neurogastroenterol Motil. 2010;22:e256.

2. de Oliveira RB, Rezende Filho J, Dantas RO, Iazigi N. The spectrum of esophageal motor disorders in Chagas' disease. Am J Gastroentetol. 1995;90:1119.

3. Costigan DJ, Clouse RE. Achalasia-like esophagus from amyloidosis. Successful treatment with pneumatic bag dilatation. Dig Dis Sci. 1983;28:763.

4. Dufrense CR, Jeyasingham K, Baker RR. Achalasia of the cardia associated with pulmonary sarcoidosis. Surgery. 1983;94:32.

5. Foster PN, Stewart M, Lowe JS, Atkinson M. Achalasia like disorders of the oesophagus in Von Recklinghausen's neurofibromatosis. Gut. 1987;28:1522.

6. Cuthbert JA, Gallagher ND, Turtle JR. Colonic and oesophageal disturbance in a patient with multiple endocrine neoplasia, type 2b. Aust NZ J Med. 1978;8:1522.

7. Similä S, Kokkonen J, Kaski M. Achalasia sicca-juvenile Sjögren syndrome with achalasia and gastric hyposecretion. Eur J Pediatr. 1978;129:175.

8. Schuffer MD. Chronic intestinal pseudo-obstruction syndromes. Med Clin North Am. 1981;65:1331.

9. Roberts DH, Gilmore IT. Achalasia in Anderson-Fabry's disease. J R Soc Med. 1984;77:430.

10. Eckardt VF, Stauf B, Bernhard G. Chest pain in achalasia: patient characteristics and clinical course. Gastroenterology. 1999;116:1300.

11. Fisichella PM, Raz D, Palazzo F, et al. Clinical, radiological and manometric profile in 145 patients with untreated achalasia. World J Surg. 2008;32:1974.

12. Leeuwenburgh I, Scholten P, Alderliesten J, et al. Long-term esophageal cancer risk in patients with primary achalasia: a prospective study. Am J Gastroenterol. 2010;105:2144.

13. Howard PJ, Maher L, Pryde A, et al. Five year prospective study of the incidence, clinical features, and diagnosis of achalasia in Edinburgh. Gut. 1992;33:1011.

14. Heller E. Extra mucous cardioplasty in chronic cardiospasm with dilation of the esophagus (Extramukose Cardiaplastik mit dilatation des oesophagus). Mirr Grenzgels Med Chir. 1913;27:141.

15. Zaninotto G, Constantini M, Rizzetto C, et al. Four hundred laparoscopic myotomies for esophageal achalasia: a single Centre experience. Ann Surg. 2008;248:986.

16. Richards WO, Torquati A, Holzman MD, et al. Heller myotomy versus Heller myotomy with dor fundoplication for achalasia: a prospective randomized double-blind clinical trial. Ann Surg. 2004;240:405.

17. Spiess AE, Kahrilas PJ. Treating achalasia: from whalebone to laparoscope. JAMA. 1998;280:638.

18. Arreola-Risa C, Sinanan M, Pellegrini CA. Thoracoscopic Heller's myotomy. Treatment of achalasia by videoendoscopic approach. Chest Surg Clin N Am. 1995;5:459.

19. Campos GM, Vittinghoff E, Rabl C, et al. Endoscopic and surgical treatments for achalasia: a systematic review and meta-analysis. Ann Surg. 2009;249:45.

20. Rosemurgy AS, Morton CA, Rosas M, et al. A single institution's experience with more than 500 laparoscopic Heller myotomies for achalasia. J Am Coll Surg. 2010;210:637.

21. Torquati A, Richards WO, Holzman MD, Sharp KW. Laparoscopic myotomy for achalasia: predictors of successful outcome after 200 cases. Ann Surg. 2006;243:587.

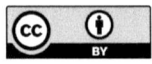

Resection of Gastroesophageal Junction Submucosal Tumors (SMTs)

Jun Liang Teh and Asim Shabbir

Introduction

- Gastroesophageal submucosal tumors are a heterogeneous group of tumors comprising of leiomyomas, gastrointestinal stroma tumors (GIST), or neurogenic tumors such as schwannoma or neurofibroma. Other possible differentials include congenital causes such as duplication cysts.
- Leiomyomas account for two-thirds of benign tumors in the esophagus and stomach. One-third of these tumors are located in the gastroesophageal junction.
- Leiomyomas are benign mesenchymal tumors and arise in the smooth muscle cells.
- Symptomatically, gastroesophageal submucosal tumors may result in dysphagia, vague chest discomfort, reflux, occasional regurgitation, or bleeding. In most other instances, asymptomatic tumors may be diagnosed following screening gastroscopy or incidentally as mediastinal masses or abdominal masses on CT scan.
- Operative technique for gastroesophageal include laparoscopic approach with or without fundoplication, laparoscopic transgastric approach, transthoracic approach, and combined laparoscopic and endoscopic approach.

Indications

- Patient factors
  - Patients fit enough to tolerate general anesthesia and undergo laparoscopy; patients who require resection of the submucosal tumor via a transthoracic approach may require single lung ventilation during the procedure.
- Disease factors
  - Symptomatic patients.
  - Giant leiomyoma measuring greater than 10 cm.
  - Submucosal lesions measuring greater than 2 cm, where histology is not available.
  - Benign submucosal tumors demonstrating an increase in size on follow-up imaging (> 1 cm/year).
  - Indeterminate histology on histology after endoscopic ultrasound (EUS) guided fine needle biopsy (FNA) has been performed.

Contraindications

- Patient factors
  - Patients with severe comorbidities (American Society of Anesthesiologists (ASA) score IV and V).

J. L. Teh
Ng Teng Fong General Hospital, National University Health System, Singapore, Singapore

A. Shabbir (✉)
National University of Singapore, Singapore, Singapore
e-mail: cfsasim@nus.edu.sg

D. Lomanto et al. (eds.), *Mastering Endo-Laparoscopic and Thoracoscopic Surgery*,
https://doi.org/10.1007/978-981-19-3755-2_32

- Patients who are unable to tolerate laparoscopy (relative contraindication consider open surgery).
- Disease factors
  - Small submucosal tumors measuring lesser than 2 cm.

Pre-op Assessment

- Upper gastrointestinal gastroscopy:
  - The size and location of the lesion is recorded.
  - The relationship of the lesion to the gastroesophageal junction and lower esophageal sphincter is assessed in order to decide the operative technique.
  - In the case of leiomyoma, rounded, mobile lesions with normal overlying mucosa are observed.
- Barium contrast swallow study is an alternative where gastroscopy is not available.
- Endoscopic Ultrasound to assess-which layer the tumor arises from,
  - the ultrasonic features of the lesion,-any acoustic shadowing
  - assess the presence of any mediastinal lymph nodes.
  - EUS—FNA can be used to biopsy the lesion.
- CT thorax/abdomen: assessment of the lesion in relation to the gastroesophageal junction, assess for metastases in the case of malignant submucosal tumors.
  - Leiomyomas are classically intramural and solitary on CT scan with smooth outlines and are multilobulated. The presence of calcifications is pathognomonic for leiomyomas.

OT Setup

Operation Room set up and patient positioning

1. The patient is placed in supine position in the reverse Trendelenburg position. Bilateral arms can be placed on arm boards if IV access

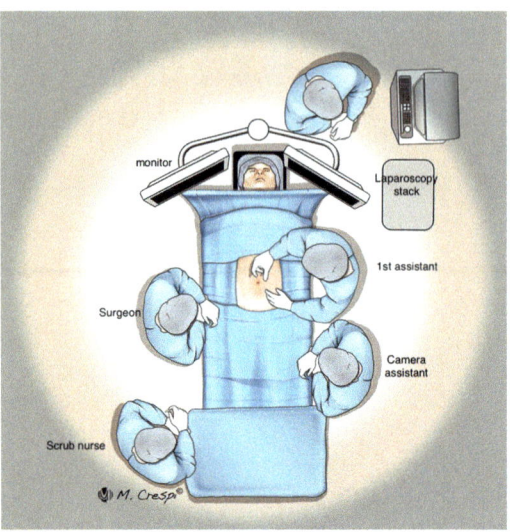

Fig. 1 OT set up and patient position

is required, or they can be tucked in bilaterally (Fig. 1).

2. A footboard is placed, and the bilateral ankles are padded with gel pads. Crepe bandages are applied to secure the feet to the footboard as well as over bilateral knees to secure the patient.
3. Mechanical deep vein thrombosis prophylaxis in the form of calf compressors or TED stockings should be instituted.
4. The operating surgeon stands on the right of the patient and the first assistant opposite the operating surgeon. The laparoscopy stack is placed to the left of the patient at the level of the shoulder of the patient.

Surgical Technique

- Essential Steps in Synthesis.
  - Safe entry and pneumoperitoneum creation.
  - Port placement.
  - Liver retraction for adequate visualization of the hiatus.
  - Hiatal dissection and mobilization of the distal esophagus.
  - Excision of the GEJ SMT.
  - Crural repair.
  - Fundoplication.

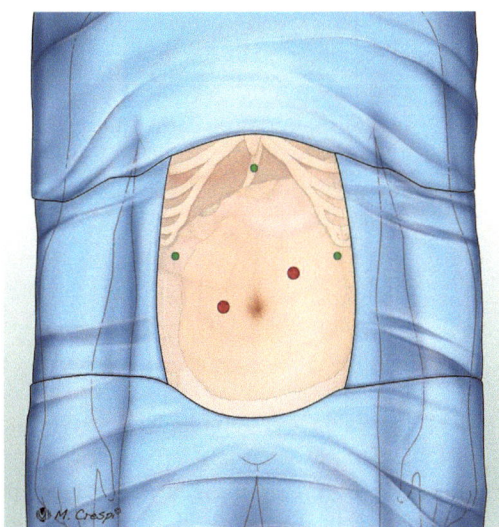

Fig. 2 Port placement

- Description of the technique.

  - Abdominal access for pneumoperitoneum.
    Pneumoperitoneum is established using the surgeon's preferred method for abdominal entry. Options include the use of a Veress needle at the Palmar's point, open Hasson technique, or the use of optical entry.
  - We perform optical entry using a 12 mm disposable optical entry port. Port Placement (Fig. 2).
    The initial trocar site for pneumoperitoneum is made 1/3 the distance up between the umbilicus and the xiphoid process, about three finger breaths to the left of the midline, this corresponds to the left mid clavicular line.
    A 12 mm port is placed to the right of the umbilicus (surgeon's right hand) and another 5 mm port (surgeon's left hand) is placed in the right subcostal area. Triangulation provided by these two working ports should allow the operating surgeon good access to the fundus of the stomach.
    A 5 mm port is placed in the left subcostal area as the assistant port to aid retraction if necessary.

  - Liver retraction.
    Liver retraction can be provided either with a Nathanson retractor/a snake retractor placed in the epigastric area or the use of OR bowel forceps to retract the liver for visualization of the hiatus.
  - Hiatal dissection and mobilization of distal esophagus.
    Entry in the lesser sac: The lesser omentum is divided and dissection taken to the level of the right crus. Any hepatic branches of the vagi or accessory left hepatic artery should be preserved as much as possible.
    Division of the phrenoesophageal membrane: The phrenoesophageal membrane is divided from the right crus toward the left crus.
    Blunt dissection of the hiatus and mobilization of the esophagus: The areolar tissue between the esophagus and the diaphragmatic crus can easily be mobilized by blunt dissection or using an energy device. When dissecting the hiatus, care must be taken to avoid injury to the abdominal aorta which lies just posterior to the esophagus.
    Creation of retroesophageal window (only required if performing posterior fundoplication or lesion is located posteriorly): Using a suction device or a grasper, a posterior esophageal window is created by bluntly dissecting the posterior adventitia tissue. Care must be taken not to injure the posterior vagus. Once the window is created, a nylon tap helps sling the esophagus and used for retraction by the assistant to facilitate exposure and dissection.
  - *Excision of the GEJ SMT.*
    For submucosal tumors that are away from the GEJ along the lesser curve, wedge resection can be performed provided narrowing the GEJ can be avoided.
    Prevention of stenosis: A orogastric Bougie inserted into the stomach helps to prevent stenosis at the gastroesophageal junction.

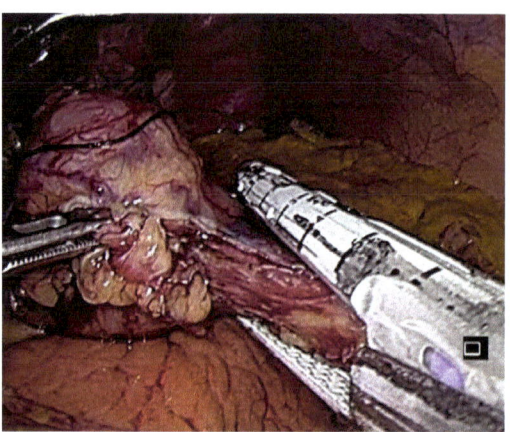

Fig. 3 Stapling of the lesser curve submucosal tumor

Excision of the tumor (Fig. 3)*:*Once isolated, excision of the tumor can then be performed with a laparoscopic linear cutter stapler. When performing tumor excision using the stapler technique, a 30 mm stapler can be utilized for the first fire as it is of a smaller profile and offers better maneuverability. Subsequent stapler fires may be performed with 45 mm or 60 mm staplers.

In cases where a full-thickness excision of the lesion is performed with an energy device, the resultant defect is closed in a single layer using an absorbable 3/0 barbed suture run continuously.

Leak test: an optional leak test can then be performed using air insufflation with gastroscopy or injection of methylene blue via the orogastric bougie.

Where the tumor encroaches upon GEJ and the lower esophageal sphincter (LES), local excision may not be possible due to high likelihood of stenosis and injury to LES under such circumstance proximal gastrectomy should be considered.

– Crural repair and reconstruction of the phrenoesophageal ligament.

Posterior crural repair: simple interrupted or figure of eight sutures using 2/0 nonabsorbable sutures like ethibond are used to approximate the left and right crus.

The esophagus is fixed to the central tendon of the diaphragm with absorbable suture.

– Fundoplication.

In patients with GEJ SMT, excision of the lesion will result in disruption of the lower esophageal sphincter fibers thereby predisposing to reflux postoperatively. Fundoplication is performed to reduce the incidence and severity of reflux post GEJ lesion excision. A wrap commensurate to the site of excision may offer the additional advantage of mitigating the effects of leakage from the repair of the GEJ excision site.

Please refer to the chapter on gastroesophageal reflux disease for details on fundoplication.

– Conclusion

Careful hemostasis.

Removal of the esophageal sling if used.

Removal of all laparoscopic ports under vision and evacuation of pneumoperitoneum.

Typically, surgical drain placement is not required.

Complications and Management

• Postoperative hemorrhage.

– Hemostasis must be observed intraoperatively and bleeding of the stapler line secured with either diathermy or suture ligation prior to ending the procedure.

- Postoperative bleeding is usually reactive in nature and is either from cut edge of the omentum or the stapler line. A trial of conservative therapy may be attempted in hemodynamically stable patients with packed cell transfusion as necessary. Reexploration may be required if there is evidence of ongoing hemorrhage, hemodynamic instability, or low hemoglobin counts despite transfusion.
- Leakage from the repair site.
  - Perforation and leakage resulting from the stapler line or repair site may happen infrequently (1–3%).
  - In most cases, expedient reexploration is necessary. Surgical principles include fashioning of the defect, repairing the defect, abdominal washout, and placement of drains. In cases not amenable to repair, a proximal gastrectomy and distal esophagectomy may be required.
- Postoperative dysphagia: managed initially with conservative therapy with a liquid diet. Consider endoscopy and balloon dilatation or revision surgery if symptoms are severe and persistent.

- Gas Bloat syndrome: conservative management and routine counseling to avoid excessive aerophagia.

Post-op Care

- Regular and adequate analgesia is prescribed. In our unit, we typically prescribe intravenous paracetamol 1 g q.d.s. Breakthrough pain is managed with opiates on PRN basis. Aggressive prophylaxis against postoperative nausea and vomiting.
- The patient is started on proton pump inhibitor therapy. PPI therapy can be discontinued after 4 weeks if the patient has symptoms of reflux or dyspepsia following surgery.
- The patient is started on clear liquids on the day of surgery and liquid diet on postoperative day 1 and minced diet on postoperative day 2.
- Patients who are clinically well and able to tolerate diet on postoperative day 2 can be safely discharged.
- The patients were reviewed in the outpatient clinic 2 weeks and 1 month after surgery.

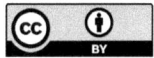

Transoral Endoscopic Zenker Diverticulotomy

Christina H. L. Ng and Chwee Ming Lim

Introduction

Zenker's diverticulum is an outpouching that emerges from Killian's triangle dehiscence, formed by oblique fibers of the inferior pharyngeal constrictor muscle and cricopharyngeus muscle. The reported prevalence lies between 0.01 and 0.11% and affects predominantly middle-aged and elderly patients [1].

Pathophysiology

The development of Zenker's diverticulum is proposed to be due to cricopharyngeal dysfunction (CPD). In CPD, repeated discoordination between the upper esophageal relaxation and pharyngeal contraction during deglutition results in perpetual increased intra-esophageal pressure contributing to the development of the outpouching over the anatomic weakness of the Killian dehiscence [2]. Similarly, patients with Zenker's diverticulum may have coexisting gastroesophageal reflux disease (GERD) and hiatus hernia, although the causal relationship between these conditions has not been established [3, 4].

Clinical Features

- Small diverticula are typically asymptomatic and may be detected incidentally on cross-sectional imaging such as computed tomography of the neck (CT neck).
- Larger diverticulum (typically more than 1 cm)—patients may present with halitosis, gurgling in the throat, regurgitation of food into the mouth, dysphagia, and even frank aspiration symptoms. In those with longstanding dysphagia, they may present with significant weight loss and malnourishment [5]. Examination of the head and neck region is usually unremarkable. On flexible nasopharyngoscopy, there may be pooling of saliva in the hypopharynx. Occasionally, a soft swelling in the neck with a positive Boyce's sign may be present. Boyce's sign refers to the presence of a splashing sound during palpation over the soft swelling in the neck. This is due to accumulated fluid within the diverticulum.

Investigations

1. Barium swallow test.
2. CT neck.

C. H. L. Ng
Department of Otorhinolaryngology-Head and Neck Surgery, Singapore General Hospital, Singapore, Singapore

C. M. Lim (✉)
Department of Otorhinolaryngology-Head and Neck Surgery, Singapore General Hospital, Singapore, Singapore

Surgery Academic Clinical Programme, Duke-NUS Medical School, Singapore, Singapore

© The Author(s) 2023
D. Lomanto et al. (eds.), *Mastering Endo-Laparoscopic and Thoracoscopic Surgery*,
https://doi.org/10.1007/978-981-19-3755-2_33

3. Functional endoscopic evaluation of swallowing (FEES) and/or Video fluoroscopy (VFS).

These investigations are performed when the clinical suspicion of aspiration is high. VFS can also be used to assess the narrowing of pharyngoesophageal sphincter and persistent prominence of cricopharyngeus muscle termed as the cricopharyngeal bar [6].

Treatment Options

Surgery is indicated for patients with symptomatic Zenker's diverticulum. Most patients with a small diverticulum (usually less than 1 cm) are usually asymptomatic.

Surgery can be broadly divided into endoscopic transoral versus an open transcervical approach. In the transoral endoscopic assisted approach, the aim of surgery is to divide the "party septal wall" between neck of the diverticulum and true esophageal opening. This procedure creates a common cavity between the esophageal lumen and diverticulum. Table 1 summarizes the pros and cons of these two approaches.

Overall, transoral endoscopic approach has lower morbidity of 8.7% as compared to open approach of 10.5%. The most common complications associated with transoral approach are cervical emphysema (2.2%), perforation (1.4%), and dental injury (1.1%); whereas complications

associated with an open approach were more severe including recurrent laryngeal nerve injury (3.3%) and esophageal perforation (3.3%) [8]. Transoral approach has a shorter operation time and shorter length of stay [9]. However, failures associated with a transoral approach lie in the difficulty of adequate visualization of the surgical field; and incomplete division of party wall resulting in an inferior ridge [10].

Contraindications

Incidental small Zenker's diverticulum of less than 1 cm does not require any surgical intervention as these patients are usually asymptomatic.

Contraindications for a transoral approach include factors that preclude adequate exposure of the hypopharynx. These factors can be summarized according to the 8 Ts of endoscopic access: teeth, trismus, transverse dimensions (mandibular), tori (mandibular), tongue, tilt (atlanto-occipital extension), treatment (prior radiotherapy), and tumor [11].

Preoperative Assessment

A barium swallow test should be done to confirm the diagnosis of a Zenker diverticulum, and to assess swallowing and the length of diverticulum (Fig. 1). Additionally, staging system can be

Table 1 Summary of the pros and cons of open versus endoscopic approach

	Open approach	Transoral endoscopic approach
Pros	Lower risk of symptom recurrence	Less invasive Shorter operating time Shorter length of hospitalization Earlier diet introduction Lower rate of complications Easy access in case of recurrence
Cons	More invasive Longer operating time (standardized mean difference 78.06 min, 95% CI 90.63,65.48) [7]. Longer length of hospitalization Longer time to diet introduction Higher rate of complications including recurrent laryngeal nerve injury	Higher rates of symptom recurrence

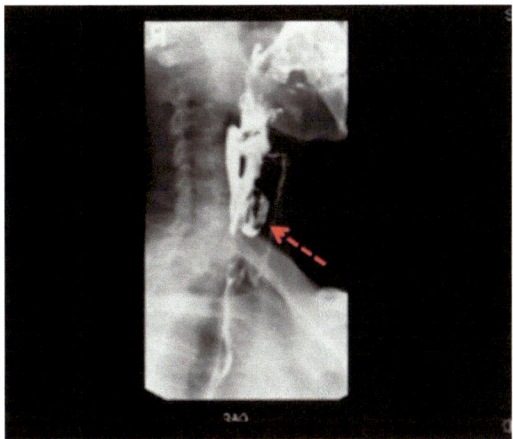

Fig. 1 Barium swallow (lateral view) demonstrating Zenker's diverticulum

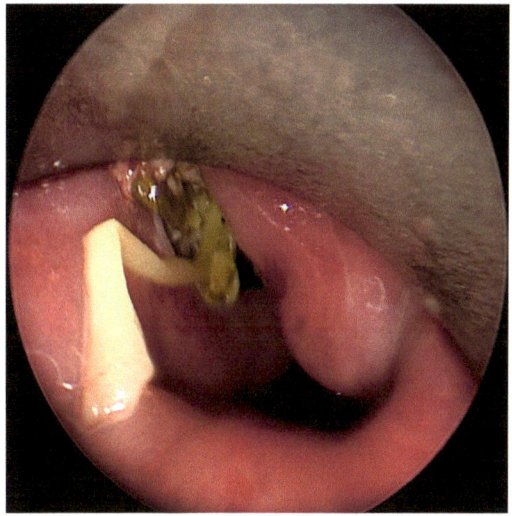

Fig. 2 Endoscopic exposure of Zenker's diverticulum sac and septum between the diverticular sac and cervical esophagus—with food debris seen in diverticulum sac

assessed on barium swallow test using Morton's staging system [12].

1. Small sacs are less than 2 cm in length.
2. Intermediate sacs are 2–4 cm in length.
3. Large sacs are greater than 4 cm in length.

OT Setup and Equipment Required

- Supine position with head donut and no shoulder roll.
- TV tower system monitor at the patient's foot.
- Weerda diverticuloscope.
- Long suction device.

Surgical Technique

- Patient is put under general anesthesia with complete muscle paralysis.
- Rigid esophagoscopy is performed to examine the entire length of the cervical esophagus.
- The scope is then slowly removed until the diverticulum is encountered at the level of cricopharyngeus before removing completely. This allows confirmation of the diagnosis and facilitated the identification of the true esophageal lumen and the lumen of the diverticulum.

- The rigid Weerda diverticuloscope (Karl Storz, Tuttlingen, Germany) is placed with anterior blade into the lumen of esophagus and posterior blade in the diverticular sac. The diverticuloscope is opened proximally sufficiently in order to allow a zero-degree 4 mm telescope and stapler insertion.
- Once a good exposure of the party wall is accomplished, the 12 mm endo-GIA 30 stapler (US Surgical Corp, Norwalk, CT) is inserted to engage septum between diverticulum sac and esophagus under direct vision. Some surgeons recommend two stay sutures to be applied on both sides of the cricopharyngeus muscle in order to retract the party wall for ease of stapling. This step can also minimize any remnant inferior ridge left in situ after the stapling process.
- Once endo-stapling of the party wall is accomplished, the divided party wall is inspected using an endoscope to ensure that there is no residual inferior ridge. The stapler line is also inspected to ensure complete closure and hemostasis.
- The summary of the surgical steps is presented in (Figs. 2, 3, and 4)

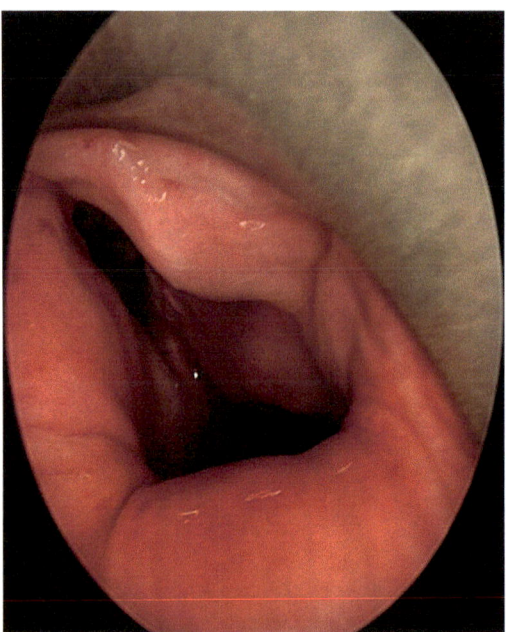

Fig. 3 Endoscopic exposure of Zenker's diverticulum sac and septum between the diverticular sac and cervical esophagus

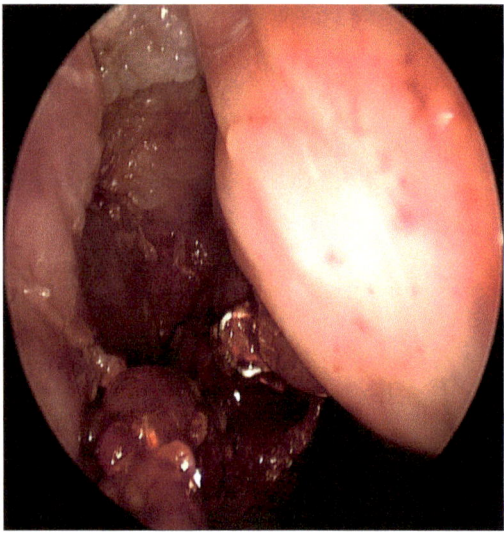

Fig. 4 Septum stapled to the inferior end of the diverticulum

Complications and Management

- Pain or discomfort of the throat—usually temporary and resolve by 1–2 days.
- Esophageal perforation leading to subcutane-

ous emphysema and possibly mediastinitis if undiagnosed intraoperatively.
- Bleeding—endolaryngeal bipolar diathermy can be used to achieve hemostasis.

Postoperative care

1. Keep nil by mouth for 24–48 h.
2. Gastrograffin swallow to be performed 24–48 h postoperatively. If there is no esophageal leak noted, oral liquid diet can be started for approximately 1 week before progressing to semi-solid diet in the next 2–4 weeks.
3. Antibiotics coverage for 1 week (covering broad spectrum bacteria including anaerobes. Clindamycin is a good alternative for those patients who are allergic to pencillin-based antibiotic.
4. Adequate analgesia.

Conclusion

Transoral endoscopic Zenker diverticulotomy is a minimally invasive approach that is effective and safe to improve symptom control among patients with this condition. Appropriate patient selection and complete division of the septal party wall between the diverticulum and true esophageal lumen are key pointers towards a successful clinical outcome.

References

1. Bizzotto A, Iacopini F, Landi R, Costamagna G. Zenker's diverticulum: exploring treatment options. Acta Otorhinolaryngol Ital. 2013;33(4):219–29.
2. Westrin KM, And SE, Carlsöö B. Zenker's diverticulum–a historical review and trends in therapy. Acta Otolaryngol. 1996;116(3):351–60. https://doi.org/10.3109/00016489609137857.
3. Sasaki CT, Ross DA, Hundal J. Association between Zenker diverticulum and gastroesophageal reflux disease: development of a working hypothesis. Am J Med. 2003;115(Suppl 3A):169S–71S. https://doi.org/10.1016/s0002-9343(03)00218-3.
4. Gage-White L. Incidence of Zenker's diverticulum with hiatus hernia. Laryngoscope. 1988;98(5):527–30. https://doi.org/10.1288/00005537-198805000-00010.

5. Prisman E, Genden EM. Zenker diverticulum. Otolaryngol Clin N Am. 2013;46(6):1101–11. https://doi.org/10.1016/j.otc.2013.08.011.

6. Muñoz AA, Shapiro J, Cuddy LD, Misono S, Bhattacharyya N. Videofluoroscopic findings in dysphagic patients with cricopharyngeal dysfunction: before and after open cricopharyngeal myotomy. Ann Otol Rhinol Laryngol. 2007;116(1):49–56. https://doi.org/10.1177/000348940711600109.

7. Albers DV, Kondo A, Bernardo WM, et al. Endoscopic versus surgical approach in the treatment of Zenker's diverticulum: systematic review and meta-analysis. Endosc Int Open. 2016;4(6):E678–86. https://doi.org/10.1055/s-0042-106203.

8. Yuan Y, Zhao YF, Hu Y, Chen LQ. Surgical treatment of Zenker's diverticulum. Dig Surg. 2013;30(3):207–18. https://doi.org/10.1159/000351433.

9. Leong SC, Wilkie MD, Webb CJ. Endoscopic stapling of Zenker's diverticulum: establishing national baselines for auditing clinical outcomes in the United Kingdom. Eur Arch Otorhinolaryngol. 2012;269(8):1877–84. https://doi.org/10.1007/s00405-012-1945-3.

10. Verdonck J, Morton RP. Systematic review on treatment of Zenker's diverticulum. Eur Arch Otorhinolaryngol. 2015;272(11):3095–107. https://doi.org/10.1007/s00405-014-3267-0.

11. Rich JT, Milov S, Lewis JS Jr, Thorstad WL, Adkins DR, Haughey BH. Transoral laser microsurgery (TLM) +/− adjuvant therapy for advanced stage oropharyngeal cancer: outcomes and prognostic factors. Laryngoscope. 2009;119(9):1709–19. https://doi.org/10.1002/lary.20552.

12. Ernster JA, Meyers AD. Zenker Diverticulum. 2020. https://emedicine.medscape.com/article/836858-overview#a1. Accessed 28 June 2020.

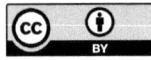

Gastroesophageal Reflux Disease

Adam Frankel and B. Mark Smithers

Introduction

Gastroesophageal reflux disease (GORD) is defined as troublesome symptoms and/or injury to the esophageal mucosa consistent with acid exposure [1]. GORD is common, with an age-adjusted global prevalence of 9% but significant variation across the world [2]. The diagnosis can often be made on clinical grounds and is more likely if there is at least a partial response to a proton pump inhibitor (PPI) [3]. Indications for oesophageal testing have been recently updated in international consensus guidelines, which include guidelines where diagnosis is not clearly established [4]. Fundoplication is the use of the gastric fundus to create a high-pressure zone on or around the lower oesophagus and is usually performed laparoscopically. It can be considered in terms of the completeness of the wrap (generally from 90 to 360°), and if less than 360°, whether the wrap is brought anterior to the oesophagus, posterior, or both. The efficacy and side effect profiles of many of the approaches have been subjected to randomised trials: anterior 90 vs 360° [5]; anterior 180 vs 360° [6]; and pos-terior 270 vs 360° [7]. The relative merits of each have been recently reviewed by Morino and colleagues [8]. Fundoplication is at least as safe and effective as PPI in relieving the symptoms of GORD [9]. For PPI-refractory GORD, fundoplication is more effective than escalating medical therapy [10].

Indications

- Established GORD, with ongoing trouble-some symptoms or complications (e.g., reflux esophagitis).
- Trial of maximal medical therapy (MMT) or intolerance of medical therapy [11]. (MMT often interpreted as twice daily proton pump inhibitor (PPI)).

Contraindications (Relative)

- Unfit for general anaesthetic (e.g., major medical comorbidity).
- Unsafe (e.g., prior complex upper abdominal surgery or injury).
- Severe oesophageal dysmotility.

Pre-op Assessment (Diagnosis Established)

Assess safety to undergo GA/operation.

A. Frankel (✉) · B. M. Smithers
Upper Gastro-intestinal and Soft Tissue Unit, Princess Alexandra Hospital, Brisbane, Australia

Academy of Surgery, The University of Queensland, Brisbane, Australia

Preoperative education on the procedure and the likely postoperative course

- all patients will experience port site pain,
- many will get referred shoulder pain (capno-peritoneum and diaphragmatic manipulation/suturing),
- some get chest pain (oesophageal spasm, extensive hiatal dissection),
- likely one night as inpatient,
- diet upgraded from liquid to soft over time (weeks),
- in-depth discussion on possible side effects (especially gas-bloat and flatulence).

OT Setup

Instrumentation

- 3× 5 mm ports (one replaced with 12 mm if cut-down approach preferred or 10 mm camera required), 1× 8 mm port
- 5 mm 30 deg laparoscope (10 mm if using 12 mm port)
- Nathanson retractor—alternative is a ratcheted toothed grasper (requires via an additional 5 mm port in the epigastrium).
- 2× laparoscopic atraumatic graspers (e.g., Johan, DeBakey)
- Advanced energy device—author preference is Ligasure with Maryland-tip.
- Laparoscopic scissors, needle holder, and suction.
- Portex sling.
- Mechanical and chemical prophylaxis and antibiotics per local guidelines.

Surgical Technique

Essential Steps in Synthesis

- Optimal positioning.
- Consider patient safety, operative access, and surgeon ergonomics.
- Safe entry and appropriate port placement.
- Adequate view.

- Liver retraction to expose the entire hiatus.
- Fat retraction suture to expose the entire fundus and the superior pole of spleen.
- Mobilise fundus to allow a loose wrap. Separate from left diaphragm, usually with division of superior short gastrics.
- Dissect the hiatus, by dividing phrenoesophageal ligament, and mobilise the distal esophagus to achieve an adequate intra-abdominal length.
- Restore the normal anatomy, perform cruroplasty, reconstitute the phrenoesophageal attachment.
- Create the wrap. Fix the fundus to the diaphragm and oesophagus.

Description of the Technique

Patient's Position

Lithotomy
- We favor the ergonomics of lithotomy with both arms out; Allen's stirrups (padded leg supports) with reverse Trendelenburg; thighs horizontal.
- Surgeon between legs, camera operator seated on patient's left, instrument nurse +/− assistant on right.

Alternative, Patient supine
- Surgeon on the patient's left, assistant right side.
- Bed mount for Nathanson retractor on patient's right.

Entry (Site for the Laparoscope)

- Approximately 5 cm below the costal margin in midclavicular line. Excellent view of the gastro-splenic region and the left crus of the diaphragm especially in obese patients. (Fig. 1).
- Optical entry or open cut-down with Hasson's cannula.

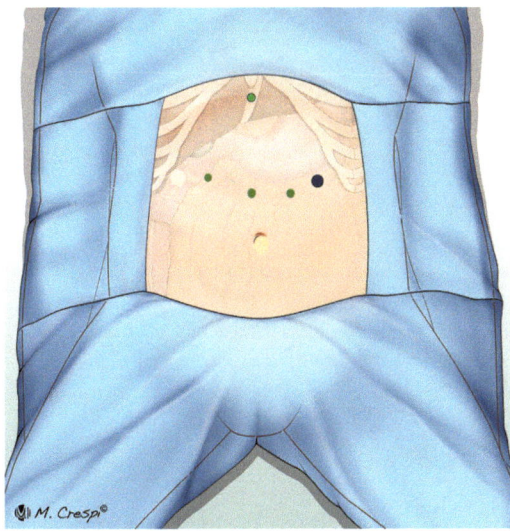

Fig. 1 Port placement

Other Ports

Placed under vision after local anaesthetic infiltration.

Precise location per surgeon preference and varied slightly for patient anatomy.

We use:

Surgeon's ports: 5 mm port—just right of midline for left hand; 8 (or 12) mm port left lateral upper quadrant, anterior to the tip of ninth rib for right hand.

- This port is used for needle and sling introduction and removal and as the exit site of the fat retraction suture.

Retraction port (assistant): 5 mm right upper quadrant

- Retraction and oesophageal sling manoeuvering,
- Liver retraction port: 5 mm sub-xiphisternal incision for Nathanson retractor. Alternatively, 5 mm port for ratcheted toothed grasper placed under left lobe of liver, attached to diaphragm 2 cm above the right crus.

Exposure to Commence Fundal Short Gastric Division (Fig. 2)

Liver retraction—Nathanson retractor or grasper (as above).

Omental retraction—Omental suture

- Via left lateral port, full length 2/0 polypropylene, artery clip on free end outside the body, multiple bites of omental fa, attached to superior greater curve overlying/covering the short gastric vessels. Needle removed via same port, port removed then reinserted with both arms of suture outside the port. Both suture arms secured with artery clip at skin level once adequate retraction. Retraction under vision monitoring the spleen, with cessation of retraction if any splenic movement.
- For obese patients, a retraction suture can be helpful on the lesser omentum to improve visualisation of the right crus and posterior hiatus.

Dissection

Limited division of superior short gastric vessels with Ligasure to allow sufficient mobility of fundus for the wrap.

- Assistant retracts the fundus to the right to expose short gastric vessels.
- If the gastro-splenic distance is very short, divide the peritoneum overlying the vessels as well as the peritoneal reflection from the fundus to the diaphragm first. This allows the vessels to lengthen and be divided with safety, avoiding physical or thermal injury to the stomach wall or splenic capsule.

Exposure and sharp division of the left phrenoesophageal ligament.

- Continue phrenoesophgeal ligament division anteriorly as far as possible to the right.

Expose the right crus.

- Assistant grasps anterior cardia fat pad and pushes to the left.
- Divide the superior lesser omentum with the Ligasure. It is rare to need to divide as low as the pars flaccida; open a few centimeters superiorly and preserve the hepatic branch/es of the vagus). Similarly, an aberrant left hepatic artery, if present, should be preserved.

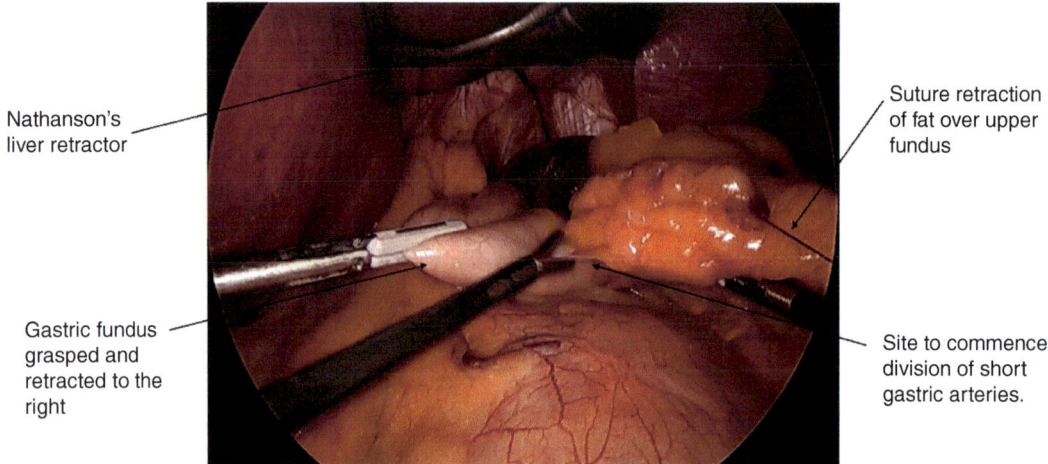

Nathanson's
liver retractor

Suture retraction
of fat over upper
fundus

Gastric fundus
grasped and
retracted to the
right

Site to commence
division of short
gastric arteries.

Fig. 2 Fat retraction and site of commencement of short gastric division

Complete dissection of the right phrenoesophageal ligament

- Sharp and blunt dissection to meet the dissection from the left.
- Anterior and posterior vagi must be identified and preserved.

Bluntly dissect posteriorly.

- Typically, with the suction device using blunt dissection, aiming to be between the posterior oesophageal wall and the posterior vagus so that it is excluded from the wrap. This is because unlike the anterior vagus, the posterior vagus is not closely applied to the oesophageal wall. After coming through the hiatus it turns abruptly posteriorly so that the majority of its fibres can join the coeliac and superior mesenteric plexuses. In the uncommon scenario of the posterior vagus not easily separating from the oesophagus it can be included in the wrap.

Pass a sling around the esophagus

- Pass a blunt grasper behind the oesophagus from right to left. View the grasper tip anterior to the left crus and bring in the sling via the left lateral port, passing it behind the oesophagus but in front of the posterior vagus

(see above). Both ends of the sling are taken out of the port and an artery forceps applied without tension.

- The two segments of the sling can be grasped close to the anterior oesophago-gastric junction by the assistant allowing the lower oesophagus to be manipulated.

Complete the anterior hiatal dissection

- With distal sling retraction, dissect the loose areolar tissue off the oesophagus. The anterior vagus usually runs on the oesophageal wall and is preserved.

Complete the posterior hiatal dissection

- Assistant lifts the sling anteriorly. Approach from the right aspect with the 30 deg scope angled to look to the left.
- Clear tissue posteriorly to identify the left crus through the window.
- If the posterior vagus was not included in the sling, it should be identified and pushed posteriorly.
- There should be a window for the wrap to be brought through.

Relax the sling and ensure an adequate intra-abdominal length of esophagus, which should be around 2 cm.

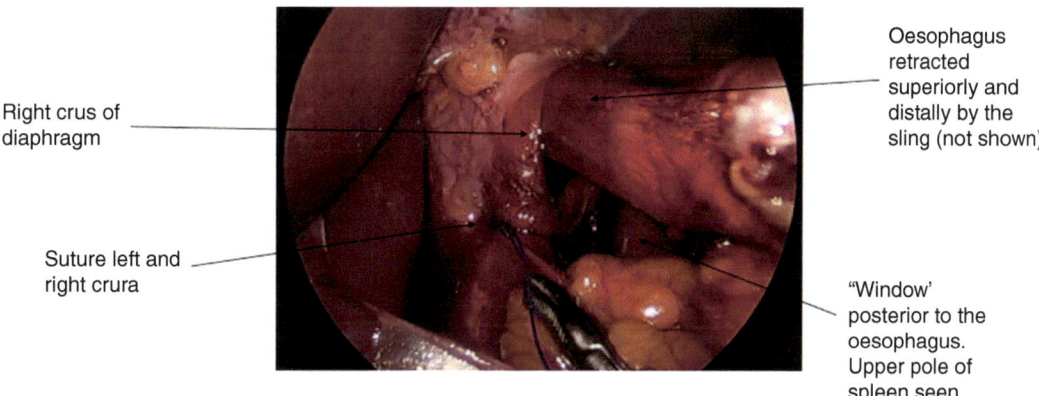

Right crus of diaphragm

Suture left and right crura

Oesophagus retracted superiorly and distally by the sling (not shown)

"Window' posterior to the oesophagus. Upper pole of spleen seen

Fig. 3 Approximation of the right and left crus posterior to oesophagus

Closure of the Hiatus (Fig. 3)

Approximate the posterior right and left crura

- Use interrupted 2/0 Novofil incorporating crural muscle and overlying connective tissue (otherwise at risk of the suture cutting through). Note that the bulk of the left crus is anterior requiring only a modest bite with the suture, while the right crus is thinner and a larger bite should be considered (ensuring no injury to the inferior vena cava). The left crus is usually also longer (semi-circular) than the more vertical and straight right crus, often necessitating asymmetric bites to ensure an appropriately-shaped hiatus is created.
- Closure should be enough for an anterior hiatal space that would allow two blunt graspers to be placed (without difficulty).
- Typically, one posterior suture is all that is required, if no hiatus hernia or minimal herniation is present. (Anterior hiatal suture closure is typically only required for giant hiatus hernias with large hiatal defect and attenuated left crus.)

Reconstruction of the Left Phrenoesophageal Ligament

This helps maintain an adequate intra-abdominal length of oesophagus and discourages herniation through the space, which, in our early experience, was the most common site for fundal hiatal herniation.

Assistant retracts the sling to the patient's right to identify the left crus.

Approximate the oesophagus muscle wall to the left crus.

- 3/0 Prolene or PDS continuous suture from 6 o'clock to 1 o'clock position
- Modest bites of the left crural pillar and the oesophageal muscularis propria.

Fundoplication—Nissen or Toupet (Fig. 4)

Conceptually, the fundus is taken behind the oesophagus with the angle of His being the pivot point and not rotated or displaced

- Loosen the left omental retraction suture/s.
- Left-hand grasper posterior to the oesophagus, right-hand grasper places the apex of the fundus into the left grasper.
- Bring the left grasper through the window to position the fundus on the right aspect of the intra-abdominal oesophagus.
- The segment of fundus is brought through more easily by grasping along the line of the superior/greater curve portion rather than the lower/distal portion of the fundus as it appears on the right side of the oesophagus.

A two-handed "toweling" maneuver can help to set the fundus in position.

- The divided short gastric vessels should lie anteriorly on the right, and the wrap should sit

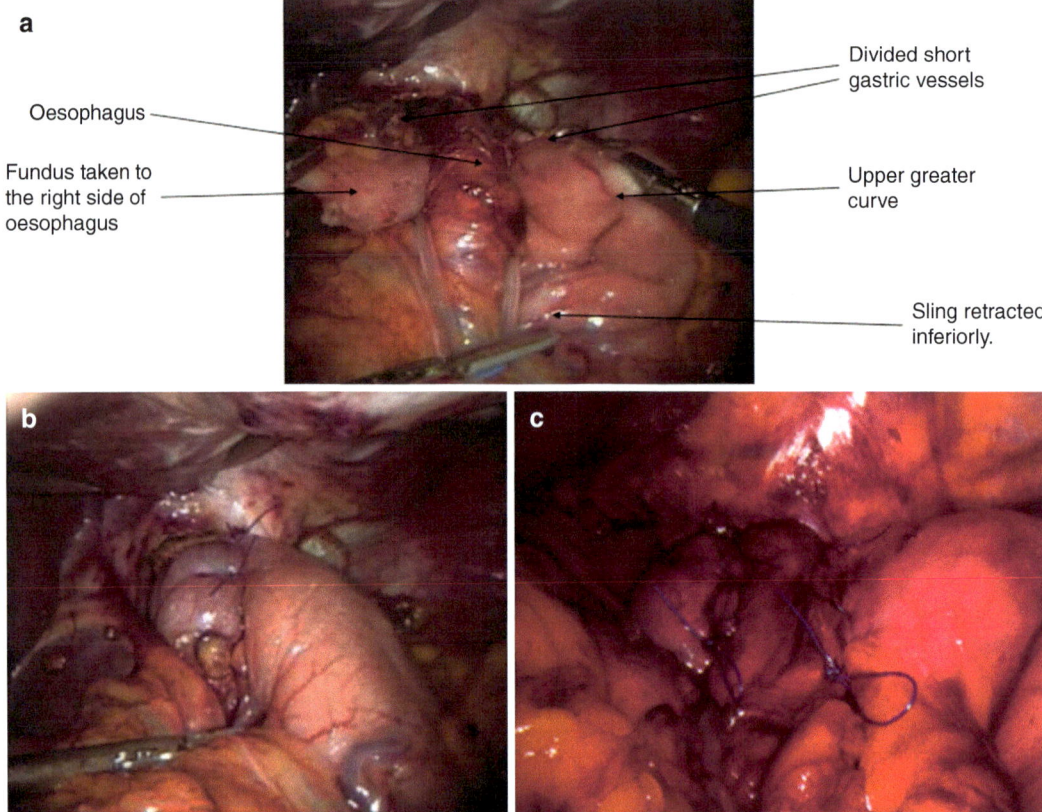

Fig. 4 (**a**) Fundus taken posterior to the oesophagus to the right—"toweling" maneuver to ensure no tension. (**b**) Completed fundoplication—Nissen (360). (**c**) Completed fundoplication—Toupet (270)

in position without tension. (If not, consider dividing another short gastric vessel).

- The assistant grasps the right portion of the fundus while surgeon gets the sutures. At this time, a bougie can also be passed by the anaesthetist.

Oesophageal bougie passed by anaesthetist.

- We routinely calibrate the hiatal closure with a 48Fr (small female) to 54Fr (large male) bougie.
- Any tension on the sling is released. The anaesthetist announces that it is being pushed distally with slow, cautious passage through the distal oesophagus into the stomach, carefully watched by the surgeon with close communication.
- Bougie is left in place while suturing the fundus.

Nissen Fundoplication

Left and right fundus sutured together anterior to the oesophagus with 2 x nonabsorbable sutures (2/0 Novofil)

- Bites of the seromuscular layer of the stomach, the muscularis propria of the esophagus (avoiding the anterior vagus nerve), and the seromuscular layer of the right fundus that had been held by the assistant.
- The assistant grasps the cardial fat pad to push posteriorly and retract distally after the suture is placed and before the suture is tied.
- The suture is tied. There should be minimal to no tension. If there is high tension then the suture should be removed and redone following manipulation of the fundal wrap.
- A second interrupted suture, 2 cm distal to the first, performed in the same manner.

Toupet Fundoplication (the authors' preferred option)

The right fundus is fixed to the hiatus and oesophagus followed by the left fundus fixed in the same way.

- At the 10 o'clock position, using a nonabsorbable suture (2/0 Novofil), a bite is taken of the oesophageal muscularis propria, the right crus and the fundus and tied.
- The assistant grasps the cardial fat pad to retract distally and push posteriorly to allow a good view of both fundal components and anterior oesophagus.
- A continuous suture is run picking up oesophagus and fundus for 2 cm and tied.
- This is then repeated on the left commencing at the 1 o'clock position.
- The anterior vagus is avoided and should lie between the two suture lines.
- Remove bougie.
- Gastropexy (after Nissan or Toupet fundoplication) using 2/0 Novofil interrupted suture to fix the fundus to the crura (7 o'clock on the right crus and 5 o'clock on the left crus). This may help to prevent recurrence, which usually occurs on the left and posteriorly.

Fundoplication—Anterior

Mobilization of oesophagus from the hiatus as described earlier

- There is rarely a need for the division of the short gastric branches.
- Ensure an adequate length of intra-abdominal oesophagus.
- There is no need for an oesophageal bougie.

Trial of wrapping anterior fundus across the oesophagus.

Fixation of the angle of His and left oesophagus

- Using a continuous nonabsorbable suture (2/0 Novofil), the angle of His is recreated by tak-

ing a bite of the lower antero-medial fundus and the left oesophago-gastric junction.
- The suture is progressed superiorly, between the antero-medial fundus and the left lateral oesophagus, up to the hiatus with the last bite including the left crus.

The fundus is folded 180° over the anterior oesophagus

- Starting superiorly, using a new nonabsorbable suture (2/0 Novofil), take a bite of stomach, oesophagus, and upper right crus at apex and suture tied.
- A continuous suture is progressed inferiorly, picking up the fundus, the right lateral oesophagus, and two further bites of the right crus.
- This is continued on the right lateral esophagus to the oesophago-gastric junction where the suture is tied.

Conclusion

Remove sling, retraction suture/s, Nathanson retractor under vision.

Complete evacuation of capnoperitoneum (reduces postoperative pain).

Ports removed under vision.

Skin closure and dressings per surgeon preference.

Complications and Management

Subcutaneous emphysema—ensure no airway compromise prior to extubation, then simple observation.

Capnothorax—due to pleural injury; observation is usually sufficient but evacuate capnothorax and capnoperitoneum if intra-operative cardiovascular or respiratory compromise.

Oesophageal spasm—see below (presents as severe chest pain in recovery or in the first few postoperative days).

Early dysphagia—best avoided with careful patient selection and intra-operative calibration of the wrap around a bougie; manage with restriction of diet (liquids); if severe then consider early endoscopy and/or reoperation.

Gas bloating—preoperative counseling (avoidance of excessive swallowing/aerophagia), postoperative counseling, cognitive behavioral therapy.

Excessive flatulence—as above.

Late dysphagia—possible causes include hiatus hernia or wrap failure allowing erosive oesophageal injury or stricture; at clinician's discretion, swallow study, CT, or endoscopy. Also, consider non-GORD diagnoses such as oesophageal dysmotility or malignancy.

Post-op Care

Regular simple analgesia, stronger analgesia (e.g. opiate) as required but this isn't common.

Dull central chest pain is usually from oesophageal spasm.

- In patients with risk factors for ischaemic heart disease, exclude acute coronary syndrome.
- Treat with reassurance, sitting upright, slow deep breathing, and a trial of IV hyoscine butylbromide (Buscopan), sublingual glyceryl trinitrate, or an oral calcium channel blocker if no contraindications exist. Opiates are not always helpful and can cause vomiting; consider a small dose of anxiolytic (e.g., 1 mg midazolam).

Smooth extubation and aggressive prophylaxis against postoperative nausea and vomiting

- Avoid retching which may contribute to early failure of the repair.
- Respiratory exercises (e.g., incentive spirometry), chest physiotherapy.
- Mechanical and chemical prophylaxis for venous thromboembolism.

Liquid diet for 24 h, upgrade if tolerating to a minced and moist diet for 4 weeks, then cautious reintroduction of solids.

References

1. Vakil N, van Zanten SV, Kahrilas P, Dent J, Jones R. The Montreal definition and classification of gastroesophageal reflux disease: a global evidence-based consensus. Am J Gastroenterol. 2006;101(8):1900–20. quiz 43
2. Dirac MA, Safiri S, Tsoi D, Adedoyin RA, Afshin A, Akhlaghi N, et al. The global, regional, and national burden of gastro-oesophageal reflux disease in 195 countries and territories, 1990–2017: a systematic analysis for the global burden of disease study 2017. Lancet Gastroenterol Hepatol. 2020;5(6):561–81.
3. Savarino E, Bredenoord AJ, Fox M, Pandolfino JE, Roman S, Gyawali CP, et al. Advances in the physiological assessment and diagnosis of GERD. Nat Rev Gastroenterol Hepatol. 2017;14(11):665–76.
4. Gyawali CP, Kahrilas PJ, Savarino E, Zerbib F, Mion F, Smout AJPM, et al. Modern diagnosis of GERD: the Lyon consensus. Gut. 2018;67(7):1351–62.
5. Hopkins RJ, Irvine T, Jamieson GG, Devitt PG, Watson DI. Long-term follow-up of two randomized trials comparing laparoscopic Nissen 360° with anterior 90° partial fundoplication. BJS (British Journal of Surgery). 2020;107(1):56–63.
6. Cai W, Watson DI, Lally CJ, Devitt PG, Game PA, Jamieson GG. Ten-year clinical outcome of a prospective randomized clinical trial of laparoscopic Nissen versus anterior 180(degrees) partial fundoplication. Br J Surg. 2008;95(12):1501–5.
7. Du X, Hu Z, Yan C, Zhang C, Wang Z, Wu J. A meta-analysis of long follow-up outcomes of laparoscopic Nissen (total) versus Toupet (270°) fundoplication for gastro-esophageal reflux disease based on randomized controlled trials in adults. BMC Gastroenterol. 2016;16(1):88.
8. Morino M, Ugliono E, Allaix ME, Rebecchi F. Laparoscopic surgery for gastroesophageal reflux disease: Nissen, Toupet or anterior fundoplication Ann Laparosc Endosc Surgery 2019;4.
9. Galmiche J-P, Hatlebakk J, Attwood S, Ell C, Fiocca R, Eklund S, et al. Laparoscopic Antireflux surgery vs esomeprazole treatment for chronic GERD: the LOTUS randomized clinical trial. JAMA. 2011;305(19):1969–77.
10. Spechler SJ, Hunter JG, Jones KM, Lee R, Smith BR, Mashimo H, et al. Randomized trial of medical versus surgical treatment for refractory heartburn. N Engl J Med. 2019;381(16):1513–23.
11. Kim D, Velanovich V. Surgical treatment of GERD: where have we been and where are we going? Gastroenterol Clin. 2014;43(1):135–45.

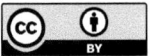

Hiatal Hernia: Update and Technical Aspects

Andrea Zanoni, Alberto Sartori, and Enrico Lauro

Introduction

Hiatal hernia is defined as the herniation of the stomach, possibly with other abdominal cavity elements, through the esophageal hiatus of the diaphragm. The most used classification describes four types of hernia: type I is the sliding hiatus hernia; type II the rolling hernia, where the gastric fundus herniate, while the gastroesophageal junction remains in the abdomen; type III the mixed hernia: with elements of both types I and II hernias; type IV is characterized by the presence of organs other than the stomach in the hernia sac. Types II–IV hernias as a group are referred to as paraesophageal hernias. Type I is the most common (95% of the cases), followed by type III, which comprises almost all paraesophageal hernias. Type II and IV are rare. Gastric volvulus is commonly associated with paraesophageal hiatal hernias. During sac reduction, the content is also retracted into the abdomen and the volvulus is automatically derotated. Natural history of hiatal hernias is not really known, but preliminary studies suggest that, like all other types of hernia, they tend to increase in size over time [1]. The anatomic disruption of the gastroesophageal junction, due to

hiatal hernia, leads to the disruption of natural anti-reflux mechanisms and hernia size is one of the main determinant of reflux severity [2]. Indeed, symptoms of hiatal hernia can be distinguished into GERD-related and Non-GERD-related. GERD symptoms are described in another chapter. Non-GERD symptoms include all those related to compression of mediastinal structures and to damage of herniated organs. A particular case is that of asymptomatic paraesophageal hernias. In those patients, prophylactic paraesophageal hernia repair is debated among experts. Although there is no consensus, most would agree that very old or debilitated patients should not undergo surgery, while younger and healthier patients, with a life expectancy of at least 10 years, should consider surgery to prevent both the risk of acute complications and potentially progressive symptoms [3].

We here describe hiatal hernia repair associated with floppy Nissen fundoplication. This procedure appears to be the most effective one and is considered the gold standard [4, 5] but it is also associated with nonnegligible potential for dysphagia and gas bloat syndrome. Adding a fundoplication after crural repair is strongly suggested by experts to stabilize the repair and reduce postoperative GERD; however, this step is not considered strictly necessary in the literature. The use of meshes is debated, but it can be useful, if not even necessary, in some cases of difficult direct repair. Both absorbable and nonabsorbable meshes have been used. We prefer absorbable meshes, which disappear and create a scaffold for tissue repair, reduc-

A. Zanoni (✉) · E. Lauro
General Surgery Division, Santa Maria del Carmine Hospital, Rovereto, Italy
e-mail: andrea.zanoni@apss.tn.it

A. Sartori
U.O. General and Emergency Surgery, San Valentino Hospital, Montebelluna, Treviso, Italy

© The Author(s) 2023
D. Lomanto et al. (eds.), *Mastering Endo-Laparoscopic and Thoracoscopic Surgery*,
https://doi.org/10.1007/978-981-19-3755-2_35

ing if not eliminating the risk of esophageal erosion. This dreaded complication has been instead reported for nonabsorbable meshes.

Moreover, the pressure gradient across the abdominal and thoracic cavities predisposes the patient to recurrence. The clinical recurrence rate is much lower than radiographic recurrence (assessed by a barium esophagram). Most patients with radiographic recurrence after repair are asymptomatic. Only a small fraction of patients will require a re-repair for complications or intractable symptoms (around 15% of patients). Since complications are not negligible, meticulous selection of patients, good indications, and careful application of surgical principles and techniques are mandatory to increase the chance of successful results. In this chapter, we will mainly focus on indications for surgery and surgical steps, since we strongly believe that these are the keys for a successful operation.

Indications

GERD-Related Esophageal Indications

- Failed optimal medical management (persistent symptoms on PPI).
- Noncompliance (unwillingness or intolerance/side effects) with chronic medical therapy.
- High volume/severe regurgitation (liquid or solid) and regurgitation as main complaint.
- Nonacid reflux.
- Severe esophagitis by endoscopy (Los Angeles C & D) and stricture.
- Barrett's columnar-lined epithelium (short Barrett & without severe dysplasia or carcinoma).

GERD-Related Extra-esophageal Indications (If Condition Is Surely Related to Reflux)

- hoarseness.
- cough.
- globus (lump sensation in the throat).

- laryngitis and laryngospasm.
- asthma.
- recurrent aspiration pneumonia.
- cardiac conduction defects.
- dental erosions and gingivitis.
- symptomatic or complicated paraesophageal hernia.

Non-GERD Indications

- Emergency repair: acute gastric volvulus, uncontrolled bleeding, obstruction, strangulation, perforation, or respiratory compromise secondary to a paraesophageal hernia.
- Elective repair: subacute symptoms, like respiratory complications from mechanical compression of the lungs (post-prandial chest fullness, shortness of breath), dysphagia, post-prandial thoracic pain, anemia or chronic bleeding, cardiac problems from compression of the heart.
- Prophylactic repair in asymptomatic patients: suggested in fit patients.

Contraindications

- Unstable or incurable preexisting comorbidities.
- Unable to tolerate general anesthesia.
- Morbidly obese patients (BMI >40 kg/m^2) (relative, consider bariatric surgery).
- Advanced age (relative).
- Coagulopathy (relative).
- Previous extensive abdominal surgery (relative).

Preoperative Workup

- EGD (to detect esophagitis, hiatal hernia, Barrett's esophagus, or neoplastic lesions).
- 24 hours pH-impedence test (only in case of GERD symptoms)
- Barium swallow (to measure the size of hiatal hernia, to describe if hernia is stable or intermittent, to detect and describe the degree of regurgitation of contrast medium).

- Manometry (to rule out dismotility, like achalasia).
- CT scan (to study the anatomy of esophago-gastric junction-EGJ region and rule out extrinsic compression of the esophagus and EGJ).

Laparoscopic Instrumentations

- Laparoscopic gauzes and epinephrine (water-diluted epinephrine-soaked gauzes can help stop minimal bleeding).
- Veress needle.
- Three 10–12 mm trocars and two 5 mm trocars.
- Bipolar laparoscopic forceps.
- Energy device: ultrasonic or radiofrequency dissector.
- Laparoscopic curved scissor.
- Laparoscopic needle holder.
- 2/0 or 0 nonabsorbable braided suture.
- Endoscopic liver retractor and table-mounted retractor holder.
- Endoclip applier.
- Atraumatic graspers.
- Cotton surgical tape or Penrose drain.
- Suction/irrigation device.
- Mesh (absorbable or nonabsorbable).

Patient Setup and Position

- Standard supine position.
- Split legs "French Position" (suggested, but optional) or Standard Supine "American Position."
- Reverse Trendelenburg position.
- Surgeon between patient's legs or on the patient's left side.

Trocars Placement (Fig.1)

- Port A (10 mm): camera port. Initial access is gained with an open or closed technique approximately 12–14 cm from the xiphoid process, slightly on the left side of the patient.

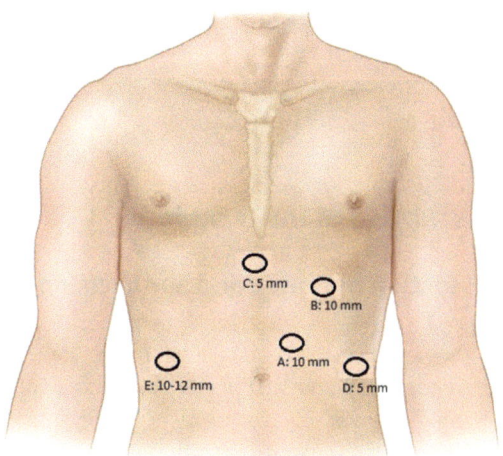

Fig. 1 Port placement

The distance from midline increases in patients with higher BMI.
- Port B (10 mm): surgeon's right-hand working port. Placed on the midclavicular line on the left side of the patient, immediately below the costal margin.
- Port C (5 mm): surgeon's left-hand working port. Below the xiphoid process, slightly higher than port B to better access the mediastinum. It is preferable to place this port immediately left to the falciform ligament to avoid interference during instrument exchanges.
- Port D (5 mm): first assistant port, placed just below the left costal margin.
- Port E (5–12 mm): liver retractor port, placed below the right costal margin.

Surgical Technique

There are several controversies in the surgical repair of a hiatal hernia but some steps are still critical for a successful outcome [3].

Essential Steps

Dissection of hiatus and sac excision.
Mobilization of esophagus.
Mobilization of gastric fundus and short gastric vessel division.

Crural closure with or without mesh reinforcement.

Floppy Nissen fundoplication.

Control endoscopy (optional).

Description of the Technique

Dissection of Hiatus and Sac Excision

- After trocars placement, abdominal exploration is carried out and liver is retracted, exposing the hiatus (Fig. 2).
- The procedure starts with the division of the pars flaccida and condensa of lesser omentum, possibly preserving the left vagal branch of the anterior vagus, with right crus identification.
- Then, the right crus is dissected starting at the 11 o'clock position, bluntly entering the mediastinum. A gentle reduction of the hernia contents is initially attempted, but only for the part that can be easily reduced: the critical step is to reduce the entire sac into the abdomen, which will bring together the content. Sac dissection facilitates reduction of the hernia, protects the esophagus from iatrogenic damage, and decreases early recurrence.
- The sac dissection is bluntly carried out with the assistant grasping the sac margin and pulling it downwards. It is important to completely dissect and reduce the sac into the abdomen, possibly without tearing it. The dissection will need to go down to the decussation of the crural fibers of the left crus. The peritoneal cover-

age of the crus should be preserved to provide some support at the time of crural closure.

- Care should be taken to identify and preserve the anterior and posterior vagus nerves, remembering that the anterior one traverses along the anterior esophagus from the left of the patient, while the posterior one comes from the right.
- When the sac and its contents are successfully reduced, a retroesophageal passage is created and a cotton surgical tape or Penrose drain is placed around the esophagus, to provide atraumatic retraction by the first assistant for safe esophageal dissection (Fig. 3).

Mobilization of Esophagus

- Retracting the surgical tape inferiorly, dissection around the esophagus is carried out. Since it is a mainly an avascular plane, blunt dissection should be preferred as much as possible, with the exception of a few esophageal aortic branches that need division with the energy device.
- The esophagus should be freed and mobilized extensively up to the inferior pulmonary veins. It is important to gain at least 3 cm of intra-abdominal esophagus, which should be mobile and should remain in the abdomen without tension.
- Important structures surround the esophagus in the mediastinum, care should be taken to identify and preserve both vagus nerves and avoid injury of pleura, pericardium, inferior pulmonary veins, and aorta. Injury of the pleura during mediastinal dissection is fre-

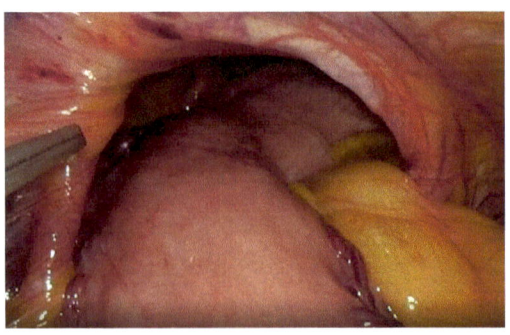

Fig. 2 Large Hiatal Hernia at diagnostic laparoscopy

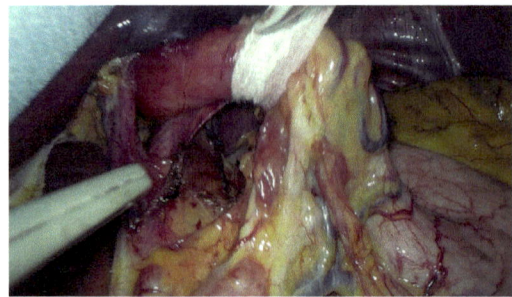

Fig. 3 A Retro-esophageal window is created to facilitate dissection and mobilization of the lower esophagus

quent in big hernias, nevertheless it does not require to be repaired to avoid causing tension pneumothorax. At the end of the procedure, the Valsalva maneuver at extubation will evacuate CO_2. Rarely, in case of severe respiratory distress, a chest drain can be placed.

Mobilization of Gastric Fundus and Short Gastric Vessels Division

– When the esophagus is well mobilized, the gastric fundus mobilization begins. The key to successful floppy Nissen consists in the division of the short gastric vessels necessary for the fundoplication, avoiding excessive gastrolysis on the greater curvature, which might be involved in "gas bloat syndrome."
– The first assistant grasps the apex of the gastrosplenic ligament and the surgeon the anterior wall of the stomach for countertraction. Then the lesser sac is entered approximately above the lower limit of the spleen, used as a caudal landmark. The dissection proceeds upwards close to the gastric wall, avoiding inadvertent thermal injuries to the stomach, up to the left crus (Fig. 4).
– The fundus must be freed completely on the posterior wall, dividing all short gastric vessels. High Frequency bipolar or ultrasonic dissectors normally provide good hemostasis without the need for clipping.
– Mobilization of the gastric fundus ends the first part of the procedure. Correct mobilization of esophagus and gastric fundus is mandatory to obtain an adequate retroesophageal window for a floppy Nissen.

Crural Closure with or Without Mesh Reinforcement

– The crus should be closed posteriorly, with possible addition of anterior closure in case of wide hiatus.
– The crus should be repaired with 0 or 2/0 braided nonabsorbable sutures. Normally a direct closure is sufficient to repair the defect. Nevertheless, in case of a huge hiatal defect (normally more than 5 cm) or weak and fragile crural muscles, a mesh can be placed onlay after direct repair. "Figure of 8" sutures or simple interrupted sutures are the best options for crural repair (Fig. 5). Both absorbable and nonabsorbable meshes have been used. We prefer absorbable meshes, which disappear and create a scaffold for tissue repair, reducing if not eliminating the risk of esophageal erosion (Fig. 6). This dreaded complication has been instead reported for nonabsorbable meshes. The mesh is fixed laterally to the pillars with single stitches or absorbable tacks, avoiding to place tacks on the anterior and

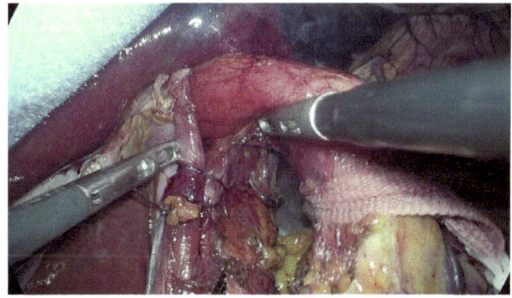

Fig. 5 Crural Closure using breaded nonabsorbable suture

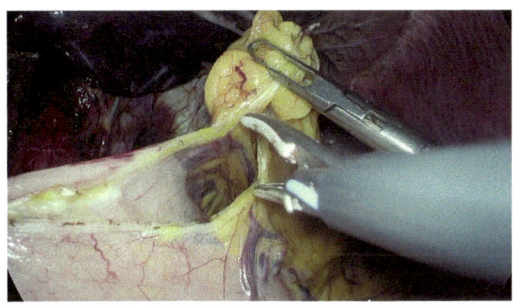

Fig. 4 Gastric Fundus mobilization along the greater curvature

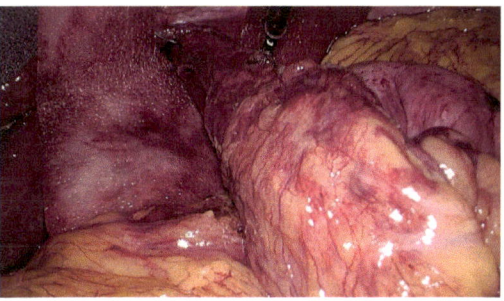

Fig. 6 Mesh used for crural reinforcement (optional)

posterior hiatus, for the high risk of damage to pericardium and aorta, respectively.

- The crural closure should neither strangulate nor shred the muscle.
- Once the hiatus is repaired, the esophagus should comfortably occupy the defect, without being angulated or compressed. The closure should permit easy passage of a 5 mm-tip instrument.

Floppy Nissen Fundoplication

- The last step of the procedure consists of the construction of a floppy fundoplication. This is 360° fundoplication positioned around the distal esophagus and esophagogastric junction (at the level of the Z line). It must be short (2 cm long) and tension-free.
- The reduced sac should be excised in order to have a more clean gastric wall to properly perform a correct fundoplication.
- The stomach is replaced in anatomical position and the assistant retracts the esophagus with the surgical cotton tape to expose the retroesophageal window and the posterior wall of the stomach.
- The surgeon brings the posterior fundus through the retroesophageal window. Then the so-called *shoeshine maneuver* is used to confirm that the fundus remains comfortably in position and is not retracted to the left of the patient (Fig. 7).
- The fundoplication is created with 2 or 3 interrupted nonabsorbable braided sutures (0 or 2/0). One or more sutures can incorporate the anterior esophageal wall. Nonetheless, we prefer to avoid including the esophagus, obtaining a more floppy wrap, and avoid damaging the anterior vagus nerve (Fig. 8). We prefer fixing the fundoplication with a lateral suture from the inferior left border of the wrap to the anterolateral esophageal wall at the level of the dissected phrenoesophageal membrane, in order to avoid telescoping or slippage of the wrap (Fig. 9). Other sutures can be added on the right side or cranially

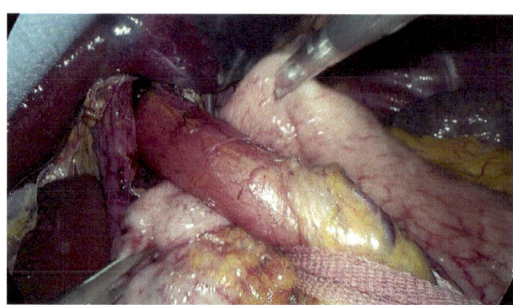

Fig. 7 The so-called *shoeshine maneuver* to confirm that the fundus is sliding loose around the esophagus

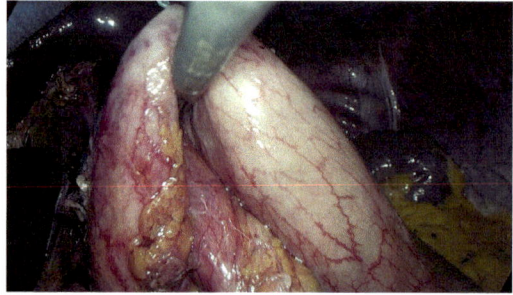

Fig. 8 A floppy fundoplication is made

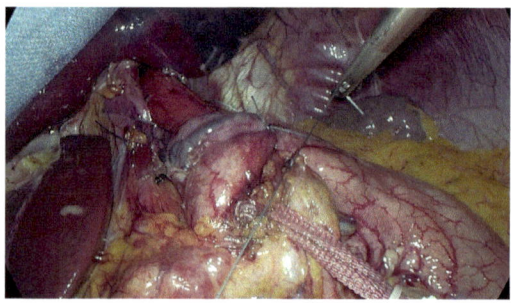

Fig. 9 To avoid slippage, additional suture may be useful to fix the wrap inferiorly

above the fundoplication if needed. Posterior or anterior gastropexy sutures can be further added.
- Intraoperative control endoscopy can be performed to confirm correct position and patency of the fundoplication and absence of twisting.
- No drain is normally necessary. The trocars are removed and the incisions are closed in standard fashion.

Postoperative Care and Follow-Up

- Upper GI Gastrografin study [1] on the first postoperative day is possible but not mandatory.
- Clear liquids are allowed on the first postoperative day (POD1).
- Soft mashed diet is started on POD2 and it is suggested until POD7.
- Soft fractionated diet is started on POD8 and suggested for 4–8 weeks, followed by return to regular diet.
- Postoperative dysphagia and delayed gastric emptying are common, but patients should be instructed that these symptoms are typically self-limiting and should disappear approximately 2 months after surgery.
- Antiemetics are given at scheduled times for the first 24 h, to avoid early retching and early recurrence, and then on demand.
- PPI are normally used in the first 15–30 days and then suspended.
- Discharged with prescription for antiemetics.
- Follow-up at 1 week with clinical evaluation, then at 1 month with a barium swallow study. We normally suggest further clinical evaluation at 6 months after surgery and then on demand.

References

1. Abdelmoaty W, Dunst C, Fletcher R, et al. The development and natural history of hiatal hernias: a study using sequential barium upper gastrointestinal series. Ann Surg. 2020;275(3):534–8. https://doi.org/10.1097/SLA.0000000000004140.
2. Jones MP, Sloan SS, Rabine JC, Ebert CC, Huang CF, Kahrilas PJ. Hiatal hernia size is the dominant determinant of esophagitis presence and severity in gastroesophageal reflux disease. Am J Gastroenterol. 2001;96(6):1711–7.
3. Bonrath EM, Grantcharov TP. Contemporary management of paraesophageal hernias: establishing a European expert consensus. Surg Endosc. 2015;29(8):2180–95.
4. Guidelines for surgical treatment of gastroesophageal reflux disease (GERD). Society of American Gastrointestinal and Endoscopic Surgeons (SAGES). https://www.sages.org/publications/guidelines/guidelines-for-surgical-treatment-of-gastroesophageal-reflux-disease-gerd/.
5. Guidelines for the management of hiatal hernia. Society of American Gastrointestinal and Endoscopic Surgeons (SAGES). https://www.sages.org/publications/guidelines/guidelines-for-the-management-of-hiatal-hernia/.

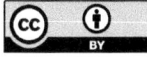

Esophageal Cysts

Aung Myint Oo

Introduction

Esophageal cysts are rare congenital anomalies of gastrointestinal tract first described by Blasius in 1711. In 1881, Roth also described esophageal cysts and there are two categories namely simple epithelial lined cysts and esophageal duplication cysts. Esophageal duplication cysts are embryologic duplication of part of the esophageal mucosa and submucosa without epithelial duplication. The prevalence of esophageal duplication cysts is 0.0122% and accounts for 10–15% of duplication cysts in the gastrointestinal tract [1]. Esophageal cysts and duplications usually do not have communication with the lumen and they can be found in the neck, chest, and abdomen. Most of the esophageal duplication cysts (two-thirds) are found in the lower esophagus in the right posteroinferior mediastinum while 1/3 in the upper/middle third of esophagus and sometimes lesions can be found in the intra-abdominal esophagus.

Presentation

67% of esophageal duplication cysts in adults can be presented with symptoms and chest pain is the most common symptom followed by dysphagia. Some other symptoms include epigastric discomfort, vomiting, stridor, cough, bleeding, and hematemesis. Presentation of hematemesis is associated with the presence of gastric epithelium in the cyst. Rarely they can present as malignant transformation. Sometimes esophageal cysts are diagnosed incidentally.

Diagnosis

Diagnosis can be made mainly by computed tomography (CT) and endoscopic ultrasound (EUS). Fluid-filled cystic lesion arising from esophagus in CT scan usually represents the diagnosis of esophageal cysts which can be confirmed by EUS. On EUS examination, the duplication cysts appear as periesophageal homogenous hypoechoic mass with multilayered wall and well-defined margins or sometimes as anechoic cysts due to a considerable amount of central fluid. EUS-guided FNA aspiration is associated with risks of infection as high as 14% and thus EUS FNA/FNAB with appropriate antibiotics cover should be considered only when the diagnosis is in doubt or any suspicious features of malignant transformation. Esophageal cysts/duplication cysts are usually found as submucosal lesions during upper gastro-

A. M. Oo (✉)
Upper Gastrointestinal, Bariatric and Metabolic Surgery, Department of General Surgery, Tan Tock Seng Hospital, Singapore, Singapore
e-mail: myint_oo_aung@ttsh.com.sg

© The Author(s) 2023
D. Lomanto et al. (eds.), *Mastering Endo-Laparoscopic and Thoracoscopic Surgery*,
https://doi.org/10.1007/978-981-19-3755-2_36

intestinal endoscopy without involving the mucosa. If there is involvement of mucosa then biopsies can be taken during endoscopy.

Indications and Contraindications

Surgical removal is the treatment of choice for symptomatic patients. While asymptomatic patients can be opted for surveillance and follow up, surgical removal can also be considered due to the potential risks of complications including mucosal ulceration, bleeding, perforation, and rarely the malignant transformation. Simple cysts can be enucleated, the duplication cysts are excised. With the advancement in minimally invasive surgeries including endoscopic intervention, the outcomes are quite satisfactory and excellent. As surgical intervention is associated with long-term complications such as heartburn, reflux esophagitis, balancing the risks and benefits of surgical intervention is very important and needed to be carefully considered and counseled in asymptomatic patients without worrisome features. Endoscopic intervention by draining the cyst into the esophageal lumen or submucosal tunneling dissection can be considered for suitable patients including those with high risk for surgery.

Pre-op Assessment

Pre-op assessment is the same for those who need esophageal surgery. Those patients who need transthoracic approach will need their pulmonary function to be evaluated. Patient's fitness for general anesthesia and surgery will also be assessed preoperatively by anesthesiologists and optimization of comorbidities by respective specialists accordingly. Pre-op optimization of nutrition and rehabilitation with pulmonary physiotherapy will also be helpful for better postoperative outcomes.

OT Setup

Except for the intra-abdominal esophageal cysts which can be approached by laparoscopy most of the esophageal cysts are approached by thoracoscopy.

For laparoscopic approach, monitor for surgeon and scopist is at the eye level on the patient's left side and the monitor for the assistant on the right side. The energy devices are set up at the patient's foot, suction and irrigation at the patient's right near the head (Fig. 1).

For thoracoscopic approach with left lateral position, monitor for the surgeon and scopist at the eye level in front of the patient (surgeon and scopist positioned at the patient's back), while the assistant position at the front with the monitor facing him from the patient's back.

For thoracoscopic approach with semi-prone/prone position, monitor for the surgeon and scopist at the eye level facing the patient's back (surgeon and scopist position at the patient's front) while the assistant stands from the patient's back with monitor at the eye level from patient's front.

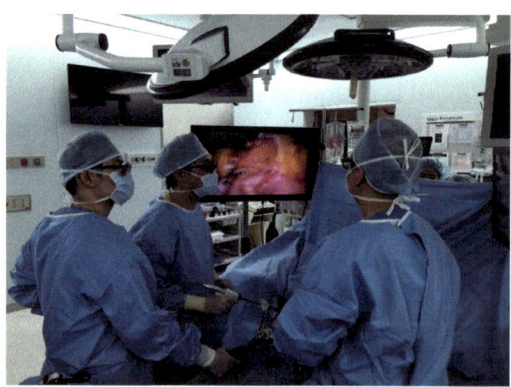

Fig. 1 OT setup for laparoscopic approach

Instrumentations

The following instruments are mostly used in the procedures.

30° telescope with camera system.
Short bowel grasper.
Mary land grasper.
Hook.
Energy device (ultrasonic dissector or advanced bipolar dissector).
Laparoscopic needle holder.
Scissors.
Lung retractor.
Liver retractor.

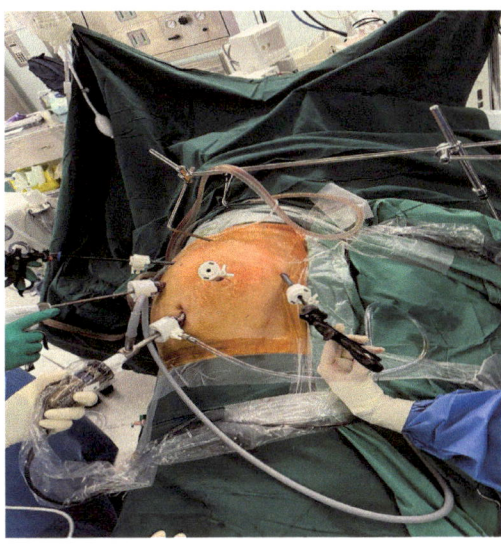

Fig. 2 Port positions for laparoscopic procedure

Patient's Position

For laparoscopic approach, patient is put in the supine position with reverse Trendelenburg and right side down position (Fig. 2).

For thoracoscopic left approach, patient is put in the left lateral position with both ventral and dorsal support with operating table bent at 30° at the level of pelvis to open the rib spaces as well as in the best position if open conversion is needed (Fig. 3).

For thoracoscopic semi-prone or prone approach, the support is put under the abdomen as well as at the level of the shoulder blade in to widen the rib spaces (Fig. 4a).

Regardless of the position, it is important to make sure that patient is well supported securely, and all the presser points are supported with soft pads/cushions.

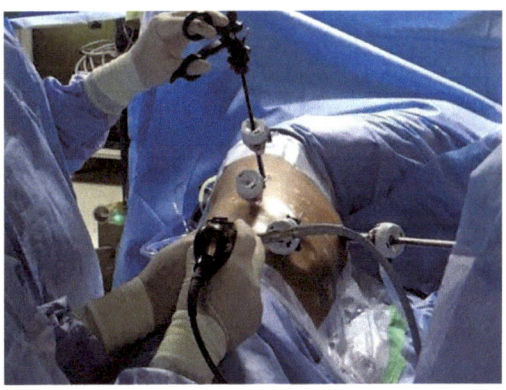

Fig. 3 Port positions for thoracoscopic procedure in left lateral position

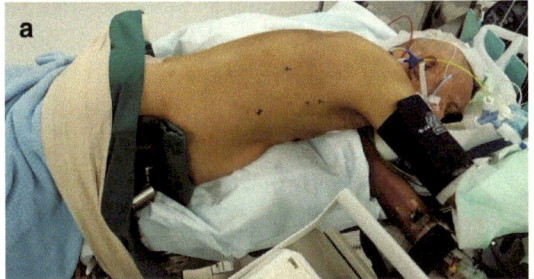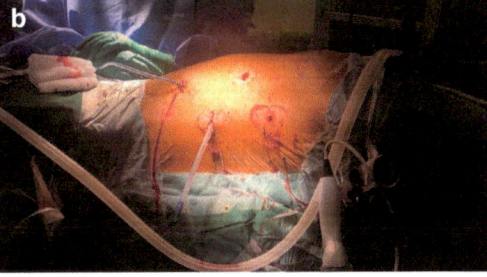

Fig. 4 (**a**) Patient is prone/semi prone position. (**b**) Ports positions in semi prone/prone position

Surgical Technique

Thoracoscopic Procedures for Thoracic Esophageal Cyst

After general anesthesia with one lung ventilation either using double lumen tubes or bronchial blocker, patient is positioned in left lateral position or semi-prone/prone position as per surgeon's preference. For left lateral position, 10 mm camera port is inserted at seventh or eighth intercostal space anterior axillary line. Working ports for surgeons are $1 \times 10 \times 12$ mm port at seventh or eighth intercostal space at posterior axillary line and 1×5 mm at third or fourth intercostal space mid axillary line. One assistant port either 5 or 10 mm depending on the availability of the lung retractor is inserted at fifth intercostal place ventral to the anterior axillary line (Fig. 3).

For semi-prone or prone position, $1 \times 10 \times 12$ mm camera port at seventh intercostal space posterior axillary line. 2×5 mm surgeon ports one at third or fourth intercostal space posterior axillary line and one just below the tip of the scapula. 1×5 mm assistant port at eighth or ninth intercostal space along the scapula line (Fig. 4b).

Laparoscopic Surgery for Intra-abdominal Esophageal Cyst

After general anesthesia, patient is positioned in the supine position, 10 mm camera port is inserted infra umbilicus, the 1×10 mm working port is inserted at right hypochondrium along the lateral border of rectus abdominus muscle and just lateral and superior to the camera port. 1×5 mm working port is inserted just 3–4 finger breadth above and slightly lateral to the 10 mm working port (Fig. 5) If needed the additional one or two assistant 5 mm ports can be inserted in the left upper abdomen (Fig. 2). The Nathanson liver retractor is inserted from the small 5 mm incision at the epigastrium just below the xiphisternum.

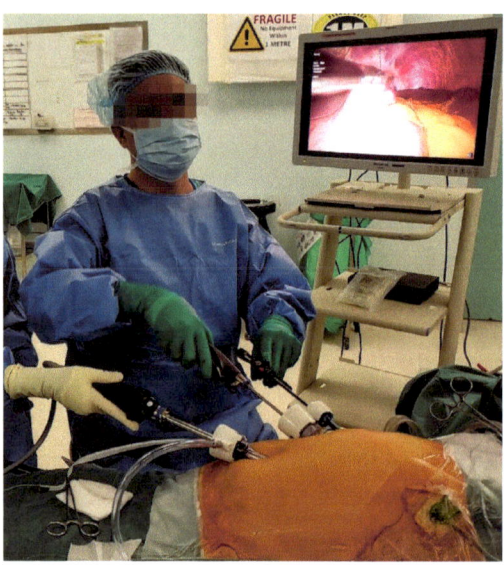

Fig. 5 Reduced Ports(three ports) position for laparoscopic procedure

Enucleation/Resection of Esophageal Cysts

After ports are inserted, the esophageal cyst is identified and mobilized carefully from mediastinal pleura by dissecting around the cyst using the energy device and hook diathermy. Dissection of the hiatus will be needed for intra-abdominal esophageal cysts. After dissecting the longitudinal and circular fibers of the esophageal wall, the enucleation/resection of the cyst is performed by dissecting the cyst completely off from the mucosa wall without injuring the cyst wall and mucosa. Care must also be taken not to injure the nerves during the dissection. After completion of the enucleation/resection of the cyst, on-table endoscopic examination with air sufflation under water is done to check for any mucosal injury and repair with 3/0 absorbable suture if needed. The dissected muscle fibers and pleura are then closed with 3/0 absorbable sutures to reinforce the defect as well as to prevent the pseudodiverticulum formation. After checking the hemostasis and suctioning of the fluid, the excised cyst is put into the retrieving bag and extracted by enlarging the camera port wound at the end of the surgery. For thoracoscopic procedure, one underwater seal chest tube drain is placed via one of the thoracoscopic port sites. The chest drain is kept for 1 or 2 days for post-op pneumothorax. However, drain is usually not needed for laparoscopic enucleation/resection of abdominal esophageal cyst.

Complications and Management

Even though complications are rare, the possible complications and their prevention/management include.

- Pneumonia—managed by pre- and post-op chest physiotherapy with incentive spirometry.
- Air leak and pneumothorax—may need a chest tube.
- Esophageal injury and leak—adequate drainage of the collection and nasogastric tube (NGT) decompression, application of endoscopic over the scope clip/esophageal stent, or rarely the surgical intervention.
- Injuries to vagus nerves and/or phrenic nerve—careful dissection during the excision/enucleation is very important to prevent injuries to the nerves.
- Formation of pseudodiverticulum—it is important to suture the muscle layers to prevent pseudodiverticulum formation.

- Bleeding—endoscopic hemostasis if intraluminal, or surgical hemostasis if bleeding did not stop spontaneously.
- Wound infection—less with the minimally invasive approach compared with open approach.

Post-op Care

Postoperatively patients will be monitored in the ward. The chest tube if inserted can be removed in the next 1 or 2 days if there is no pneumothorax. Patient can start oral liquid the next day followed by diet if tolerating well and most of the patients can be discharged on POD (Postoperative Day) 2 or 3. Chest physiotherapy with incentive spirometry and ambulatory physiotherapy can start on POD 1. After discharge, the patient is followed up in outpatient clinic.

Reference

1. Olajide AR, Yisau A, et al. Gastrointestinal duplications: experience in seven children and a review of the literature. Saudi J Gastroenterol. 2010;16(2):105–9. https://doi.org/10.4103/1319-3767.61237.

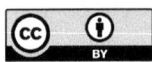

McKeown Esophagectomy

Koji Kono

Introduction

Esophageal cancer is the sixth most frequent cause of cancer death worldwide and affects more than 450,000 people all over the world [1]. Most patients with esophageal cancer in Asian countries such as Japan and China have squamous cell carcinoma (SCC), while most of those in Western countries have adenocarcinoma [2, 3]. In particular, the incidence of esophageal adenocarcinoma in the USA and the UK is rapidly increasing, in which the age-adjusted incidence has risen by 39·6% for men and 37·5% for women every 5 years in the UK [3]. Despite improvements in surgical techniques and perioperative management [4, 5] and surgery combined with chemotherapy and/or radiotherapy [6, 7], the prognosis of esophageal cancer at advanced stage remains poor with 30–40% in a 5-year survival globally [8] and the 5-year survival rate for the patients receiving esophagectomy in Japan was 55.5% [9].

It is generally accepted that conventional open surgical procedures for esophageal cancer are traumatic and invasive, despite continuous advances in perioperative management and surgical techniques. Since Cuschieri et al. reported thoracoscopic surgery in minimally invasive esophagectomy (MIE) in 1992 [10], MIE has become one of the standard surgical approach for esophageal cancer. A randomized trial of MIE compared with open esophagectomy showed a lower incidence of pulmonary infections, a shorter hospital stay, and better short-term quality of life than did open esophagectomy, with no compromise in the quality of the resected specimen [11]. Moreover, treatment in high-volume centers with experienced surgeons and the availability of critical-care support is associated with improved outcomes [12].

McKeown Esophagectomy

The common surgical approaches to curatively resect esophageal cancer include trans-hiatal, Ivor Lewis, and McKeown (three incision) esophagogastrectomy [13]. McKeown esophagectomy is defined as consisting of thoracic esophageal mobilization with lymph node dissection (thoracoscopic or open), abdominal exploration (laparoscopic or open), and stomach mobilization with lymph node dissection, and subsequently left cervical incision for anastomosis. Potential advantages of the McKeown approach compared to the Ivor Lewis include less incidence of local recurrence, applicable to the tumors at or above the level of carina, and anastomosis in neck easier to manage if anastomotic leak occurs [13]. The issue of two-field (thoracic

K. Kono (✉)
Department of Gastrointestinal Tract Surgery,
Fukushima Medical University, Fukushima, Japan
e-mail: kojikono@fmu.ac.jp

© The Author(s) 2023
D. Lomanto et al. (eds.), *Mastering Endo-Laparoscopic and Thoracoscopic Surgery*,
https://doi.org/10.1007/978-981-19-3755-2_37

+ abdomen) vs. three-field (thoracic + abdomen + neck) lymph node dissection is still debatable.

McKeown esophagectomy is appropriate for all patients with Siewert type I and II patients, as well as all patients with tumor above the gastroesophageal junction, up to the level of the clavicle. Most importantly, Ivor Lewis should not be applied to tumors at or above the level of carina due to the risk of a positive esophageal surgical margin.

Indications for McKeown Esophagectomy

- Carcinoma of the upper, middle, and lower third of the esophagus, especially applicable to the tumors above the level of carina.
- T1a carcinoma not amenable to endoscopic resection, T1b, T2, T3, and T4a.
- Salvage esophagectomy after definitive chemoradiation.
- End-stage benign strictures of the esophagus are not amenable to trans-oral dilations (caustic injury, peptic structures).

Contraindications

- Tracheobronchial, mediastinal, and intra-abdominal structures invasion (T4b).
- Stage IVb disease.
- Advanced physiologic age and frailty.
- Prohibitive comorbidities.

OT Setup

Device

The basic surgical device uses a spatula-type monopolar electric scalpel and LigaSure™ Maryland 37, and a microline scissors for manipulating around the recurrent laryngeal nerve.

Position/Port Position

Raise both hands, and take a prone position with the face fixed by Prone View® and the trunk fixed by a spine surgery operation frame (Spine Table) (Fig. 1). By using the position, interference between the forceps and the operating table is prevented. After intubation of a single lumen spiral tracheal tube, a blocker is placed in the right main bronchus for left single lung ventilation in order to make surgical field stable. Alternatively, both lung ventilation with artificial pneumothorax also can be possible.

Port placement starts with four ports as shown in Fig. 2 and 6 mmHg pressure under artificial pneumothorax. First, a 12 mm trocar is inserted into fifth intercostal space (ICS), while observing with a 0° rigid endoscope, and the pleural incision is safely observed under direct vision to prevent lung injury. After confirming the proper insertion of the port into the chest cavity, pneumothorax is initiated and a complete collapse of the right lung is obtained. Thereafter, the endoscope is changed to a 30° rigid endoscope to perform intrathoracic operation. Next, insert a 12 mm port into the ninth ICS as a camera port, and insert a 5 mm port into the seventh ICS and a 5 mm port into the third ICS. The operator uses

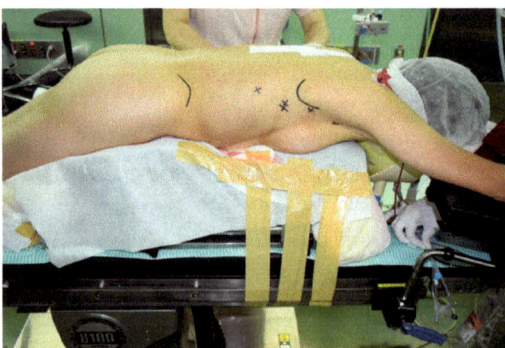

Fig. 1 Position of the patients. Raise both hands, and take a prone position with the face fixed by Prone View® and the trunk fixed by a spine surgery operation frame (Spine Table)

the fifth and seventh ICS port, and the assistant uses the third ICS port (Figs. 2 and 3).

First, a 12 mm trocar is inserted into V intercostal space (ICS), while observing with a 0°degree rigid endoscope, and the pleural incision is observed under direct vision to prevent lung injury. After confirming the proper insertion of the port into the chest cavity, pneumothorax is initiated and a complete collapse of the right lung is obtained. Thereafter, the endoscope is changed to a 30° rigid endoscope to perform intrathoracic operation. Next, insert a 12 mm port into the ninth ICS as a camera port, and insert a 5 mm port into the seventh ICS and a 5 mm port into the third ICS. The operator uses the fifth and seventh intercostal space port, and the assistant uses the third intercostal space port.

Insert a 12 mm port into the ninth intercostal space as a camera port and the operator uses the 5th (12 mm) and 7th (5 mm) intercostal space port, and the assistant uses the third intercostal space port (5 mm).

Description of the Technique

Dissection of the Azygos Vein

An incision is made in the mediastinum pleura and the azygos vein is isolated with preservation of the right bronchial artery at the backside of the azygos vein. The azygos vein is dissected with Powered ECHELON FLEX® 7 (Fig. 4) and confirm the preservation of the right bronchial artery (Fig. 5). At this point, the camera is moved to the fifth ICS port, and the Powered ECHELON is inserted from the ninth ICS to adjust the axis of the device. The dorsal stump of the azygos vein is grasped by the end loop PDSII® and lifted outward to ensure a visual field near the root of the right bronchial artery.

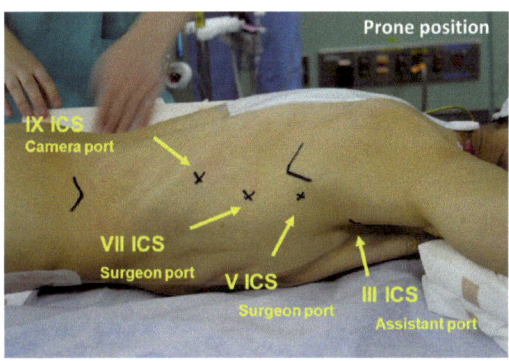

Fig. 2 Port insertion

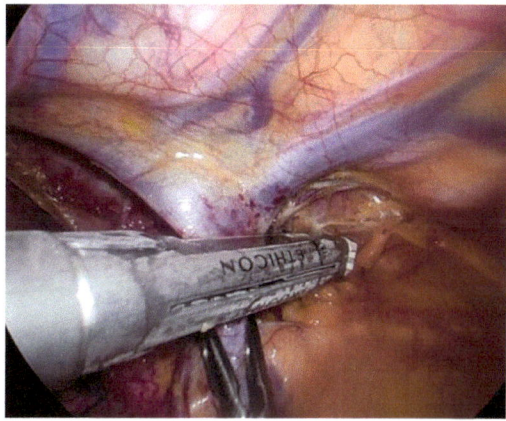

Fig. 4 Azygos vein transection

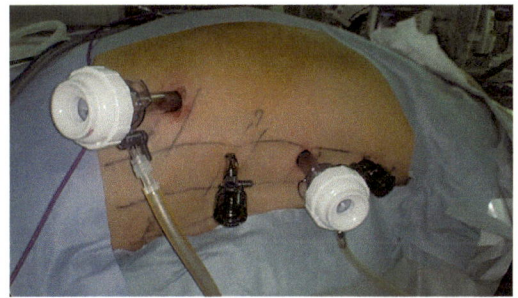

Fig. 3 Port

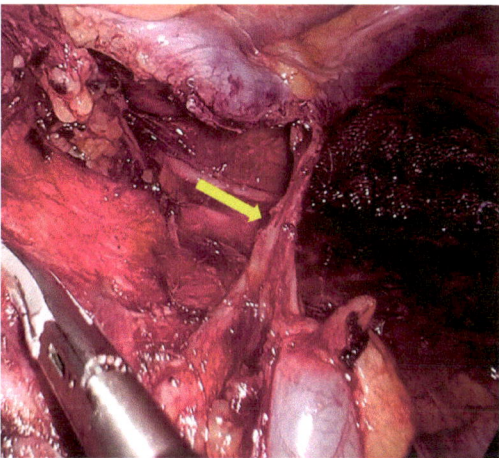

Fig. 5 Preservation of the right bronchial artery

Dissection of Lymph Node Along the Rt-recurrent Nerve

The mediastinal pleura is dissected along the right vagus nerve until the right subclavian artery, and the pleura is dissected posteriorly on the right subclavian artery to expose the front surface of the right subclavian artery (Fig. 6). Next, along the right wall of the trachea, the tissue containing the right recurrent laryngeal nerve is mobilized. At this time, the blood vessel plexus on the side wall of the trachea should be preserved to maintain the blood flow for the trachea. This lymphatic tissue is sharply and bluntly dissected with a Microline® scissor to identify and preserve the right recurrent laryngeal nerve and to dissect the lymph node, which is mainly located on the dorsal side (Fig. 6). In the area around the Rt-recurrent laryngeal nerve, the use of an electric scalpel or a vessel sealer should be avoided. Lymph node dissection is performed until the back side of the right subclavian artery and there is a branch of the inferior thyroid artery in the area, so it is essential to prevent bleeding and keep the surgical site dry.

Dissection of the Thoracic Duct

In the mediastinum, the ventral side of the azygos vein is mobilized from the Aorta, and the thoracic duct is identified on the ventral side. The ligation of the thoracic duct is based on the collective ligation including the surrounding tissue with the end loop PDSII® or clip (Fig. 7). On the oral side, the thoracic duct was attached to the esophagus. The mid-thoracic and upper thoracic esophagus are separated from the Aortic Arch and the left pleura. In some cases depending on the T- or N-factors, we are preserving the thoracic duct.

Dissection of Subcarinal Lymph Node

The lower right pulmonary ligament is dissected, and the pleura, the pericardium, and the right pulmonary vein are identified. The right main bronchus is identified near the right hilum, lymph node along Rt-main bronchus, and subcarinal lymph node are dissected at the tracheal bifurcation (Fig. 8), while preserving lung branches from the right vagus nerve. The right vagus nerve is dissected on the peripheral side after the pulmonary branch to maintain the cough reflux (Fig. 9).

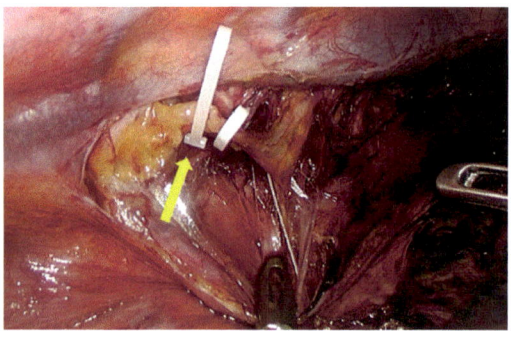

Fig. 7 Dissection of the thoracic duct

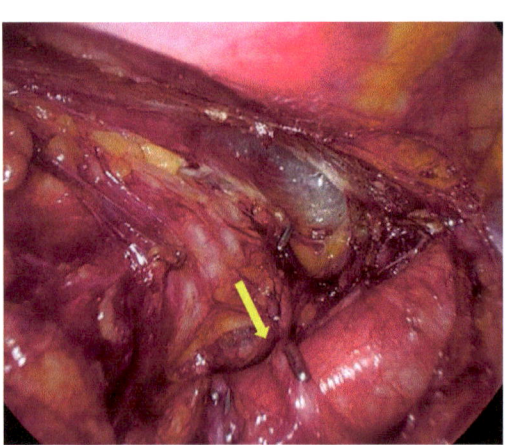

Fig. 6 Dissection of lymph node along the Rt-recurrent nerve

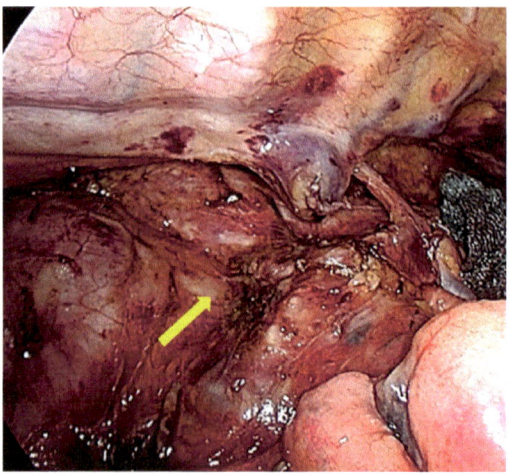

Fig. 8 Subcarinal lymph node dissection

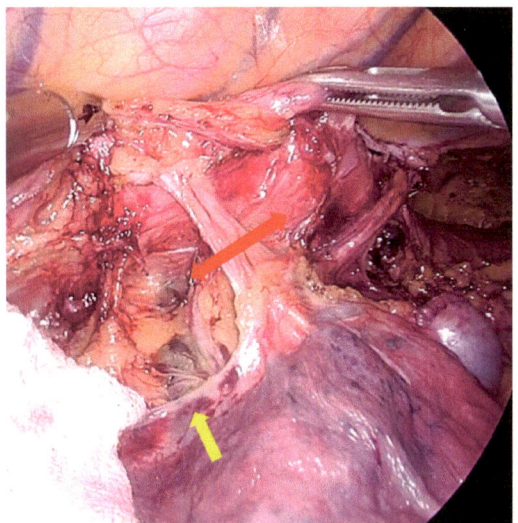

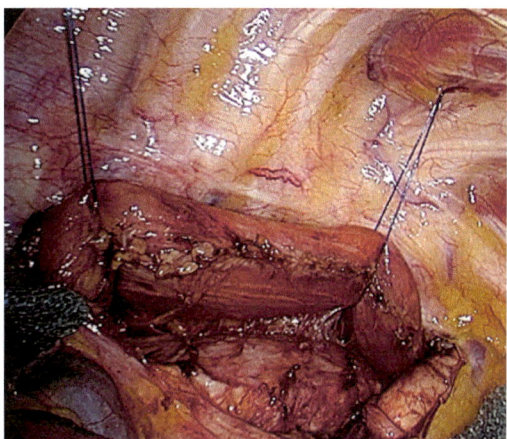

Fig. 10 Encircle the upper thoracic esophagus

Fig. 9 Preservation of the pulmonary branch of the Rt-vagus nerve

Dissection of the Lymph Node Along Lt-recurrent Nerve

The upper thoracic esophagus is detached from the left side wall of the trachea and encircles the esophagus at the height of the Aortic Arch and Rt-subclavian artery, by guiding with Endomini Retract®, and stretch the upper thoracic esophagus to upper direction at two positions (Fig. 10). The surrounding tissue including Lt-recurrent laryngeal nerve is mobilized from the trachea and easily identifies the Lt-recurrent laryngeal nerve. Then, using a microline scissors, the left recurrent laryngeal nerve is exposed, and the lymph nodes along the Lt-recurrent nerve are sharply and bluntly dissected (Fig. 11). Thereafter, dissect the esophagus using the Powered ECHELON FLEX® GST system (Fig. 12) and pulling up the oral side of the esophagus to upper direction, lymph node dissection along the Lt-recurrent nerve is performed until the oral side as much as possible, but the dissection from the mediastinum side is completed at the site where adipose tissue is found on the trachea side (pre-tracheal fat), and the lymph node dissection along the Lt-recurrent nerve is continued to the subsequent neck procedure. Over-stretch of the recurrent nerve and use of an electric scalpel or a vessel sealer should be avoided.

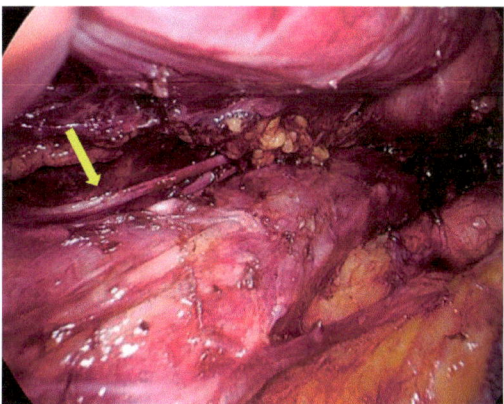

Fig. 11 Dissection of lymph node along Lt-recurrent laryngeal nerve

By securing the Lt-recurrent laryngeal nerve toward Aortic Arch, and the lymph node surrounded by the left main trachea, the left pulmonary artery wall, the Aortic Arch, and the left vagus nerve is dissected. The left bronchial artery can be identified and it is securely preserved. Care should be taken as damage to the left bronchial artery can lead to major bleeding.

Dissection of Lymph Node in the Mid Mediastinum

By exposing the left main bronchus, pericardium, and left pulmonary vein, lymph node in the mid mediastinum is dissected and attached to the caudal side of the esophagus (Fig. 13). The left vagus nerve is dissected caudally beyond the left main

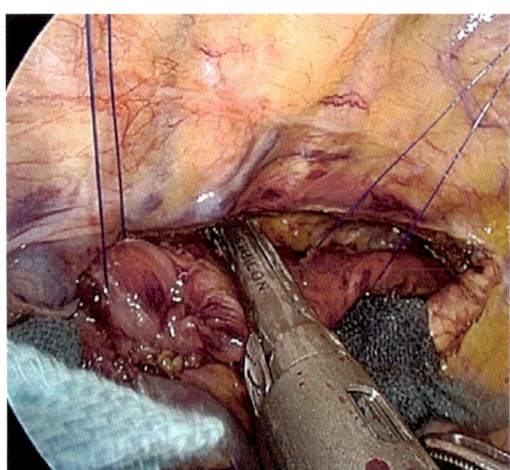

Fig. 12 Transection of the upper thoracic esophagus

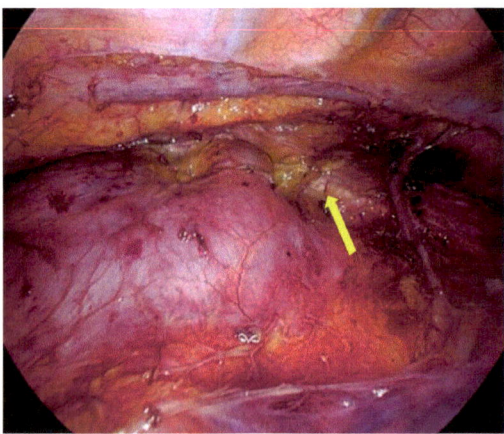

Fig. 13 Dissection of lymph node in the mid mediastinum

bronchus to preserve the left vagal pulmonary branch.

Lower Mediastinal Lymph Node Dissection

The pericardium, left lung pleura, diaphragmatic limb, and inferior vena cava are exposed and lower mediastinal lymph node is dissected. Several esophageal arteries branched from the descending aorta can be identified and dissected with a vessel sealer.

Drainage for the Chest Cavity

After washing, confirm hemostasis, insert Thoracic drain (24Fr) from the ninth ICS port site.

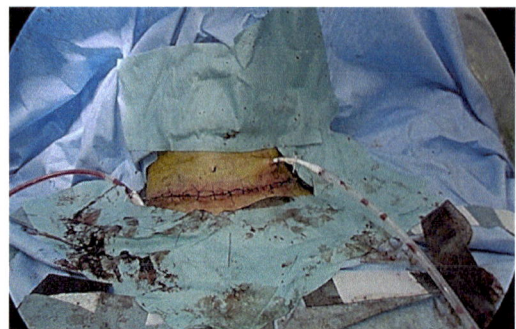

Fig. 14 Collar incision for neck dissection and anastomosis

Neck Lymph Node Dissection

The neck skin incision is based on a collar incision (Fig. 14). The sternocleidomastoid muscle and anterior cervical muscle group are preserved. Supraclavicular lymph node, lymph node along carotid sheath, and lymph node along recurrent laryngeal nerve are dissected on the both left and right sides. The omohyoid muscle is resected, and the transverse carotid artery and vein, and phrenic nerve should be preserved.

Reconstruction

Our department basically uses the retro-sternal route for reconstruction of the gastric tube, but in cases where the gastric tube cannot be used for reconstruction, such as in cases after gastrectomy, reconstruction of the pedicled jejunum with a vascular anastomosis through the anterior chest wall.

The retro-sternal space is manually separated from caudal side and thereafter, under visual guidance by laparoscopy, the retro-sternal route is made. At the same time, blunt dissection is done from the cervical wound and completes the retro-sternal route. The gastric tube is covered with a sterilized probe cover for ultrasonic waves. While paying attention to the direction so that the gastric tube does not twist, pull the silk thread from the cervical wound and raise the gastric tube. In order to confirm blood supply for the gastric tube, the ICG fluorography is routinely performed (Fig. 15), and it is important to check if the demarcation line is present or not.

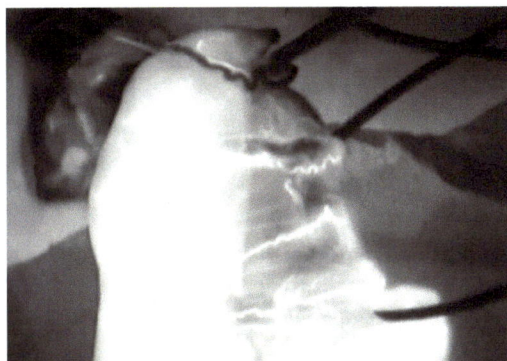

Fig. 15 ICG fluorography of the gastric tube

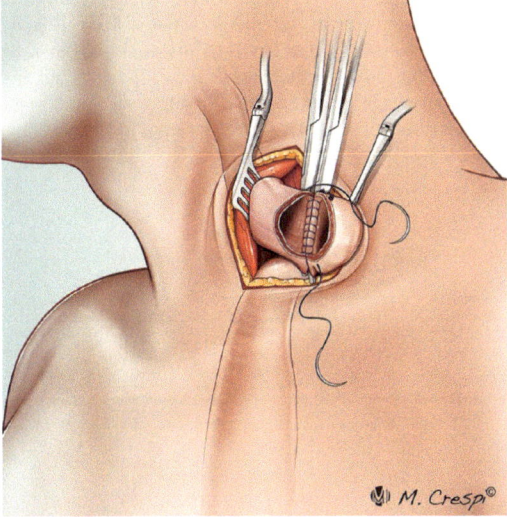

Fig. 16 Neck anastomosis

Apply pediatric intestinal forceps to both ends of the planned cervical esophageal anastomosis, and perform layer-to layer anastomosis with 4–0 monofilament absorbent thread in the interrupted suture fashion (Fig. 16). After completion of the anastomosis, the gastric tube was pulled slightly caudally from the abdomen to straighten the reconstruction route as much as possible, and the excess omentum was dropped into the posterior mediastinum to fill in the posterior mediastinum route so that we can prevent pyothorax when cervical anastomosis leakage occurred.

Postoperative Management

It is generally accepted that the McKeown esophagectomy in high-volume centers with experienced surgeons and the availability of critical-care support is associated with improved outcomes [12].

When necessary, bronchoscopy or a mini-tracheostomy can be used to ensure adequate bronchial toilet. Fluid balance and oxygen saturation should be closely monitored and oxygen supplementation is essential. It is also important to provide nutritional support by enteral feeding through jejunostomy routinely placed at the time of surgery.

Thrombosis prophylaxis should be performed by sequential pneumatic compression devices for the first two postoperative days (POD) and subcutaneous injection of low molecular weight heparins. Prophylactic antibiotics are given for 24 h.

Physiotherapy with gradual breathing exercises and general condition exercises is performed from the day of surgery to the day of discharge at least twice a day.

A contrast study to check the integrity of the anastomosis is routinely performed at 5–7 POD. The chest drain will be removed when the effluent amounts to less than 200 mL of fluids.

Patients are discharged when they are able to tolerate the soft diet and the pain is sufficiently controlled to permit normal mobilization. The patient is then seen in the outpatient clinic 1 month after discharge.

References

1. Ferlay J, Colombet M, Soerjomataram I, Mathers C, Parkin DM, Pineros M, et al. Estimating the global cancer incidence and mortality in 2018: GLOBOCAN sources and methods. Int J Cancer. 2019;144(8):1941–53.
2. Pohl H, Welch HG. The role of overdiagnosis and reclassification in the marked increase of esophageal adenocarcinoma incidence. J Natl Cancer Inst. 2005;97(2):142–6.

3. Lepage C, Rachet B, Jooste V, Faivre J, Coleman MP. Continuing rapid increase in esophageal adenocarcinoma in England and Wales. Am J Gastroenterol. 2008;103(11):2694–9.

4. Pennathur A, Zhang J, Chen H, Luketich JD. The "best operation" for esophageal cancer? Ann Thorac Surg. 2010;89(6):S2163–7.

5. Wu PC, Posner MC. The role of surgery in the management of oesophageal cancer. Lancet Oncol. 2003;4(8):481–8.

6. van Hagen P, Hulshof MC, van Lanschot JJ, Steyerberg EW, van Berge Henegouwen MI, Wijnhoven BP, et al. Preoperative chemoradiotherapy for esophageal or junctional cancer. N Engl J Med. 2012;366(22):2074–84.

7. Cunningham D, Allum WH, Stenning SP, Thompson JN, Van de Velde CJ, Nicolson M, et al. Perioperative chemotherapy versus surgery alone for resectable gastroesophageal cancer. N Engl J Med. 2006;355(1):11–20.

8. Ferlay J, Soerjomataram I, Dikshit R, Eser S, Mathers C, Rebelo M, et al. Cancer incidence and mortality worldwide: sources, methods and major patterns in GLOBOCAN 2012. Int J Cancer. 2015;136(5):E359–86.

9. Tachimori Y, Ozawa S, Numasaki H, Ishihara R, Matsubara H, Muro K, et al. Comprehensive registry of esophageal cancer in Japan, 2010. Esophagus. 2017;14(3):189–214.

10. Cuschieri A, Shimi S, Banting S. Endoscopic oesophagectomy through a right thoracoscopic approach. J R Coll Surg Edinb. 1992;37(1):7–11.

11. Biere SS, van Berge Henegouwen MI, Maas KW, Bonavina L, Rosman C, Garcia JR, et al. Minimally invasive versus open oesophagectomy for patients with oesophageal cancer: a multicentre, open-label, randomised controlled trial. Lancet. 2012;379(9829):1887–92.

12. Birkmeyer JD, Siewers AE, Finlayson EV, Stukel TA, Lucas FL, Batista I, et al. Hospital volume and surgical mortality in the United States. N Engl J Med. 2002;346(15):1128–37.

13. van Workum F, Berkelmans GH, Klarenbeek BR, Nieuwenhuijzen GAP, Luyer MDP, Rosman C. McKeown or Ivor Lewis totally minimally invasive esophagectomy for cancer of the esophagus and gastroesophageal junction: systematic review and meta-analysis. J Thorac Dis. 2017;9(Suppl 8):S826–S33.

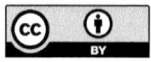

Part IX

Upper Gastrointestinal Surgery: Gastric Surgery

Gastric Gastrointestinal Stromal Tumor

Danson Yeo and Jaideep Rao

Introduction

Gastrointestinal stromal tumor (GIST) is the most common mesenchymal tumor originating in the gastrointestinal tract, originating from the interstitial cells of Cajal. GISTs occur most commonly in the stomach (60%), followed by the small intestine (30%) [1].

The standard of care for localized GISTs is complete surgical resection without dissection of clinically negative lymph nodes [2]. Any GIST is considered potentially malignant, indications for surgery for gastric GISTs are as listed below. For non-gastric GISTs, surgical resection is recommended regardless of tumor size or morphology [3].

Indications for Surgery for Gastric GISTs

1. Tumor >2 cm.
2. Increase in size on follow-up.
3. Signs of malignancy; irregular margins, cystic changes, necrosis, and heterogenous echogenicity.
4. Symptomatic; ulceration and bleeding, gastric outlet obstruction (large antral GISTs).

The goal of surgery is R0 surgery (i.e., excision margins are clear of tumor cells). While laparoscopic surgery for gastric GISTs resection is associated with superior postoperative outcomes, the decision to undertake laparoscopic versus open surgery should be made at the discretion of the surgeon. The European Society for Medical Oncology (ESMO) guidelines discourage laparoscopy for patients with large tumors due to the risk of tumor rupture [2], while Otani et al. [4] suggest 5 cm as the limit for laparoscopic wedge resection. Intraoperative tumor rupture is associated with a very high risk of peritoneal relapse [5].

The initial diagnosis of a GIST is usually suggested by endoscopy, endoscopic ultrasound (EUS), or computed tomography (CT) of the abdomen. Preoperative histological diagnosis is not necessary unless considering neoadjuvant imatinib therapy [3]. Neoadjuvant imatinib therapy should be considered for localized GISTs when R0 resection is not feasible or for organ preservation [3]. En bloc resection of a GIST that has invaded surrounding organs may be necessary to achieve negative margins and to avoid tumor rupture [6]. The principles of surgery for GIST are negative margins, and resection without rupture of the tumor.

D. Yeo (✉)
Department of General Surgery, Tan Tock Seng Hospital, Singapore, Singapore
e-mail: danson_xw_yeo@ttsh.com.sg

J. Rao
Mount Elizabeth Novena Hospital, Singapore, Singapore

© The Author(s) 2023
D. Lomanto et al. (eds.), *Mastering Endo-Laparoscopic and Thoracoscopic Surgery*,
https://doi.org/10.1007/978-981-19-3755-2_38

Surgical Technique

Instruments
- 12 mm ports, 5 mm ports
- Nathanson retractor (for proximal gastric GISTs if liver retraction is required. Alternative methods of liver retraction may be used).
- 10 mm 30° laparoscope
- Advanced energy device—author preference is the Harmonic 1000I.
- Atraumatic graspers.
- Clip applicator.
- Suction/irrigation device.
- Laparoscopic stapler.

Operating Room Setup and Patient Position

The patient is placed in the supine position with both arms out and a footboard. The laparoscopic stack is placed on the patient's left, the machines for the energy devices are placed at the patient's feet, and the suction machines are placed on the patient's right.

The main surgeon stands on the patient's right along with the camera assistant, while the first assistant stands on the patient's left.

After the subumbilical port is placed, the abdominal cavity is inspected for evidence of peritoneal metastasis. Pneumoperitoneum is maintained at 12 mmHg. Location of the ports depends on the location of the tumor, but is generally similar to that used in laparoscopic gastrectomy.

Operative Steps

Stapled wedge resection can be easily performed for most anterior wall gastric GISTs. Tumor rupture must be avoided at all cost. The tumor should be handled gently if at all, while and the surrounding tissues can be sutured or handled for traction. To avoid stenosis, the tumor should be elevated and the stapler fired perpendicular to the long axis of the stomach.

An extraction bag is recommended for retrieval of the specimen.

For tumors in the posterior gastric wall, the greater omentum may need to be incised in the avascular portion away from the gastroepiploic arcade in order to enter the lesser sac to reach the tumor.

For tumors near the greater or lesser curve, the omentum and feeding vessels will need to be ligated and dissected free in order to perform a wedge resection. This is best done with an energy device.

The most challenging gastric GIST surgeries are for endophytic tumors, or tumors located in the fundus, lesser curve, and the antrum.

Endophytic Gastric GIST on the Anterior Gastric Wall

Endophytic Tumors Located on the Anterior Gastric Wall (Fig. 1)

- An incision is made on the anterior gastric wall adjacent to the tumor.
- The tumor is then everted through the gastrostomy and lifted anteriorly (Fig. 2).
- Lift both edges of the gastrostomy and staple across, resecting the tumor and stapling close the gastrostomy at the same time. Alternatively, the tumor can be excised with a stapler and the gastrostomy subsequently closed with sutures.

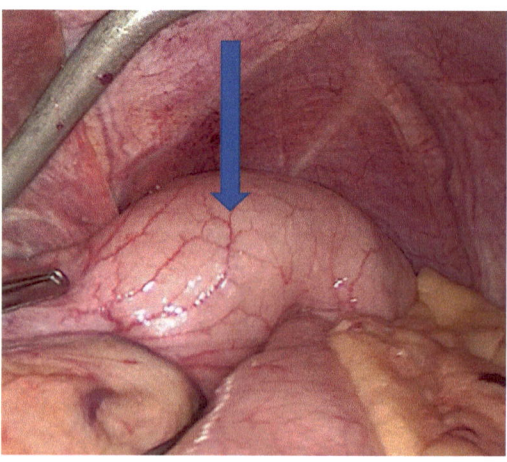

Fig. 1 Endophytic GIST on the anterior gastric wall

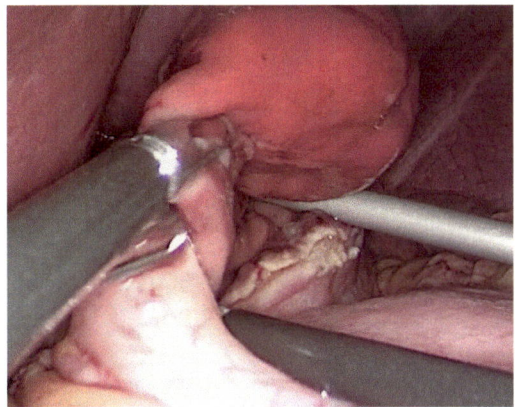

Fig. 2 Eversion of tumor through an adjacent gastrostomy

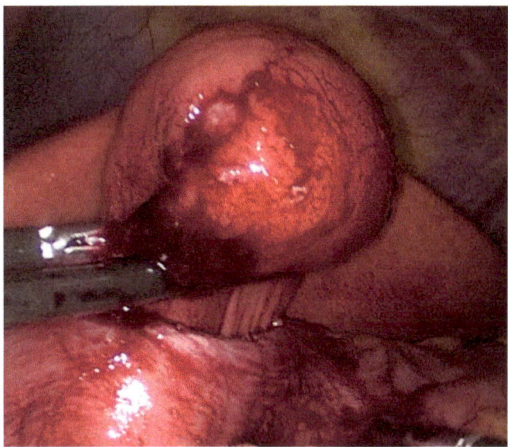

Fig. 4 Posterior wall tumor lifted through a gastrostomy on the anterior wall

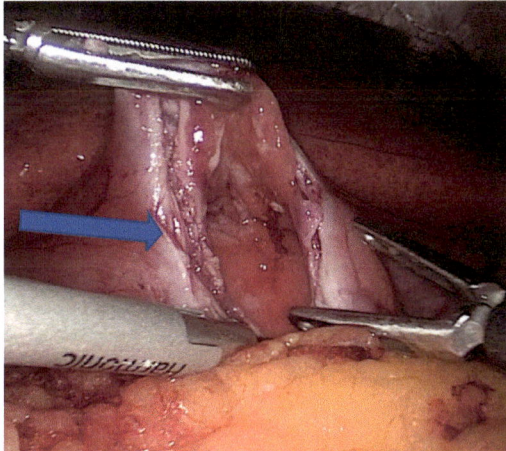

Fig. 3 Anterior gastrostomy overlying the tumor

Endophytic Gastric GIST on the Posterior Gastric Wall

- An incision is made on the anterior gastric wall overlying the tumor (Fig. 3).
- The posterior wall tumor is lifted up through the gastrostomy and resected with a stapler (Fig. 4).
- The anterior wall gastrostomy is closed with a stapler or with sutures.

Antral GISTs

- Stapled wedge resection of broad antral tumors may be difficult to perform due to the thickened musculature of the antrum, making it less mobile.
- Anterior wall tumors may be excised with an energy source, such as harmonic, and the gastrostomy closed transversely to prevent strictures. A gastrojejunostomy can be performed if there is concern of stenosis of the antrum/pylorus after excision.
- In cases of large antral GISTs, it may not be possible to perform a wedge resection. A distal gastrectomy may be required to achieve negative resection margins.

Fundal/Lesser Curve/ Cardioesophageal Junction (CEJ) GISTs

- Resection of a fundal or lesser curve tumor should be performed over a bougie or gastroscope to ensure that the CEJ is not narrowed.
- Intragastric resection may be performed for tumors located in the posterior wall near the CEJ, whereby laparoscopic ports are placed through the anterior gastric wall into the gastric lumen, and stapler resection is performed.

Other methods such as endoscopic submucosal dissection have been described. However, enucleation of GISTs is not considered standard treatment as GISTs do not form a true capsule, originates from the muscle layer (unlike early gastric cancer), and disruption of the pseudocapsule and perforation of the gastric wall may happen simultaneously resulting in peritoneal dissemination [7].

Postoperative Management

Margin status may not be a significant prognostic factor for GIST recurrence [8]. In cases where the resection margin has microscopic tumor cells (R1), postoperative imatinib therapy is recommended when the malignant potential is high (based on size and mitotic index). Routine surveillance can be performed for low-risk GISTs [3].

References

1. Soreide K, Sandvik OM, Soreide JA, Giljaca V, Jureckova A, Bulusu VR. Global epidemiology of gastrointestinal stromal tumours (GIST): a systematic review of population-based cohort studies. Cancer Epidemiol. 2016;40:39–46.

2. Casali PG, Abecassis N, Aro HT, et al. Gastrointestinal stromal tumours: ESMO-EURACAN clinical practice guidelines for diagnosis, treatment and follow-up. Ann Oncol. 2018;29(Suppl 4):iv267–iv78.

3. Koo DH, Ryu MH, Kim KM, et al. Asian consensus guidelines for the diagnosis and management of gastrointestinal stromal tumor. Cancer Res Treat. 2016;48(4):1155–66.

4. Otani Y, Furukawa T, Yoshida M, et al. Operative indications for relatively small (2-5 cm) gastrointestinal stromal tumor of the stomach based on analysis of 60 operated cases. Surgery. 2006;139(4):484–92.

5. Hohenberger P, Ronellenfitsch U, Oladeji O, et al. Pattern of recurrence in patients with ruptured primary gastrointestinal stromal tumour. Br J Surg. 2010;97(12):1854–9.

6. Gold JS, Dematteo RP. Combined surgical and molecular therapy: the gastrointestinal stromal tumor model. Ann Surg. 2006;244(2):176–84.

7. Kong SH, Yang HK. Surgical treatment of gastric gastrointestinal stromal tumor. J Gastric Cancer. 2013;13(1):3–18.

8. McCarter MD, Antonescu CR, Ballman KV, et al. Microscopically positive margins for primary gastrointestinal stromal tumors: analysis of risk factors and tumor recurrence. J Am Coll Surg. 2012;215(1):53–9. discussion 59–60

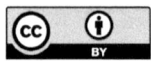

Gastric Carcinoma: Subtotal and Total Gastrectomy

Danson Yeo

Introduction

Gastric cancer is the fourth most common malignancy and the second most common cause of death among all malignancies worldwide [1]. More than half of new gastric cancer cases come from Eastern Asia (China and Japan), while Korea and Japan have the highest incidence rate in the world [2].

Risk factors for gastric cancer include tobacco smoking [3], alcohol consumption [4] and a high intake of salt and preserved foods [5]. *Helicobacter pylori* infection is an important risk factor for gastric cancer having been classified as a class I carcinogen [6], although only 1–3% of patients with *H. pylori* infection go on to develop gastric cancer [7].

The mainstay of curative treatment for gastric cancer is complete resection with lymphadenectomy.

Anatomy of the Stomach

The stomach has a rich anastomotic blood supply. The blood supply to the uppermost portion of the stomach and the lower esophagus is from a branch of the left inferior phrenic artery. The upper stomach is also supplied by the short gastric vessels in the gastrosplenic ligament, as well as small arteries arising from branches of the splenic artery towards the posterior wall of the fundus. If one of these vessels predominates, it is called the posterior gastric artery.

The largest blood supply comes from the left gastric artery arising from the celiac axis. The left gastric artery runs along the lesser curve of the stomach and joins with the right gastric artery. The right gastric artery is a branch of the common hepatic artery and supplies the region of the pylorus and lesser curve.

The blood supply along the greater curve comprises of the right gastroepiploic artery arising from the gastroduodenal artery, and the left gastroepiploic artery arising from the splenic artery.

Type of Surgery and Lymph Node Dissection

Surgical resection with lymphadenectomy is the gold standard of treatment for gastric cancer. Early cancers that meet the following criteria may be suitable for endoscopic resection; T1a lesion, differentiated-type adenocarcinoma without ulceration, diameter < 2 cm [8].

The standard surgery for either clinically node-positive (cN+) or > T2 tumors is either a total or distal gastrectomy. Distal gastrectomy may be performed when a satisfactory proximal resection margin can be obtained, otherwise total gastrectomy is performed. Tumors located along the greater curve with potential lymph node metastasis to station 4sb

D. Yeo (✉)
Upper Gastrointestinal and Bariatric Surgery, Department of General Surgery, Tan Tock Seng Hospital, Singapore, Singapore
e-mail: danson_xw_yeo@ttsh.com.sg

© The Author(s) 2023
D. Lomanto et al. (eds.), *Mastering Endo-Laparoscopic and Thoracoscopic Surgery*,
https://doi.org/10.1007/978-981-19-3755-2_39

may require a total gastrectomy with splenectomy. For T1 tumors, a resection margin of 2 cm is recommended, for T2 tumors with expansive growth patterns, a proximal margin of at least 3 cm is recommended, while a proximal margin of at least 5 cm is recommended for tumors with an infiltrative growth pattern. If the above cannot be satisfied, frozen section examination of the proximal margin may be performed to ensure an R0 resection.

D2 lymphadenectomy is indicated for cN+ or > cT2 tumors while D1 or D1+ lymphadenectomy is sufficient for cT1N0 tumors. D2 lymphadenectomy should be performed whenever the possibility of nodal involvement cannot be excluded or the depth of tumor invasion is uncertain [8]. The Japanese Gastric Cancer Association defined the lymph nodes of the stomach and assigned station numbers [9]. Lymph node stations 1–12 and 14v are considered regional gastric lymph nodes, while metastasis to any other nodes is considered metastatic. The regional lymph node stations should be excised according to the type of gastric resection and the extent of lymphadenectomy as detailed in Table 1.

Contraindications

Gastrectomy as a reduction surgery for advanced gastric cancer with incurable factors such as unresectable liver metastasis and peritoneal metastasis is not recommended [8, 10]. Staging laparoscopy may be performed for patients at high risk of peritoneal dissemination, especially if neoadjuvant chemotherapy is being considered.

Surgical Technique

Instruments
- 3 × 12 mm ports, 2 × 5 mm ports
- Nathanson retractor (not required if alternative methods of liver retraction are used).
- 10 mm 30° laparoscope

- Advanced energy device—author preference is the Harmonic 1000I.
- Atraumatic graspers.
- Clip applicator.
- Suction/irrigation device.
- Laparoscopic stapler.

Operating Room Setup and Patient Position

The patient is placed in the supine position with both arms out and a footboard. The laparoscopic stack is placed on the patient's left, the machines for the energy devices are placed at the patient's feet, and the suction machine is placed on the patient's right.

The main surgeon stands on the patient's right along with the camera assistant, while the first assistant stands on the patient's left.

After the sub umbilical port is placed, the abdominal cavity is inspected for evidence of peritoneal metastasis. Pneumoperitoneum is maintained at 12 mmHg. Rest of the ports are placed as shown in Fig. 1. Retract the liver to expose the hiatus; author's preference is to use

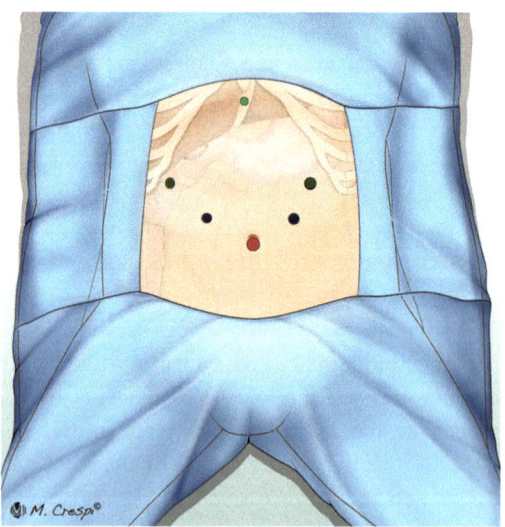

Fig. 1 Trocar placement

Table 1 Extent of lymphadenectomy according to the type of gastric resection

Gastrectomy	D1	D1+	D2
Subtotal gastrectomy	1, 3, 4sb, 4d, 5, 6, 7	(D1) + 8a, 9	(D1) + 8a, 9, 11p, 12a
Total gastrectomy	1, 2, 3, 4, 5, 6,7	(D1) + 8a, 9, 11p	(D1) + 8a, 9, 11p, 11d, 12a

the Nathanson liver retractor, others may use tape or sutures to sling the liver or a fan retractor.

Operative Steps: Distal Gastrectomy (Fig. 2)

Dissection of the Greater Omentum/ Left Gastrocolic Ligament (Station 4d)

- The surgeon's left hand and the assistant lifts the greater omentum/greater curve of the stomach.

- Incise the gastrocolic ligament at a transparent part of the omental bursa at least 3 cm away from the gastroepiploic arcade (Fig. 3).
- Continue the dissection towards the splenic flexure until the root of the left gastroepiploic artery/vein is reached (Fig. 4).
  - Be aware of the transverse colon and transverse mesocolon at all times.

Ligation of Left Gastroepiploic Vessels (Station 4sb)

- The surgeon's left hand grasps the left gastroepiploic vessels and lifts superiorly.

Fig. 2 Distal gastrectomy operative steps

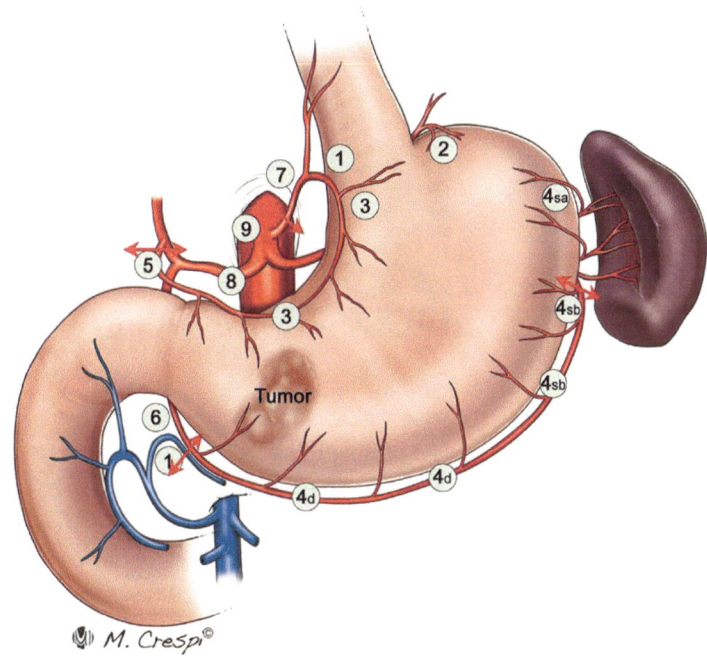

M. Crespi©

Fig. 3 Dissection of the greater omentum/left gastrocolic ligament

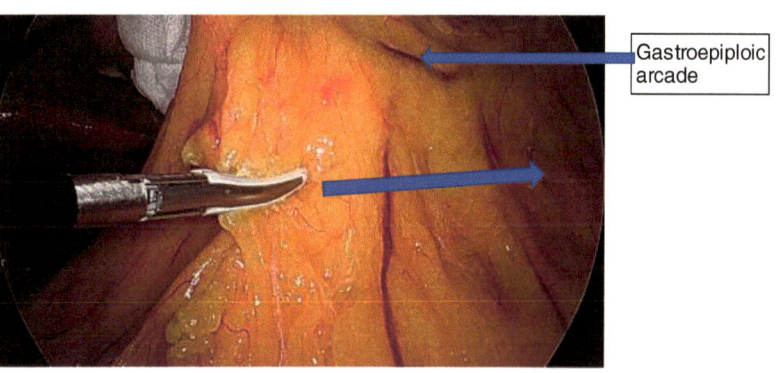

Gastroepiploic arcade

Fig. 4 Dissection of the greater omentum/left gastrocolic ligament

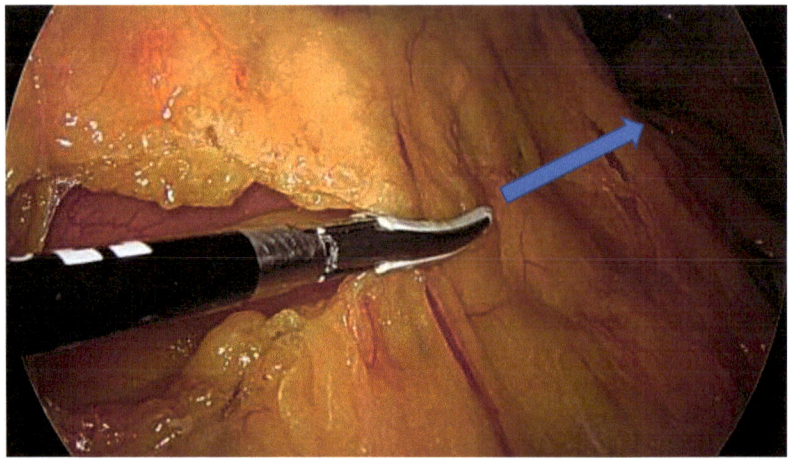

Fig. 5 Ligation of the left gastroepiploic vessels

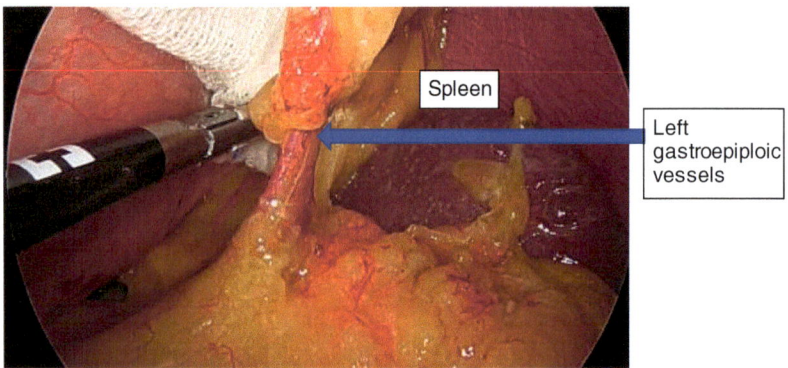

Fig. 6 Ligation of the left gastroepiploic vessels

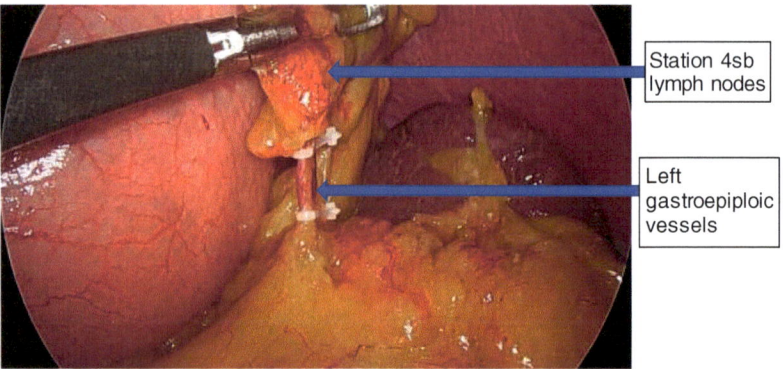

- A gauze may be placed behind the stomach to aid in retraction and visualization of the vascular pedicle (Fig. 5).
- The left gastroepiploic artery may give off 2 branches; the omental and splenic branch. The left gastroepiploic vessels are divided distal to the omental and splenic branches between clips using the energy device (Fig. 6).
- The greater curvature vessels are divided close to the stomach until the avascular area is reached just before the short gastric vessels.

Dissection of the Greater Omentum/Right Gastrocolic Ligament (Station 4d)

- The surgeon's left hand holds up the gastroepiploic arcade, while the assistant lifts up the stomach.
- The dissection is continued along the gastrocolic ligament towards the right gastroepiploic vessels and head of pancreas (Fig. 7).
- Adhesions between the gastrocolic ligament and the transverse mesocolon are best divided with blunt dissection to avoid injury to the middle colic vessels within the transverse mesocolon.
- Take down any adhesions between the posterior stomach and pancreas/transverse mesocolon until the gastroduodenal artery is exposed (Fig. 8).
  - Be aware of the middle colic vessels that may be adherent to the gastrocolic ligament.

Ligation of the Right Gastroepiploic Artery (Station 6)

- Surgeon's left hand holds up the right gastroepiploic vessels while the assistant lifts up the posterior stomach and provides countertraction (Fig. 9).
- The right gastroepiploic vein is clipped while preserving the anterior superior pancreaticoduodenal vein (Fig. 10), while the right gastroepiploic artery is clipped at the junction of the gastroduodenal artery (Fig. 11).
- The omentum is dissected off the duodenum/pylorus (Fig. 12).
  - Be careful to avoid injury to the pancreas.

Dissection of the Hepatoduodenal Ligament

- Place a gauze below duodenum and the hepatoduodenal ligament.

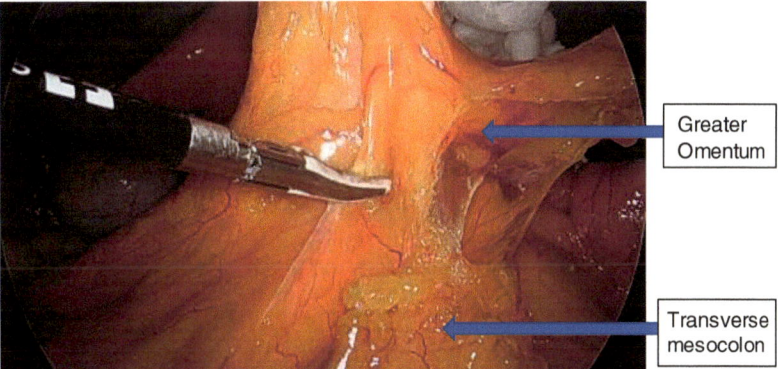

Fig. 7 Dissection of the greater omentum/right gastrocolic ligament

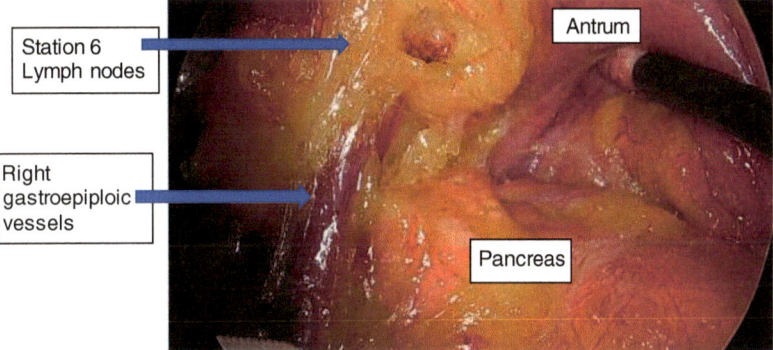

Fig. 8 Dissection of the greater omentum/right gastrocolic ligament

Fig. 9 Right gastroepiploic vessels

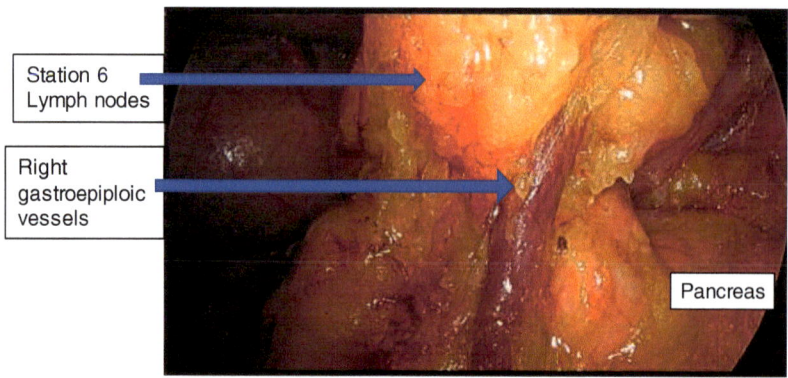

Station 6 Lymph nodes

Right gastroepiploic vessels

Pancreas

Fig. 10 Right gastroepiploic vein

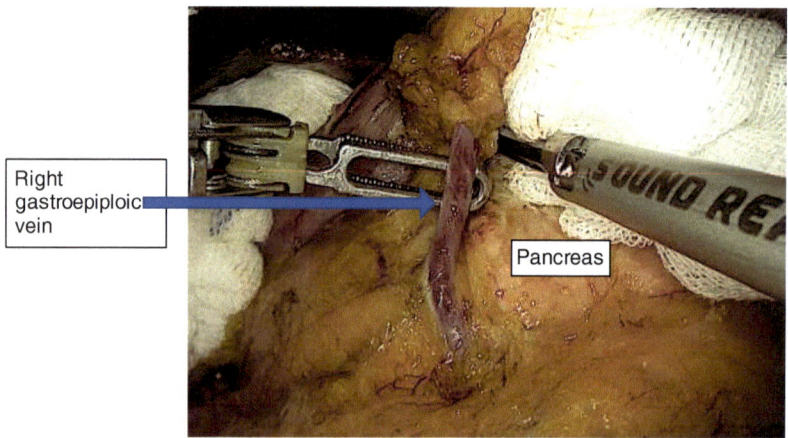

Right gastroepiploic vein

Pancreas

Fig. 11 Right gastroepiploic artery

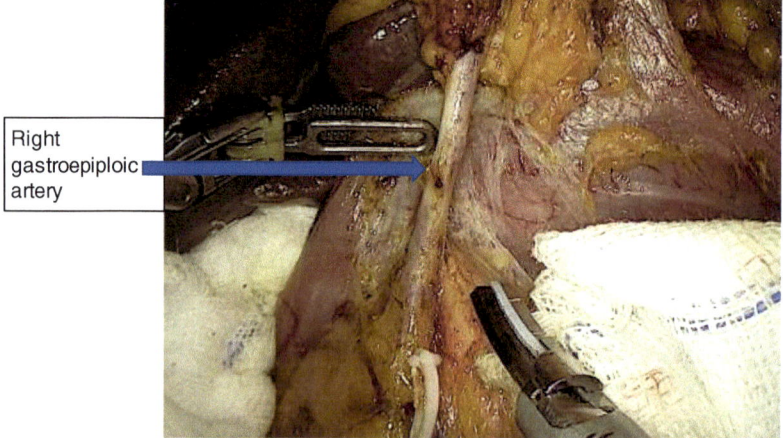

Right gastroepiploic artery

- Incise the hepatoduodenal ligament (Fig. 13).
- Surgeon's left hand holds up the right gastric vessels while the assistant retracts the pylorus inferiorly.
- Dissect the right gastric vessels off the pylorus with an energy device, small feeding vessels

may be encountered during this dissection. Hemostasis can be achieved with the energy device.

– The gauze placed posterior protects the pancreas and the common hepatic artery from injury.

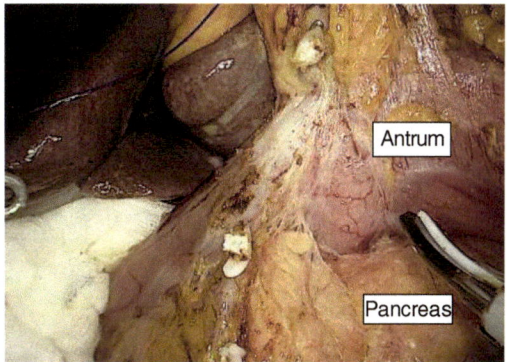

Fig. 12 Post ligation of the right gastroepiploic vessels

Ligation of the Right Gastric Artery and Dissection Along the Hepatic Artery Proper (Station 5)

- Hold up the right gastric vessels superiorly, exposing its origins from the hepatic artery proper. The lymph nodes at the root of the right gastric vessels are dissected (station 5 lymph nodes) (Fig. 14).
- The right gastric vessels are divided between clips at the root (Fig. 15).

Transection of the Duodenum

- The duodenum is transected with a stapler (Fig. 16).

Fig. 13 Dissection of the hepatoduodenal ligament

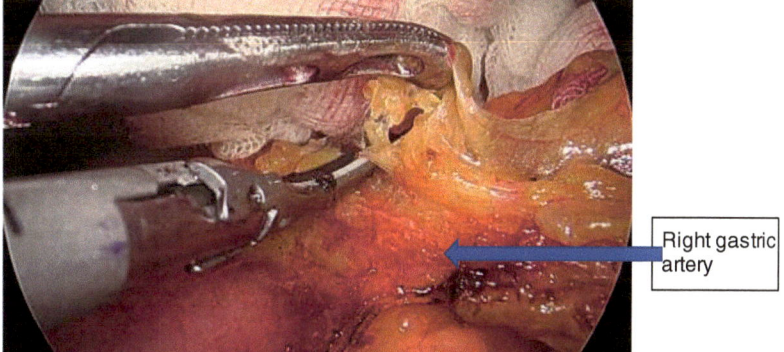

Fig. 14 Exposing the right gastric artery at the root

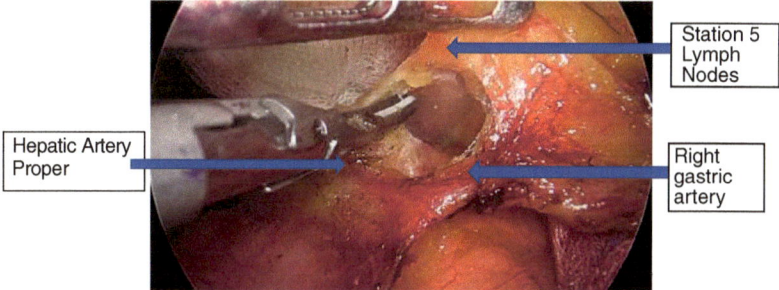

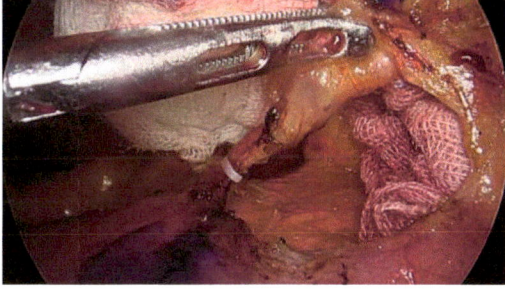

Fig. 15 Ligation of the right gastric vessels

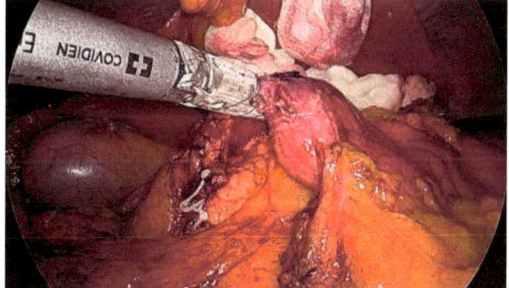

Fig. 16 Transection of the duodenum

– Ensure that the vascular clips are not caught in the stapler jaws prior to firing the stapler.

• After transection, the stomach is flipped away to the left to expose the celiac axis (Fig. 17).

Opening of the Hepatogastric Ligament/Lesser Omentum

• The lesser omentum is opened up until the right crus (Fig. 18).

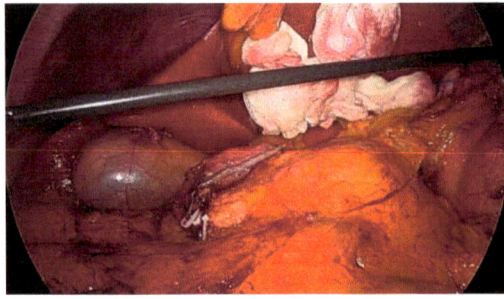

Fig. 17 Expose the celiac axis

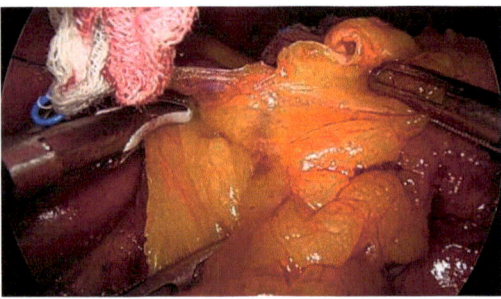

Fig. 18 Opening of the hepatogastric ligament/lesser omentum

Fig. 19 Dissection along the common hepatic artery and splenic artery

– Beware of a replaced left hepatic artery arising from the left gastric artery that may be traversing the lesser omentum.

Dissection Along the Common Hepatic Artery and Splenic Artery (Station 8a, 12a and 11)

• The assistant holds up the left gastric vessels superiorly while gently retracting the pancreas inferiorly. Surgeon's left hand holds up the fatty tissue over the superior border of the pancreas (Station 8a lymph node) and dissects it off the common hepatic artery. The dissection may be continued posteriorly along the hepatic artery to expose the portal vein, thereby taking Station 12a lymph nodes as well.

• The dissection is continued along the upper border of the pancreas from the common hepatic artery (Fig. 19), across the celiac axis onto the splenic artery to excise Station 11p lymph nodes along the splenic artery (Fig. 20).

Ligation of the Left Gastric Artery (Station 7, 9)

• The assistant lifts the left gastric vessels and pulls the pancreas downwards to expose the celiac axis.

• Dissect out the coronary vein (Fig. 21) and the left gastric artery (Fig. 22), dividing the vessels between clips (Fig. 23) (The coronary vein usually lies anterior to the left gastric artery).

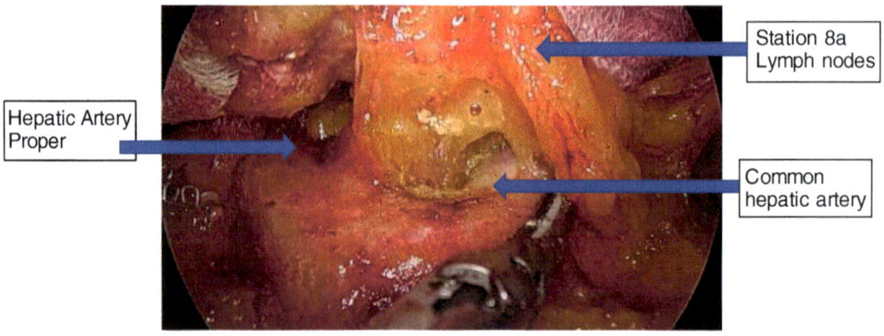

Fig. 20 Dissection of Station 11p Lymph Nodes

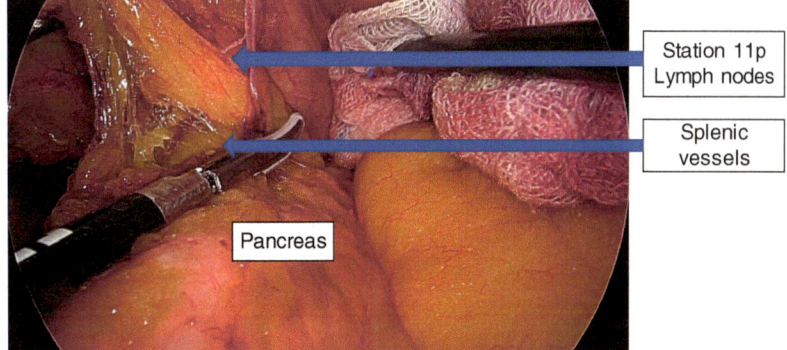

Fig. 21 Coronary vein

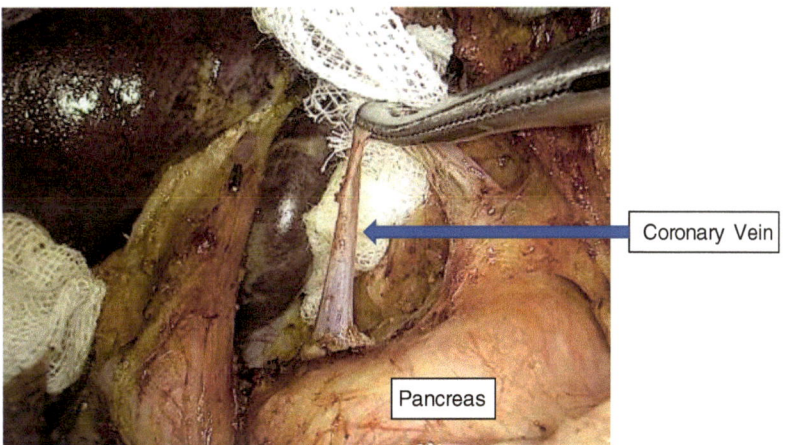

Fig. 22 Left gastric artery

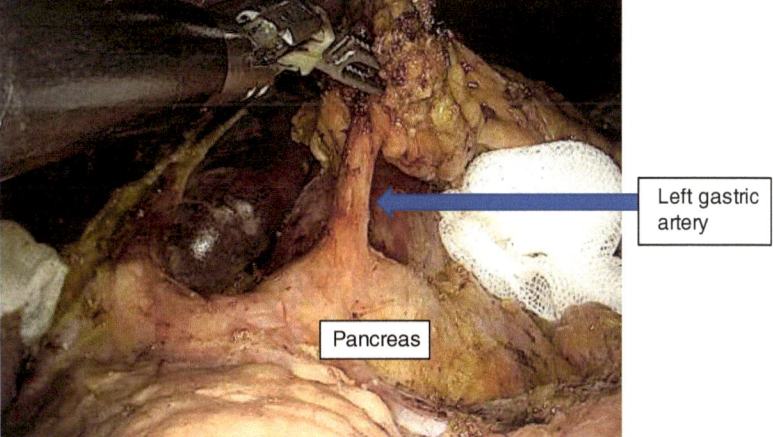

Dissection of the Proximal Lesser Curve (Station 1)

- The lesser omentum is divided until the esophagus is reached (Fig. 24).
- The surgeon's left hand and the assistant holds up Station 1 lymph nodes to provide traction.
- Station 1 lymph nodes are excised off the right crus, the cardio-esophageal junction, and thereafter the lesser curve of the stomach (Fig. 25).

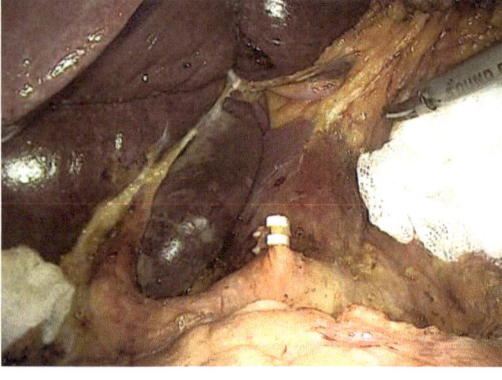

Fig. 23 Ligation of left gastric vessels

- The anterior vagus nerve is transected during this step.
  - Avoid injury to the distal esophagus during dissection.

Transection of the Proximal Stomach

- Transection of the proximal stomach is performed with a stapler (Fig. 26).
  - Ensure that any nasogastric tube in the stomach is removed prior to stapling.
  - In cases where there is a concern of cancer invasion of the proximal staple line, remove the specimen first for inspection with consideration of frozen section examination of the proximal staple line.

Figure 27 shows the vessels of the celiac axis stripped of lymph nodes, and proximal transection of the stomach completed.

Fig. 24 Dissection of the proximal lesser curve

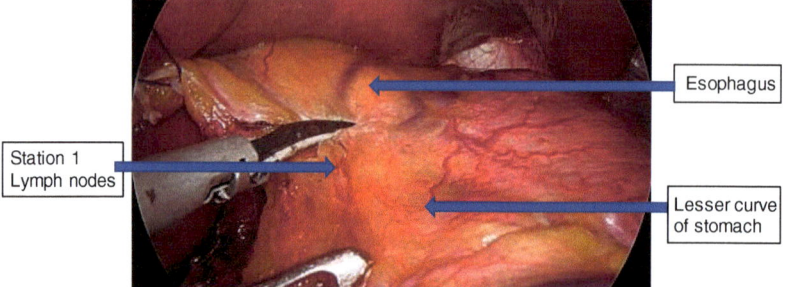

Fig. 25 Dissection of Station 1 Lymph nodes

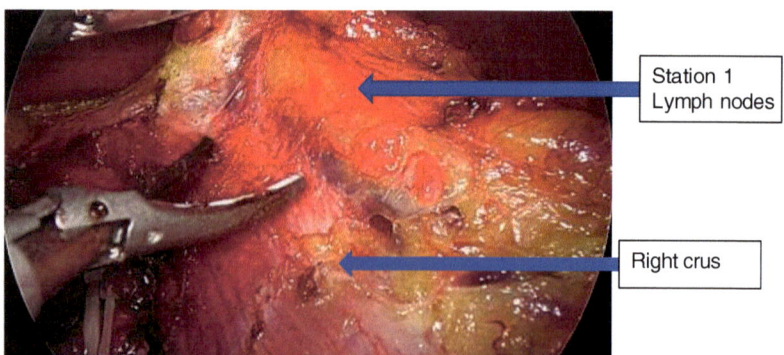

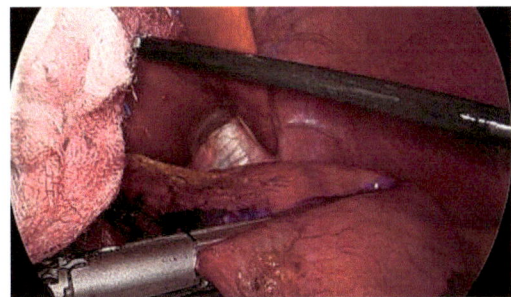

Fig. 26 Transection of the proximal stomach

Anastomosis

– Possible anastomosis includes a Billroth II anastomosis, Roux-En-Y anastomosis (Figs. 28 and 29), or Delta anastomosis.
– Type of anastomosis performed depends on the surgeon's experience and patient factors.

Fig. 27 Post dissection of lymph nodes around the celiac axis

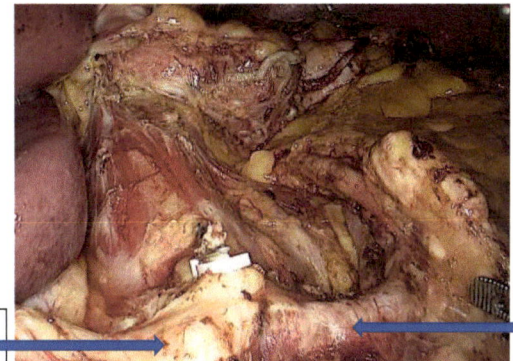

Common hepatic artery

Splenic artery

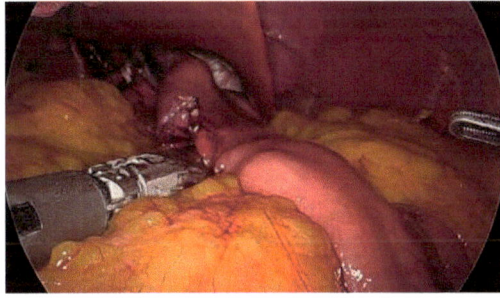

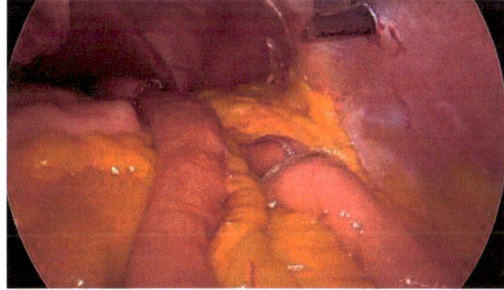

Fig. 28 Stapled Roux-En-Y gastrojejunal anastamosis

Fig. 29 Stapled Jejunal-jejunal anastamosis

Operative Steps: Total Gastrectomy

Additional Steps

- After ligation of the left gastroepiploic vessels (Step 2 of distal gastrectomy), the dissection is continued cephalad dividing the short gastric vessels until the left crus is reached.
- Lymph node station 4sa is taken along with the short gastric vessels (Fig. 30).

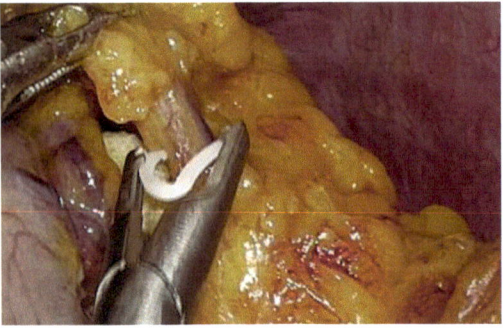

Fig. 30 Short gastric vessels

- Lymph node station 2 dissected off the angle of His to expose the cardioesophageal junction on the left (Fig. 31).
- Station 1 lymph nodes are dissected off the esophagus until the level of the cardioesophageal junction (Fig. 32).
- A short distance of the thoracic esophagus may be dissected through the hiatus in order to reduce tension in the subsequent anastomosis (Fig. 33).

Anastomosis

- Perform a Roux-en-Y esophageal-jejunal anastomosis.
- Anastomosis can be a side-to-side linear stapled anastomosis (Fig. 34), an end-to-side circular stapled anastomosis with an orvil (Fig. 35), or a handsewn anastomosis.

Fig. 31 Dissection of Station 2 lymph nodes

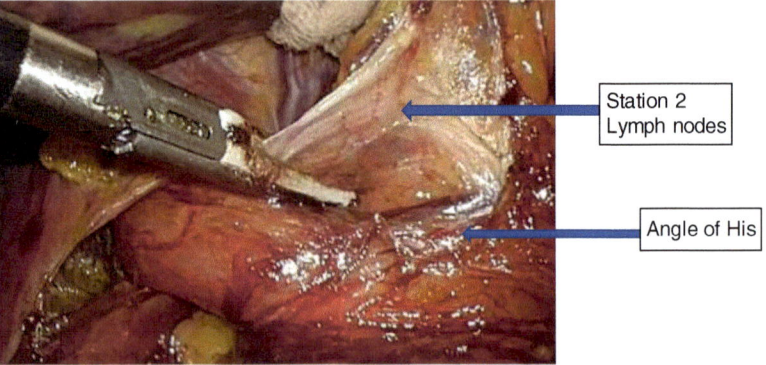

Fig. 32 Dissection of station 1 lymph nodes

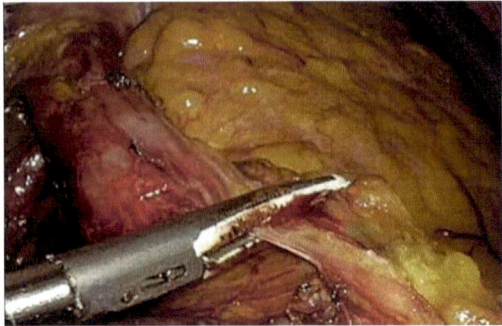

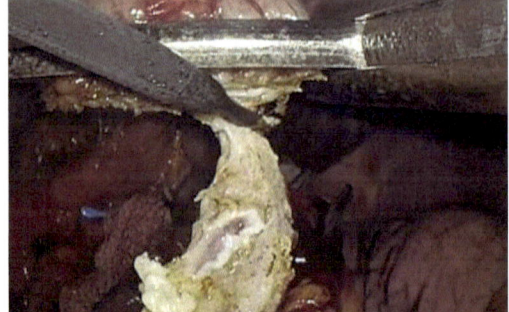

Fig. 33 Transection of the esophagus

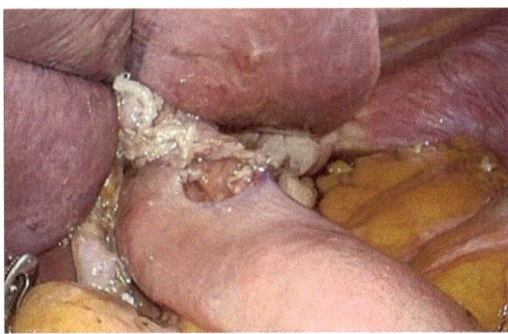

Fig. 34 Linear Stapled side-side anastamosis

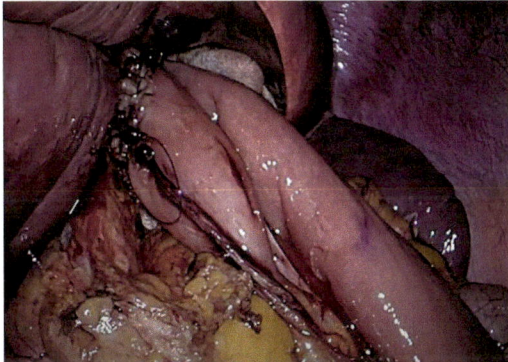

Fig. 35 End-side Circular anastomosis

Complications

Patients who are septic post-gastrectomy should undergo a Computed Tomographic scan of the abdomen and pelvis with intravenous and oral contrast. Potential sources of sepsis include pneumonia, intra-abdominal collections, leak from the anastomosis, or duodenal stump.

Long-term complications after total gastrectomy include dumping syndrome and Vitamin B12 deficiency. Patients with vitamin B12 deficiency may require regular intramuscular vitamin B12 injections.

References

1. Sitarz R, Skierucha M, Mielko J, Offerhaus GJA, Maciejewski R, Polkowski WP. Gastric cancer: epidemiology, prevention, classification, and treatment. Cancer Manag Res. 2018;10:239–48.
2. Inoue M, Tsugane S. Epidemiology of gastric cancer in Japan. Postgrad Med J. 2005;81(957):419–24.
3. Humans IWGotEoCRt and IARC Working Group. Tobacco smoke and involuntary smoking. IARC Monogr Eval Carcinog Risks Hum. 2004;83:1–1438.
4. Glade MJ. Food, nutrition, and the prevention of cancer: a global perspective. American Institute for Cancer Research/World Cancer Research Fund, American Institute for Cancer Research, 1997. Nutrition. 1999;15(6):523–6.
5. WHO, Joint, and FAO Expert Consultation. Diet, nutrition and the prevention of chronic diseases. World Health Organ Tech Rep Ser 2003;916(i-viii), 1–149, backcover.
6. International Agency for Research on Cancer. Schistosomes, liver flukes and Helicobacter pylori. IARC Working Group on the Evaluation of Carcinogenic Risks to Humans. Lyon, 7–14 June 1994. IARC Monogr Eval Carcinog Risks Hum. 1994;61:1–241.
7. Suerbaum S, Michetti P. Helicobacter pylori infection. N Engl J Med. 2002;347(15):1175–86.
8. Japanese Gastric Cancer Association. Japanese gastric cancer treatment guidelines 2018 (5th edition). Gastric Cancer. 2020.
9. Japanese Gastric Cancer A. Japanese classification of gastric carcinoma: 3rd English edition. Gastric Cancer. 2011;14(2):101–12.
10. Fujitani K, Yang HK, Mizusawa J, et al. Gastrectomy plus chemotherapy versus chemotherapy alone for advanced gastric cancer with a single non-curable factor (REGATTA): a phase 3, randomised controlled trial. Lancet Oncol. 2016;17(3):309–18.

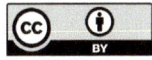

Part X

Bariatric Procedures

Laparoscopic Gastric Banding for Morbid Obesity

Davide Lomanto, Emre Gundogdu, and Mehmet Mahir Ozmen

Obesity is a rapidly rising problem worldwide in both developed and developing countries. It is not only reducing the quality of life but also shortens the duration of life with the comorbidities it brings [1]. Studies show that a two-point rise in the Body Mass Index (BMI) reduces one's life expectancy by almost 10 years, and it also significantly affects the quality of life in morbidly obese patients [2]. Obesity is a serious medical problem as it links directly to many common comorbidities such as:

- Type II diabetes mellitus.
- Hypertension.
- Coronary heart disease.
- Hyperlipidemia.
- Asthma.
- Sleep apnea.
- Reflux esophagitis.
- Gallstones.
- Osteoarthritis and spine problems.
- Certain cancers, e.g., breast cancer.

D. Lomanto (✉)
Department of Surgery, YLL School of Medicine, National University Singapore, Singapore, Singapore
e-mail: surdl@nus.edu.sg

E. Gundogdu
Department of Surgery, Liv Hospital, Ankara, Turkey

M. M. Ozmen
Department of Surgery, Medical School, Istinye University, Istanbul, Turkey

There is no single effective treatment that fits all obese patients. Today, there are treatment options where behavioral therapies, medical treatments, endoscopic interventions, and surgical treatment options are applied alone or in combination. There is inconsistency in success rates and a high rate of regaining weight after treatments where nonsurgical weight-loss methods are applied alone or in combination [3]. Bariatric surgery (BS) often reduces premature mortality relative to morbidly obese individuals who have not undergone weight-loss intervention [4]. Therefore, surgical options are increasingly considered in the treatment of morbid obesity. Dietary modification, physiotherapy, drugs, and obesity surgery (if required) is the key approach.

Surgery for weight loss has been devised and practiced over the last 40 to 50 years. Bariatric surgical procedures cause weight loss by restricting the amount of food the stomach can hold, causing malabsorption of nutrients, or by a combination of both gastric restriction and malabsorption. Bariatric procedures also often cause hormonal changes. In this context the type of surgery falls into two broad categories:

- *Restrictive*—reduce the size of the gastrointestinal tract, e.g., laparoscopic gastric banding, sleeve gastrectomy, vertical gastroplasty.
- *Malabsorptive*—alter metabolism and reduce absorption, e.g., gastric bypass, biliopancreatic diversion, etc.

© The Author(s) 2023
D. Lomanto et al. (eds.), *Mastering Endo-Laparoscopic and Thoracoscopic Surgery*,
https://doi.org/10.1007/978-981-19-3755-2_40

Bariatric or obesity surgery is recommended for the severely obese, in cases where weight reduction through medical therapy has been unsuccessful or where patients suffer from serious complications of obesity. According to the 1991 National Institutes of Health (NIH) consensus conference on gastrointestinal surgery for severe obesity [5], those who are suitable for obesity surgery are:

- Patients with a Body Mass Index (BMI)* of more than 40 kg/m².
- Patients with a BMI* of more than 35 kg/m² and obesity-related comorbidities.

While in the Asian population several studies have shown higher abdominal fat (5–10%) compared to others, so the Indication for Surgical treatment is 2.5–point BMI less:

- Patients with a Body Mass Index (BMI)* of more than 37.5 kg/m².
- Patients with a BMI* of more than 32.5 kg/m² with obesity-related comorbidities.

* BMI = weight (kg)/height (m) × height (m)

Surgery has become increasingly popular as they are usually performed via a laparoscopic approach. Several procedures like sleeve gastrectomy, gastric banding, and gastric bypass have been proven to be very effective not only in weight reduction but also in treating all comorbidities [6]. On average, patients can lose about 50–60% of their excess weight. More importantly, surgery can result in improvement or complete resolution of the various obesity complications like Diabetes mellitus type II, Hypertension, Obstructive Sleep Apnea, etc.

New guidelines on metabolic surgery in type II diabetes treatment algorithm have been published by international diabetes organizations due to the increasing data supporting the use of metabolic surgery for diabetes treatment [7]. Accordingly, they concluded that bariatric surgery should be recommended for patients with a BMI 40 kg/ m2 and those with inadequately controlled hyperglycemia and BMI 35 kg/m2 regardless of glycemic control. In addition, surgery should be considered for patients with a BMI of 30–34.9 kg/m2 and poorly controlled hyperglycemia, and for Asian patients with poorly controlled hyperglycemia with a BMI as low as 27.5 kg/m2 [7, 8].

Laparoscopic Gastric Banding (LAGB)

Gastric banding is a pure restrictive and reversible procedure and it is based on the principle of forming a small volume pouch near the stomach by wrapping the fundus with various synthetic grafts and limiting the passage to the distal part of the stomach. Food intake of patient is reduced by its restrictive and satiety effects. With LAGB, patients, experience early and prolonged satiety as well as reduced appetite. For this purpose, Wilkinson performed the first study on this subject in 1976 using the Marlex graft wrapped around the stomach [9]. Later, Hallberg and Forsell defined the device, which is now called the Swedish Adjustable Gastric Band (SAGB), in 1976 [10]. Also, during this period, an inflatable silicone-based gastric band, known today as the American Lap-Band, was defined by Kuzmak [11]. The first laparoscopic use of AGB was reported by Dr. Belachew in 1993 [12].

It is minimally invasive, and the diameter of the band is adjustable through an access port which is implanted under the skin. Adjustments of the band are usually carried out at an outpatient clinic during follow-up visits and are critical for successful outcomes.

On the technical point of view after the initial experience with Belachew's original technique for band placement which is so-called perigastric technique, higher rate of complications like slippage and pouch dilatation were reported. Subsequently with the modified "pars flaccida technique" several studies and RCTS showed a significant reduction of these complications [13, 14].

Indications

The indications to undergo bariatric surgery are based on body mass index (BMI) as well as the presence of comorbidity.

- BMI $\geq$ 40 kg/m², or body weight $\geq$ 100lbs above ideal body weight.

- BMI ≥ 35–<40 kg/m^2 and $\geq$ 1 high-risk comorbid condition, or body weight $\geq$ 80lbs above ideal body weight + 1 comorbidity.
- Failure to respond to, low likelihood of responding to, or refusal to undergo medically sound weight-loss program.
- Well informed and motivated and accepts operative risk.

Contraindications

- Absolute.
  - Mentally impaired, unable to weigh the risk and benefits of surgery.
  - Active neoplastic disease.
  - Cirrhosis with portal hypertension.
  - Unstable or incurable preexisting comorbidities (CAD, DM, asthma, AIDS, etc.), or uncontrolled psychiatric condition.
  - Pregnancy.
  - Immobility.
  - Inability or refusal to comply with postoperative regimens.
  - Active substance abuse.
  - Lack of social support.
  - Unable to tolerate general anesthesia.
- Relative.
  - Age.
  - Coagulopathy.
  - Previous abdominal surgery.

Preoperative Preparations

Preoperative planning is very important in order to achieve a successful result in patients who have undergone bariatric surgery. A group of qualified medical professionals, such as psychiatrists/psychologists, nutritionists, cardiologists, pulmonologists, endocrinologists, surgeons, and social workers, are an integral part of patient optimization. Patients often attend group classes designed to educate them about lifestyle changes they should follow after surgery and what to expect during and after surgery. The technical details of the surgery and the physical changes that will occur, as well as the adaptation to the nutritional and psychological aspects of the sur-

gery, are equally important. It is also important to examine patients before the operation in terms of excluding other diseases that may cause weight gain and to perform laboratory tests. Preoperative upper gastrointestinal system endoscopy is useful for the exclusion of gastric pathologies. At the same time, the presence of preoperative cholelithiasis should be evaluated with hepatobiliary ultrasound.

- Patient education.
- Psychological evaluation.
- Thorough history and physical examination.
- Referral to appropriate specialty.
- Screening laboratory tests (FBC, liver function, HgbA1c, iron, total iron-binding capacity, vit B$_{12}$, folate, vit D, calcium, thyroid function, serum lipid).
- Gallbladder ultrasound.
- Upper GI evaluation.
- Dietary counseling.
- Preoperative weight loss, esp. BMI >60 kg/m^2.

OT Setup, Patient Position, and Operative Team Position (Fig.1)

- Video monitor over at patient's left and right shoulders.

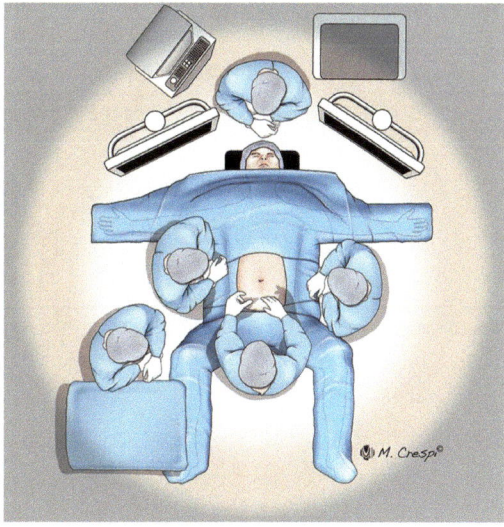

Fig. 1 Common operating room setup for bariatric surgery

- Patient supine with arms out, preferably split leg, secured to operative table, reverse Trendelenburg (about 25°).
- Surgeon between patient's legs or on the patient's right side if not split leg; assistant on either side of the patient or on the patient's left side if not split leg.

Instrumentation

- Optical Trocar or Veress needle for access.
- 5 mm ports (3 or 4)
- 15– 18 mm port (1)
- 30–45° scope, 5 or 10 mm (1)
- Nathanson liver retractor or Snake Retractor (1).
- Atraumatic graspers, 5 mm (2).
- Maryland dissector, 5 mm (1).
- Curved scissors, 5 mm (1).
- Hook diathermy, 5 mm (1).
- Energy-based scalpel (Thunderbeat, Olympus; Harmonic™ Ethicon, Ligasure™ Medtronic, etc.), 5 mm (1).
- Goldfinger (Obtech, Ethicon) (1).
- Band placer (1).
- Needle holder (2).
- Permanent sutures.
- Gastric band with access port (1).
- Suction/irrigation device (1).

Trocar/Port Placement (Fig. 2)

The places of incision and the number of trocars to be used are determined in a way that the surgeon feels comfortable. Generally, a total of four trocars are sufficient for this surgery. According to this;

- Port 1
  - 12–15 mm port
  - Midline 8–10 cm supra umbilical, placed optimally to view the operative field/working space (For initiation of working field, for the laparoscope/camera, for passage of gastric band).
- Port 2
  - 5 mm port
  - Just below the xiphoid for Nathanson liver retractor, or
  - Right Subcostal if a Snake Liver Retractor is utilized.
- Port 3
  - 5 mm or 10 mm port
  - Four finger breath below left costal margin, at the anterior axillary line (For left-hand assisting instruments).
- Port 4
  - 5 mm or 10 mm port
  - Below the right costal margin, at the anterior axillary line (For right-hand instruments).

Surgical Technique (Pars Flaccida Technique: (Figs. 3, 4, and 5)

- Dissection at the Angle of His.
  - Retract the liver up and to the right with a Nathanson retractor, exposing the diaphragm at the esophageal hiatus.
  - Using graspers draw down the fundus.

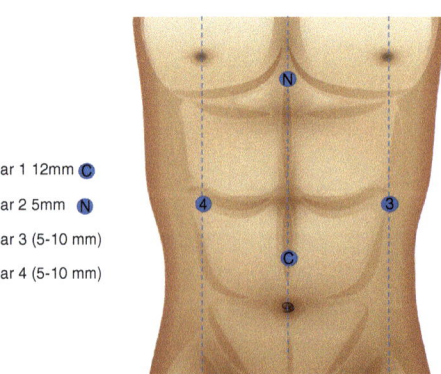
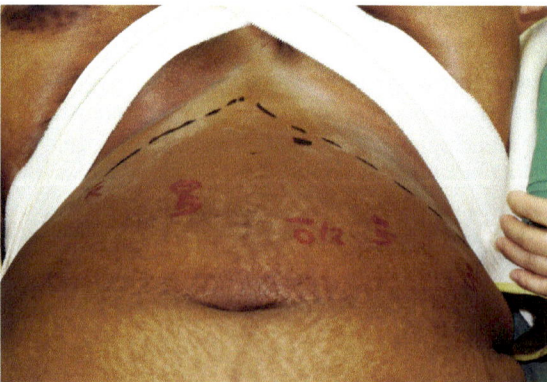

Trocar 1 12mm
Trocar 2 5mm
Trocar 3 (5-10 mm)
Trocar 4 (5-10 mm)

Fig. 2 Position of the trocars (**left**: illustration of the trocar positions, **right**: anterior view)

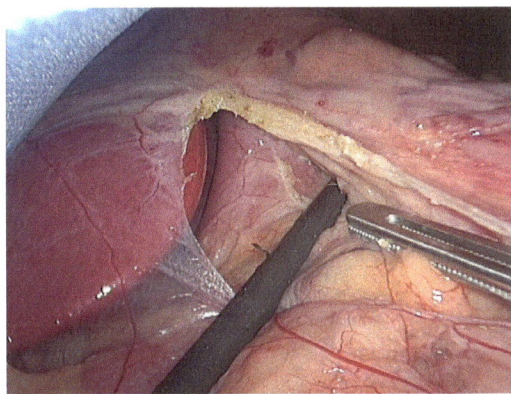

Fig. 3 First step of the pars flaccida approach: opening of the lesser omentum

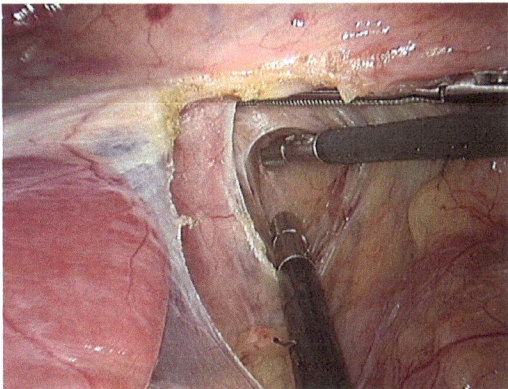

Fig. 4 Second step of the pars flaccida approach: dissection of the right crus and retrogastric tunnel using avascular plane dissection

- Dissect the gastrophrenic peritoneal attachment to expose the left crus, using hook diathermy or energy-based scalpel (Harmonic™, Ligasure™).
- Dissection at the Lesser Curve.
  - Draw the mid-lesser curve to the patient's left, with graspers.
  - Divide the pars flaccida of the lesser omentum.
  - Retract the posterior wall of the lesser sac to expose the anterior margin of the right crus.
  - Make a small opening in the peritoneum about 5 mm in front of the anterior margin of the right crus.
  - Dissect the retroesophagogastric opening using a blunt instrument or articulating dissector "Goldfinger" (Obtech, Ethicon) until it exits at the left crus.
- Band Placement and Calibration of Gastric Pouch (Figs. 6, 7, 8, and 9).
  - Band placer passed gently through the retroesophagogastric tunnel in a counterclockwise advancement until it exits at the left crus.
  - Band tubing is inserted into the slot of the placer.
  - Band placer withdrawn along its path to the lesser curve and retrieve the tubing.

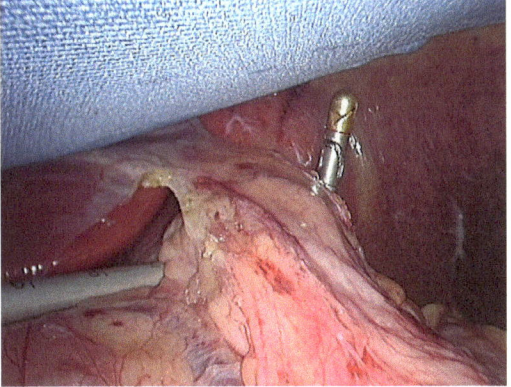

Fig. 5 The retrogastric tunnel is completed reaching the left crus using a dedicated instrument called "goldfinger"

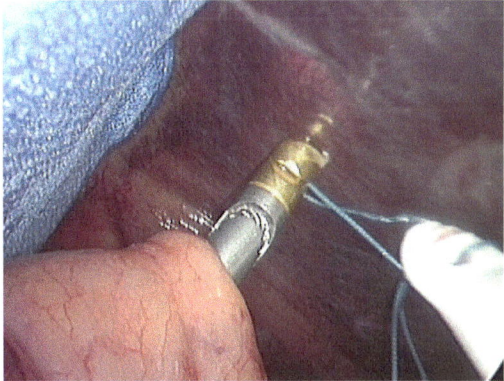

Fig. 6 The goldfinger is utilized to create the retrogastric tunnel

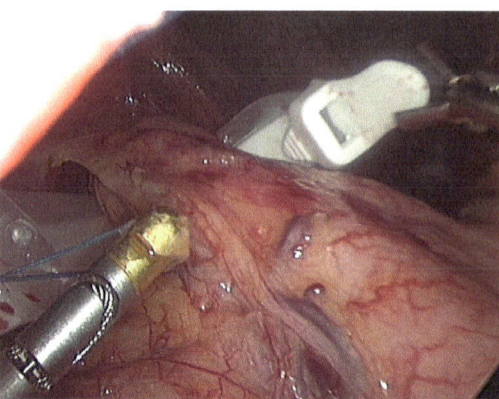

Fig. 7 The goldfinger is utilized to pass the gastric banding behind the stomach

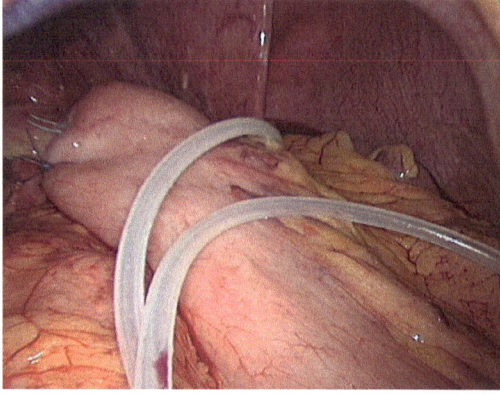

Fig. 8 The gastric band is then covered by a gastro-gastric flap using 3–4 nonabsorbable seromuscular stitches. The flap must cover completely the anterior part of the band

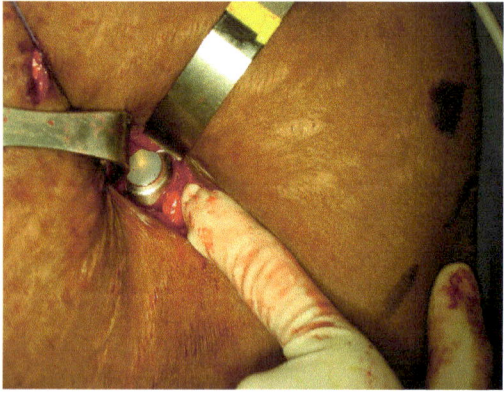

Fig. 9 Then the port reservoir is sutured at the abdominal fascia

- Draw the tubing until the band is in place, and partially close the buckle.
- Inflate the calibration balloon with 25 ml of air, withdraw the calibration tube until it touches the esophagogastric junction.
- Position the band over the equator of the balloon.
- Deflate the calibration balloon, and bring band to complete closure.
- Anterior fixation of the fundus and anterior gastric wall over the band, with three to four ventro-ventral sutures.
- Withdraw the calibration balloon.
• Placement of Gastric Band Calibration Port.
  - Bring out band tubing through a port site, with a large loop remaining within to prevent the tube from ripping off the calibration port due to extensive movement of patient.
  - Connect band tubing to access port, and secure to anterior rectus sheath with permanent sutures.

Surgical Technique Descriptive

The patient is positioned in the anti-Trendelenburg position (20–30°) with a slight inclination to the right and legs apart. The endo-laparoscopic monitor is placed on the head of the patient. The operation is started with the surgeon between the legs of the patient and the assistant surgeon on the side of the patient. Pneumoperitoneum can be created either using a Veress needle Technique (at umbilicus or Palmer Point), open Hasson technique, or using an Optical Trocar for an easy access under vision. The 12–15 mm optical trocar is inserted on the midaxillary line four fingers below the left costal margin. Then, one 5 mm and two other 5–10 mm cannulas were inserted as in Fig. 2. Two are the working port and the right subcostal utilized for liver retraction if not a subxiphoid Nathanson Retractor is used. The left lobe of the liver is elevated to expose the cardia of the stomach and the diaphragmatic crus. The dissection starts from the greater curvature and continues towards the diaphragm, and, at this stage, the left paraesophageal ligament dissection is completed, and the left crus is exposed. Then, the pars flacida is opened and the peritoneal sheet close to the edge of the right crus is opened to enter the retrogastric area. A retrogastric tunnel is created using a "Goldfinger instrument" or an atraumatic grasper till reaching the left crus and the phrenogastric ligament. During this step, we avoid the use of calibrated tube or balloon to avoid injury of the posterior GE wall. The band is inserted and passed through the retrogastric tunnel and closed over the bucket, then secured by anterior gastrogastric sutures using three or four nonabsorbable seromuscular stitches. This is to cover the anterior part of the band completely. If any injury or laceration of the posterior gastric wall is suspected, a methylene blue dye test is carried out. The connecting tube is passed through the subxiphoid port and connected to the port placed and anchored over the left rectus abdominis. The gastric band can be calibrated if needed after 3–4 weeks, with water/saline injection. Additional calibrations were later considered based on clinical evaluation of symptoms and weight loss during follow-up.

Postoperative Care

In order to keep the gastric band in the optimal position, it is very important to follow the patients with an appropriate diet program. The gastric passage may be narrowed due to postoperative edema of the gastric mucosa. Patients are started on the postoperative diet with liquids and continue with pureed, soft, and solid foods for a period of 3–4 weeks. These dietary guidelines should be given to patients in writing with the support of a dietician in the clinic. Patients may not be able to lose weight in this early period because the feeling of satiety caused by the band has not yet formed. When they start eating solids, they will often need reassurance that they will start losing weight [15].

- Upper GI gastrografin study on the first postoperative day; if normal findings, patient allowed to take fluids then structured diet.

- Adjustment of gastric band usually starts 4–6 weeks after operation and every 4–6 weeks thereafter based on the patient's rate of weight loss and food-fluid tolerance.
- Goal of gastric band adjustment.
  - Loss of excess weight within 18 months to 3 years.
  - Weight loss of 0.5–1.0 kg per week.
  - Sensation of prolonged satiety.
  - No negative symptoms.
- Adjustment of Gastric Band (two different type).
  - SAGB (high volume, low pressure).
    3–4 cc of fluid added at first adjustment
    1–1.5 cc of fluid on subsequent adjustment
    Final total volume of 6–8.5 cc.
  - LAP-BAND (low volume, high pressure).
    0.5–1.0 cc of fluid added at first adjustment
    0.3–0.5 cc of fluid on subsequent adjustment
    Final total volume of 3–5 cc.
- Adjustment Guidelines.
  - Adjustment not necessary.
    Adequate rate of weight loss.
    No negative symptoms.
    Eating reasonable range of food.
  - Consider adding fluid.
    Inadequate weight loss.
    Rapid loss of satiety after meals.
    Hunger between meals.
    Increased volume of meals.
  - Consider removing fluid.
    Vomiting, heartburn, reflux into the mouth.
    Choking, coughing spells, wheezing; especially at night.
    Difficulty with a broad range of food.
    Maladaptive eating behavior.

Side-Effect and Complications after LAGB (Table 1)

Band patients require long-term follow-up and are likely to require adjustments to the band on a regular basis. Even in the experienced hands

Table 1 Complications after LAGB

Minor complications
• Acute stomal obstruction
• Minimal bleeding
• Port infection
• Delayed gastric emptying
Major complications
• Gastric/esophageal perforation
• Hemorrhage
• Band erosion
• Band slippage/prolapse
• Port/tubing malfunction
• Port/tube leakage
• Esophageal dilatation

10–20% of patients who have weight-loss operations require follow-up operations to correct complications [16]. The majority of revision surgeries are minor revisions due to minor complications such as port revision and repositioning. Abdominal hernias are the most common complications requiring follow-up surgery. More than one-third of obese patients who have gastric surgery develop gallstones [17]. During rapid or substantial weight loss a person's risk of developing gallstones is increased. Gallstones can be prevented with supplemental bile salts taken for the first 6 months after surgery [18].

Nearly 30% of patients who have weight-loss surgery develop nutritional deficiencies such as anemia, osteoporosis, and metabolic bone disease. These deficiencies can be avoided if vitamin and mineral intake are maintained. Women of childbearing age should avoid pregnancy until their weight becomes stable because rapid weight loss and nutritional deficiencies can harm a developing fetus [19, 20].

Regarding the complications, LAGB is the obesity surgery with lowest rate of complications and mortality (0.2–0.4%) [21, 22]. The most common complications that require an intervention are band slippage, erosion and perforation, and port/tube dysfunction or infection.

Early complications are seen in the immediate postoperative period and include misplacement of the band, perforation, and early slippage with secondary acute pouch dilatation. Late complications include pouch dilatation, band herniation, spontaneous variation in volume, erosion of the gastric wall, and migration of the band.

Slippage

A gastric band can migrate distally along the stomach or the stomach proximally above the band. Most gastric band slippages are anterior and present chronically [23]. A posterior band slippage is rare but can occur if the gastric band has been placed within the lesser sac of the stomach. Misplacement of the band is usually caused by the surgeon's lack of experience and rarely occurs when the surgeon is experienced. The band may be placed in the perigastric fat not a constant finding, and the diagnosis may be delayed for a few days. The use of barium has been controversial because it may cause inflammation and fibrosis in these critically ill patients or in the lower part of the stomach, the latter causing severe gastric outlet obstruction.

Perforation

As with any laparoscopic surgery, hollow organ perforations can be seen after LAGB, but specific to this procedure, perforations usually develop in the cardia of the stomach [24]. This early gastric perforation is usually due to surgical trauma to the stomach wall. The patient presents with fever, pain, and leukocytosis. Water-soluble contrast imaging may reveal the leakage from the stomach. However, leakage is not a constant finding, and the diagnosis may be delayed for a few days. The use of barium has been controversial because it may cause inflammation and fibrosis in these critically ill patients and is probably better avoided if there is definite evidence of leakage. Gastrografin is an alternative option. CT is also diagnostic, showing the leakage and the possible associated subphrenic abscess.

Pouch Dilation

Early pouch dilatation has been described in low-positioned bands. Pouch dilatation is also a common late complication. After surgery, the pouch gradually increases in volume but retains a grossly concentric shape. It may also be secondary to overinflation of the band or to eccentric band herniation that results from focal band weakness. A contrast X-ray swallow test will identify the gastric pouch enlargement, diagnostic of a pouch dilatation. Management of a pouch dilatation should consist of initial band deflation with the pars flaccida approach, where with minimal dissection and higher position of the band, there is less risk for dilation. Slippage of the band can cause eccentric pouch dilation [25].

Erosion

The clinical presentation of chronic gastric erosion varies between asymptomatic conditions and acute abdominal emergency. Mechanical damage to the wall may be secondary to intraoperative trauma to the muscular layers, inflammatory reaction to foreign bodies, infection, and use of nonsteroidal anti-inflammatory medication. it is eventually a consequence of local gastric ischemia secondary to a tight band and the incidence of erosion following gastric band surgery remains currently at around 1% [26]. The passage of the contrast out of the lumen around the band is a certain indication of band erosion. Gastric erosion is highly likely if an open band is seen. Findings may be associated with a change in band position.

Leakage of the Banding System

Leakage is typically a late complication. It may occur at the level of the band or the connector tube or at the access port. It is first suspected when filling and insufficient deflating volume of the banding system combined with loss of eating restriction are observed Leakage of contrast material is usually detected while adjusting the band diameter. The incidence of port-related revisions is around 6% and the majority of these are for the management of leaks [27].

Infection

As around any foreign body, soft-tissue infection around the access port is possible. In addition, even the sterile puncture and adjustment of the stoma size may introduce infection, which then extends along the connector tube and along the band, with possible abscess formation. Infection increases the risk of perforation and fistulization and may necessitate surgical debridement and removal of the band.

Since its introduction in 1993, laparoscopic adjustable gastric banding has been the subject of many studies and evaluations. The continuous progress in surgical technique and increasing experience of surgeons have decreased the rate of many complications. LAGB procedure has been a very popular procedure for a while due to the relatively low learning curve, being technically easy, the duration of hospitalization is short, it can be applied as outpatient operations in some places, the early complication rates are low, and the desired level of weight loss can be achieved due to the adjustment of the band [28, 29]. The popularity of Gastric Banding was at the peak around 2008–2010 (about 40% of bariatric procedures worldwide) and then due to the high number of long-term and serious complications such as weight gain, obstructive symptoms, dysphagia, band slippage, esophageal dilatation, esophagitis, and gastric erosion and also the advent of other restrictive procedures like sleeve gastrectomy the frequency of LAGB procedures went down dramatically worldwide [30, 31]. Many patients and surgeons today prefer procedures like Laparoscopic Sleeve Gastrectomy or Roux-en-Y gastric bypass as an alternative to gastric banding. However, even though results have shown the efficacy of the banding in weight loss, controlling comorbidities such as diabetes mellitus II, hypertension, and OSA when the long-term results showed failure in weight loss, weight regain, long-term complications, banding becomes less and less utilized today [25, 28, 32, 33].

References

1. Gundogdu E, Moran M. Adjustable gastric banding. Ann Laparosc Endosc Surg. 2020. https://doi.org/10.21037/ales-2019-bms-06.
2. Angrisani L, Santonicola A, Iovino P, Vitiello A, Higa K, Himpens J, Buchwald H, Scopinaro N. IFSO worldwide survey 2016: primary, Endoluminal, and Revisional procedures. Obes Surg. 2018;28(12):3783–94. https://doi.org/10.1007/s11695-018-3450-2.
3. Bond DS, Phelan S, Leahey TM, Hill JO, Wing RR. Weight-loss maintenance in successful weight losers: surgical vs non-surgical methods. Int J Obes. 2009;33(1):173–80. https://doi.org/10.1038/ijo.2008.256.
4. Flum DR, Dellinger EP. Impact of gastric bypass operation on survival: a population-based analysis. J Am Coll Surg. 2004;199(4):543–51. https://doi.org/10.1016/j.jamcollsurg.2004.06.014.
5. NIH conference. Gastrointestinal surgery for severe obesity. Consensus development conference panel. Ann Intern Med. 1991;115(12):956–61.
6. Golzarand M, Toolabi K, Farid R. The bariatric surgery and weight losing: a meta-analysis in the long- and very long-term effects of laparoscopic adjustable gastric banding, laparoscopic roux-en-Y gastric bypass and laparoscopic sleeve gastrectomy on weight loss in adults. Surg Endosc. 2017;31(11):4331–45. https://doi.org/10.1007/s00464-017-5505-1. Epub 2017 Apr 4.
7. Rubino F, Nathan DM, Eckel RH, Schauer PR, Alberti KG, Zimmet PZ, Del Prato S, Ji L, Sadikot SM, Herman WH, Amiel SA, Kaplan LM, Taroncher-Oldenburg G, Cummings DE, Delegates of the 2nd Diabetes Surgery Summit. Metabolic surgery in the treatment algorithm for type 2 diabetes: a joint statement by international diabetes organizations. Diabetes Care. 2016;39(6):861–77. https://doi.org/10.2337/dc16-0236.
8. American Diabetes Association. 7. Obesity management for the treatment of type 2 diabetes. Diabetes Care. 2017;40(Suppl 1):S57–63. https://doi.org/10.2337/dc17-S010.
9. Wilkinson LH, Peloso OA. Gastric (reservoir) reduction for morbid obesity. Arch Surg. 1981;116(5):602–5. https://doi.org/10.1001/archsurg.1981.01380170082014.
10. Hallberg D, Forsell I. Ballongband vid behandling av massiv overvikt (balloon band for the treatment of massive obesity). Svensk Kirwgi. 1985:43–106.
11. Kuzmak LI. Silicone gastric banding: a simple and effective operation for morbid obesity. Contemp Surg. 1986;28:13–8.
12. Belachew M, Legrand M, Vincenti VV, Deffechereux T, Jourdan JL, Monami B, Jacquet N. Laparoscopic placement of adjustable silicone gastric band in the treatment of morbid obesity: how to do it. Obes Surg. 1995;5(1):66–70. https://doi.org/10.1381/096089295765558196.
13. O'Brien PE, Dixon JB, Laurie C, Anderson M. A prospective randomized trial of placement of the laparoscopic adjustable gastric band: comparison of the perigastric and pars flaccida pathways. Obes Surg. 2005;15(6):820–6. https://doi.org/10.1381/0960892054222858.
14. Di Lorenzo N, Furbetta F, Favretti F, et al. Laparoscopic adjustable gastric banding via pars flaccida versus perigastric positioning: technique, complications, and results in 2,549 patients. Surg Endosc. 2010;24(7):1519–23. https://doi.org/10.1007/s00464-009-0669-y.
15. Cobourn Chris S, Dixon JB. LAGB: the technique. In: Obesity, bariatric and metabolic surgery. Cham: Springer; 2016. p. 299–306.
16. Carelli AM, Youn HA, Kurian MS, Ren CJ, Fielding GA. Safety of the laparoscopic adjustable gastric band: 7-year data from a U.S. center of excellence. Surg Endosc. 2010;24(8):1819–23. https://doi.org/10.1007/s00464-009-0858-8.
17. Gustafsson U, Benthin L, Granström L, Groen AK, Sahlin S, Einarsson C. Changes in gallbladder bile composition and crystal detection time in morbidly obese subjects after bariatric surgery. Hepatology. 2005 Jun;41(6):1322–8. https://doi.org/10.1002/hep.20686.
18. Uy MC, Talingdan-Te MC, Espinosa WZ, Daez ML, Ong JP. Ursodeoxycholic acid in the prevention of gallstone formation after bariatric surgery: a meta-analysis. Obes Surg. 2008;18(12):1532–8. https://doi.org/10.1007/s11695-008-9587-7.
19. Dixon JB, Dixon ME, O'Brien PE. Pregnancy after lap-band surgery: management of the band to achieve healthy weight outcomes. Obes Surg. 2001;11(1):59–65. https://doi.org/10.1381/096089201321454123.
20. Jefferys AE, Siassakos D, Draycott T, Akande VA, Fox R. Deflation of gastric band balloon in pregnancy for improving outcomes. Cochrane Database Syst Rev. 2013;4:CD010048. https://doi.org/10.1002/14651858.CD010048.pub2.
21. Chakravarty PD, McLaughlin E, Whittaker D, Byrne E, Cowan E, Xu K, Bruce DM, Ford JA. Comparison of laparoscopic adjustable gastric banding (LAGB) with other bariatric procedures; a systematic review of the randomised controlled trials. Surgeon. 2012;10(3):172–82. https://doi.org/10.1016/j.surge.2012.02.001. Epub 2012 Mar 8.
22. O'Brien PE, MacDonald L, Anderson M, Brennan L, Brown WA. Long-term outcomes after bariatric surgery: fifteen-year follow-up of adjustable gastric banding and a systematic review of the bariatric surgical literature. Ann Surg. 2013;257(1):87–94. https://doi.org/10.1097/SLA.0b013e31827b6c02.
23. Boschi S, Fogli L, Berta RD, Patrizi P, Di Domenico M, Vetere F, Capizzi D, Capizzi FD. Avoiding complications after laparoscopic esophago-gastric banding: experience with 400 consecutive patients. Obes Surg. 2006;16(9):1166–70. https://doi.org/10.1381/096089206778392329.
24. Soto FC, Szomstein S, Higa-Sansone G, Mehran A, Blandon RJ, Zundel N, Rosenthal RJ. Esophageal

perforation during laparoscopic gastric band placement. Obes Surg. 2004;14(3):422–5. https://doi.org/10.1381/096089204322917981.

25. O'Brien PE, Hindle A, Brennan L, Skinner S, Burton P, Smith A, Crosthwaite G, Brown W. Long-term outcomes after bariatric surgery: a systematic review and meta-analysis of weight loss at 10 or more years for all bariatric procedures and a single-Centre review of 20-year outcomes after adjustable gastric banding. Obes Surg. 2019;29(1):3–14. https://doi.org/10.1007/s11695-018-3525-0.

26. Brown WA, Egberts KJ, Franke-Richard D, Thodiyil P, Anderson ML, O'Brien PE. Erosions after laparoscopic adjustable gastric banding: diagnosis and management. Ann Surg. 2013;257(6):1047–52. https://doi.org/10.1097/SLA.0b013e31826bc21b.

27. Tog CH, Halliday J, Khor Y, Yong T, Wilkinson S. Evolving pattern of laparoscopic gastric band access port complications. Obes Surg. 2012;22(6):863–5. https://doi.org/10.1007/s11695-011-0567-y.

28. Chang SH, Stoll CR, Song J, Varela JE, Eagon CJ, Colditz GA. The effectiveness and risks of bariatric surgery: an updated systematic review and meta-analysis, 2003-2012. JAMA Surg. 2014;149(3):275–87. https://doi.org/10.1001/jamasurg.2013.3654.

29. Chapman AE, Kiroff G, Game P, Foster B, O'Brien P, Ham J, Maddern GJ. Laparoscopic adjustable gastric banding in the treatment of obesity: a systematic literature review. Surgery. 2004;135(3):326–51. https://doi.org/10.1016/S0039-6060(03)00392-1.

30. Gündoğdu E, Bilgiç Cİ, Moran M, Güldoğan CE, Dilektaşli E, Özmen MM. Evaluation of the effects of laparoscopic adjustable gastric banding versus laparoscopic sleeve gastrectomy on weight loss. Eur Res J. 2019;6(1):36–42.

31. English WJ, DeMaria EJ, Brethauer SA, Mattar SG, Rosenthal RJ, Morton JM. American Society for Metabolic and Bariatric Surgery estimation of metabolic and bariatric procedures performed in the United States in 2016. Surg Obes Relat Dis. 2018;14(3):259–63. https://doi.org/10.1016/j.soard.2017.12.013. Epub 2017 Dec 16.

32. Himpens J, Cadière GB, Bazi M, Vouche M, Cadière B, Dapri G. Long-term outcomes of laparoscopic adjustable gastric banding. Arch Surg. 2011;146(7):802–7. https://doi.org/10.1001/archsurg.2011.45.

33. Chevallier JM, Zinzindohoué F, Douard R, Blanche JP, Berta JL, Altman JJ, Cugnenc PH. Complications after laparoscopic adjustable gastric banding for morbid obesity: experience with 1,000 patients over 7 years. Obes Surg. 2004;14(3):407–14. https://doi.org/10.1381/096089204322917954.

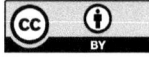

Laparoscopic Sleeve Gastrectomy

Sajid Malik and Sujith Wijerathne

Bariatric surgery (BS) has proved its role in treating obesity and related comorbidities. The number of Laparoscopic Sleeve Gastrectomies (LSGs) performed globally has increased markedly and has become "trendy" among bariatric surgeons in the last few years [1]. LSG has attained its position as the primary procedure of choice in bariatric surgery for morbid obesity. In this procedure, 80% of the stomach, mainly the body and fundus are removed longitudinally, leaving behind a sleeve of the stomach along the lesser curve [2, 3]. The procedure can be performed by minimally invasive approaches as well as single incision access or even robotic surgery with comparable results [4, 5]. The weight loss is achieved by restricting the food entering the stomach. Another factor in the effectiveness of weight loss in sleeve gastrectomy is the decrease in blood levels of ghrelin, "the hormone that stimulates hunger," and a majority of cells responsible for producing this hormone is found in the fundus which is removed during this procedure. This procedure can be performed as the first stage in more complex bariatric cases including cases of super-obesity before procedures like Roux-en-Y gastric bypass or the duodenal switch can be performed [6]. The objective is to achieve an initial weight loss that would help to perform more extensive mixed restrictive or malabsorptive procedures safely and effectively [7–9].

Indications

- First stage procedure before a more complex procedure for BMI > 60.
- Preferred bariatric procedure for the high-risk obese BMI 35–40.
- Revision of previous laparoscopic adjustable gastric banding (LAGB).
- Redo LSG.

Contraindications

- Extensive previous surgery.
- Crohn's Disease.
- Elderly patients with extensive comorbidities.

Preoperative Preparation

- Weight and height measurement on a standard electronic scale.
- Nutritional parameters.
- Evaluate cardiopulmonary function.
- Obstructive sleep apnea tests.

S. Malik (✉)
Department of General Surgery, Allama Iqbal Medical College, Jinnah Hospital, Lahore, Pakistan

S. Wijerathne
Department of Surgery, National University Health System, Singapore, Singapore

General Surgery Services, Alexandra Hospital Singapore, Queenstown, Singapore

© The Author(s) 2023

D. Lomanto et al. (eds.), *Mastering Endo-Laparoscopic and Thoracoscopic Surgery*, https://doi.org/10.1007/978-981-19-3755-2_41

- 2 weeks on low or very low caloric diet
- Upper GI endoscopy.
- Testing for Helicobacter pylori.
- Psychiatric evaluation.
- Chemoprophylaxis.
- Thromboprophylaxis.

Instruments

For LSG, Laparoscopic tray with full set of instruments is required, including endoscopic gastrointestinal anastomosis (GIA) staplers, and silk and polyglactin sutures

- Energy device (Ultrasonic or Advanced bipolar or combined).
- 3 × 5 mm ports
- 1 × 10 mm ports
- 1 × 15 mm port
- 1 × Optical-view Trocar
- 1 × Dissecting forceps
- 2 × Bowel graspers
- 1 × Babcock forceps
- 1 × Bowel Grasper Single Action
- 1 × Curved scissors
- 1 × L-hook
- 1 × Suction Irrigation 5 mm/10 mm cannula
- Nathanson/Snake liver retractor.
- Clip Applicator with Hemolock.
- 1 × Needle holder curved
- 1 × Veress Needle.

Patient and Trocar Positions

- Supine with reverse-Trendelenburg position.
- Foot support on board.
- Anti-embolic precautions.
- Prophylactic antibiotics.
- 12 mm Optical port is placed under direct vision approximately 15 cm below the xiphoid process and almost 4 cm left to the midline.
- Pneumoperitoneum is created and 30 laparoscope is introduced.
- A 5 mm port is placed in left lateral flank at the same level as the optical port.

- Another 5 mm port is placed in right epigastric region for liver retraction.
- Another 12/15 mm port is placed in mid epigastrium in the midline.
- Another 5 mm port is placed on the right side lateral to the 12/15 mm port.
- Left lobe of the liver is retracted using a snake retractor.

Operative Techniques

After the pneumoperitoneum is created, a diagnostic laparoscopy is done to exclude other pathologies. The liver is retracted cranially, and the GE junction is exposed (Fig. 1). A point in the greater curve is identified and marked at 6 cm proximal to the pylorus as the distal extent of the resection (Fig. 1).

Division of the greater omentum to enter the lesser sac and division of short gastric vessels is achieved by using an energy device along the gastrocolic and gastrosplenic ligaments from the greater curvature up to the angle of His (Figs. 2, 3, and 4). Be aware of gastroduodenal and right gastric artery at pylorus and stop dissection about 5 cm proximal to it to prevent injury to these vessels and to preserve perfusion of the pylorus and the distal antrum [7]. Make sure to dissect closely along the greater curvature leaving no fat behind.

Next step is to lift and pull the stomach to the right of patient to have a better view of gastro-

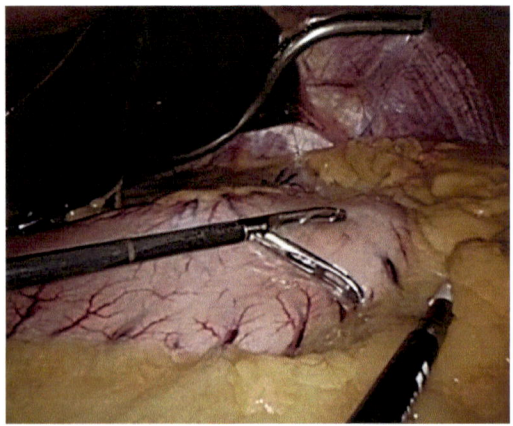

Fig. 1 Placement of boogie and placing it on suction

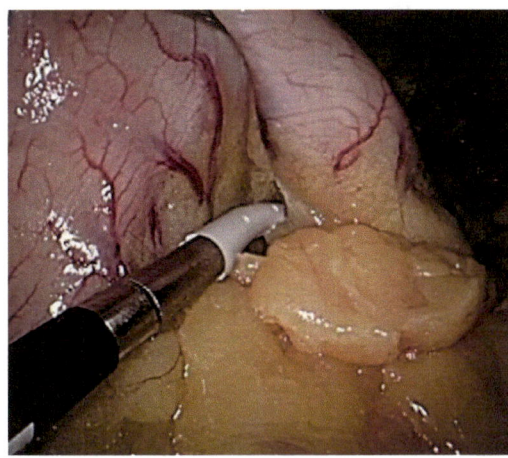

Fig. 2 Dissection started at 6 cm proximal to pylorus to enter lesser sac

esophageal (GE) junction along with left crus and spleen to dissect down any adhesions on posterior wall of stomach (Fig. 4). Last of few short gastric vessels in this area can be divided along the left crus. The greater curvature must be completely freed up to the left crus of the diaphragm.

Next step is to position the bougie (size 36 Fr) in the stomach before using stapler. Afterward linear cutting staples are used to vertically transect the stomach creating a narrow gastric tube with an estimated capacity of less than 150 ml. Check location of anvil and cartridge both anteriorly and posteriorly to achieve optimized stapling (Figs. 5 and 6). It is important to compress the line of transection of the gastric tissue with the

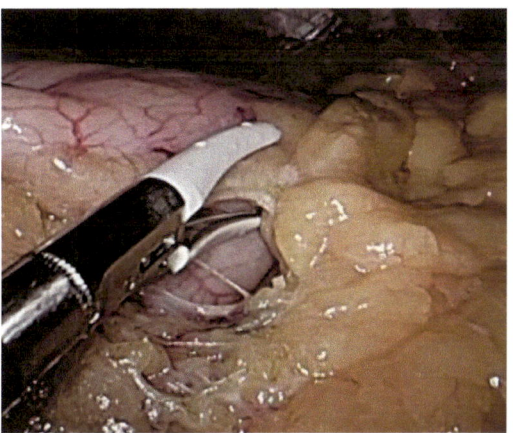

Fig. 3 Lesser sac entry

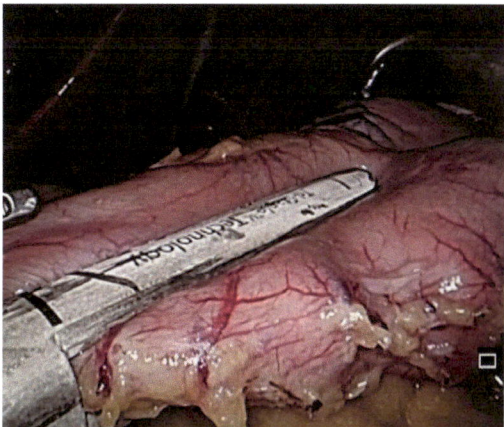

Fig. 5 First cutting staples

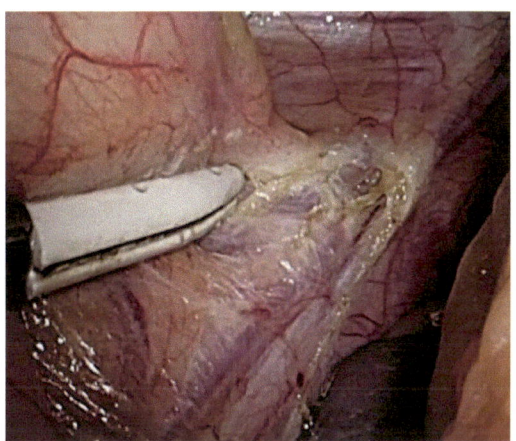

Fig. 4 Posterior wall of stomach

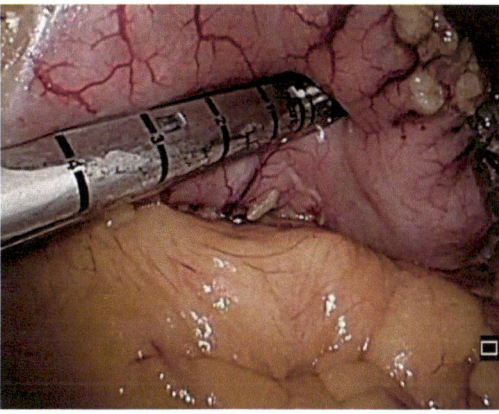

Fig. 6 View of posterior wall and less curve to check the position of stapler

staple for 15 s prior to firing, to get adequate hemostasis and stapling of gastric tissues. First, stapler is usually 60 mm black or green cartridge for the antrum. Gold cartridges can be used together with Seamguards to prevent staple line bleeding and leaks. Second, cartridge should be green, black, or purple depending on the surgeon's choice, but smaller cartridges than those mentioned above are not recommended in this region. Care must be taken to avoid stenosis at incisura (Fig. 7). It is good practice to rotate the stomach and stapler anteriorly to have a look at the posterior wall before firing the stapler and distal end must be at least 2 cm from GE junction (Fig. 8). Hold the "new" stomach and ask anesthetist to off the suction and remove the bougie, observe for few minutes for any bleed or leak at

this point. Next reinforcement sutures can be applied to any areas of bleeding and omentopexy to prevent volvulus; however, these measures are debatable and must be practiced as tailored approach for individual cases.

Role of drains in the subhepatic space adjacent to the gastric tube is controversial and is not recommended. The resected stomach is placed in a specimen bag or even can be directly extracted through the epigastric 15 mm port site. Fascial sutures are not routinely used for 5 mm or 10 mm port sites, but 15 mm port site fascia should be closed to prevent future port site hernia.

When to Convert

- Massive blood loss.
- Dense adhesions.

Major Post-op Complications and Management

Hemorrhage

Risk of postoperative bleeding is from 1–5% and the source could be intraluminal or extraluminal. Intraluminal bleeds can present as melena or hematemesis due to bleeding from staple line. Upper GI bleeding protocol should be followed. Large-bore IV cannula, fluid resuscitation, Input/output monitoring, and blood transfusion if needed should be practiced. Urgent Upper GI endoscopy to locate and control the bleeding is warranted.

Extraluminal bleeding is commonly from staple line, injury to abdominal viscera, or from port site. These patients presents with drop of serial hemoglobin, tachycardia, or occasionally hypotension. Urgent diagnostic laparoscopy helps to make the diagnosis and to evacuate hematoma along with control of source of bleeding. Even if source is not identified, hematoma evacuation and drain placement serve as a treatment.

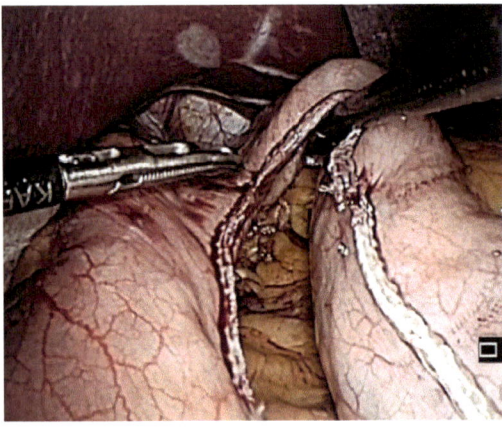

Fig. 7   Observe staple line

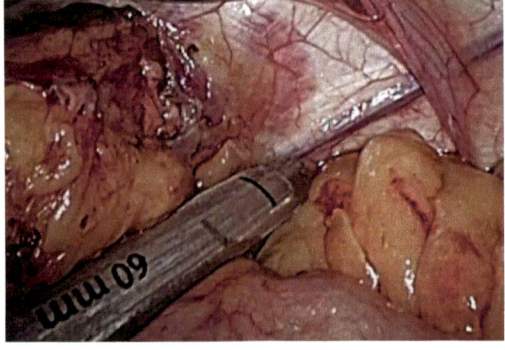

Fig. 8   last stapler 2 cm from GE junction

Staple Line Leak

Staple line leak is the most dreadful complication of LSG which can occur in approximately 2–3% of patients [10]. Based on upper GI contrast studies and radiological findings, leaks are divided into two types: Type I is a controlled leak and could be easily managed with aspiration, drainage, or through a natural fistulous tract formation; Type II is a disseminated variety and needs an urgent diagnostic laparoscopy, wash out and surgical repair of leak if technically feasible. Enteral nutrition with feeding jejunostomy is preferred as the mode of feeding in these patients. Early and delayed presentations are classified based on the time of presentation after surgery (either within 3 days or after 8 days, respectively).

Treatment of delayed and disseminated variety is challenging because of hemodynamic instability of patient and inflammatory reaction leading to sepsis [11]. Treatment in this condition involves vigorous resuscitation with fluids, IV antibiotics, holding off oral feeding, aspiration/drainage under radiological guidance, followed by surgical repair of leak as a definitive procedure [12].

Stenosis

This rare complication is observed in less than 2% of patients and needs urgent attention once diagnosed. Patients present with vomiting, regurgitation, or feeling of fullness [13]. It is further subdivided into two subtypes anatomical or functional stenosis which determines the treatment options in both groups. Upper GI endoscopy is a good initial investigation to diagnose anatomical variety but tridimensional *CT with 3D reconstruction* is a diagnostic modality with good sensitivity for functional groups [14].

Intraoperatively to prevent stenosis, the endoluminal bougie should be placed along the lesser curvature going all the way distal to the antrum and avoid excessive lateral traction and twisting of the stomach. Avoid pushing the bougie too distally which can result in shorter and larger than expected gastric tube when bougie is removed. Endoscopic balloon dilatations with multiple sessions can be used to treat stenosis with or without an alternative option of stenting. If recurrent or unresolved after dilatation then Roux-en-Y Gastric Bypass (RYGB) is a treatment option.

Portal Thrombosis

This rare complication occurs in almost 0.3–0.5% of cases. Several factors like splenic ischemia, dehydration in early postoperative period, variation in blood flow after resection of vessels along greater curvature, and thrombophilia can contribute to this. Clinical severity is the predictor of the outcome of treatment which includes holding off oral feeding and providing IV fluids for rehydration. Anticoagulation should be considered even on slightest suspicion. Treatment with therapeutic dose of low molecular weight heparin for 5–7 days and bridging therapy with oral anticoagulation with Warfarin to keep INR between 2–3 for 3–6 months is needed. Surgical options for portal thrombosis are reserved for complicated cases like thrombosis leading to splanchnic ischemia [15, 16].

Postoperative Care

1. Admit to ICU or Surgical High Dependency unit for close monitoring for signs of obstructive sleep apnea.
2. Diet is maintained on general liquids for 1 week and gradually progressed by the dietician.
3. Encourage early sitting up on the bed and if possible early ambulation.
4. Chest physiotherapy.
5. Continue mechanical deep vein thrombosis prophylaxis during the rest of hospitalization.
6. Gradual exercise is started 1 month after the operation with advice from a physiotherapist.

References

1. Buchwald H, Oien D. Metabolic/bariatric surgery worldwide 2011. Obes Surg. 2013;23:427–36.
2. Young MT, Gebhart A, Phelan MJ, Nguyen NT. Use and outcomes of laparoscopic sleeve gastrectomy vs laparoscopic gastric bypass: analysis of the American College of Surgeons NSQIP. J Am Coll Surg. 2015;220:880–5.
3. ASMBS Clinical Issues Committee. Updated position statement on sleeve gastrectomy as a bariatric procedure. Surg Obes Relat Dis. 2012;8:e21–6.
4. Elli E, Gonzalez-Heredia R, Sarvepalli S, Masrur M. Laparoscopic and robotic sleeve gastrectomy: short- and long-term results. Obes Surg. 2015;25:967–74.
5. Maluenda F, Leon J, Csendes A, Burdiles P, Giordano J, Molina M. Single-incision laparoscopic sleeve gastrectomy: initial experience in 20 patients and 2-year follow-up. Eur Surg. 2014;46:32–7.
6. Silecchia G, Boru C, Pecchia A, Rizzello M, Casella G, Leonetti F, Basso N. Effectiveness of laparoscopic sleeve gastrectomy (first stage of biliopancreatic diversion with duodenal switch) on co-morbidities in super-obese high-risk patients. Obes Surg. 2006;16:1138–44.
7. Santoro S. Technical aspects in sleeve gastrectomy. Obes Surg. 2007;17(11):1534–5.
8. Himpens J, Dobbeleir J, Peeters G. Long-term results of laparoscopic sleeve gastrectomy for obesity. Ann Surg. 2010;252(2):319–24.
9. Frezza EE. Laparoscopic vertical sleeve gastrectomy for morbid obesity. The future procedure of choice? Surg Today. 2007;37:275–81.
10. Márquez MF, Ayza MF, Lozano RB, et al. Gastric leak after laparoscopic sleeve gastrectomy. Obes Surg. 2010;20:1306–11.
11. Himpens J, Dapri G, Cadiere GB. Treatment of leaks after sleeve gastrectomy. Bariatric Times. 2009. http://bariatrictimes.com/treatment-of-leaks-after-sleevegastrectomy/. Accessed 29 October 2012.
12. Oshiro T, Kasama K, Umezawa A, et al. Successful management of refractory staple line leakage at the esophagogastric junction after a sleeve gastrectomy using the HANAROSTENT. Obes Surg. 2010;20:530–4.
13. Goitein D, Matter I, Raziel A, Keidar A, Hazzan D, Rimon U, et al. Portomesenteric thrombosis following laparoscopic bariatric surgery: incidence, patterns of clinical presentation, and etiology in a bariatric patient population. JAMA Surg. 2013;148:340–6.
14. Rebibo L, Hakim S, Dhahri A, Yzet T, Delcenserie R, Regimbeau JM, et al. Gastric stenosis after laparoscopic sleeve gastrectomy: diagnosis and management. Obes Surg. 2016;26:995–1001.
15. Condat B, Pessione F, Helene Denninger M, Hillaire S, Valla D. Recent portal or mesenteric venous thrombosis: increased recognition and frequent recanalization on anticoagulant therapy. Hepatology. 2000;32:466–70.
16. Hamoui N, Anthone GJ, Kaufman HS, Crookes PF. Sleeve gastrectomy in the high-risk patient. Obes Surg. 2006;16(11):1445–9.

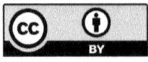

Laparoscopic Roux EN y Gastric Bypass (LRYGB)

Rajat Goel, Chih-Kun Huang, and Cem Emir Guldogan

Introduction

Edward Mason introduced a different approach to bariatric surgery (BS) in 1966, inspired by the observation that subtotal gastrectomies often cause weight loss (WL) [1]. The first gastric bypass procedure was performed by horizontal section of 10% volume of the upper stomach and anastomosis into the jejunal loop, excluding 90% of the gastric reservoir. Wittgrove and Clark established a standard technique for laparoscopic gastric bypass in 1991 [2]. Similar progressive improvement in the results of Laparoscopic Roux-en-Y Gastric Bypass (LRYGB) is reported in most large series around the world [3, 4].

BS or Metabolic Surgery (MS) has given morbidly obese patients sustainable WL and better or complete control of weight-related comorbidities like Type 2 Diabetes Mellitus (T2DM), hypertension (HT), hyperlipidemia (HL), obstructive sleep apnea, joint pain, and others. Laparoscopic Roux-en-Y (LRYGB) is considered the gold

standard BS procedure giving the above benefits for a longer period of time. LRYGB is also associated with lifelong follow-up like other bariatric surgeries and requires stringent intake of multivitamins, calcium tablets, vitamin d supplements, and Iron for long periods of time to prevent nutrition-related side effects a few years down the line.

With LRYGB method, up to 25% total body WL (68.2% excess WL) can be achieved in the long term [5, 6]. After LRYGB, WL was attributed to consuming a smaller volume and bypassing the jejunum. However, it is likely that there is a complex interplay of physiological mechanisms including food intake, food preferences, calorie restriction, and energy expenditure.

Early complications occur in approximately 4% of patients after LRYGB. The most common complications are bleeding, perforation, or leakage requiring immediate surgical intervention [7]. In 15–20% of patients, late complications such as abdominal pain, obstruction, anastomotic stricture, and marginal ulcers may occur up to 10 years after surgery [8, 9].

Patient Selection and Indications

Medical treatment can be tried in morbid obesity, but failure rates are still very high, patients can be evaluated for surgery after medical treatment fails. NIH has determined some conditions for patients who want to have BS in 1991 [10]. The

R. Goel
Supreme Superspecialty Hospital, Faridabad, India

Aakash Healthcare Superspeciality Hospital, Dwarka, New Delhi, India

C.-K. Huang
Body Science & Metabolic Disorders International Medical Center, China Medical Hospital, Taichung, Taiwan

C. E. Guldogan (✉)
Department of Surgery, Liv Hospital, Ankara, Turkey

© The Author(s) 2023
D. Lomanto et al. (eds.), *Mastering Endo-Laparoscopic and Thoracoscopic Surgery*,
https://doi.org/10.1007/978-981-19-3755-2_42

Society of American Gastrointestinal Endoscopic Surgeons (SAGES) has similar recommendations [11].

- Patients who are unlikely to respond to medical treatment.
- Patients who are motivated and informed about surgical risks.
- Patients with a body mass index (BMI) > 40 kg/m^2.
- Patients with BMI between 35 and 40 kg/m^2, with one high-risk comorbid condition.

In Asian setup, the following guidelines are followed

- BMI >37 kg/m^2 irrespective of comorbidity.
- BMI >32 kg/m^2 in the presence of T2DM or two or more obesity-related comorbidities.

These guidelines ensure that patients can be properly classified for surgery, and patients can be prepared for surgery.

Contraindications

- Contraindications of General Anesthesia.
- Intractable Coagulopathy.
- Metastatic or Inoperable Malignancy.
- Cirrhosis with Portal Hypertension (Type B and C Budd Chiari Classification).
- Inflammatory Bowel Disease.
- Previous Surgery involving small bowel resection.
- Relative contraindications include large ventral hernia, multiple previous abdominal surgeries, extremes of age (<18 and >65), alcohol/drug abuse.

Note: Surgery should be deferred if the patient plans for pregnancy within 12–18 months.

Preoperative Assessment

The most important aspect for long-term success of LRYGB is proper counseling regarding life-

style and dietary changes, regular follow-ups, and need for prolonged supplement usage.

Preoperative Investigation

Blood Investigation

Complete blood count, Blood Group, Renal Function Test, Liver Function test, PT/INR, PTTK, Lipid Profile, Thyroid Profile, Blood sugar random (Blood sugar Fasting and Postprandial, HbA1C, C peptide level if Diabetic), Vitamin B12, and Vitamin D3.

1. X-ray Chest.
2. ECG and 2D ECHO or 2D Stress Echo (If hypertensive).
3. Upper Gastrointestinal Endoscopy (to rule out H. Pylori Infection).
4. Ultrasound Examination of whole abdomen (to rule out gall stones) and if present Cholecystectomy should be planned with bariatric even if asymptomatic.
5. Urine Routine and Microscopy.
6. Ultrasound Doppler Bilateral Lower Limb Venous System (to rule out DVT).

OT Setup and Port Positioning

Patient's Position

All long instruments, Nathanson's Liver Retractor, and 45°long scope should be ready. Patient should be in Supine position or split leg according to surgeon preference with secure strapping and padding of bony points and table should be checked for reverse Trendelenburg position. We catheterize all patients routinely. (Fig. 1).

Port Positioning

Our preferred entry is by 0 telescope mounted on 12 mm 15 cm long Optiview trocar in the left midclavicular line 15–18 cm from Epigastrium.

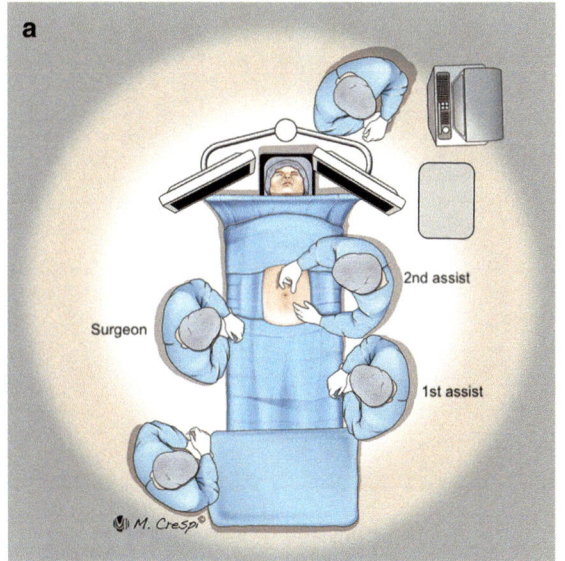
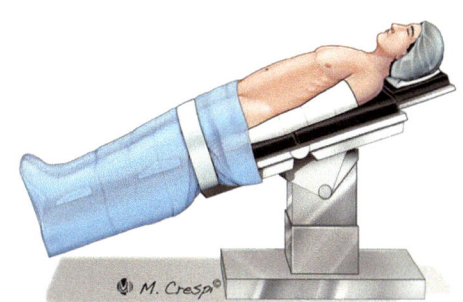

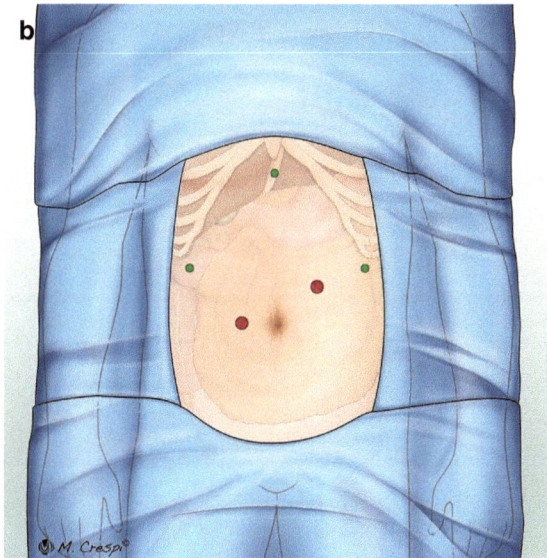

Fig. 1 (**a**) Patient's position. (**b**) Port placement

1. Second Trocar is inserted 5 or 12 mm 15–18 cm from epigastrium in right midclavicular line (Surgeon port).
2. Third 12 mm trocar is inserted a palm breadth from second trocar in right upper abdomen (Surgeon port).
3. Fourth 5 mm port through epigastrium for liver retractor.
4. Fifth 5 mm port palm breadth from first on left upper abdomen (Assistant Port) (Fig. 1b).

Surgical Technique

Step 1: Creation of gastric pouch: Patient is placed in steep reverse Trendelenburg position. Dissection is done along lesser curvature starting between first and second vessel from gastroesophageal junction. A retrogastric tunnel is created by blunt dissection and energy source. A 60 mm linear blue or purple stapler applied transversely from port 3 and followed by Vertical 60 mm Blue or Purple firings [2–3] from port 2 to create 25–30 ml pouch is created over 36 french bougies. Gastrotomy is created at distal most part of the pouch for Gastrojejunostomy (Fig. 2).

Step 2: Fashioning of Gastrojejejunostomy: Patient is made supine. Transverse Mesocolon mesentery is lifted to identify DJ Flexure (Ligament of Treitz) and small bowel is counted 70–100 cm (Depending on BMI kg/m2) and 45 cm blue or purple stapler is used and Gastrojejunostomy is fashioned and enterotomy closed by vicryl 2/0 after performing Jejuno-jejunostomy. Now Patient is again made reverse Trendelenburg. The patency of Gastrojejunostomy is checked by smooth passage of Orogastric Tube. Leakage is checked by methylene blue dye test (Fig. 3).

Step 3: Side to Side Jejuno-Jejunostomy: 60 mm white stapler is used to form BilioPancreatic limb just distal to Gastrojejunostomy. Now 100 cm Alimentary Limb is counted and Side to side Jejuno-Jejunostomy is fashioned by 60 mm white stapler and enterotomy closed by vicryl 2/0 (Fig. 4).

Step 4: Closure of Mesenterc defects: Both Jejeunojejunostomy and Petersen defects are closed by nonabsorbable 2/0 Ethibond sutures.

Step 5: Drain Insertion and closure of defects: One Jackson Pratt drain is put close to Gastrojejunostomy anastomosis and all ports are closed (12 mm ports are closed in layers and 5 mm only skin is closed).

Post-op Course

Patient is kept NPO on the day of surgery and put on pantoprazole infusion (80 mg in 50 ml normal saline at 5 ml/h). Patient is started on oral sips on post-op day1 and mobilized with chest physiotherapy and Incentive spirometry. On postoperative day 2 30–50 ml clear liquid is started and the patient is discharged with one dose of protein solution. Gradually Clear liquid fluid is escalated to 80–100 ml per hour followed by blend diet and full small meals over a period of 1–2 months. Note patient should not drink water 30 min before and 30 min after every meal. Patient should not use any straw. Most important is complete absti-

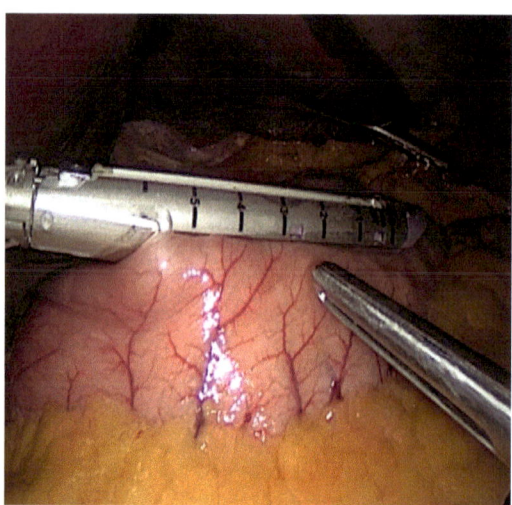
Fig. 2 Creation of Gastric pouch

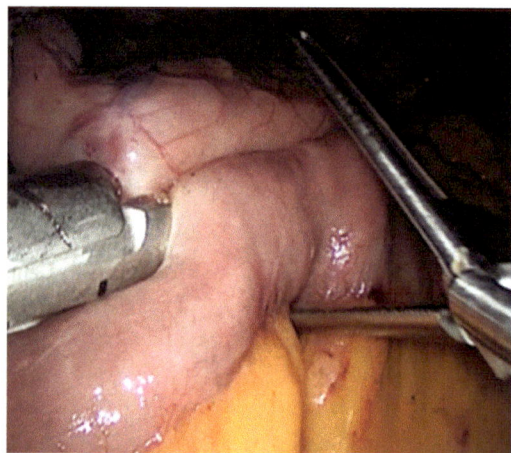
Fig. 3 Fashioning of Gastrojejunostomy

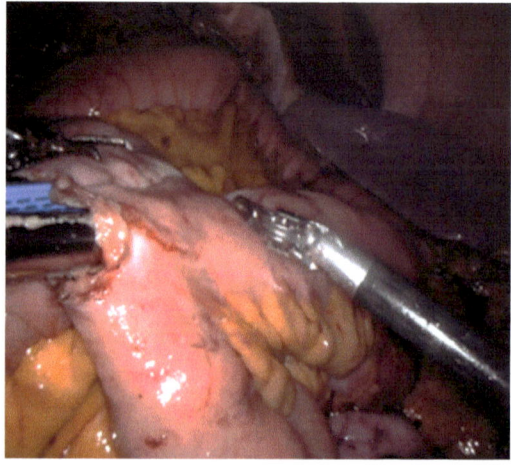
Fig. 4 Side to side Jejuno-jejunostomy

nence from Alcohol and Smoking to prevent any complications. Another important point is the continuous intake of multivitamins, Calcium, VitaminD3, and Iron throughout life. Patient is also advised for complete laboratory checks once a year and monthly meetings with the physician and should be encouraged to attend support group meetings.

Common Complications

- *Bleeding*: Any evidence of bleeding like disproportionate rise in pulse rate and drop in hemoglobin should warn for diagnostic laparoscopy even in absence of any abdominal signs. CECT abdomen may be used as an adjunct for relaparoscopy but should not be mandatory and clinical suspicion should alert the clinician to have a diagnostic check. Any bleeder should be sutured (over hemostat) and if no bleeding is seen, check endoscopy intraoperative should be done and bleeder taken care of. If still no bleeder is seen and jejeunojejunostomy is suspected oversewing the anastomosis and if required refashioning the anastomosis should be considered.
- *Leakage:* Another very important complication is leakage from anastomotic site. Re Laparoscopy with resuturing/refashioning anastomosis/Gastrostomy drainage with feeding jejeunostomy should be attempted depending on the time of redo surgery and patient general condition. Leakage from Jejeunojejunostomy should be dealt with suturing/refashioning with distal feeding jejunostomy should be done.
- *Stenosis:* Gastrojejunostomy stricture should be dealt with the removal of triggering factor (Smoking) and serial dilatations or refashioning. Jejuno-jejunostomy stricture will present with obstruction or abdominal distension and will require refashioning.
- *Others:* Deep Venous Thrombosis and Pulmonary embolism should be dealt with

standard treatment protocols. Weight regain treatment will vary from diet counseling, redosurgery (Limb lengthening/fundectomy). Internal hernias are rare if both mesenteries are closed but if any doubt exists immediate Diagnostic laparoscopy or Exploratory Laparotomy should be done. Nutritional deficiencies have to be dealt with on case to case basis and may even require reversal of procedure in extreme cases.

Late Complications

- Vitamin deficiencies and hair loss.
- Dental problems.
- Abdominal pain and discomfort.
- Dumping syndrome.
- Postprandial hypoglycemia.
- Loss of bone density.
- Kidney stones.
- Gallstones.
- Gastric remnant distension.
- Marginal ulcers.
- Stomal Stenosis [12].

Conclusion

LRYGB offers both benefits and complications, the mechanisms of which are still not fully understood. Most clinicians agree that beneficial effects outweigh harm [13, 14]. The suggestions that the LRYGB relies solely on mechanical restriction and malabsorption are no longer valid. In order to achieve positive results after LRYGB, the harmony of intestinal hormones, bile acids, nerve mechanisms, intestinal microbiota, food preferences and changes in energy expenditure is essential [15]. Complications can be seen in all bariatric surgical methods. However, many studies have been conducted in order to diagnose complications early and manage them correctly after LRYGB.

References

1. Mason EE, Ito C. Gastric bypass in obesity. Surg Clin N Am. 1967;47(6):1345–51.
2. Wittgrove AC, Clark GW, Schubert KR. Laparoscopic gastric bypass, Roux en-Y: technique and results in 75 patients with 3-30 months follow-up. Obes Surg. 1996;6(6):500–4.
3. Weiss AC, Parina R, Horgan S, Talamini M, Chang DC, Sandler B. Quality and safety in obesity surgery—15 years of Roux-en-Y gastric bypass outcomes from a longitudinal database. Surg Obes Relat Dis. 2016;12(1):33–40.
4. Maciejewski ML, Livingston EH, Smith VA, Kavee AL, Kahwati LC, Henderson WG, Arterburn DE. Survival among high-risk patients after bariatric surgery. JAMA. 2011;305(23):2419–26.
5. Olbers T, Gronowitz E, Werling M, Mårlid S, Flodmark CE, Peltonen M, Marcus C. Two-year outcome of laparoscopic Roux-en-Y gastric bypass in adolescents with severe obesity: results from a Swedish Nationwide study (AMOS). Int J Obes. 2012;36(11):1388–95.
6. Buchwald H, Avidor Y, Braunwald E, Jensen MD, Pories W, Fahrbach K, Schoelles K. Bariatric surgery: a systematic review and meta-analysis. JAMA. 2004;292(14):1724–37.
7. Hofmann W, van Koningsbruggen GM, Stroebe W, Ramanathan S, Aarts H. As pleasure unfolds: hedonic responses to tempting food. Psychol Sci. 2010;21(12):1863–70.
8. Abdeen G, Le Roux CW. Mechanism underlying the weight loss and complications of Roux-en-Y gastric bypass. Rev Obes Surg. 2016;26(2):410–21.
9. Franco J, Ruiz P, Palermo M, Gagner M. A review of studies comparing three laparoscopic procedures in bariatric surgery: sleeve gastrectomy, Roux-en-Y gastric bypass and adjustable gastric banding. Obes Surg. 2011;21:1458–68.
10. Consensus Development Conference Panel. Gastrointestinal surgery for severe obesity. Ann Intern Med. 1991;115(12):956–61.
11. Nguyen NT, DeMaria E, Ikramuddin S. In: Hutter MM, editor. The SAGES manual: a practical guide to bariatric surgery. Springer Science & Business Media; 2008.
12. le Roux CW, Sinclair P. Gastric bypass: mechanisms of functioning, In *gastric bypass*. Cham: Springer; 2020. p. 7–21.
13. Abdeen G, Le Roux CW. Mechanism underlying the weight loss and complications of Roux-en-Y gastric bypass. Review. Obesity surgery. 2016;26(2):410–21.
14. Pinkney J. Consensus at last? The international diabetes federation statement on bariatric surgery in the treatment of obese type 2 diabetes. Diabet Med. 2011;28(8):884–5.
15. le Roux CW, Welbourn R, Werling M, Osborne A, Kokkinos A, Laurenius A, Olbers T. Gut hormones as mediators of appetite and weight loss after Roux-en-Y gastric bypass. Ann Surg. 2007;246(5):780–5.

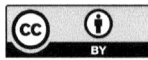

One Anastomosis Gastric Bypass (OAGB)

Hrishikesh Salgaonkar, Alistair Sharples,
Kanagaraj Marimuthu, Vittal Rao,
and Nagammapudur Balaji

One-anastomosis gastric bypass is an attractive option in the armament of a Bariatric surgeon. A relatively simple procedure, it has been effective in inducing weight loss and resolution of obesity-associated comorbidities. Easy technique, shorter operative times, and low complication rates make it an attractive alternative option, particularly in super-obese individuals. While concerns remain regarding the long-term safety profile with regards to biliary reflux, risk of esophagogastric malignancies, and marginal ulcer. For the scope of this chapter, our focus will be on the advent of the concept, the surgical technique, and tips and tricks.

Introduction

The concept of "loop" gastric bypass was first introduced by Mason in 1967, which consisted of a gastric bypass with only one anastomosis [1]. Mason's suggested a short and horizontal-shaped wide gastric pouch. This configuration exposed the esophageal mucosa to caustic bile reflux from the jejunal loop. Due to its bile reflux-inducing mechanism, this concept was abandoned quickly. Rutledge in 1997, introduced his version of one

H. Salgaonkar (✉) · A. Sharples · K. Marimuthu ·
V. Rao · N. Balaji
Department of Bariatric and Upper GI Surgery,
University Hospitals North Midlands,
Stoke-on-Trent, UK

anastomosis gastric bypass naming it "mini-gastric bypass" (MGB). This was mainly because the original technique was described through a mini-laparotomy [2]. In his technique, the gastric pouch was a lesser curvature-based long sleeve starting 2–3 cm distal to the crow's feet and extending slightly to the left of the "angle of His" proximally. A single ante-colic anastomosis between the gastric pouch and jejunum, about 3–5 cm wide was constructed 180–220 cm distal to the ligament of Treitz. This distance from the ligament of Treitz was modified marginally in selected cases based on the obesity class, age, and dietary preferences.

In order to reduce bile reflux, in 2002 Carbajo and Caballero proposed a variation to this technique wherein a latero-lateral anastomosis was performed between the gastric pouch and jejunal loop, averagely 250–350 cm from the ligament of Treitz. They named the technique "one anastomosis gastric bypass" (OAGB) or "bypass gastrico de una anastomosis" in Spanish (BAGUA) [3].

Over the years a variety of names like "omega loop gastric bypass" (OLGB) or "single anastomosis gastric bypass" (SAGB) have been used to describe the procedure [4, 5]. Finally, in 2013, a group of surgeons proposed the term "mini-gastric bypass-one anastomosis gastric bypass" (MGB-OAGB) to standardize the nomenclature and reduced the confusion created by multiple names for essentially the same procedure [6]. This nomenclature was later approved by the International Federation for the Surgery of

D. Lomanto et al. (eds.), *Mastering Endo-Laparoscopic and Thoracoscopic Surgery*,
https://doi.org/10.1007/978-981-19-3755-2_43

Obesity and Metabolic disorders (IFSO) MGB-OAGB task force and recommended that OAGB should be the identifier for this procedure in future publications [7]. Over the last decade, although the popularity of the procedure is on the rise particularly in Asia Pacific and Europe region, [8] concerns regarding the possibility of bilio-enteric reflux and its long-term implications mainly the theoretical risk of gastric and esophageal cancer persists.

Indications

Suitability for bariatric surgery is based on body mass index (BMI) and the presence of comorbidity. These indications remain the same for offering OAGB

- BMI of 40 kg/m^2 or greater without coexisting medical problems.
- Patients with a BMI greater than or equal to 35 kg/m^2 and one or more obesity-related comorbidities, e.g., type 2 diabetes, hypertension, severe debilitating arthritis, hyperlipidemia, obstructive sleep apnoea (OSA), nonalcoholic fatty liver disease (NAFLD), gastroesophageal reflux disease (GERD), etc.
- Patients with BMI between 30 and 34.9 kg/m^2 with recent onset type 2 diabetes or metabolic syndrome also may undergo weight loss surgery, although there is a lack of sufficient data to demonstrate long-term benefits in such patients [9, 10].

Contraindications

As OAGB is performed under general anesthesia, any contraindications for giving general anesthesia automatically is a contraindication to proceed with surgery. From a surgical perspective, there are no absolute contraindications to OAGB, although relative contraindications do exist. These are drug/alcohol dependency, unstable coronary artery disease, end-stage lung disorders, severe heart failure, patients receiving active cancer treatment, portal hypertension, Crohn's dis-

ease, and impaired intellectual capacity which prevents the patient from understanding the long-term implications and postoperative care. Preoperative reflux has been found to have an increased risk with the development of postoperative bile reflux [11] and hence it is the author's opinion that OAGB should be deferred in these groups of patients.

Preoperative Assessment and Work-Up

Patients should be evaluated by a multidisciplinary team comprising of surgeon, physician, psychologist/psychiatrist, and nutritionist. These teams should work in close collaboration with the general practitioners and community healthcare/social workers. A thorough preoperative psychological, nutritional, and medical evaluation including assessment of comorbidities and fitness for surgery should be done. Patient education with regards to the lifestyle changes they need to undergo, what to expect before, during, and after surgery, nutritional and psychological changes postsurgery is paramount. We routinely prescribe 2 weeks of low-calorie high protein diet preoperatively. This is particularly helpful to shrink the liver size and assist during the surgery with liver retraction.

Operative Technique

Operation theater layout—The patient is placed supine position with split leg (Fig. 1). In bariatric surgery securing patient to the operative table is of paramount importance with straps at mid-thigh levels, to both legs separately and foot support.

Test this preoperatively by placing patient in anti-Trendelenburg position before starting the surgery. Both the arms are tucked by the patient side. Compression stockings and pneumatic compression devices are applied to both legs until unless contraindicated. The surgeon stands in between the legs, camera operator on the right side, and another assistant on the left. Standard 5

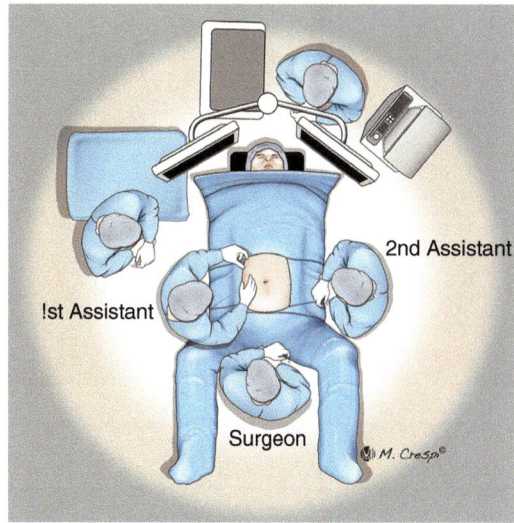

Fig. 1 Theater setup and patient position

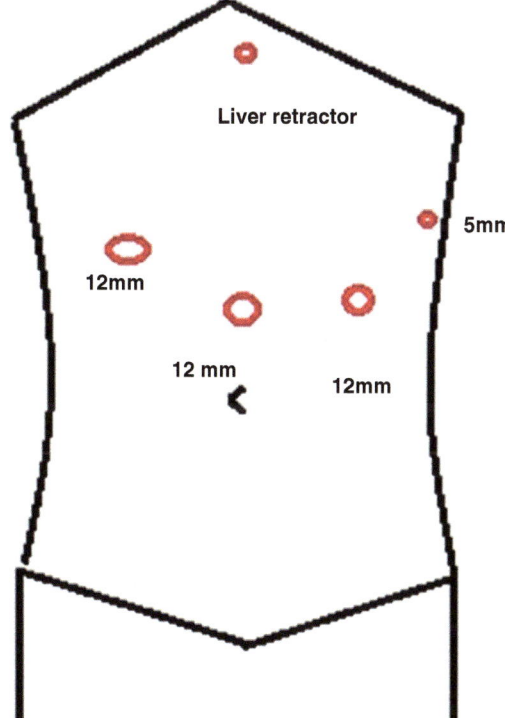

Fig. 2 Port placement

trocars technique is used (Fig. 2). While techniques for performing various bariatric procedures have a reasonable amount of variation based upon surgeon preference and training, the objectives are relatively uniform.

Instrumentation—Over the years with advances in instrument technology many types of nontraumatic bowel graspers, energy devices, needle holders, suturing devices, liver retractors, suction-irrigation devices and tools designed for dissecting the abdominal cavity have been developed. Based on surgeon preference these can vary, important factor when using any device or instrument is its safety profile, simplicity of use, cost, easy availability, and reusability.

Abdominal access and technique—Creation of pneumoperitoneum can be done using a Veress needle or by direct trocar entry (Optical entry) and insufflating the abdomen to 12–15 mm of Hg. The table is then placed in anti-Trendelenburg position 30–40°. This allows better visualization of the stomach and tissue spaces that need to be dissected. Rest trocars are placed under vision. A liver retraction device is placed through one of these port sites, usually substernal to expose the hiatal, stomach, and surrounding areas.

Always start by performing a general examination of the peritoneal cavity to exclude any other pathology, e.g., abdominal wall hernia, adhesions, etc.

Phase 1—The angle of His and fundal fat pad is identified. While some surgeons just delineate the fundal fat pad, others prefer to dissect off the same to expose the left crus of the diaphragm explicitly in order for optimal positional of the stapling device at this extremely critical location. Always look out for a hiatal hernia which is not an uncommon occurrence in morbidly obese. If present, dissect the phreno-esophageal membrane and peri-esophageal adhesions to reduce the hernia. Post reduction, at least 2–3 cm of intra-abdominal length of esophagus should be achieved. Hiatal closure is performed using standard principles and care.

Phase 2—The most important step in OAGB is creation of a "long gastric pouch" to keep the bile stream as far away from the esophagus as possible. Identify the crow's foot and just distal to it, dissect the gastro-hepatic omentum adjacent to the lesser curvature to enter the retro-gastric space. Care should be taken so that the entry point is always distal to the crow's foot and proximal to the pylorus. Avoid unnecessary dissection medially along the lesser curvature posteriorly, so as to avoid injury to the left gastric artery. Based upon sur-

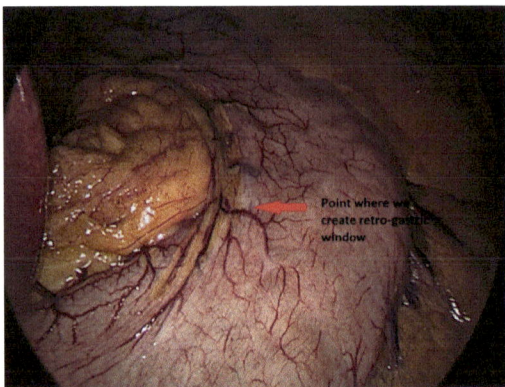
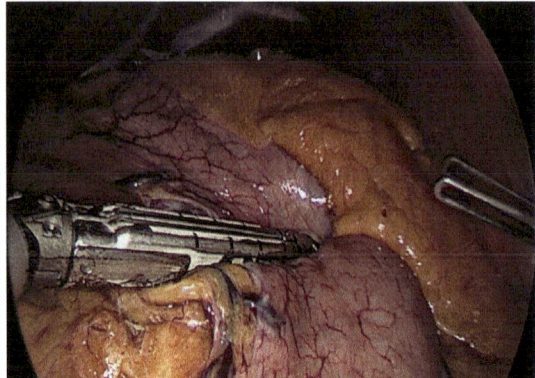

Fig. 3 Identification of "crow's feet" and first endo-stapler fire horizontally in distal gastric region perpendicular to the lesser curvature

geon preference different stapling devices can be used. Using a 45 mm/3–4 mm stapler the first fire is performed from the right-side working trocar in a relatively perpendicular direction to the lesser curvature (Fig. 3). Any gastric pouch shorter than 9 cm has been correlated with an increased risk of postoperative duodeno-gastroesophageal reflux.

Lee et al. [12] long pouch also reduces the tension on the future anastomosis. At this moment the anesthetist passes a 36–40 Fr bougie under vision and narrow pouch is created over this. Vertical sectioning is next and using a 60 mm/3–4 mm stapler introduced through the left working trocar, fired from the crotch of the first fire parallel to the lesser curve and vertically up towards the angle of His. The endo-stapler is adjusted close to the bougie but not very tight. When in doubt ask the anesthetist to pull back the bougie by a few centimeters and reinsert to make sure it is not caught in the endo-stapler. After every staple fire, migratory staples if any should be removed. This reduces the risk of endo-stapler misfiring. Before every staple fire, check for posterior wall redundancy and do necessary adjustments. As you progress cranially towards the angle of His, posterior adhesions if any should be dissected. Once close to the angle of His, connection with the anterior dissection done at the onset is possible. Make sure to create a wide retro-gastric window so as to visualize the left crus of diaphragm. Stay well away "1–2 cm" lateral to the esophagogastric junction. This step is extremely critical to avoid complications namely leaks. Also, take care that the tip of the endo-

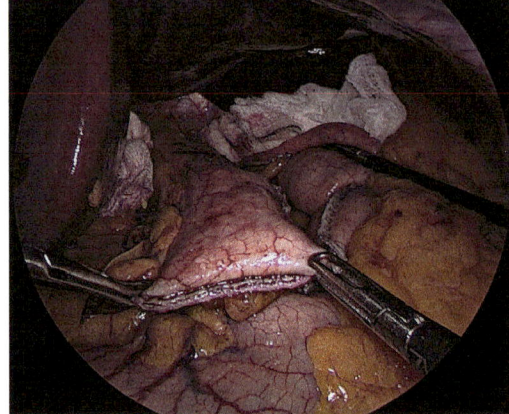

Fig. 4 Tension-free long gastric pouch

stapler jaw does not injure the spleen or splenic vessels. Verify complete gastric transection, any terminal tissue connections do not hesitate to use an additional endo-staple fire. It is important to achieve hemostasis along the gastric staple lines on pouch as well as the remnant stomach, as these areas may become difficult to visualize once you perform gastro-jejunal anastomosis. A good gastric pouch should be long (15–18 cm), narrow, well vascularized without any torsion. It should be easy to bring the pouch caudally without any undue tension (Fig. 4).

Phase 2—Reduce the anti-Trendelenburg tilt and if required we can do a slight Trendelenburg so as to help visualize and measure entire small bowel. The first step is to visualize the ligament of Treitz, which is achieved by lifting the gastro-colic omentum above the transverse colon. Jejunal counting is done with atraumatic bowel graspers, sequentially by grasping and running segments in increments of 5–10 cm. Once we reach a point of 150–200 cm distally, the assistant grasps the bowel as an indicator. The point varies based upon the patient's obesity class, BMI, and comorbidities profile. In certain specific scenarios, this point may be extended beyond 200 cm. Although longer limb lengths can give better weight loss results, it also increases the risk of malnutrition and excess weight loss, especially beyond 250 cm [11, 13]. It is the author's preference to continue running the bowel distally to count the entire small bowel upto the ileocecal junction, so as to assess the common channel (CC) length. Maintaining at least 300–350 cm of common channel is a prudent strategy.

Once the measurement is complete the assistant grasps the small bowel and holds it in place. Based upon surgeon preference if needed we can put a serosal stitch with vicryl keeping long ends or encircle the small bowel by a soft rubber drain (e.g., Jaques catheter) through a small opening in the mesentery. The assistant grasps the drain or vicryl stitch ends which helps in fixing the point as well as helps in providing traction during the gastro-jejunal (GJ) anastomosis. If any difficulty or tension while bringing the small bowel loop towards the gastric pouch should warrant an omental split.

Phase 3—Using an ultrasonic shear or a diathermy hook, small apertures are made in the distal gastric pouch and the small bowel (usually about 5 mm). Confirm that we have entered the lumen by passing a tip of nontraumatic bowel grasper into the lumen through the aperture or aspiration of intraluminal contents. Secure hemostasis and rule out any mechanical injury on the posterior or lateral wall. Using a 30 mm or 45 mm/3–4 mm stapler an ante-colic GJ anastomosis is performed. The gastro-enteric opening is then closed using 2–0 reabsorbable sutures or Stratafix or V-loc continuous closure. The authors prefer re-enforcing with a second sero-muscular layer (Two-layered technique). During learning curve, it may be advisable to perform the anastomosis over a gastric bougie by asking the anesthetist to pass the same distally into the efferent limb. The authors prefer performing a latero-lateral anastomosis so as to maintain an isoperistaltic pattern of food bolus flow (Fig. 5).

Bile reflux is a major criticism of OAGB, and hence some surgeons prefer adding an "anti-reflux mechanism" wherein a continuous latero-lateral suture between the small bowel loop (along the antimesenteric border) and the staple line of gastric pouch performed. This should be done ideally before the GJ anastomosis is done

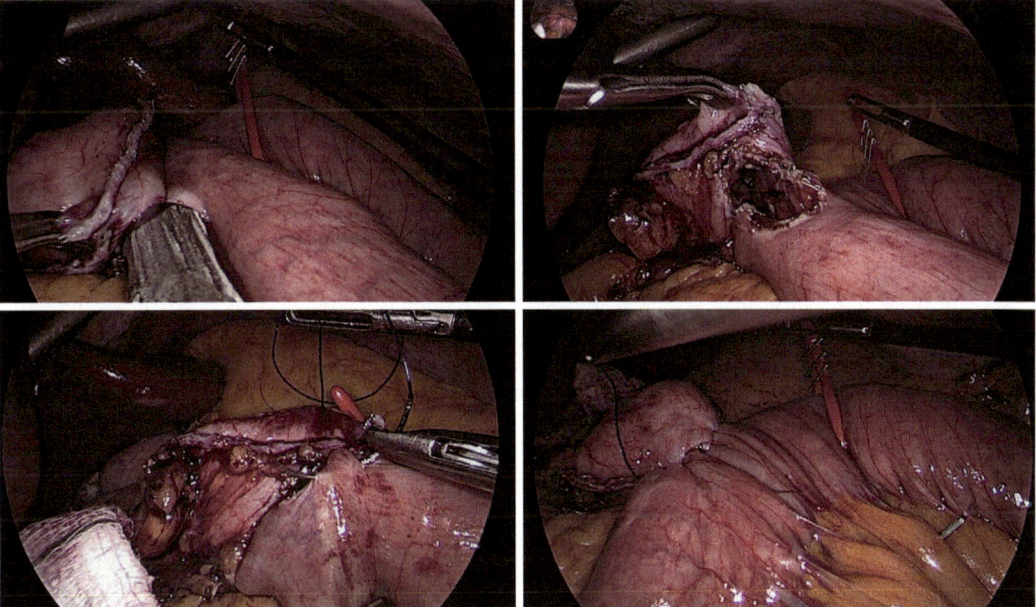

Fig. 5 Steps of gastro-jejunal anastomosis

performed starting from between the junction of first and second vertical staple firing on the gastric pouch and 8–10 cm caudally up to the tip of gastric pouch as described in the "Spanish BAGUA technique" [14].

Phase 4—Competency of the anastomosis is tested using a leak test "methylene blue" or "pneumatic test" with help of the anesthetist. This can be done through a nasogastric tube or calibration tube respectively positioned just proximal to the anastomosis. Visualize all the staple lines and potential sites for bleeding and secure hemostasis using titanium clips. We routinely do not place intra-abdominal drain. All trocars are removed under vision to rule out any port site bleeding.

Postoperative Care

As per the ERAS protocol (Early recovery after surgery), adequate analgesics and anti-emetics are prescribed. Early mobilization and free fluids (clear liquid diet) starting initially with 20–30 ml swallows of water are recommended once patient is fully awake. Most patients usually tolerate this regimen well and are discharged 24h postoperatively with specific advice on diet, physical activity, medications, and red flag signs. We routinely discharge patients with anti-thrombotic prophylaxis (also given during hospital stay) based on the hospital recommendations. The bariatric team is always contactable by telephone for consultation if needed and there is a very low threshold to call the patient back for evaluation if any issues.

Complications

Although there is paucity of evidence from randomised control trials, early and late complication rates following OAGB are acceptable and comparable [7]. Complications such as staple line bleeding, anastomotic leak, stricture, marginal ulcer, surgical site infections, port site hernia, conversion rates, diarrhoea, dumping syndrome etc are similar to any other bariatric procedure. Risk of internal hernia is lower in OAGB compared to RYGB, as also is the occurrence of small bowel obstruction. Inadequate weight loss is relatively

uncommon in OAGB [12]. This is mainly due to the greater effect of malabsorption, which may be a favourable effect in super-obese. The same may also lead to theoretically higher risk of nutritional deficiencies. There is lack of long-term data with regards to nutritional complications. Hence, lifelong follow up is paramount, and in the event of excessive weight loss or specific nutritional deficiency treatment with additional supplements is necessary. Unattended, risk of life-threatening malnutrition, Wernicke encephalopathy, iron deficiency anaemia and hypo-albuminemia is high. In cases where despite of active intervention excessive weight loss and deficiencies persists, reversal of OAGB to a RYGB or a sleeve gastrectomy is a valuable option. The two major criticism of OAGB are bile reflux and possible risk of cancer. Bile reflux – Overall incidence of bile reflux after OAGB is 1–4%, with a statistical correlation with pouches shorter than 9 cm and presence of preoperative GERD [11]. In symptomatic reflux, the initial treatment consists of trial with probiotics e.g. yogurt, avoiding fatty and high-volume meals and proton-pump inhibitors (PPI). However, in severe and intractable cases, a reversal or revision to RYGB may be considered with a Roux-limb of 50 cm or more. Risk of cancer – Potential risk of gastric or esophageal cancer following OAGB is derived from the fact that exposure of GE junction and esophagus to alkaline bile reflux is a risk factor for Barrett's esophagus. Till date only 4 cases of gastric cancer have been reported after loop gastric bypass (not OAGB), 3 of which were in the remnant stomach which are basically not related to OAGB. Only 1 case of cancer at gastric cardia following OAGB has been published. In conclusion definitive correlation of gastric cancer to OAGB has not yet been proven. The OAGB technique of Carbajo is an excellent modification to decrease or eliminate bile reflux after OAGB.

Conclusion

OAGB is one of the simpler bariatric procedure with a shorter learning curve and hence is an important addition to the armament of any bariatric surgeon. It provides durable weight loss and metabolic results with lower perioperative morbidity and hence holds promise for the future. Proper patient selection and standardization of technique are paramount so that in future OAGB forms an equivalent alternative to routinely performed bariatric and metabolic surgery.

Tips

- Secure the patient well to the operating table, this allows us to maneuver the operating table to suit us when we operate in the supra or infra-colic compartments. Assess before scrubbing for the case.
- Have a good team assisting during the surgery. A team well versed with the procedure reduces operative times and complications.
- Do not hesitate to introduce additional trocars, struggling to reach the area of interest may lead to unnecessary complications.
- Take care while manipulating the calibration tube or bougie, avoid any forceful intervention while inserting the same.
- Always keep a long gastric pouch.
- Always measure the entire bowel length namely the Biliopancreatic limb and the common channel. Maintain at least 300–350 cm of common channel.

Disclosure

Author's institutional practice The primary bariatric procedure of choice in the institution of the author is a Roux Y Gastric bypass (RYGB) with the OAGB being reserved for patients with BMI > 55 or 60. However all patients are consented for a OAGB as a backup procedure if there are any technical factors that may hinder the safe performance of a RYGB. It is also to be noted that OAGB is an equally safe and effective procedure with frequently reported weight loss and co-morbidity resolution being better than a RYGB. However, in spite of being a simpler procedure, the author's institution has dealt with complications related to troublesome gastric reflux, bile reflux, malabsorption and excess weight loss needing conversion to a RYGB. Internal hernias (Peterson's hernia)

although rare have been seen and dealt with in addition to rare twists seen with the long gastric pouch. These are to be borne in mind when the technique is adopted and advised to patients.

References

1. Mason EE, Ito C. Gastric bypass in obesity. Surg Clin North Am. 1967;47(6):1345–51.
2. Rutledge R. The mini-gastric bypass: experience with the first 1, 274 cases. Obes Surg. 2001;11(3):276–80.
3. Carbajo M, García-Caballero M, Toledano M, et al. Oneanastomosis gastric bypass by laparoscopy: results of the first 209 patients. Obes Surg. 2005;15(3):398–404.
4. Lee WJ, Lin YH. Single-anastomosis gastric bypass (SAGB): appraisal of clinical evidence. Obes Surg. 2014;24(10):1749–56.
5. Chevallier JM, Arman GA, Guenzi M, et al. One thousand single anastomosis (omega loop) gastric bypasses to treat morbid obesity in a 7-year period: outcomes show few complications and good efficacy. Obes Surg. 2015;25(6):951–8.
6. Musella M, Milone M. Still "controversies" about the mini gastric bypass? Obes Surg. 2014;24(4):643–4.
7. De Luca M, Tie T, Ooi G, et al. Mini gastric bypass-one anastomosis gastric bypass (MGB-OAGB)-IFSO position statement. Obes Surg. 2018;28:1188–206.
8. Angrisani L, et al. Bariatric surgery and Endoluminal procedures: IFSO worldwide survey 2014. Obes Surg. 2017;27(9):2279–89.
9. Dimitrov DV, Ivanov V, Atanasova M. Advantages of bariatric medicine for individualized prevention and treatments: multidisciplinary approach in body culture and prevention of obesity and diabetes. EPMA J. 2011;2(3):271–6.
10. Mancini MC. Bariatric surgery--an update for the endocrinologist. Arq Bras Endocrinol Metabol. 2014;58(9):875–88.
11. Musella M, Susa A, Manno E, De Luca M, Greco F, Raffaelli M, et al. Complications following the mini/one anastomosis gastric bypass (MGB/OAGB): a multi-institutional survey on 2678 patients with a mid-term (5 years) follow-up. Obes Surg. 2017;27:2956–67.
12. Lee WJ, Lee YC, Ser KH, Chen SC, Chen JC, Su YH, et al. Revisional surgery for laparoscopic minigastric bypass. Surg Obes Relat Dis. 2011;7:486–91.
13. Lee WJ, Wang W, Lee YC, Huang MT, Ser KH, Chen JC, et al. Laparoscopic mini-gastric bypass: experience with tailored bypass limb according to body weight. Obes Surg. 2008;18:294–9.
14. Carbajo MA, Luque-de-León E, Valdez-Hashimoto JF, Ruiz-Tovar J. Anti-reflux one-anastomosis gastric bypass (OAGB)—(Spanish BAGUA): step-by-step technique, rationale and bowel lengths. In: Deitel M, editor. Essentials of mini – one anastomosis gastric bypass. Cham: Springer; 2018.

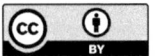

Part XI

Hepatobiliary Surgery: Gallbladder

Elective Cholecystectomy

Arnel Abatayo

Introduction

Cholecystectomy is one of the most commonly performed abdominal surgery to date. In the last few decades, it is increasingly performed laparoscopically, even with third-world countries in Asia. In Mongolia for example, where there are limited resources, they have found a 62% increase in laparoscopic cholecystectomy being performed for 9 years since 2005 [1]. At present, the "gold standard" in gallbladder (GB) surgery is laparoscopic cholecystectomy (LC). This is because of its associated advantages over conventional open technique that includes less postoperative pain, better cosmesis, and shorter hospital stays [2–8]. However, despite the advances in technology, the complications associated with laparoscopic cholecystectomy remain the same. It is therefore necessary for surgeons to be familiar with the basic principles and techniques in performing a safe and efficient procedure. Below is the anatomy of Gallbladder (Fig. 1).

A. Abatayo (✉)
Department of Surgery, Chong Hua Hospital
Mandaue, Cebu, Philippines

© The Author(s) 2023 307
D. Lomanto et al. (eds.), *Mastering Endo-Laparoscopic and Thoracoscopic Surgery*,
https://doi.org/10.1007/978-981-19-3755-2_44

Fig. 1 Gallbladder anatomy

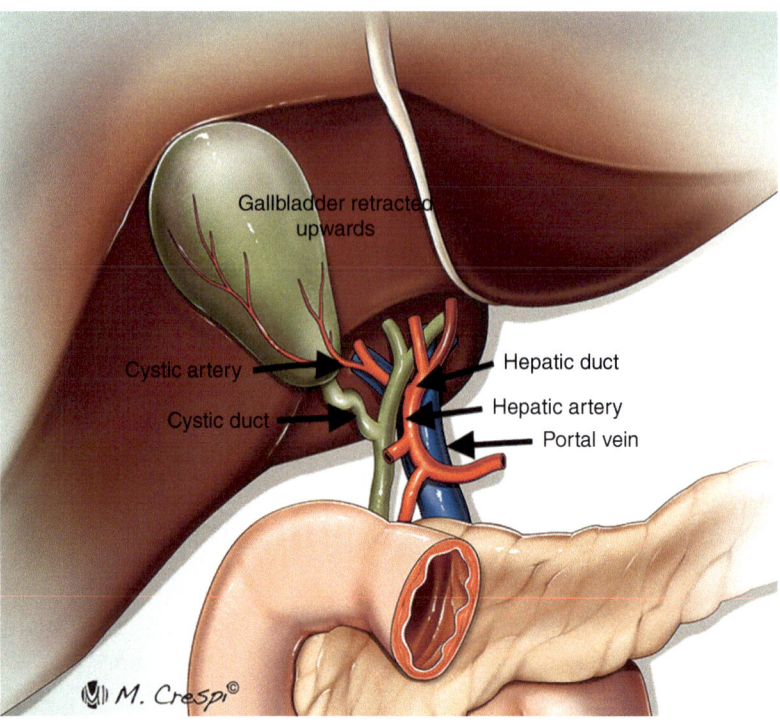

Gallbladder retracted upwards

Cystic artery

Cystic duct

Hepatic duct

Hepatic artery

Portal vein

M. Crespi©

Indications

The indications for laparoscopic cholecystectomy are the same as for open cholecystectomy [9]:

- Symptomatic GB stones.
- Asymptomatic GB stones in patients with certain conditions (elderly patients with diabetes, patients with increased risk for GB cancer, and individuals isolated from medical care for extended periods of time).
- Acalculous cholecystitis.
- Gallbladder polyps >0.8 cm or lesser in symptomatic patients.
- Porcelain gallbladder.

Contraindications

The contraindications of laparoscopic cholecystectomy include the following:

- Generalized peritonitis.
- Septic shock from cholangitis.
- Severe acute pancreatitis.

- Untreated coagulopathy.
- Cholecystoenteric fistulas.
- Previous abdominal operations.
- End-stage cirrhosis of the liver with portal hypertension.
- Suspected or known gallbladder cancer.

However, some would consider these as relative contraindications nowadays because of surgeon experience and judgment. Absolute contraindications of LC are usually related to the anesthetic risks.

Preoperative Assessment

Laboratory Work-Up

The basic blood work-up needed in evaluating GB disease generally includes complete blood count and liver enzymes such as SGPT, Alkaline Phosphatase, and Bilirubin levels. Uncomplicated GB disease generally shows normal or unremarkable results. However, if any of these blood tests are elevated, a more complicated disease should be considered, such as acute cholecystitis, or in cases where bile duct obstruction (e.g., Mirizzi syndrome, CBD stone) may be present. A study using multivariate analysis showed that neutrophil count was the only independent predictor of acute cholecystitis [10]. Also, the role of procalcitonin in determining disease severity has been discussed in some literature especially with regards to inflammatory response; however, its value in determining GB disease severity still needs further investigation. Aside from assessing for GB disease severity, it is important to evaluate for the presence of other related conditions. Serum amylase and lipase may be requested to rule out the presence of pancreatitis, especially in a patient complaining of severe epigastric pain.

Imaging

Ultrasonography

Despite the newer and more advanced imaging modality now available, ultrasonography (US) remains the first-line imaging modality in the evaluation of gallbladder disease. It is cost-effective, less invasive, widely available, and easy to use [11]. A comparison among different diagnostic imaging for acute cholecystitis reported that US has 81% sensitivity (95% CI: 0.75–0.87) and 83% specificity (95% CI: 0.74–0.89) [12].

MRI/MRCP

Magnetic Resonance Imaging (MRI) generally gives a better picture of the GB compared to US. It is the recommended imaging modality next to US, especially in cases where US report is inconclusive. The diagnostic yield of MRI for acute cholecystitis showed an 85% sensitivity (95% CI: 0.66–0.95) and 81% specificity (95% CI: 0.69–0.90) based on a 2012 meta-analysis [12]. One advantage of MRCP is that it can define the anatomy of the biliary system, which makes it very useful in assessing other related conditions.

CT Scan

Contrast-enhanced computed tomography (CT) may have a limited role in gallbladder disease. It is generally used to evaluate other organ systems to rule out other conditions. However, CT is the imaging of choice in determining an emphysematous GB. It can accurately assess the presence of gas within the gallbladder wall or lumen, indicative of GB emphysema, which appears clearly as a hypodense area on CT [13].

When to Do Surgery?

The timing of surgery depends on the overall condition of the patient. Generally, patients who are well with no signs of complicated GB disease can be scheduled electively. Otherwise, for those with more complicated GB disease, such as acute cholecystitis, an emergent or urgent surgery within 72 h is advised which is discussed in the section of emergency laparoscopic surgery.

Operating theater Setup

Below are the operating room setup (Fig. 2) and port placement (Fig. 3).

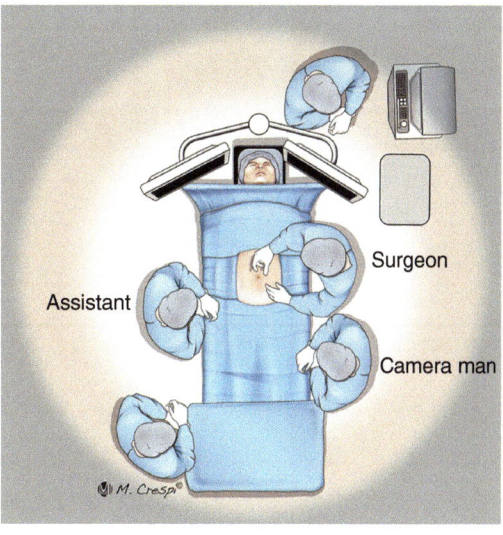

Fig. 2 Operating room setup

Port Placement

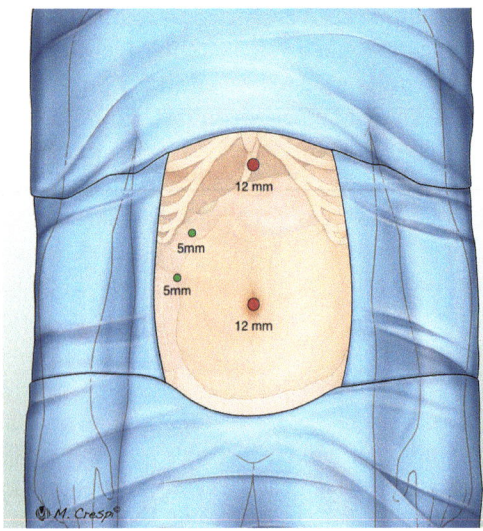

Fig. 3 Port placement

Standard Technique

1. Retract the GB fundus supero-laterally, exposing the infundibulo-cystic junction (IC) and hepatocystic triangle.
2. Open the peritoneal membrane around the IC junction, anteriorly and posteriorly, extending towards the GB body. This will open the Hepatocystic triangle.
3. Continue dissecting and clear the hepatocystic triangle to expose the cystic artery, cystic duct, and cystic plate. By doing this, you have already achieved the "critical view of safety" (Fig. 4).
4. Ligate the cystic artery using clips/suture and cut. This step sometimes helps lengthen the cystic duct, especially in cases where the IC junction is close to the CBD.
5. Intraoperative assessment of the biliary tree using intraoperative cholangiogram may be

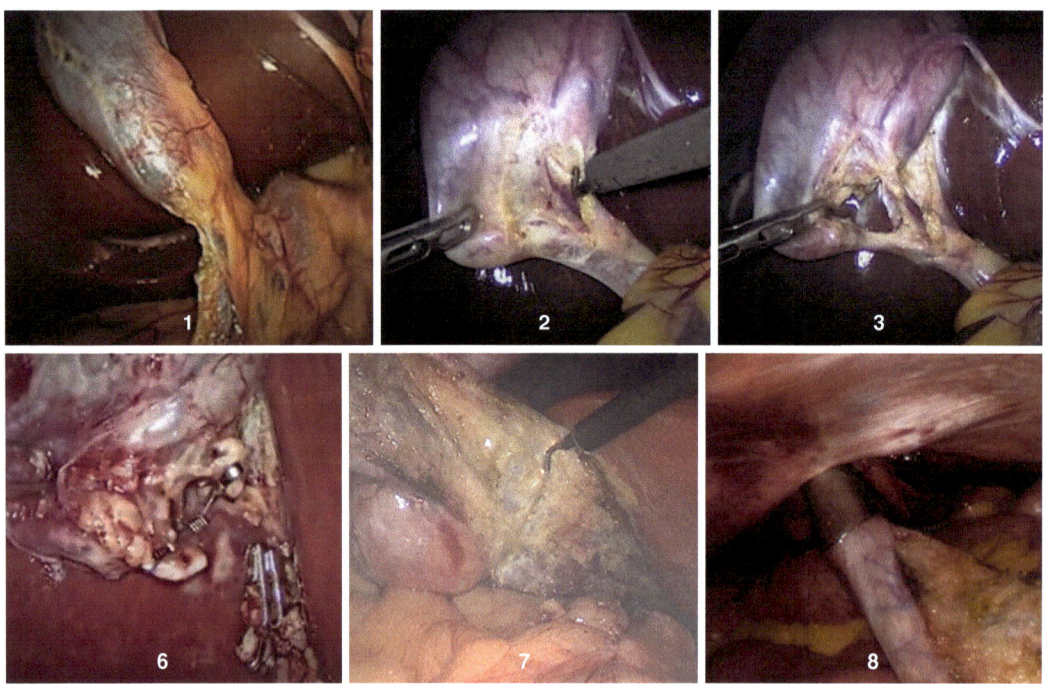

Fig. 4 Steps in doing laparoscopic cholecystectomy

selectively done depending on surgeon preference or when clinically indicated during this time.

6. Ligate the cystic duct using clips/suture and cut.
7. Completely remove the remaining part of the GB from the liver bed.
8. Extract the GB through the umbilical port. Another option is to extract the GB through the epigastric region if a larger port was used.

Complications and Management

Laparoscopic cholecystectomy is generally a safe procedure, especially in uncomplicated cases. However, in rare situations, complications occur due to several factors such as unusual anatomy, presence of inflammation and adhesions, and many others. Intraoperative complications include vascular injuries, bowel perforation, mesenteric injuries, and bile duct injuries which are usually managed successfully through laparoscopy. Although other serious complications have been reported, they will not be discussed here since they are beyond the scope of this section.

Postoperative Care

Majority of patients can start general liquids once fully awake and their diet progressed as tolerated. A low-fat diet in the early postoperative period is advised but may vary widely depending on the surgeon's experience. Some evidence demonstrated that some post-cholecystectomy patients experience food intolerance to fatty food [14, 15]. Pain in the umbilical incision can easily be managed with oral analgesics and generally resolves after 2–3 days. There are patients who may experience pain in the right shoulder which is due to the irritation of CO_2 to the diaphragm, but this usually improves within 24h post-op. Patients may freely ambulate with no restrictions. In certain situations however the limitation of lifting heavy objects may be prudent for a few weeks in cases where the umbilical incision is enlarged during specimen extraction.

Laparoscopic Cholecystectomy in Obesity

Obesity used to be considered a relative contraindication to LC due to the technical difficulties associated with this condition. This resulted in a higher morbidity and mortality as well as higher rate of conversion [16]. However, due to advances in technology, improved instrumentation and increase in surgical experience, the practice of LC has become safer and more feasible among obese patients [17–19]. Majority of the issues encountered in an obese patient are due the increase in abdominal wall thickness as well as increase in intra-abdominal fat resulting in a cramped operative field. Here are a few tips that can help you achieve a safe and successful LC in this group of patients.

1. Use of longer trocars, laparoscope, and instruments.
2. When inserting trocars, it is important to angulate its direction towards the area of the gallbladder. This is because obese patients naturally have thicker abdominal wall restricting its movement.
3. In situations where long laparoscope and instruments are not available. Umbilical trocar can be inserted at the supraumbilical region to keep it close to the operative site.
4. Judicious use of additional trocars to facilitate retraction of the liver and the omentum. This can improve the operative field and provide better access to the GB and other critical structures.

References

1. Expansion of Laparoscopic Cholecystectomy in a Resource Limited Setting, Mongolia: a 9-year cross-sectional retrospective review.
2. Soper NJ, Stockmann PT, Dunnegan DL, Ashley SW. Laparoscopic cholecystectomy. The new 'gold standard'? Arch Surg. 1992;127:917.

3. Schirmer BD, Edge SB, Dix J, et al. Laparoscopic cholecystectomy. Treatment of choice for symptomatic cholelithiasis. Ann Surg. 1991;213:665–7.
4. Wiesen SM, Unger SW, Barkin JS, et al. Laparoscopic cholecystectomy: the procedure of choice for acute cholecystitis. Am J Gastroenterol. 1993;88:334.
5. Wilson RG, Macintyre IM, Nixon SJ, et al. Laparoscopic cholecystectomy as a safe and effective treatment for severe acute cholecystitis. BMJ. 1992;305:394.
6. Rattner DW, Ferguson C, Warshaw AL. Factors associated with successful laparoscopic cholecystectomy for acute cholecystitis. Ann Surg. 1993; 217:233.
7. Johansson M, Thune A, Nelvin L, et al. Randomized clinical trial of open versus laparoscopic cholecystectomy in the treatment of acute cholecystitis. Br J Surg. 2005;92:44.
8. Yamashita Y, Takada T, Kawarada Y, et al. Surgical treatment of patients with acute cholecystitis: Tokyo guidelines. J Hepato-Biliary-Pancreat Surg. 2007;14:91.
9. NIH releases consensus statement on gallstones. bile duct stones and laparoscopic cholecystectomy. Am Fam Physician. 1992;46:1571–4.
10. Naidu K, Beenen E, Gananadha S, Mosse C. The yield of fever, inflammatory markers and ultrasound in the diagnosis of acute cholecystitis: a validation of the 2013 Tokyo guidelines. World J Surg. 2016;40:2892–7.
11. Kiriyama S, Kozaka K, Takada T, et al. Tokyo guidelines 2018: diagnostic criteria and severity grading of acute cholangitis (with videos). J Hepatobiliary Pancreat Sci. 2018;25(1):17–30. https://doi.org/10.1002/jhbp.512.
12. Kiewiet JJ, Leeuwenburgh MM, Bipat S, Bossuyt PM, Stoker J, Fuks D, Mouly C, Robert B, Hajji H, Yzet T, Regimbeau J-M, Boermeester MA. A systematic review and meta-analysis of diagnostic performance of imaging in acute cholecystitis. Radiology. 2012;264:708–20.
13. Patel NB, Oto A, Thomas S. Multidetector CT of emergent biliary pathologic conditions. Radiographics. 2013;33:1867–88.
14. Fisher M, Spilias DC, Tong LK. Diarrhoea after laparoscopic cholecystectomy: incidence and main determinants. ANZ J Surg. 2008;78:482–6.
15. Johnson AG. Gallstones and flatulent dyspepsia: cause or coincidence? Postgrad Med J. 1971;47:767–72.
16. Liu CL, Fan ST, Lai EC, Lo CM, Chu KM. Factors affecting conversion of laparoscopic cholecystectomy to open surgery. Arch Surg. 1996;131:98–101.
17. Simopoulos C, Polychronidis A, Botaitis S, Perente S, Pitiakoudis M. Laparoscopic cholecystectomy in obese patients. Obes Surg. 2005;15:243–6.
18. Ammori BJ, Vezakis A, Davides D, Martin IG, Larvin M, McMahon MJ. Laparoscopic cholecystectomy in morbidly obese patients. Surg Endosc. 2001;15:1336–9.
19. Paajanen H, Kakela P, Suuronen S, Paajanen J, Juvonen P, Pihlajamaki J. Impact of obesity and associated diseases on outcome after laparoscopic cholecystectomy. Surg Laparosc Endosc Percutan Tech. 2012;22:509–13.

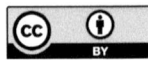

Part XII

Hepatobiliary Surgery: Common Bile Duct Stones

Laparoscopic Choledochotomy for Bile Duct Stones

Nguyen Hoang Bac, Pham Minh Hai, and Le Quan Anh Tuan

Introduction

Laparoscopic common bile duct exploration was first reported in the early 90′. Although this procedure has proved beneficial, the widespread adoption of laparoscopic common bile duct exploration is limited because of the technical complex, the need for specialized instruments (choledochoscope), and limited exposure and training of the surgical team to LCBDE.

Most of CBD stones can be managed by ERCP. LCBDE is mostly performed in patients with concomitant gallstones and CBD stones.

Patient Selection

Laparoscopic choledochotomy (LCD) is indicated for:

N. H. Bac
Department of Surgery, University of Medicine and Pharmacy, Ho Chi Minh city, Vietnam

P. M. Hai
Department of Hepatobiliary and Pancreatic Surgery, University Medical Center, Ho Chi Minh city, Vietnam

L. Q. A. Tuan (✉)
Department of Surgery, University of Medicine and Pharmacy, Ho Chi Minh city, Vietnam

Department of Hepatobiliary and Pancreatic Surgery, University Medical Center, Ho Chi Minh city, Vietnam
e-mail: tuan.lqa@umc.edu.vn

- Gallstones with concomitant CBD stones.
- CBD stones detected during cholecystectomy.
- CBD stones that failed to endoscopic approach (inaccessibility of the scope, large CBD stones, multiple CBD stones).
- Multiple primary CBD stones and intrahepatic stones.

Laparoscopic choledochotomy is recommended for patients with CBDs diameter more than 7 mm to reduce risk of postoperative stricture [1].

Procedure

Operating Room Setup, Patient Positioning, and Setting Surgical Team

Patient is placed in supine reverse Trendelenburg position. The arms should be tucked at the patient's sides.

10 mm laparoscope of 30° or 45° is used.

Operating room setup is as in Fig. 1.

Technique

Trocar Placement
Trocar sites are as in (Fig. 2).

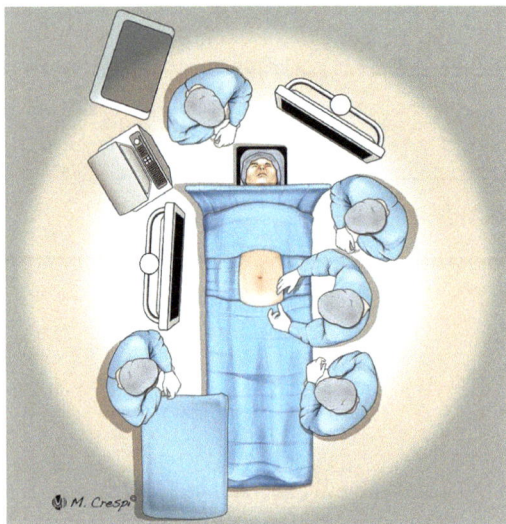

Fig. 1 OR setup

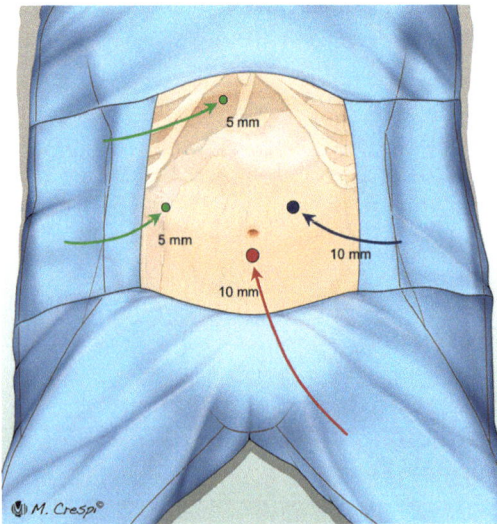

Fig. 2 Trocar position

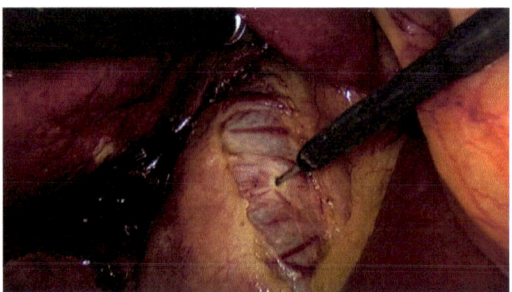

Fig. 3 crossing vessels on CBD anterior wall

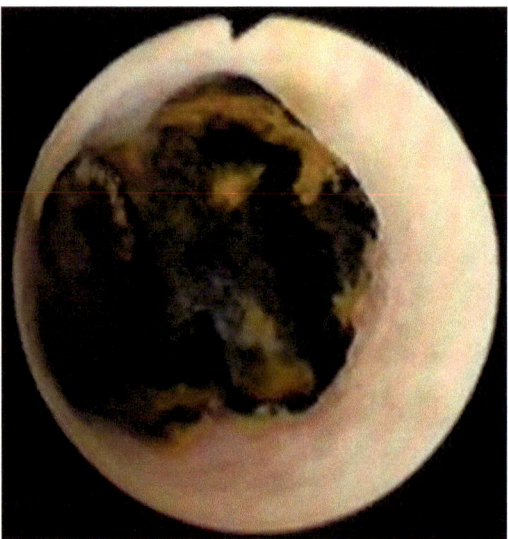

Fig. 4 Choledochoscopy

Choledochotomy

First, hepatoduodenal ligament is exposed. CBD is the most lateral and superficial tubular structure in hepatoduodenal ligament. It is recommended that we should clear fat tissue to expose anterior CBD wall. If the location of CBD is not clear, aspiration of bile by a narrow-gauge needle may help. A longitudinal incision of 1–2 cm is made on the anterior CBD wall. Limitation of using surgical energy when opening the CBD is essential to avoid late stricture of CBD due to thermal injury. We often use needle tip electrocautery as in Fig. 3. Scissors without cautery is an alternative choice. Stay sutures may facilitate CBD exposure for opening. Bile culture should be done when necessary.

Exploration of Bile Ducts and Stone Removal

After choledochotomy, small stones can be washed out using an irrigator or flushing water through a rubber catheter. High pressure during irrigation should be avoided in case of cholangitis.

Choledochoscope is very useful to inspect the CBD and intrahepatic bile ducts for stones and stricture (Fig. 4). The choledochoscope

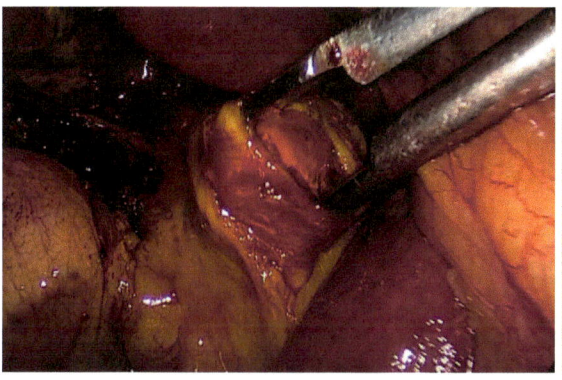 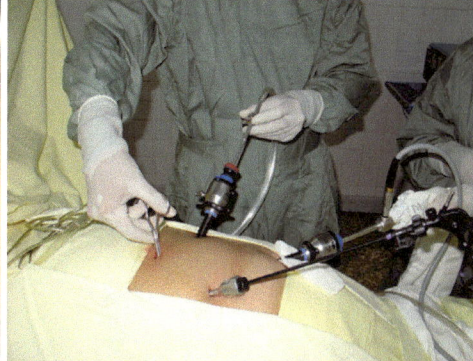

Fig. 5 Stones extraction by forceps

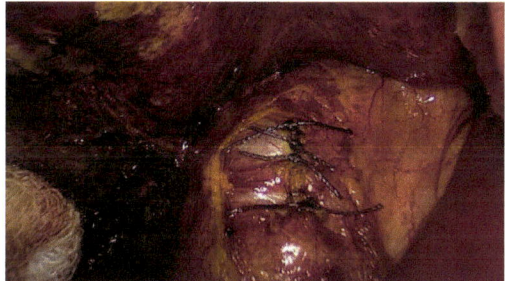

Fig. 6 Primary closure of CBD

should be introduced through a plastic trocar located at the epigastric region, above the opening of the CBD to minimize excessive angulation of the choledochoscope during manipulation. When exploration demonstrates stones, basket or balloon catheter will be used to extract stones. In case of large or impacted stones, fragmentation is necessary. Electro-hydraulic lithotripsy or laser lithotripsy can be used. We prefer to use electro-hydrolic litho-tripsy for fragmentation of bile duct stones because it is faster and less expensive compared to laser. Fragments will be removed by basket or balloon or flushing via a plastic catheter. With respect to acute cholangitis, there is higher risk of hemobilia when performing multiple litho-tripsy. Hence, we should only address stones that cause obstruction. Residual stones should be removed via T-tube tract after 3–4 weeks by percutaneous cholangioscopy.

Stone forceps can be applied through 5 mm epigastric opening after removing the trocar to extract CBD stones as in Fig. 5. This modifica-tion facilitates the extraction of CBD stones espe-cially large stones or multiple stones which is more common in Asia. Stones extracted are placed in a plastic bag. Gas loss when using stone forceps is insignificant.

Closure of CBD

Closure of CBD incision can be done with or without biliary drainage. CBD closure without biliary drainage is called primary closure. Biliary drainage can be performed with T-tube (external drainage) or internal stent (internal drainage). With regard to internal stent placement, a subse-quent endoscopic session is required to remove it. T-tube placement provides a T-tube tract through which postoperative percutaneous explo-ration of the bile ducts or residual stone manage-ment by choledochoscopy is enabled.

Primary closure: There is evidence that this technique has benefits as compared to biliary drainage such as reducing hospital stay, operating time, and overall cost. Primary closure is indi-cated in selected patients without acute cholangi-tis, without distal CBD obstruction, and complete clearance of bile duct stones [2].

Suturing in a continuous or interrupted fash-ion with absorbable 3.0 or 4.0 suture is usually used for primary closure (Fig. 6). After that, a white gauze is used to inspect bile leak.

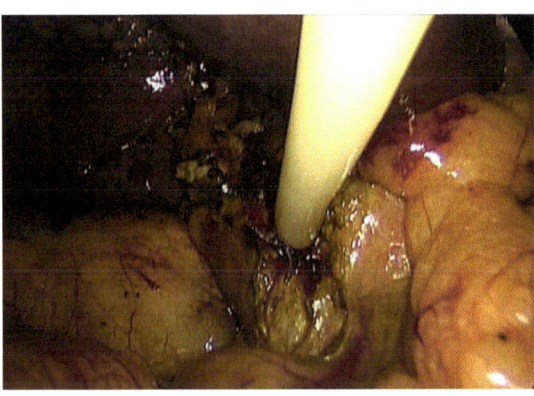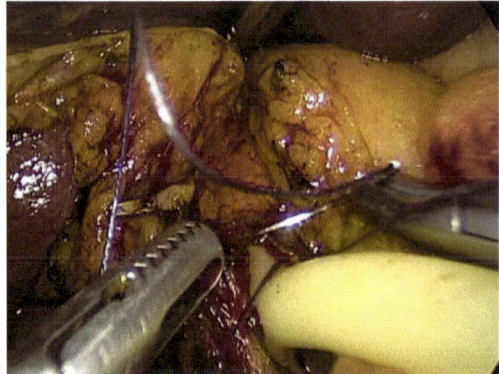

Fig. 7 Closure of CBD around T-tube

T-tube placement: A suitable T-tube size is selected according to the size of the CBD. Suturing in a continuous or interrupted fashion with absorbable 3.0 or 4.0 suture is performed around the T-tube (Fig. 7). Flushing water through T-tube helps detect a leak that needs to be reinforced.

Drainage and Closure of Trocar Sites

A subhepatic drain is routinely placed and usually removed after 2–3 days if there is no bile leak.

All trocar sites are closed.

Complications and Management

Bile leak rate was reported around 5–7% [2]. Bile leak is usually mild and self-limited.

Complications specific to primary closure are persistent cholangitis or biliary obstruction. This happens when there are retained stones or distal obstruction of the CBD or ascending acute cholangitis.

Late stricture of CBD may occur and less than 1%, mostly because of inappropriate closure technique or choledochotomy in a CBD less than 7 mm.

Summary

Laparoscopic choledochotomy is feasible and safe. Complication rate is low. Complications are usually mild and self-limited. Appropriate indication of laparoscopic choledochotomy is important.

References

1. Zerey M, Haggerty S, Richardson W, Santos B, Fanelli R, Brunt LM, et al. Laparoscopic common bile duct exploration. Surg Endosc. 2018;32(6):2603–12.
2. Lambour A, Santos BF. Common bile duct exploration. 2020.

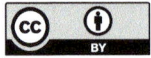

Part XIII

Hepatobiliary Surgery: Liver

Hepatic Cyst/Abscess

Rakesh Kumar Gupta

Introduction

Hepatic cysts are common, occurring in at least 2–7% of the population, and are typically discovered incidentally with the frequent use of ultrasonography and computed tomography. Only about 16% of such cysts are symptomatic [1]. They may be either congenital or acquired. The more common congenital variety may represent malformed bile ducts while the acquired type of hepatic cyst usually arises as sequelae of inflammation, trauma or parasitic disease, and sometimes neoplastic disease [2].

Classification of cystic liver lesions according to etiology

Congenital
• Ductal (dilatation of intrahepatic duct)
– Ductal cyst
– Caroli's disease(cystic dilatation of intrahepatic bile ducts)
• Parenchymal (solitary or polycystic)

Acquired
• Infectious
– Bacterial—Pyogenic liver abscess
– Parasitic—Hydatid cyst, amoebic liver abscess
• Traumatic
• Neoplastic (biliary cystadenoma, cystadenocarcinoma)

R. K. Gupta (✉)
Department of Surgery, B.P. Koirala Institute of Health Sciences, Dharan, Nepal

There has been a significant improvement in diagnosis, treatment, and outcome of these hepatic lesions.

Congenital Cyst

- Presentation: They are usually asymptomatic. They can cause right upper quadrant pain due to stretching of Glisson's capsule and bloating if large due to pressure effect. If very large, they may be palpable abdominally. Acute abdominal pain may occur due to hemorrhage in cyst or its rupture. Sometimes they may cause jaundice due to compression effect.
- Investigations: Ultrasound, CT scanning, and MRI can show cyst anatomy. LFT may be slightly abnormal.
- Treatment: Options include watchful monitoring if asymptomatic and aspiration/sclerotherapy if symptomatic.Laparoscopic/open fenestration may be effective in certain cases. Liver transplantation is occasionally needed in case of polycystic liver disease or Caroli's disease with liver failure [3].

Neoplastic Cysts

- Presentation: usually asymptomatic or vague symptoms including bloating, nausea, and fullness can occur. Abdominal pain and biliary obstruction can result as they enlarge.
- Investigation: LFT may be normal. Carbohydrate antigen (CA)—19–9 may be

raised. Typical pattern may be seen on CT-scan.
- Treatment: The definitive treatment is complete surgical resection.

Liver Abscess

- Liver abscesses are caused by bacterial (pyogenic abscess), parasitic (amoebic abscess), or fungal organisms. In developed countries pyogenic abscesses are the most common but worldwide, amoebic abscesses are the most common [4].
- Pyogenic liver abscesses(PLA) are usually multiple but may be single too, affecting right lobe of liver in 74% cases [5]. Most are secondary to infection originating in the abdomen. It may be iatrogenic secondary to liver biopsy or a blocked biliary stent. Bacterial endocarditis and dental infection are other causes. It is more common in immunocompromised. It can be a complication of umbilical vein catheterization in infants. It tends to be polymicrobial. Organisms are usually of bowel origin. Klebsiella pneumoniae has emerged as the most common organism [6]. Other organisms include E. coli, Bacteroid species, enterococci, streptococci, and staphylococci.
- Amoebic liver abscesses (ALA), caused by Entamoeba histolyticais usually single, common in tropical and subtropical areas and more likely if there is poor sanitation and overcrowding. Transmission is via feco-oral route. Amoebae invade intestinal mucosa and gain access to portal venous system. It affects right lobe in 80% cases [7].
- Presentation: Multiple abscesses tend to present more acutely while single ones are more indolent. Patients usually present with right upper quadrant pain which may refer to the right shoulder, associated with swinging fever, night sweats, nausea, vomiting, anorexia, and weight loss. Patients may have cough and dyspnea due to diaphragmatic irritation. Jaundice may be present in 6–29% of cases [8]. Examination may reveal tender hepatomegaly.
- Investigation: Total leucocyte count and ESR will be raised. Mild normochromic normo-

cytic anemia may be present. LFT may be deranged (raised transaminase, raised alkaline phosphatase, raised bilirubin, low albumin). Blood culture will be positive in 50% of cases of PLA [9]. Stool may contain cysts or trophozoites of E. histolytica in ALA. Serology will be helpful in ALA. Chest x-ray may reveal raised right hemidiaphragm, atelectasis, or pleural effusion. Ultrasonography can show abscess (usually single central location in ALA, multiple peripheral location in PLA). CT scan is good for detecting small abscesses as well as for detecting the intra-abdominal cause.

- Treatment: Most of the cases of liver abscesses are managed by either antibiotics alone or combination of antibiotics and drainage guided by ultrasonography or CT. Percutaneous Catheter Drainage (PCD) is more effective than Percutaneous Needle Aspiration (PNA) because it facilitates a higher success rate, reduces the time required to achieve clinical relief, and supports a 50% reduction in abscess cavity size [10]. The combination of third-generation cephalosporin and metronidazole is the first-line choice of antibiotics in PLA. Treatment may be needed for upto 12 weeks and should be guided by the clinical picture, culture, and radiological evidence. Metronidazole is the treatment of choice in ALA. Use of percutaneous drainage has steadily increased whereas the use of surgical drainage has declined [11]. Surgery is needed if the abscess has ruptured or if there is known pathology such as appendicitis.

Hydatid Cysts

- Aetiopathogenesis: It is caused by infection with metacystode (larval stage) of Echinococcus tapeworms (E. granulosus and E. multilocularis). Canine, carnivores such as dogs, and wolves act as definitive hosts where adult form of parasites live and sexual cycle occurs. They give eggs which are passed into feces of these hosts. These eggs are ingested by herbivores such as sheep, an intermediate host. These eggs are turned into larval stage (child form). Herbivores are intermediate hosts because they are eaten by the definitive hosts. This is how cycle of parasitic zoonoses completes. Human are not supposed to come in between these two hosts. But if accidentally, human ingest these eggs by ingestion of food/water contaminated with eggs or through close contact with infected dogs, human acts as intermediate host and is a dead end because they are not further eaten up by carnivores. In humans the eggs reach small intestine, invade the intestinal wall with three pairs of hooks and reach portal vein. Since right portal branch is small in length and course is relatively straight, and mostly going to the right upper segments of liver. That is why most common site of hydatid cyst in liver is segment 7/8. Larvae that escape hepatic filtering are carried to the lung. From the lung, larvae may disseminate to other distant body parts such as brain, bone, spleen, and kidney.

- Initially, when eggs attach to capillary in liver, they proliferate and are active. But as immunity starts fighting with these eggs, they may become dead. Hence, the fate of eggs is determined by immunity [12]. Larvae that escape the host's defense, develop into small cysts surrounded by a fibrous capsule. These cysts grow at a rate of 1–3 cm/year and may remain undetected for years [13]. Thus, they can reach very large sizes before they become clinically evident. A cyst in liver is composed of three layers:
  - Adventia (pericyst): consists of compressed liver parenchyma and fibrous tissue induced by expanding parasitic cyst.
  - Laminated membrane (ectocyst): is elastic white covering, easily separable from the adventitia.
  - Germinal epithelium (endocyst): is a single layer of cells lining the inner aspect of the cyst and is the only living component, being responsible for the formation of other layers as well as hydatid fluid and brood capsules within the cyst. In some cysts, laminated membrane may eventually disintegrate and brood capsules are freed and grow into daughter cysts.
- Presentation: There is usually no symptom in acute stage when eggs just infect the liver.

When a cyst is formed, this will produce pressure symptoms most commonly as the right upper abdominal heaviness or pain [14]. Hepatomegaly may be present. If cyst becomes so large, it may produce portal hypertension and obstructive jaundice. Sometimes acute abdominal pain may occur and this is because of complications (such as perforation, infection), not just because of cyst formation. Very rarely anaphylaxis can also occur following perforation.

- Investigation: There will be eosinophilia, slightly deranged LFT. Serological test is of use for diagnosis. ELISA (Enzyme-linked Immunosorbent assay) has sensitivity above 90% and is useful in mass-scale screening. The counter-immunoelectrophoresis has the highest specificity (100%) and high sensitivity (80–90%). CASONI test has been used most frequently in the past but is at present considered only of historical importance because of low sensitivity. The sensitivity and specificity of ELISA are highly dependent on the method of antigen preparation, and cross-reactions with other helminthic diseases occur if crude antigen is used. Purified fraction may yield high sensitivity and specificity [15]. Ultrasound is the imaging modality of choice for diagnosis. CT and MRI are modalities of choice for number, site, and identification of complications. CT is better than MRI to look for calcification while MRI is better to look for biliary involvement. Indirect signs of biliary communication are deformed cyst, Crampledhydatid membrane, dilatation of biliary tree, close contact between cyst and biliary branch, interrupted calcified wall, and fluid-fat level in the cyst. WHO has developed a standardized classification system [16], originally developed by Gharbi and colleagues in 1981, and is currently the screening method of choice (Table 1).
- Treatment: All of the four modalities (chemotherapy, interventional radiology, endoscopic procedure, and surgery) have a role in its management. The choice of an optimal treatment should be carefully assessed in each case [17].
- Chemotherapy (albendazole 400 mg twice a day): It is useful in type 1 and 3a WHO cysts,

Table 1 Classification of hydatid cyst of liver

WHO-2001	Gharbi-1981	Description	Stage
CE1	Type I	Unilocular, unechoic, Hydatid sand, snow storm	Active
CE2	Type III	Multi-septated, rosette like, honeycomb cyst, spoke wheel sign	Active
CE3A	Type II	Cyst with detached membrane(water lily sign)	Transitional
CE3B	Type III	Cyst with daughter cysts in solid matrix	Transitional
CE4	Type IV	Cyst with heterogeneously/hyper-echoic contents. No daughter cysts, ball of wool sign	Inactive
CE5	Type V	Solid cyst with calcified wall	Inactive

where the cyst is single, less than 5 cm. The rationale is that the drug can penetrate the cyst wall. But when the cyst has predominant solid component or daughter cysts, the drug may not penetrate even after long-term use of chemotherapy and drugs should not be used. However, it can be used as adjuvant or neoadjuvant to PAIR or surgery to prevent recurrence. Four days to 1 month of preoperative therapy and 4–6 months postoperative therapy with albendazole are recommended. As per WHO, 3 months preoperative therapy is most effective. It is of no use in calcified dead cyst.

• Interventional radiology:

Treatment options are
– PAIR (Percutaneous Aspiration Injection Reaspiration):
Indications are [18]:

• CE1, CE2, CE3.
• Multiple cysts if accessible to puncture.
• Infected cyst.
• Patients who fail to respond to medical management.
• Patients in whom surgery is contraindicated.
• Patients who relapse after surgery.

Contraindications

• noncooperative patient,
• inaccessible to puncture,
• cyst communicating with biliary tree,
• inactive/calcified cyst.

– PAIR-D (D=Drainage) is a variant of PAIR associated with insertion of intracystic catheter at the end of the procedure and drained for 24 h.

– D-PAI (Double Puncture Aspiration Injection): It is used for univesicular cyst. With ultrasound guidance, fine needle drainage of cyst was performed, 95% alcohol was injected, and left in situ partly filling the cyst cavity. The same procedure is performed 3 days later [19].

– PEVAC (Percutaneous Evacuation of cyst contents): It is used for multivesicular cysts. It involves the following steps: ultrasound-guided cyst puncture and aspiration of cyst fluid to release intracystic pressure and thereby avoid leakage; insertion of a large bore catheter; aspiration and evacuation of daughter and endocyst by injection and reaspiration of isotonic saline; cystography; injection of scolicidal only if no cystobiliary fistula is present; external drainage of cystobiliary fistula combined with sphincterotomy; and catheter removal after complete cyst collapse and closure of cystobiliary fistula [20].

Complications of Interventional radiology procedures are

• Same risk as of any puncture such as hemorrhage and infection.
• Secondary echinococcosis caused by spillage.
• Anaphylactic shock or allergic reaction.
• Chemical cholangitis if cyst communicates with biliary tree.
• Systemic toxicity of scolicidal agent if cyst is large.

Advantages of Interventional radiology procedures are

- Minimal invasiveness.
- Require less expertise.
- Reduced risk compared to surgery.
- Reduced hospital time.
- Cost effective.
- Can be performed in remote areas with less infrastructures
- Surgery.

Preoperative evaluation includes

- Complete blood count and blood grouping.
- Electrocardiogram.
- Electrolytes.
- PT/INR.
- Renal and Liver function test.
- Review of imaging—triphasic CT or MRI

Indications of surgery are

- Complicated cysts.
- Large CE2-CE3b cysts.
- Single liver cyst located superficial and carries risk of perforation (such as following trauma).
- Cyst communicating biliary tree.
- Infected cyst.
- Cyst exerting pressure effects on adjacent vital organ

Contraindication for surgery are

- General contraindication such as multiple medical comorbidities.
- Multiple cysts in multiple organs.
- Cysts that are difficult to access.
- Dead calcified cyst.
- Very small cyst

Aims of surgery are

- Complete extirpation of the parasites.
- Obliteration of residual cavity.
- Identification and management of biliary fistula and other complications

Surgical procedures can be *conservative procedures* (partial cystectomy or deroofing, marsupialization, and external drainage) or *radical procedures* (pericystectomy, subadvential cystectomy, and formal liver resection). These procedures can be performed laparoscopically or via open surgery. There are a few contraindications of laparoscopic procedure and these are

- Severe cardiopulmonary disease is unlikely to tolerate prolonged CO_2-induced pneumoperitoneum and deemed unfit for laparoscopy by the anesthesiologists.
- Previous multiple upper abdominal surgery likely to have adhesions and thus limiting vision and increasing the difficulty level of laparoscopic dissection.
- Recurrent hydatid cysts.
- Deep located cysts.
- Rupture of cyst in biliary tree.

Conservative procedures are safe and technically simple. However, their disadvantages are high postoperative complications and recurrence rate as shown in Table 2. Radical procedures have a lower rate of recurrence [21] but many authors still consider them inappropriate, claiming that intraoperative risks are too high for benign disease [22].

Table. 2 Complications of conservative surgery

Early	Late

• Liver-related complications
  – Bile leakage
  – Residual cavity infection/abscess
  – Perihepatic collection/hematoma
  – Hepatic abscess
• Spillage-related complications
  – Secondary hydatosis
  – Anaphylaxis
• Scolicidal-induced complication
  – Chemical sclerosing cholangitis
  – Methemoglobinemia
	• Biliary fistula
	• Biliary stricture
	• Recurrence

Endoscopic management: ERCP will be helpful for major biliary communication with dilated bile duct [23].

Operative Details of Various Surgical Procedures

Laparoscopic Deroofing, a conservative procedure Iis most common surgery being performed for hydatid cyst.

Recommended instruments
- One 10 mm trocar.
- A 30° angled laparoscope.
- Two 5 mm trocar.
- One 10 mm trocar.
- One 5 mm grasping forceps.
- One generated grasping forceps.
- A 5 mm hook.
- Irrigation and aspiration probe.
- Energy devise: (Harmonic scalpel, ligasure, etc.).
- Specimen retrieval bag.
- Liver detractors (may be required to retract liver)

Figure1 describes operation theater setup and position of surgeon and the assistants. The surgeon usually stands on the left-hand side of the patient but may stand between the legs of the patient placed in a "Y" position.

Technique
- All patients are operated under General anesthesia with a Foley's catheter and nasogastric tube placed immediately after induction in either supine position or the French position
- A 10 mm port at the umbilicus houses the 30° telescope. A 5 mm trocar is placed just below the xiphoid process to the right or the left of the falciform ligament, depending on the location of the cyst. This port is used to expose the liver. One 5 mm and one 10 mm ports, in the right and left flank, allow the surgeon to puncture the cyst dome, aspirated its contents, and excise the cyst wall in a careful sequential fashion to facilitate homeostasis (Fig. 2.
- A gauge soaked with 3% saline or 10% betadine is kept around the cyst to prevent contamination by spillage before puncture of the cyst (Fig. 3).
- Decompression of the cyst by aspiration of the cyst fluid using a wide bore needle through one of the 5-mm ports or by direct percutaneous entry under laparoscopic guidance taking care to avoid spillage and by the use of at least

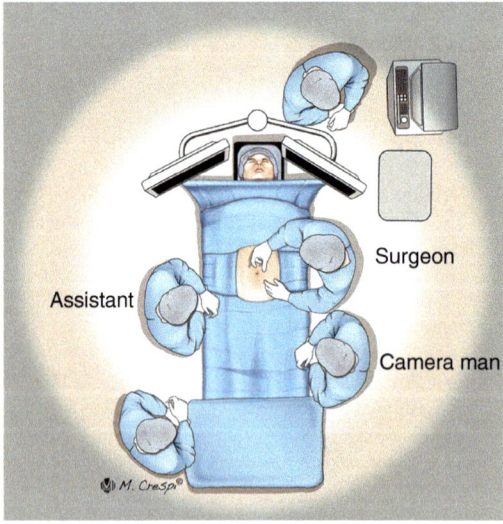

Fig. 1 Operation theater setup and position of surgeon and the assistants

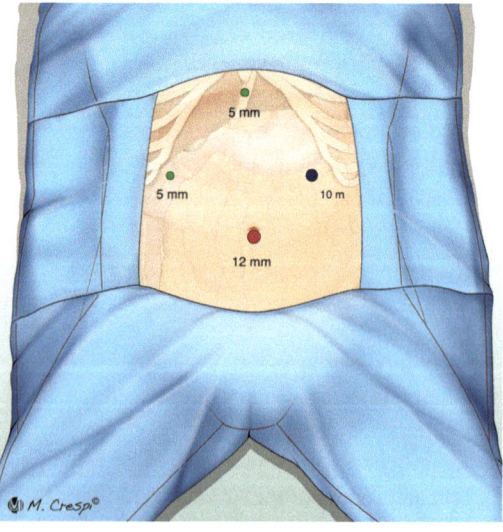

Fig. 2 Port placement

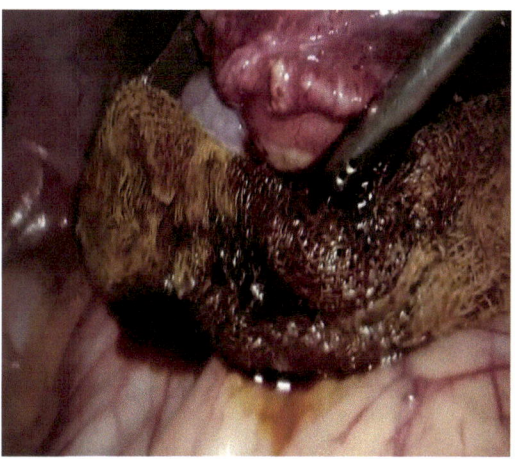 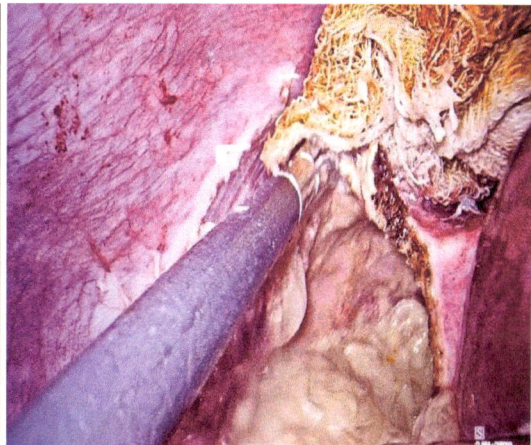

Fig. 3 Cystic lesion isolated from rest of abdominal cavity with Betadine-soaked gauge

one continuous suction cannula around the needle puncture site.

- Once cyst is punctured, cyst content should be examined as further step depends on it. In a typical viable cyst, the content will be clear with sand and debris of broad capsules. The content will be initially clear and later turns bilious in case of cyst with biliary communication due to valvular mechanism. (Biliary system pressure is 15–20 cm of H2O while intracystic pressure is 30–80 cm of H2O) Infected cyst has purulent content with flakes. Dead cyst has toothpaste-like content.

- Aspiration of as much of the cyst fluid and injection of equal amounts of scolicidal agents (10% povidone iodine or hypertonic saline) into the cyst cavity without removing the needle. Hypersonic saline is preferred because stain of providing iodine may mimick bile leak. In case of biliary communication, avoid injection of scolicidal agent 10% betadine because of fear of chemical cholangitis.

- Aspiration of the cyst contents after 10 min using high-powered suction at a negative pressure via 10 mm trocar introduced directly into the cyst under vision (Fig. 4).

- Scoring of Glisson's capsule of area to be deroofed with high-frequency electrosurgery.

- Mesenchymal dissection can be performed using ultrasonic dissector.

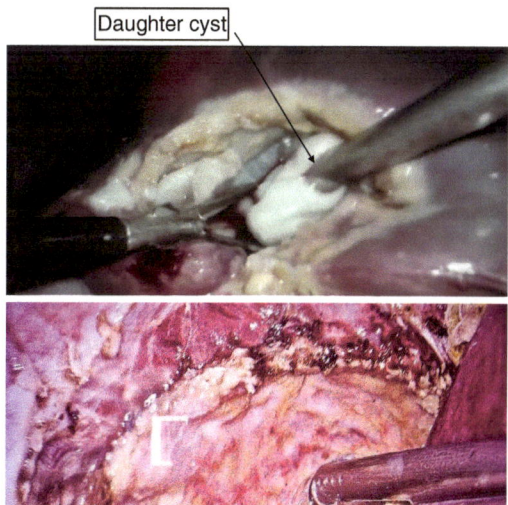

Fig. 4 Aspiration of cyst content with 10 mm suction

- Once the dome of cyst is deroofed, all residual elements should be evacuated until the cavity is clear.

- Direct inspection of the interior of the cyst by introducing the scope into the cyst to look for remaining cyst elements and biliary leakage, if any, for subsequent attention.

- Removal of the cyst wall and cyst elements by using an impermeable specimen bag.
- The specimen is extracted either by partial morcellation, dilatation at the umbilicus, enlarging another port site or by a small MC Burney or subcostal incision.
- Cholangiography or ICG (Fig. 5) is useful to detect bile leak.
- Inspection of raw surface of liver, and if required it is covered with fibrin glue.
- Management of Residual cavity: Various options are
  - Water-tight suturing without drain.
  - Marsupialization.
  - Capsulorrhaphy and Capitonnage.

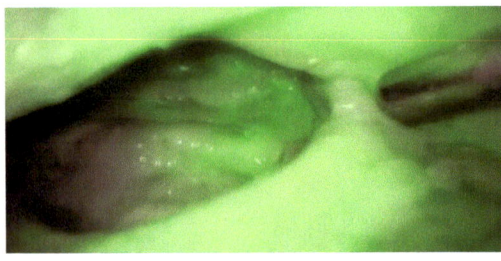

Fig. 5 Indocyanine Green (ICG) imaging showing no biliary communication of cyst

  - Omentoplasty: It is the option of choice nowadays. A viable flap of omentum is sutured to cyst cavity and drain is kept.
- Sending scolices for confirmation by microscopy or for culture, if deemed infected.

Other Operative Procedures

Radical procedures include pericystectomy, subadvential cystectomy, and formal liver resection (Fig. 6). Radical surgery has pros and cons shown in Table 3.

Indications of radical procedure are:

  - Large cystobiliary communication—unable to manage by Roux-en-Y anastomosis.
  - Hydatid cyst with biliary obstruction leading to atrophy of segment.

Complications of Hydatid cysts of liver: The most common complications in order of frequency are infection, biliary communication, rupture into peritoneal cavity/pleural cavity, and portal hypertension [24].

Fig. 6 (**a**) various layers of hydatid cyst (**b**) total cystectomy (**c**) subtotal cystectomy (**d**) hepatectomy

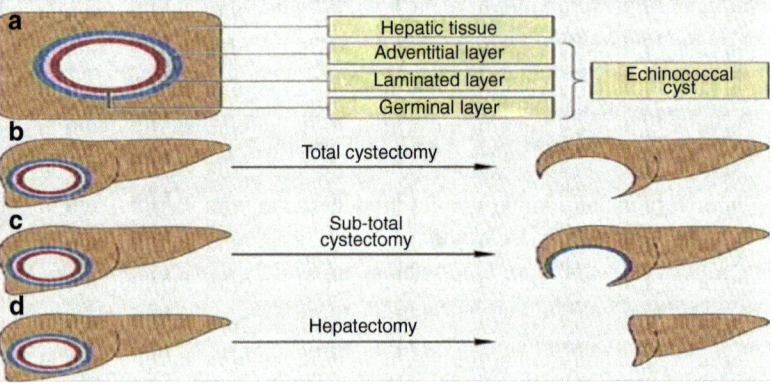

Table 3 Pros and cons of radicle procedure

Pros	Cons
Complete eradication of cyst	Expertise required
	Time-consuming
Less recurrence	More morbidity
Less biliary complication	Too radical for cystic
No residual cavity	hydatid

Biliary Communication and its Management

The incidence of cysto-biliary communication ranges between 3 and17% [25]. The rupture of hydatid cysts into biliary ducts and the migration of the hydatid material in the biliary tree lead to other biliary complications such as cholangitis, sclerosis odditis, and hydatid biliary lithiasis. The diagnosis of this complication can usually be made by using ultrasound and abdominal CT scan. The presence of dilated common bile duct, jaundice, close proximity of cystic lesion to major ducts are strongly suggestive of cystobiliary communication. The various treatment options are as follows:

- Direct suturing of fistula orifice with the absorbable suture is indicated if perifistulous cyst wall is not calcified or too fibrotic. If calcified, suturing with omentoplasty may be helpful.
- In case of hydatid cyst in main biliary tree, CBD exploration with removal of cyst material with T-tube drainage is indicated if ERCP is not available.
- Cyst communication with a large duct may require drainage with Roux-en-Y hepaticojejunostomy.
- Radical surgery is the best procedure for large biliary-cyst fistula.

References

1. Gloor B, Ly Q, Candinas D. Role of laparoscopy in hepatic cyst surgery. Dig Surg. 2002;19:494–9.
2. Gamblin TC, Holloway SE, Heckman JT, GellerDA. Laparoscopic resection of benign hepatic cysts: a new standard. J Am Coll Surg. 2008;207:731–6.
3. Lantinga MA, Gevers TJ, Drenth JP. Evaluation of hepatic cystic lesions. World J Gastroenterol. 2013;2119(23):3543–54.
4. LiX,ZhangJL,WangYH,etal.Hepatobiliarycystadenoma and acstadenocarcinoma: a single center experience. Tumori. 2013;99(2):261–5.
5. Giorgio A, Esposito V, Farella N, et al. Amoebic liver abscesses: a new epidemiological trend in a non-endemic area. In Vivo. 2009;23(6):1027–30.
6. Bosanko N, et al. Presentations of pyogenic liver abscess in one UK centre over a 15 year period. JR Coll Physicians Edinb. 2011;41:13–7.
7. Nazir NT, Penfield JD, Hajjar V. Pyogenic liver abscess. Cleve Clin J Med. 2010;77(7):426–7.
8. Jha AK, Das G, Maitra S, et al. Management of large amoebic liver abscess- a comparative study of needle aspiration and catheter drainage. J Indian Med Assoc. 2012;110(1):13–5.
9. Singh V, Bhalla A, Sharma N, et al. Pathophysiology of jaundice in amoebic liver abscess. Am J Trop MedHyg. 2008;8(4):556–9.
10. Abbas MT, Khan FY, Muhsin SA, et al. Epidemiology, clinical feature and outcome of liver abscess: a single reference center experience in Qatar. Oman Med J. 2014;29(4):260–3.
11. Cai YL, Xiong XZ, Lu J, et al. Percutaneous needle aspiration versus catheter drainage in the management of liver abscess: a systemic review and meta-analysis. HPB(Oxford). 2015;17(3):195–201.
12. Levin DC, Eschelman D, Parker L, Rao VM. Trends in use of percutaneous versus open surgical grainage of abdominal abscesses. J Am CollRadiol. 2015;12(12 PtA):1247–50.
13. Zhang W, Ross AG, McManus DP. Mechanisms of immunity in hydatid disease: implication for vaccine development. L Immunol. 2008;15181(10):6679–85.
14. Wenbao Z, Li J, McManus DP. Concepts in immunology and diagnosis of hydatid disease. Clin Microbiol Rev. 2003;16(1):18–36.
15. Moro P, Schantz PM. Echinococcosis: a review. International Journal of Infectious Disease. 2009;13:125–33.
16. Fadel SA, Asmar K, Faraj W, Khalife M, Haddad M, El-Merhi F. Clinical review of liver hydatid disease and its unusual presentations in developing countries. AbdomRadiol (NY). 2019;44(4):1331–9.
17. Magistrelli P, Massetti R, Coppola R, Messia A. Surgical treatment of hydatid disease of liver: a 20 year experience. Arch Surg. 1991;126:518–23.
18. PAIR: Puncture, Aspiration, Injection, Re-aspiration- An option for the treatment of Cystic Echinococcosis. WHO/CDS/CSR/APH/2001.6.
19. Giorgio A, Tarantino L, Francica G, et al. Unilocularhydatid liver cysts: treatment with US-guided, double percutaneous aspiration and alcohol injection. Radiology. 1992;184(3):705–10.
20. Schipper HG, Lameris JS, van Delden OM, Rauws EA, Kager PA. Percutaneous evacuation of multivesicular

echinococcal cysts with or without cystobiliary fistula which contain non-drainable material: first results of a modified PAIR method. Gut. 2002;50(5):718–23.

21. Deo KB, et al. Surgical management of hepatic hydatid cyst- conservative versus radical surgery. HPB.2020.03.003.

22. Balik A, et al. Surgical treatment of hydatid disease of liver review of 304 cases. Arch Surg. 1999;134:166–9.

23. Ersan O, Yusuf B. Endoscopic therapy in the management of hepatobiliaryhydatid disease. J ClinGatroenterol. 2002;35:16–174.

24. Khanfar N. Hydatid disease: a review and update. Current Anaesthesia& Critical Care. 2004;15:173–83.

25. Eckert J, Deplazes P. Biological, epidemiological, and clinical aspects of echinococcosis, a zoonosis of increasing Cancer. ClinMicrobiol Rev. 2004;17(1):107–35.

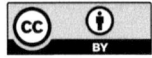

Laparoscopic Wedge Liver Resection

Ahmad Ramzi Yusoff and Davide Lomanto

Introduction

Laparoscopic liver resection was introduced as a surgical technique more than two decades ago. The initial successful laparoscopic anatomical hepatectomy was reported in 1996 by Azagra et al., who performed a left-lateral segmentectomy in a patient with a benign adenoma of segments II and III [1, 2]. The technique has grown from a novel procedure to an essential component of the highly specialised hepatobiliary unit armamentarium. Amongst the advantages of laparoscopic liver surgery are: reduced hospital stay, reduced postoperative pain, lowered risk of peritoneal adhesions, better cosmetic outcomes, and much shorter convalescence [3].

Laparoscopic wedge liver resection is often selected as the starting point for most hepatobiliary surgeons during their laparoscopic liver surgery endeavour. It is commonly a nonanatomical resection performed for benign or malignant indication [1].

Indications for Laparoscopic Wedge Liver Resection [1, 3]

1. Superficial lesion of 5 cm or less in diameter.
2. Small peripherally located lesions [left-lateral segments, segment VI, or the anterior segment of the right liver (segment V)].
3. Lesions of 3 cm or less in diameter in other segments.

Peripherally located lesions are desirable for laparoscopic resection as they are often devoid of large venous structures, require less mobilisation and dissection, and easily controlled should bleeding occur [4]. Nonetheless, sound oncologic principles as in open surgery must be observed during laparoscopic wedge resection for malignancy which are radical resection, and at least 1 cm free surgical margin. Owing to the lack of digital palpation during laparoscopic wedge resection, routine use of intraoperative ultrasonography to precisely locate the tumour and to plan the division of liver parenchyma has become mandatory [4].

Contraindications

These are mainly related to the anatomy, size, and location of the lesions. (Some could be of relative contraindication in a good, high-volume center) [1, 4].

A. R. Yusoff (✉)
Department of Surgery, Universiti Teknologi MARA, Sg. Buloh, Selangor, Malaysia

D. Lomanto
Department of Surgery, YLL School of Medicine, National University Singapore, Kent Ridge, Singapore

© The Author(s) 2023
D. Lomanto et al. (eds.), *Mastering Endo-Laparoscopic and Thoracoscopic Surgery*,
https://doi.org/10.1007/978-981-19-3755-2_47

331

- A large tumour (>5 cm in diameter).
- Lesions at the superior aspect of the liver, i.e., segments VII and VIII.
- Lesions near the major hepatic veins, inferior vena cava, and hepatic hilum.
- Evidence of severe portal hypertension.
- Presence of coagulopathy and thrombocytopenia.

Preoperative Assessment

Please refer to the previous text in the manual.

OT Setup

Instrumentations

- Laparoscopic trocars and cannula (2 × 12 mm, 1 × 10 mm, 2 × 5 mm).
- Hand-assisted port GelPort→ (optional).
- 10 mm 30°telescope
- Laparoscopic intraoperative ultrasound.
- Energy devices (Harmonic, Ligasure, Monopolar diathermy).
- Cotton tape, silicone snugger (For Pringle's manoeuvre—optional).
- Topical haemostatic agent (Surgicel→—optional).
- Endoscopic vascular stapler (optional).
- Endoscopic retrieval bag.

Patient's Position

- Supine position with both lower limbs in the abduction.
- The surgeon stands in between the patient's legs.
- Left-lateral position may be used for limited resection of segment VI.

Technique

(shown here is the technique for laparoscopic hand-assisted nonanatomical liver resection of segment VI tumour)

Access and Port Position

- Place a 10 mm supraumbilical port for the telescope.
- Place two 12 mm working ports in both right and left flanks. The 12 mm right flank port may be replaced with Gelport→ for hand-assisted surgery.
- Insert another 5 mm assistant port in the epigastrium or the right or left subcostal along the mid-clavicular line depending on the site of the lesion.

Scope and Pneumoperitoneum

- Use a 30° and 10mm laparoscope.
- Set CO2 pressure at 12 mmHg with medium flow at 10 L/min.

Exploration

Assess the liver by intraoperative laparoscopic ultrasound to determine the size and location of the lesion, to identify additional lesions, and to determine the feasibility of laparoscopic resection.

Mobilization

- Divide the attaching ligaments of the liver (the round, falciform, and triangular ligaments) (Fig. 1).
- Divide both the right and left triangular, and coronary ligaments according to the site of the lesion.

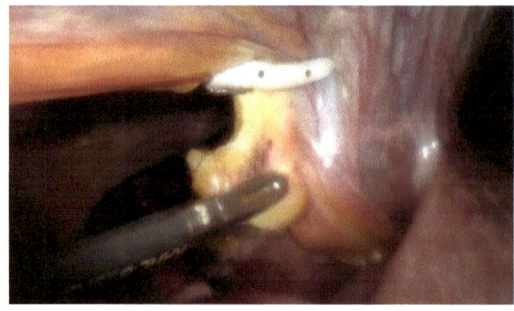

Fig. 1 Division of falciform ligament for liver mobilization

- Prepare Pringle's manoeuvre, although this is not routine for wedge resection; it is good to prepare for one in case of bleeding. Place tape around the porta hepatis and pass it into a silicone drain and secure it on the outside of the abdomen through an assistant port.

Parenchymal Transection

- Mark the surface of the liver parenchyma for transection by electrocautery, taking into account the 1 cm margin for a malignant lesion.
- Use hook electrocautery for parenchymal transection (Fig. 2).
- Alternatively, the harmonic scalpel (Ethicon, US) can be used for more convenient resection and simultaneous haemostasis (Figs. 3 and 4).

- For suitable cases, divide any pedunculated lesions with an endoscopic linear stapler.
- Pack or apply the topical haemostatic agent to the parenchymal defect or use bipolar cautery or clips to secure haemostasis (Figs. 5 and 6).

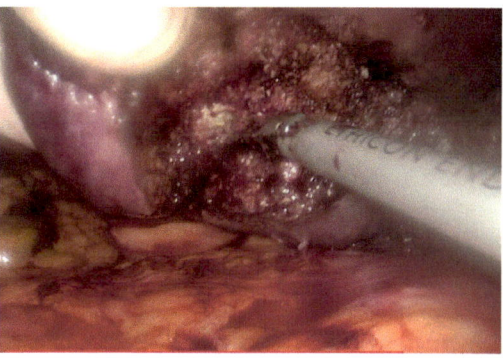

Fig. 4 Deeper parenchymal dissection with Harmonic scalpel

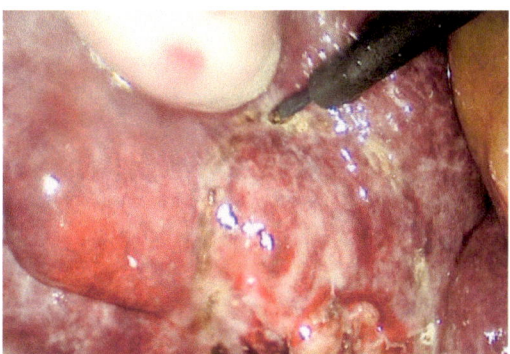

Fig. 2 Marking the area for tumour dissection with 1 cm margin using hook diathermy

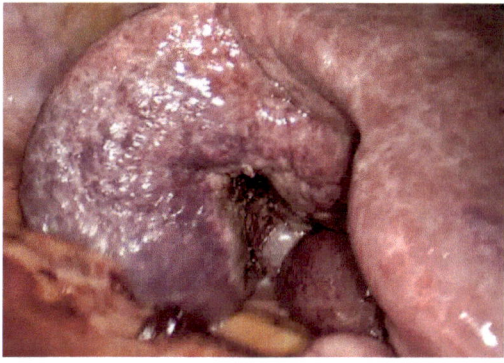

Fig. 5 Appearance of the cavity in segment VI of liver after nonanatomical resection of the tumour

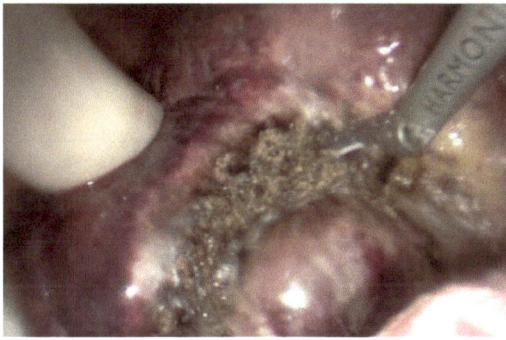

Fig. 3 Initial tumour dissection with Harmonic scalpel

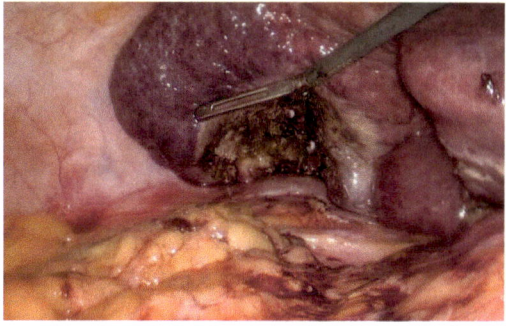

Fig. 6 The cavity left after the resection is packed with haemostatic agent

Extraction

- For small specimen, use an endopouch to retrieve it from either one of the 12 mm flank ports.
- For larger specimen, replace the 12 mm port with a 15 mm trocar for insertion of a larger endopouch. Place the specimen in the bag and extract it out with the 15 mm trocar.
- Stop the CO_2 insufflation, and incise the skin and fascia at the 15 mm trocar site to retrieve the bag and the specimen.
- Close the fascia carefully with an absorbable suture.

Complication of Laparoscopic Wedge Liver Resection

Although uncommon as this is considered minor hepatic resection, potential complications include;

Early

- Intra-abdominal haemorrhage especially in cirrhotic liver.
- Bile leak.
- Bowel ileus.
- Wound infection.

Late

- Biloma.
- Subphrenic abscess.
- Incisional hernia.

Postoperative Management

- Early feeding.
- Adequate analgesia.
- Early ambulation.
- Placement of a subhepatic drain (optional).
- Deep venous thrombosis prophylaxis.

References

1. Clavien P-A, Sarr MG, Fong Y, Miyazaki M. Atlas of upper gastrointestinal and hepato-pancreato-biliary surgery. Springer; 2015.
2. Cannon RM, Brock GN, Marvin MR, Buell JF. Laparoscopic liver resection: an examination of our first 300 patients. J Am Coll Surg. 2011;213(4):501–7.
3. Sasaki A, Nitta H, Otsuka K, Takahara T, Nishizuka S, Wakabayashi G. Ten-year experience of totally laparoscopic liver resection in a single institution. Br J Surg. 2009;96(3):274–9.
4. Gigot J-F, Glineur D, Azagra JS, Goergen M, Ceuterick M, Morino M, et al. Laparoscopic liver resection for malignant liver tumours: preliminary results of a multicenter European study. Ann Surg. 2002;236(1):90.

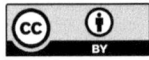

Laparoscopic Left Liver Resection

Pham Minh Hai and Le Quan Anh Tuan

Introduction

Liver resection is basically parenchymal transection and vessels, bile ducts control which is related to risk of major bleeding, bile leak, and unwanted injury of hepatic remnant. Distribution of vessels and bile ducts consists of two parts. One is hepatic veins. The other is hepatic pedicles which are covered by Glisson's capsule and located deeply in the hepatic parenchyma. This leads to technical difficulties as controlling inflow and outflow. This is explanation for limitation of applying laparoscopic surgery in major anatomical hepatectomy such as right hepatectomy and left hepatectomy.

In recent years, laparoscopic left hepatectomy (LLH) becomes more common all over the world. Its indication includes both benign and malignant liver lesions. Most of laparoscopic left hepatectomy are done in specialized centers with HBP experts. However, it is reported that this procedure is feasible and safe.

P. M. Hai
Department of Hepatobiliary and Pancreatic Surgery, University Medical Center, Ho Chi Minh city, Vietnam

L. Q. A. Tuan (✉)
Department of Hepatobiliary and Pancreatic Surgery, University Medical Center, Minimally Invasive Surgical Training Center, Ho Chi Minh City, Vietnam

Department of General Surgery, University of Medicine and Pharmacy, Ho Chi Minh City, Vietnam
e-mail: tuan.lqa@umc.edu.vn

Patient Selection

LLH is indicated for:

1. Benign or malignant lesions are located in the left liver (segments 2, 3, 4) while less resection is inappropriate.
2. Donor of the living liver transplantation.

Procedure

Generally, there are many types of laparoscopic approach in left liver resection. They are dorsal approach, Arantius-first approach, glissonean pedicle approach, and anterior approach [1–3]. In this chapter, we describe technically LLH with combination of glissonean pedicle approach and anterior approach [3, 4].

Operating Room Setup, Patient Positioning, and Surgical Team

Patient is placed in supine reverse Trendelenburg position. The arms should be tucked at the patient's sides. The legs are abducted.

Operating room setup is described in (Fig. 1)

© The Author(s) 2023

D. Lomanto et al. (eds.), *Mastering Endo-Laparoscopic and Thoracoscopic Surgery*,
https://doi.org/10.1007/978-981-19-3755-2_48

Technique

1. Trocar placement

First 12 mm trocar is placed at the umbilicus.

Another 12 mm trocar and three 5 mm trocars are placed as in (Fig. 2)

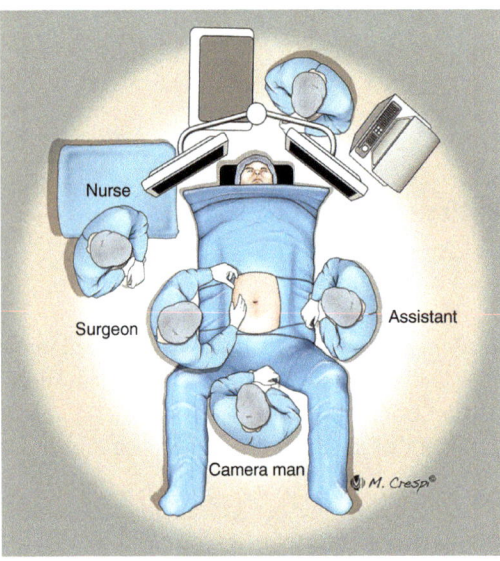

Fig. 1 OR setup

2. Exploration

Staging is very important in case of malignant or suspected malignant lesions. Abdominal inspection is performed to assess the liver, peritoneal, and mesenteric metastases.

Intraoperative ultrasonography is very useful to determine the size, location, number of the lesion, satellite nodules, and the level of liver cirrhosis. This helps to decide the resectability or an alternative surgical plan. Indocyanine green (ICG) can also be used for the purpose of exploration.

3. Mobilization of the left liver

Mobilization of left liver is performed by dividing round ligament, falciform ligament, left coronary ligament and part of right coronary ligament, left triangular ligament, and then hepatogastric ligament. A cholecystectomy is always done in our technique.

4. Hepatic hilum dissection

We perform Glissonean pedicle dissection according to Takasaki's technique. As a result, left hepatic pedicle is encircled with a tape. Then, left hepatic pedicle is temporarily clamped with bulldog clamps to confirm the efficacy of pedicle clamping and to visualize the ischemic demarcation line as well (Fig. 3)

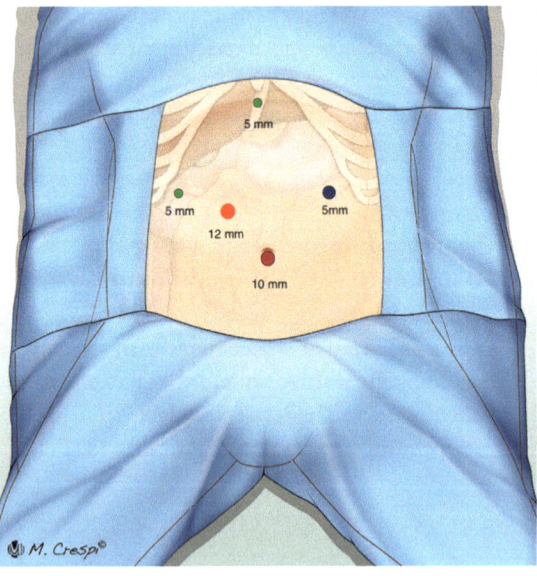

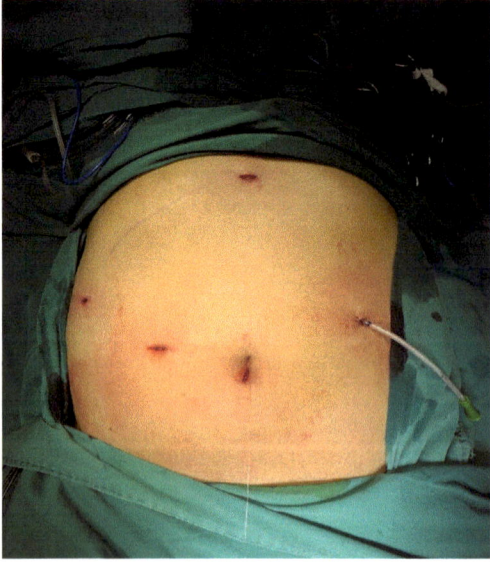

Fig. 2 Trocar position

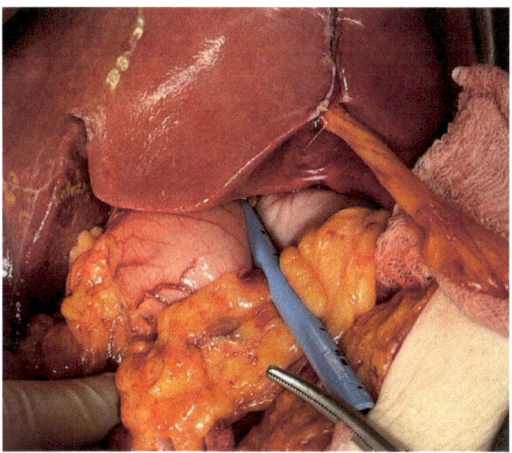

Fig. 3 Clamping of left hepatic pedicle

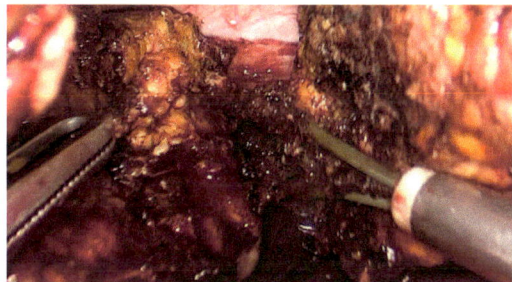

Fig. 4 Parenchymal dissection

5. **Parenchymal dissection**

According to the demarcation line on diaphragmatic surface and visceral surface of the liver, the parenchyma is dissected using ultrasonic shears or CUSA (Fig. 4).

In superficial 2 or 3 cm of liver parenchyma, there are no major vessels. Hence, we can dissect liver parenchyma safely with energy devices. When proceeding to deeper parenchyma, vascular structures should be recognized using crush-clamp technique and clipped before dividing. The parenchymal dissection should be peripheral to central direction with the left side of the middle hepatic vein as the landmark. (Fig. 5).

Hepatic parenchymal dissection is continued to caudate area. The left hepatic pedicle is then well exposed.

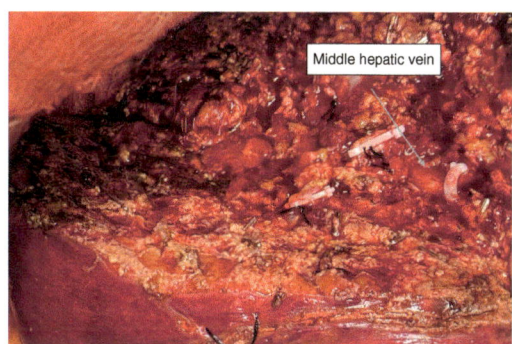

Fig. 5 Middle hepatic vein as anatomical landmark

6. **Transection of the left hepatic pedicle and left hepatic vein**

The bulldog clamps are removed and the left hepatic pedicle is divided by a vascular stapler. Other alternatives are using large clips, ligation, or suturing before transection. Care should be taken to avoid stenosis of the right hepatic duct (Fig. 5).

Although the left hepatic pedicle can be divided before parenchymal dissection, we prefer it after parenchymal dissection because of better visualization of the left hepatic pedicle and better free space around it that may lower the risk of bleeding and lower the risk of inadvertent injuries in case of anatomical variation.

Then comes the separation of the left liver from caudate area.

After that, left hepatic vein is exposed and divided. Vascular staplers, ligation, or suturing can be used. Care should be taken to avoid injury to the middle hepatic vein.

7. **Hemostasis**

Bleeding and bile leakage is carefully inspected. Clips or sutures are used for bleeding and bile leak.

8. **Removal of specimen**

Specimen is placed in a retrieval bag. A drain is usually placed close to the raw surface of the liver. The specimen is extracted through expanded incision of umbilical port or Pfannenstiel incision.

Complications

The main complication of laparoscopic left hepatectomy is bleeding. It is better to prevent bleeding than to stop bleeding. When bleeding occurs, we have many options including bipolar coagulation, vessel sealing devices, clips, staplers, and sutures. Laparoscopic suturing skill is important in laparoscopic liver resection. When there is no progress in a certain period or uncontrollable bleeding, conversion should be considered.

Summary

Laparoscopic left hepatectomy is more common but technically demanding. Parenchymal dissection should be peripheral to central with middle hepatic vein as the landmark. Bleeding is the most important issue in laparoscopic liver resection.

References

1. Okuda Y, Honda G, Kurata M, Kobayashi S, Sakamoto K. Dorsal approach to the middle hepatic vein in laparoscopic left hemihepatectomy. J Am Coll Surg. 2014;219(2):e1–4.
2. Ome Y, Honda G, Kawamoto Y. Laparoscopic left Hemihepatectomy by the Arantius-first approach: a video case report. J gastrointest Surg. 2020;24(9):2180–2.
3. Takasaki K. Glissonean pedicle transection method for hepatic resection: a new concept of liver segmentation. J Hepato-Biliary-Pancreat Surg. 1998;5(3):286–91.
4. Jamieson GG, Launois B, Cherqui D, Randone B, Gayet B, Machado MAC. Hepatectomies by laparoscopic approach: intra-Glissonian approach versus extra-Glissonian and posterior approach. In: Launois B, Jamieson GG, editors. The posterior intrahepatic approach in liver surgery. New York, NY: Springer New York; 2013. p. 143–69.

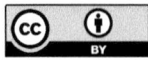

Laparoscopic Right Hepatectomy

Brian K. P. Goh

Introduction

Laparoscopic liver resection was first performed over two decades ago and is widely adopted in many institutions worldwide today [1]. However, laparoscopic liver resection especially for major hepatectomies remains a highly complicated and technically demanding procedure and is routinely performed only by specialized surgeons in high-volume centers today [2, 3]. In this chapter, we share the operative techniques adopted at our institution based on our experience with over 800 laparoscopic liver resections performed to date [1, 2, 4, 5].

Surgical Technique

Position

1. Reverse Trendelenburg position.
2. Supine position with primary operator on the right side.
3. Alternative position: Supine with both limbs abducted and surgeon stands between the legs.

B. K. P. Goh (✉)
Department of Hepatopancreatobiliary and Transplant Surgery, Singapore General Hospital and National Cancer Centre Singapore, Singapore Liver Transplant Service, SingHealth Duke-National University of Singapore Transplant Centre, Singapore, Singapore

SingHealth Duke-NUS Liver Transplant Center, Duke-National University of Singapore Medical School, Singapore, Singapore

Access and Port Position

1. Usually 5–6 ports are used (another 5 mm port may be used for application of the extracorporeal Pringles maneuver.
2. Place an initial 12 mm port for the camera at the right hypochondrium (4–5 cm from the midline).
3. Place two 12 mm working ports to the right and left of the initial port (about 5 cm from the camera port.
4. Insert another two 5 mm assistant ports at right subcostal and epigastrium.
5. Place another 5 mm port in the left hypochondrium if the extracorporeal Pringles Maneuver is used.

Scope and Pneumoperitoneum

1. A rigid 30°–10 mm laparoscope or a flexible tip 0°–10 mm laparoscope.
2. Set CO_2 pressure at 12 mmHg with high flow.
3. Two gas insufflators or the AirSeal device may be used to maintain a constant pneumoperitoneum.

Exploration

1. Use of intraoperative laparoscopic ultrasound is imperative to determine the size and

© The Author(s) 2023
D. Lomanto et al. (eds.), *Mastering Endo-Laparoscopic and Thoracoscopic Surgery*,
https://doi.org/10.1007/978-981-19-3755-2_49

location of the lesions and to identify additional lesions.

2. To identify key anatomical structures/landmarks such as the right hepatic vein, middle hepatic vein (MHV) (which is critical in guiding parenchyma transection), and the right Glissonian pedicle (including right anterior and right posterior pedicles.

Mobilization

1. Use monopolar energy to divide the ligaments of the liver (the round, falciform, and triangular ligaments).
2. Divide both the right and left triangular, and coronary ligaments according to the site of the lesion.
3. Rotating the table clockwise will allow gravity to assist in liver mobilization.
4. Mobilize the liver off the inferior vena cava (IVC) taking the short hepatic veins in a caudal to cranial direction (be aware of possible large inferior right hepatic veins which can be identified on preoperative imaging) (the IVC should be flat implying a low central venous pressure).
5. Division of the IVC ligament is critical to enable division of the right hepatic vein later.
6. It may not always be possible to mobilize the liver completely off the cava especially cranially in all patients (especially with liver having a long craniocaudal diameter). This can be done later after transection of the liver parenchyma.
7. This step of mobilization of the liver can also be performed after parenchymal transection instead of being performed as the initial step as in the medial to lateral approach. This is especially useful for patients with a large right lobe or in the presence of a bulky tumor.
8. Prepare Pringle's maneuver: encircle the porta hepatis with tape and pass it outside the abdomen through a 5 mm port.

Inflow Control

1. After cholecystectomy, proceed to dissect and identify the inflow structures (after dividing the cystic artery and duct, the gallbladder can be left attached to the liver to aid in retraction during hilar dissection).
2. Inflow control can be obtained via several approaches:
   (a) The classical extrahepatic intrafascial approach.
   (b) Extrahepatic Glissonian Approach.
   (c) Intrahepatic Glissonian Approach.
3. Extrahepatic dissection:
   (a) This approach is essential for living donor hepatectomy and tumors located close to the hilum.
   (b) Right hepatic artery is usually identified posterior to right hepatic duct and anterior to the right portal vein.
   (c) Right portal vein is dissected from the Glissonian sheath identifying the bifurcation with the left portal vein. Division of the caudate branch is useful to obtain additional length on the right portal vein. The portal vein is encircled with a tie.
   (d) Test clamping of the right portal vein and right hepatic artery should be performed to identify the ischemic line prior to ligating these structures.
   (e) Indocyanine green by negative staining may be used to aid in the identification of the ischemic line, especially in cases with chemo-damaged liver or cirrhosis.
   (f) At least two clips should be placed to the staying side of the right hepatic artery and portal vein to reduce the risk of slippage and postoperative bleeding.
   (g) The right hepatic duct is divided only after wide parenchyma transection to reduce the risk of common hepatic duct stricture.
4. In the extrahepatic Glissonian approach to the right pedicle, identification of the blood-

less space between Laennec's capsule and the Glissonian sheath as described by Suigioka et al. [6] is essential.

5. In the intrahepatic Glissonian approach, the hepatic parenchyma is transected anteriorly and posteriorly to the right pedicle or alternatively small hepatectomies as described by Machado et al. [7] can be created.

6. Both extrahepatic and intrahepatic Glissonian approaches are generally quicker to perform compared to the classical extrahepatic interfacial approach.

7. An important point to note is that a complete 360° dissection of the Glissonian pedicle is not essential and may result in troublesome bleeding as the terminal branches for the MHV are in close proximity. Usually, dissection of about 180°–270° of the right Glissonian pedicle is adequate to allow application of the laparoscopic bull-dog clamps and identification of the ischemic line.

8. Division of the Glissonian pedicle can be performed safely with vascular staplers after the liver parenchyma has been transected widely including transection of segment IX.

9. It must be ensured that the stapler is applied away from the hepatic duct bifurcation to avoid common hepatic duct stricture.

10. When feasible especially in the presence of a short right Glissonian pedicle, separate division of the right anterior and posterior pedicles will avoid accidental narrowing of the common hepatic duct.

Parenchyma Transection

1. This is usually performed with a Cavitron Ultrasonic Surgical Aspirator in combination with an energy device such as harmonic scalpel (Ethicon, USA) or Thunderbeat (Olympus, Japan). A bipolar forceps is also essential. Use intraoperative ultrasound intermittently to guide the transection plane.

2. Small (<5 mm) biliovascular structures can be divided with the energy device.

3. Larger structures are clipped with metal clips or self-locking clips.

4. Reducing the number of clips applied unnecessarily is important to minimize clip slippage.

5. It is useful to perform transection of the paracaval portion of the caudate early to allow control of the right hilar structures.

6. Transection of the hepatic parenchyma proceeds in a caudo-cranial direction along the MHV and the two lobes of the liver are gradually separated like an open book. Segment V tributaries are easily identified and divided.

7. Once the parenchyma has been widely transected, the right Glissonian pedicle can be divided with clips or vascular stapler (if this has not been done previously as with the extrahepatic or intrahepatic Glissonian approach).

8. Parenchyma transection continues cranially along the MHV and careful identification of segment VIII hepatic vein branches especially of segment VIII ventral is critical to avoid shearing of these venous tributaries from the MHV resulting in troublesome bleeding.

9. Finally, the root of the right vein is isolated and this is stapled off with the vascular (white reload).

10. Vascular clamps should always be ready at this final step as a misfire of the stapler can result in catastrophic bleeding.

11. After completion of transection, the liver surface should be inspected for bile leak and bleeding. This should be performed with a Valsalva maneuver after rehydration of the patient and with the pneumoperitoneum lowered to about 5 mmHg.

12. Hemostatic adjuncts may be used on the transected liver parenchyma surface.

13. A closed suction drain is placed in selected cases.

Extraction

1. The specimen is placed in a large bag and extracted via a lower midline or Pfannenstiel incision.
2. Usually, a 6–8 cm incision is required for extraction.

References

1. Goh BK, Lee SY, Teo JY, Kam JH, Jeyaraj PR, Cheow PC, et al. Changing trends and outcomes associated with the adoption of minimally-invasive hepatectomy: a contemporary single institution experience with 400 consecutive resections. Surg Endosc. 2018;32:4658–65.
2. Goh BK, Lee SY, Koh YX, KAm JH, Chan CY. Minimally invasive major hepatectomies: a southeast Asian single institution contemporary experience with its first 120 consecutive cases. ANZ J Surg. 2020;20:553–7.
3. Chua D, Syn N, Koh YX, Goh BK. Learning curves in minimally invasive hepatectomy: systematic review and meta-regression analysis. Br J Surg. 2021;108:351–8.
4. Goh BK, Prieto M, Syn N, Koh YX, Lim KI. Critical appraisal of the learning curve of minimally invasive hepatectomy: experience with the first 200 cases of a southeast Asian early adopter. ANZ J Surg. 2020;90(6):1092–8.
5. Kabir T, Goh BK. Contemporary techniques commonly adopted for performing laparoscopic liver resection. Laparosc Surg. 2018;2:61.
6. Sugioka A, Kato Y, Tanahashi Y. Systematic extrahepatic Glissonian pedicle isolation for anatomical liver resection based on Laennec's capsule: proposal of a novel comprehensive surgical anatomy of the liver. J Hepatobiliary Pancreat Sci. 2017;24:17–23.
7. Machado MA, Makdissi FF, Galvao FH, Machado MC. Intrahepatic Glissonian approach for laparoscopc right segmental liver resections. Am J Surg. 2008;196:e38–42.

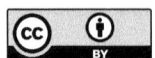

Laparoscopic Internal Drainage of Pancreatic Pseudocysts

Le Quan Anh Tuan and Pham Minh Hai

Introduction

According to revised Atlanta criteria, pancreatic pseudocyst (PP) is a chronic (>4 weeks) fluid collection within pancreatic parenchyma or adjacent space of pancreas which has no solid debris [1]. Pancreatic pseudocyst is consequence of acute pancreatitis in most cases. However, it may be consequence of chronic pancreatitis, pancreatic trauma, or pancreatic operation [2].

There are variety of clinical manifestations from asymptomatic to appearance of complications. Symptoms can be pain, nausea, and vomiting. Sometimes we can see upper gastrointestinal bleeding. Infection, hemorrhage, and rupture of cyst are the most common complications of PPs [3, 4].

Surgery has been main treatment method for PP for nearly a century from the first surgically internal drainage in 1921 [5]. Endoscopic internal drainage emerged from 1975. After being modified and developed, the latter shows that its efficacy of PP resolution was similar to that of surgery and this technique's complications were comparable to surgery. In addition, endoscopic therapy had benefits of hospitalization, mental health, and cost when compared with surgery [6–8]. Currently, surgery still plays an important role in the management of PP. Typically, surgical treatment includes surgical drainage (internal and external) and excision. Both can be done by open or laparoscopic surgery. This chapter focuses on technically laparoscopic internal drainage.

Patient Selection

Because of the benefits of nonoperative intervention, such as endoscopic internal drainage and percutaneous external drainage, indication of surgical internal drainage is limited at present. This technique is indicated when other drainage procedures are a failure or cannot perform. Patients with recurrent pseudocyst are also suitable for this technique and patients with enteric obstruction or biliary obstruction are suitable as well.

One important thing we need to check carefully before doing surgical internal drainage is the matureness of PP's wall. Appropriate time for this technique is usually after 6 weeks and thickness is more than 3 mm as well.

L. Q. A. Tuan (✉)
Department of Hepatobiliary and Pancreatic Surgery, University Medical Center, Minimally Invasive Surgical Training Center, Ho Chi Minh City, Vietnam

Department of General Surgery, University of Medicine and Pharmacy, Ho Chi Minh City, Vietnam
e-mail: tuan.lqa@umc.edu.vn

P. M. Hai
Department of Hepatobiliary and Pancreatic Surgery, University Medical Center,
Ho Chi Minh city, Vietnam

© The Author(s) 2023
D. Lomanto et al. (eds.), *Mastering Endo-Laparoscopic and Thoracoscopic Surgery*,
https://doi.org/10.1007/978-981-19-3755-2_50

Procedure

Operating Room Setup, Patient Positioning, and Surgical Team

Like other laparoscopic surgery, a flexible table is required to change the patient's position during the operation. This is necessary because it can help creating better exposure owing to gravity. Cautery system should be prepared while energy system such as harmonic scalpel or ligasure is rarely needed. Ideally, there are two monitors located at the head of the bed over both shoulders' side. One is for the surgeon and scrub nurse and another is for assistants. When lack of facility, given just one monitor, the placement should be on the left side of the patient.

Patient's position is decubitus with slight head up. As mentioned, head up help us having better view resulting from gravity retraction. Patient's legs may be split to make space for camera man or kept close to each other. Arms are usually tucked to create free spaces for surgeon, assistants, and scrub nurse's activities. Team is set up as in Fig. 1.

Technique

Trocar Placement

First trocar is 12 mm in size which is placed at infra-umbilicus by close technique or Hasson technique. However, consequence of intra-abdominal inflammation usually presents, we prefer to use Hasson technique. One more 12 mm trocar and two 5 mm trocars are placed as in Fig. 2.

Exposure of Pancreatic Pseudocyst

There are two ways to enter the lesser sac to expose PP. One is dividing gastrocolic ligament below gastroepiploic vessels. We have to free enough space for PP's wall for anastomosis. In this way, we can do either cystogastrostomy or cystojejunostomy. When inflammation does not present, exposure of PP's wall is usually performed easily. However, when inflammation still exists, this will confront with

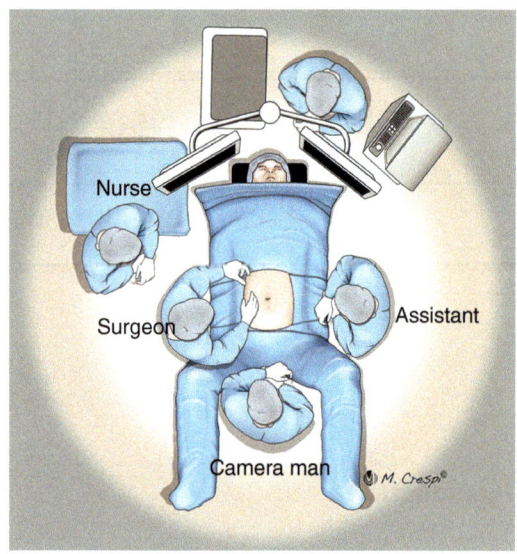

Fig. 1 Personnel setup

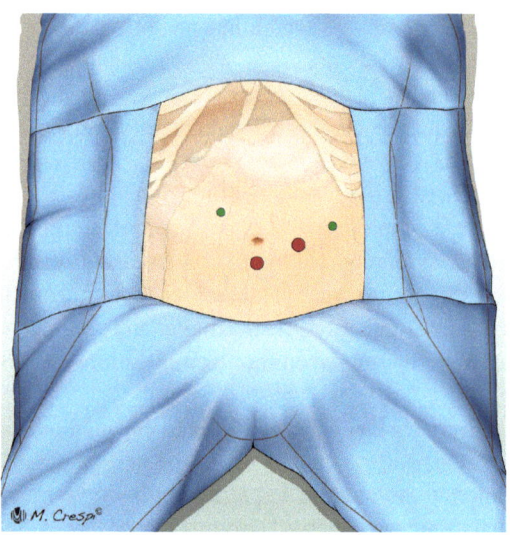

Fig. 2 Trocar position

difficulties. In this situation, we should change to the second approach. Second way is transmesenteric approach. Transverse colic mesentery usually adheres to PP's wall. Hence, one additional advantage of second way is thicker wall which will form a better anastomosis. In second way, we only open transverse colic mesentery to enter PP. With respect to transmesenteric approach, we only do cystojejunostomy.

Insight inspection of pancreatic pseudocyst and cyst wall biopsy.

Purpose of insight inspection of PP is exploring signs of bleeding and pancreatic necrosis which may lead to postoperative complications. These complications can cause consequences including reoperation or mortality. Because differentiation between PP and other types of pancreatic cysts is a challenge, cyst wall biopsy is necessary. Misdiagnosis as PP was reported in up to one-third of pancreatic cyst lesions [9].

Cystogastrostomy or Cystoduodenostomy or Cystojejunostomy

Surgical internal drainage includes cystogastrostomy, cystoduodenostomy, and cystojejunostomy depending on PP's location. Cystogastrostomy and cystoduodenostomy are performed when PP's wall is close to posterior wall of stomach. The former usually happens when PP is located in body or tail of pancreas. In contrast, the latter usually occurs when PP is located in head of pancreas. With regard to cystojejunostomy, the procedure can be done with any position of PP. Among them, pseudocystoduodenostomy seems to be rarely applied in laparoscopic drainage [10].

Technically, all surgical internal drainages have the same method. That is anastomosing PP's wall with lumen of alimentary tract such as posterior wall of stomach, wall of duodenum, and wall of small intestine. For laparoscopic drainage, anastomosis can be done by stapler or suturing. However, stapler is preferred due to saving operating time. In cystogastrostomy, there are some types of techniques such as endogastric, exogastric, and transgastric approaches [10, 11]. To pseudocystojejunostomy, Roux en Y anastomosis is usually fashioned [12]. Below, we describe technically cystojejunostomy with Roux en Y anastomosis by stapler.

After exposing, inspecting, and biopsy PP, below steps will be done one after another:

- Approaching cyst via incising through transverse mesocolon or through gastrocolic liga-

ment. The choice of approach depends on certain case. In case of through transverse mesocolon, opening should be just left of middle colic vessels. Sometimes puncturing or ultrasonography is used before opening cyst.
- Transecting jejunum at level 25–30 cm from ligament of Treitz by a linear stapler.
- Making a Y anastomosis between Y limb (proximal limb) and Rous limb (distal limb). Jejunojejunostomy is performed side to side by a linear stapler too. Distance from anastomosis to stump of distal limb is approximate 60–70 cm. we prefer to close enterotomy with continuous suture. Mesenteric defect should be closed.
- Enterotomy is performed close to the end cut of Roux limb. Cystojejunostomy is fashioned by one more linear stapler and defect of enterotomy and cyst are closed by continuous suture as well.
- Placing a drain is usually not necessary.
- Closure of trocar incision.

Outcomes

Effect of laparoscopic drainage was reached in 98% cases and recurrence rate was 2.5% in a systematic review [13].

It was also reported associating with low morbidity (<2%) [13]. Postoperative morbidities can be infection or bleeding. Most of the cases with morbidities were conservatively treated.

Summary

Laparoscopic internal drainage is technically feasible. It was associated with high rate of success and low morbidity. However, this technique should be performed when endoscopic or percutaneous drainage is failed or in case of recurrent pancreatic pseudocyst because endoscopic or percutaneous procedure is less invasive than it and has had benefits of hospitalization and mental health as well.

References

1. Banks PA, Bollen TL, Dervenis C, Gooszen HG, Johnson CD, Sarr MG, et al. Classification of acute pancreatitis--2012: revision of the Atlanta classification and definitions by international consensus. Gut. 2013;62(1):102–11.
2. Bradley EL 3rd. A clinically based classification system for acute pancreatitis. Ann Chir. 1993;47(6):537–41.
3. Bradley EL, Clements JL Jr, Gonzalez AC. The natural history of pancreatic pseudocysts: a unified concept of management. Am J Surg. 1979;137(1):135–41.
4. Sankaran S, Walt AJ. The natural and unnatural history of pancreatic pseudocysts. Br J Surg. 1975;62(1):37–44.
5. Parks RW, Tzovaras G, Diamond T, Rowlands BJ. Management of pancreatic pseudocysts. Ann R Coll Surg Engl. 2000;82(6):383–7.
6. Johnson MD, Walsh RM, Henderson JM, Brown N, Ponsky J, Dumot J, et al. Surgical versus nonsurgical management of pancreatic pseudocysts. J Clin Gastroenterol. 2009;43(6):586–90.
7. Rogers BH, Cicurel NJ, Seed RW. Transgastric needle aspiration of pancreatic pseudocyst through an endoscope. Gastrointest Endosc. 1975;21(3):133–4.
8. Varadarajulu S, Bang JY, Sutton BS, Trevino JM, Christein JD, Wilcox CM. Equal efficacy of endoscopic and surgical cystogastrostomy for pancreatic pseudocyst drainage in a randomized trial. Gastroenterology. 2013;145(3):583–90.e1.
9. Warshaw AL, Compton CC, Lewandrowski K, Cardenosa G, Mueller PR. Cystic tumors of the pancreas. New clinical, radiologic, and pathologic observations in 67 patients. Ann Surg. 1990;212(4):432–43; discussion 44–5.
10. Zerem E, Hauser G, Loga-Zec S, Kunosić S, Jovanović P, Crnkić D. Minimally invasive treatment of pancreatic pseudocysts. World J Gastroenterol. 2015;21(22):6850–60.
11. Agalianos C, Passas I, Sideris I, Davides D, Dervenis C. Review of management options for pancreatic pseudocysts. Transl Gastroenterol Hepatol. 2018;3(3):18.
12. Patel AD, Lytle NW, Sarmiento JM. Laparoscopic roux-en-Y drainage of a pancreatic pseudocyst. Curr Surg Rep. 2013;1(2):131–4.
13. Aljarabah M, Ammori BJ. Laparoscopic and endoscopic approaches for drainage of pancreatic pseudocysts: a systematic review of published series. Surg Endosc. 2007;21(11):1936–44.

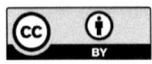

Laparoscopic Distal Pancreatectomy

Pham Minh Hai and Le Quan Anh Tuan

Introduction

Distal pancreatectomy (DP) consists of standard DP (with or without splenic preserving) and Radical antegrade modular pancreatosplenectomy (RAMPS). The former is also called DP. The latter is indicated for malignant or suspected malignant tumors. Both can be performed via laparoscopic or open approach.

Laparoscopic distal pancreatectomy (LDP) was first described and reported in 1996 by Alfred Cuschieri et al. [1]. LDP was initially indicated for chronic pancreatitis. After that, the indication was expanded to other benign and premalignant lesions located in body and tail of pancreas. In recent years, LDP has not only been developed in plenty of countries but its indication is also expanded to body and tail of pancreatic cancers [2, 3]. However, application of standard LDP for pancreatic adenocarcinoma has still been controversial, especially for medium and large tumors.

P. M. Hai
Department of Hepatobiliary and Pancreatic Surgery, University Medical Center, Ho Chi Minh city, Vietnam

L. Q. A. Tuan (✉)
Department of Hepatobiliary and Pancreatic Surgery, University Medical Center, Minimally Invasive Surgical Training Center, Ho Chi Minh City, Vietnam

Department of General Surgery, University of Medicine and Pharmacy, Ho Chi Minh City, Vietnam
e-mail: tuan.lqa@umc.edu.vn

It is lack of evidence in this condition [4]. This chapter's purpose is to describe technically standard laparoscopic distal pancreatectomy.

Procedure

Generally, standard LDP consists of LDP with splenectomy and laparoscopic spleen preserving distal pancreatectomy (LSPDP), also called SSLDP (spleen sparing laparoscopic distal pancreatectomy)

Operating Room Setup, Patient Positioning, and Surgical Team

Patient is placed in supine reverse Trendelenburg position. The arms should be tucked at the patient's sides. The legs are abducted.

10 mm laparoscope of 30° or 45° is used.

The main surgeon and scrub nurse are positioned on the patient's right side. The first assistant's (cameraman) position is between patient's legs and second assistant stands on the left side. The back table is set up on the right side of patient, above the scrub nurse (Fig. 1).

© The Author(s) 2023
D. Lomanto et al. (eds.), *Mastering Endo-Laparoscopic and Thoracoscopic Surgery*, https://doi.org/10.1007/978-981-19-3755-2_51

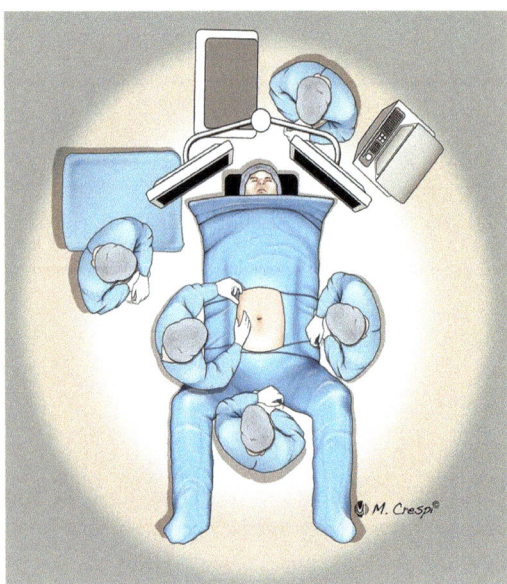

Fig. 1 Personnel setup

Surgical Technique

In this chapter, we technically describe procedure of LDP step by step. We describe both LDP with and without splenectomy. There are six main steps during procedure apart from general steps which are present in most laparoscopic surgeries. They are [1] exposure of pancreas and infra-pancreatic superior mesenteric vein, [2] mobilization of transverse mesocolon and splenic flexure of colon, [3] posterior dissection and splenic vessel exposure, [4] upper border of pancreatic neck and celiac trunk dissection, [5] pancreatic neck transection, and [6] separating specimen. LDP with splenectomy and LDP without splenectomy differ from each other at last step. The description with details will be presented below.

Trocar Placement

First trocar is 12 mm in size which is placed at infra-umbilicus by close technique or Hasson technique. One 12 mm trocar and two or three 5 mm trocars are placed as in Fig. 2.

Inspection

Staging is very important in case of malignant or suspected malignant lesions. This is a mandatory step. Abdominal inspection is performed to assess liver, peritoneal, and mesenteric metastases. Beside this, we can assess the resectability of tumor.

Pancreatic Exposure and Infra-pancreatic Superior Mesenteric Vein Exposure

After abdomen is carefully explored and signs of advanced stage are not found, the lesser sac is entered by dividing gastrocolic ligament below level of gastroepiploic vessels. Gastrocolic ligament should be divided bilaterally to duodenum and splenic flexure of colon to completely expose body and tail of pancreas. This can cause injuries to transverse mesocolic vessels, duodenum, and transverse colon, especially at the site of pancreatic head. Some tips which can help avoiding these consequences are meticulous dissection and following landmarks such as gastroepiploic vessels and duodenum. Greater omentum can become ischemic after dividing gastrocolic ligament but there is mostly no need to resect it.

Next is mobilization of the stomach. Then suturing posterior wall of stomach against anterior abdominal wall is done by 2.0 absorbable suture. We prefer to use vicryl. The direction for pulling stomach is cranial and medial. As a result, superior border of pancreas and celiac trunk may be well accessed as we act at below steps. Pancreatic lesion is also inspected.

Infra-pancreatic superior mesenteric vein (SMV) is dissected at inferior pancreatic border. Right gastroepiploic and middle colic vein are important landmarks. SMV is covered by a thin layer called adventitial tissue and loose thin connective tissue outer. Dissector forceps can be useful to dissect and enter the loose thin connective tissue around SMV to expose SMV. Middle colic vein can drain separately or join with gastroepiploic vein to SMV. We prefer to leave middle

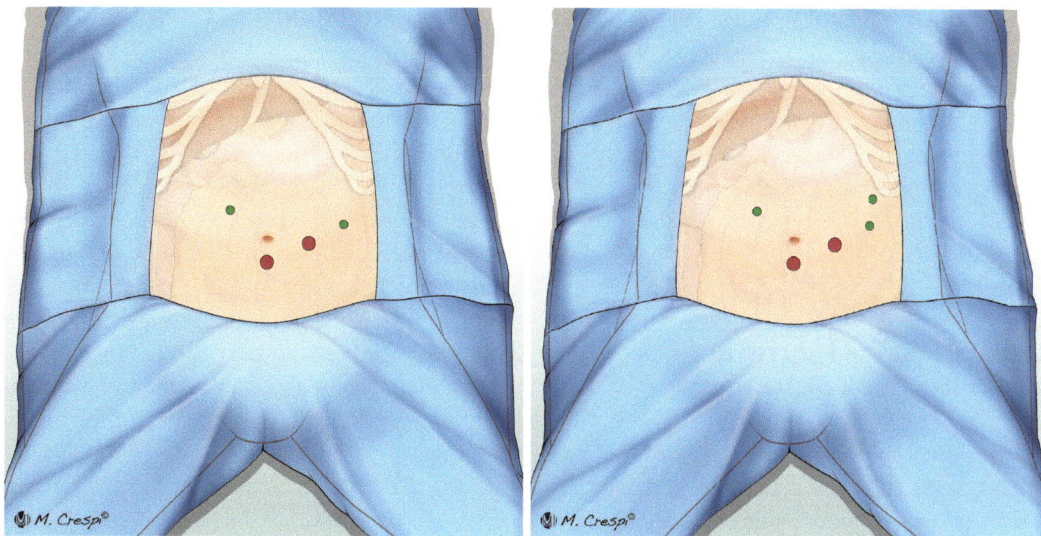

Fig. 2 Trocar position

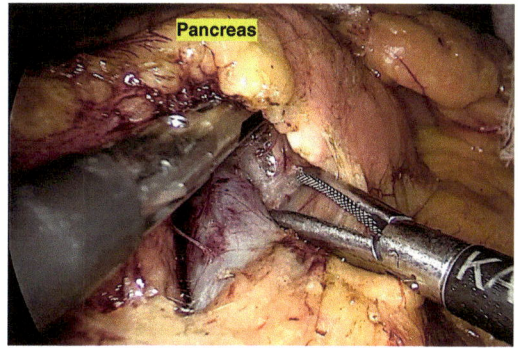

Fig. 3 SMV and PV exposure

colic vein unless it impedes such as in SMA first approach or some variations.

SMV and portal vein (PV) exposure (Fig. 3) is slowly developed upward till superior border of pancreas. This work is recommended under viewing. Expanding our dissection to the left of SMV facilitates this work. During expanding dissection, we need to consider vessels near SMV.

Transverse Mesocolic and Splenic Flexure of Colon Mobilization

Mobilization of transverse mesocolon is separating it from inferior border of pancreas. Transverse mesocolon consists of two peritoneal leaves. One passes on retroperitoneum in cranial at anterior surface or inferior border of pancreas; another runs downward. We need to incise the former at the site of inferior border of pancreas for mobilizing. Incision is usually started below pancreatic body. After that blunt forceps should be applied to identify the right plane. That is avascular plane. Mobilization will progress in left direction and then splenic flexure of colon is mobilized by dividing splenocolic omentum. Mobilized colon is retracted inferiorly to well expose both inferior border of pancreas and spleen. During mobilizing route, there are some small vessels going across dissection plane. Hence, an energy device has been usually used to provide a clean view.

Posterior Dissection and Splenic Vessel Exposure

Following right dissection plane of previous step, posterior dissection of pancreatic body and tail occurs. The aim of this step is separation of distal pancreas from retroperitoneal structures and facilitating splenic vessel exposure (Fig. 4). In open surgery, authors have begun exposing splenic vessels with anterior view from cranial border of pancreas. Splenic artery is prior exposed because splenic vein is located deeper and in caudal which is covered by pancreatic parenchyma. With laparoscopic surgery, this is preferably done with posterior view after pancreas is taken away from retroperitoneum and lifted. By doing this, splenic vein is first dissected. Circulating these vessels is usually combined with anterior dissection later in the next step.

Upper Border of Pancreatic Neck and Celiac Trunk Dissection

Dissection is started at the upper border of pancreatic neck and then proceeded left laterally. The fat and lymph nodes along common hepatic artery (CHA), left gastric artery, and splenic artery are dissected in case of malignancy. Partly exposed splenic artery of the previous step is more dissected and encircled at the site of the planned line of pancreatic transection. Then, splenic vein is dissected and encircled.

In LDP with splenectomy, splenic vessels are transected. Splenic artery should be first ligated and transected at the planned pancreatic transection line. Splenic vein is transected separately or together with the pancreas by staplers. There are various applicable kinds of vascular ligation such as vascular staplers, clip, tie, or suturing.

Pancreatic Transection

The distal pancreas is divided by a linear stapler (Fig. 5). Although none of the staplers has proved superior in terms of postoperative pancreatic fistula (POPF), short height staplers are usually used. Tissue compression when stapling relates to risk of bleeding and POPF. Gradually increasing pressure with three or four consecutive stairs should be performed with at least 3 min for each stair to achieve best tissue compression before transection.

Alternative methods of transecting the pancreas is to use ultrasonic shears or electrocautery to divide pancreatic parenchyma. Pancreatic duct

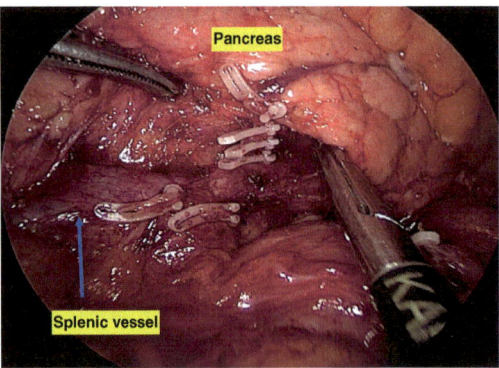

Fig. 4 Splenic vessel exposure

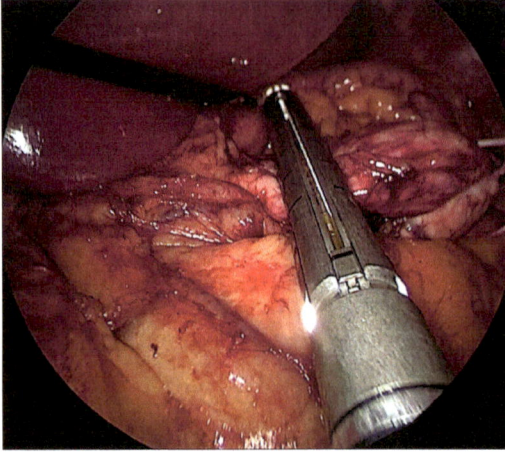
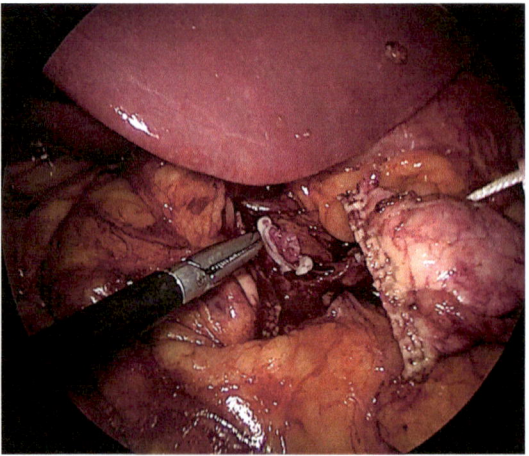

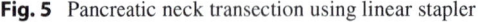
Fig. 5 Pancreatic neck transection using linear stapler

should be identified and ligated or sutured by a nonabsorbable monofilament suture. The stump is oversewn with a running suture to secure bleeding and pancreatic leakage.

Separating Specimen

In this step, LDP with splenectomy is different from LDP without splenectomy.

Laparoscopic Distal Pancreatectomy with Splenectomy

After splenic vessels and the pancreas are transected, dissection is continued further to left lateral direction. Ensuring en bloc dissection with lymph nodes and fat surrounding pancreas is necessary, especially for pancreatic cancer or high malignant potential lesion. After the body and tail of the pancreas is completely separated from retroperitoneum, splenorenal ligament is exposed and divided to mobilize the spleen. The specimen is extracted in a retrieval plastic bag (Fig. 6). Distal pancreatectomy with splenectomy, showing splenic artery ligation and spleen mobilization.

Laparoscopic Spleen Preserving Distal Pancreatectomy

This technique requires more advanced laparoscopic surgical skills (Fig. 7). Operating time is usually longer than LDP with splenectomy. However, postoperative complication rate is reported lower than LDP with splenectomy. Moreover, spleen plays a role in immunity in human body. Postoperative infection rate of spleen preserving was also reported significantly decreasing [5–9]. There are two methods of preserving spleen. They are splenic

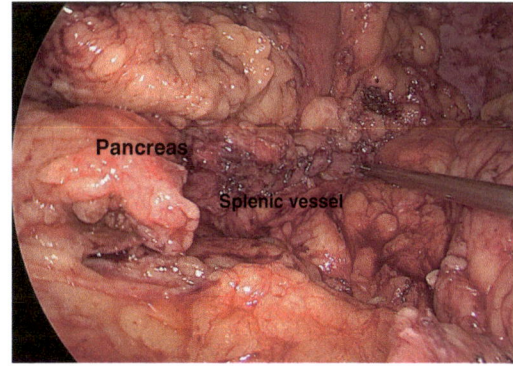

Fig. 7 Spleen preserving distal pancreatectomy

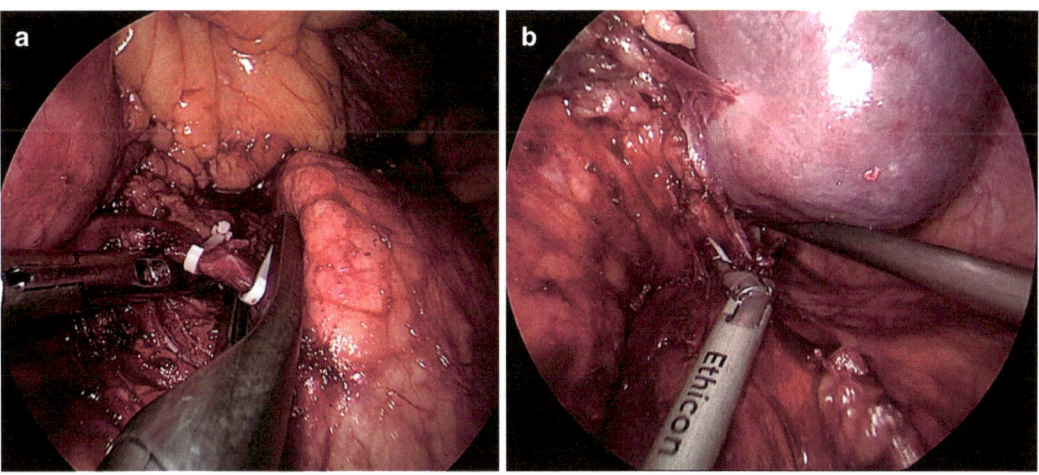

Fig. 6 Distal pancreatectomy with splenectomy. (**a**) Splenic artery ligation, (**b**) spleen mobilized

vessels saving (Kimura's technique) and sacrificing (Warshaw's technique). The former associated lower rate of ischemic spleen. In terms of technical advantages, Warshaw technique is easier to do.

With Warshaw's technique, splenic vessels are transected two times. First time of transecting is similar to LDP with splenectomy. After that mobilization of distal pancreas and splenic vessels is proceeded to splenic hilum. Then, pancreatic tail is separated from splenic hilum. Splenic artery and vein are exposed above freed pancreatic tail. These vessels are divided second time. The short gastric vessels are preserved.

In splenic vessel preserving technique, dissection is performed along splenic vein and artery. There are direct branches from splenic vessels to the pancreas. These vessels should be dissected meticulously and divided using ultrasonic shears or advanced bipolar energy, if necessary, clips are applied. When uncontrollable bleeding happens, Warshaw's technique is an alternative option.

Finally, inspection for bleeding and fluid clearance is completed. A drain is positioned close to pancreatic stump. Specimen in placed in retreival bag and exteriorized via expanded incision of umbilical port or Pfannenstiel incision.

Complication and Management

Complications are POPF, postpancreatectomy hemorrhage (PPH), and delayed gastric emptying. These complications are identified and classified according to consensus of International Study Group of Pancreatic Surgery (ISGPS). Among them, POPF and bleeding are most common [10, 11]. Management of POPF and PPH are described in "Laparoscopic pancreaticoduodenectomy."

Summary

Standard laparoscopic distal pancreatectomy is now indicated for both benign and premalignant lesions located in body or tail of pancreas. It is still controversial to indicate standard LDP for pancreatic adenocarcinoma. Standard LDP can be done with or without splenectomy.

References

1. Cuschieri A, Jakimowicz JJ, van Spreeuwel J. Laparoscopic distal 70% pancreatectomy and splenectomy for chronic pancreatitis. Ann Surg. 1996;223(3):280–5.
2. Björnsson B, Sandström P. Laparoscopic distal pancreatectomy for adenocarcinoma of the pancreas. World J Gastroenterol. 2014;20(37):13402–11.
3. Postlewait LM, Kooby DA. Laparoscopic distal pancreatectomy for adenocarcinoma: safe and reasonable? J Gastrointest Oncol. 2015;6(4):406–17.
4. Tewari M. Surgery for pancreatic and Periampullary cancer. Singapore: Springer Nature Singapore Pte Ltd; 2018.
5. Butturini G, Damoli I, Crepaz L, Malleo G, Marchegiani G, Daskalaki D, et al. A prospective non-randomised single-center study comparing laparoscopic and robotic distal pancreatectomy. Surg Endosc. 2015;29(11):3163–70.
6. Casadei R, Ricci C, D'Ambra M, Marrano N, Alagna V, Rega D, et al. Laparoscopic versus open distal pancreatectomy in pancreatic tumours: a case–control study. Updat Surg. 2010;62(3):171–4.
7. Mellemkjoer L, Olsen JH, Linet MS, Gridley G, McLaughlin JK. Cancer risk after splenectomy. Cancer. 1995;75(2):577–83.
8. Pendola F, Gadde R, Ripat C, Sharma R, Picado O, Lobo L, et al. Distal pancreatectomy for benign and low grade malignant tumors: short-term postoperative outcomes of spleen preservation-a systematic review and update meta-analysis. J Surg Oncol. 2017;115(2):137–43.
9. Shoup M, Brennan MF, McWhite K, Leung DH, Klimstra D, Conlon KC. The value of splenic preservation with distal pancreatectomy. Arch Surg (Chicago, Ill: 1960). 2002;137(2):164–8.
10. Liao CH, Wu YT, Liu YY, Wang SY, Kang SC, Yeh CN, et al. Systemic review of the feasibility and advantage of minimally invasive Pancreaticoduodenectomy. World J Surg. 2016;40(5):1218–25.
11. Chen K, Liu XL, Pan Y, Maher H, Wang XF. Expanding laparoscopic pancreaticoduodenectomy to pancreatic-head and periampullary malignancy: major findings based on systematic review and meta-analysis. BMC Gastroenterol. 2018;18(1):102.

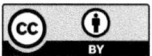

Laparoscopic Pancreaticoduodenectomy

Le Quan Anh Tuan and Pham Minh Hai

Introduction

Evolution and difficulties of Laparoscopic pancreaticoduodenectomy.

Pancreaticoduodenectomy (PD), understood as radical pancreaticoduodenal resection at present, was popularized by Allen O. Whipple and colleagues [1]. At that stage, this procedure is associated with a high rate of morbidity and mortality. With natural evolution, developments in equipment and technically surgical skill had been appearing. Gagner and Pomp [2] successfully performed laparoscopic pancreaticoduodenectomy (LPD) in 1994. The procedure's popularization was still low, especially over the next decade. This is due to high rate of postoperative complications and technical difficulties. Pancreatic head and duodenum are located deeply in retroperitoneal space and are close to major vascular structures. These result in difficulties in performing LPD. Moreover, life-threatening complications can happen if these major vascular structures are injured.

In recent years, outcome of LPD has been significantly improved owing to developments of surgical technique, medicine and equipment, and energy devices, for example. LPD has become more common all over the world. However, this is still a challenging procedure.

LPD consists typically of standard LPD, LPD with arterial first approach, and LDP with superior mesenteric-portal vein resection. This chapter's purpose is to describe technically the former.

Indications

LPD is generally indicated for below conditions:

1. Resectable and borderline resectable periampullary cancers
2. Targeting of malignant pancreatic head neoplasms (IPMN)
3. Chronic pancreatitis with inflammatory mass in pancreatic head
4. Benign periampullary neoplasms not amenable to local resection

Patient Selection

Theoretically, most indicated PD is able to perform LPD. Because of certain limitations as proceeding LPD such as higher abdominal pressure

L. Q. A. Tuan (✉)
Department of Hepatobiliary and Pancreatic Surgery, University Medical Center, Minimally Invasive Surgical Training Center, Ho Chi Minh City, Vietnam

Department of General Surgery, University of Medicine and Pharmacy, Ho Chi Minh City, Vietnam
e-mail: tuan.lqa@umc.edu.vn

P. M. Hai
Department of Hepatobiliary and Pancreatic Surgery, University Medical Center, Ho Chi Minh city, Vietnam

© The Author(s) 2023
D. Lomanto et al. (eds.), *Mastering Endo-Laparoscopic and Thoracoscopic Surgery*,
https://doi.org/10.1007/978-981-19-3755-2_52

357

which can cause consequences for respiratory and cardiac systems. Because LPD operating time is long, patients with severe respiratory and cardiac disease should be eliminated. Apart from this, vascular resection and reconstruction require a high level of laparoscopic surgical skills, longer time and they can cause more blood loss as well. Although authors can do LPD with borderline resectable tumors belong to periampullary pathologies, other authors have recommended that borderline resectable tumors are only performed at a few specialized centers; indication for LPD in cancer patients should be limited at resectable stage.

Procedure

Generally, there are two main procedures in classification. One is classic PD called Kausch-Whipple. Another one is pyloric preservation PD (PPPD) which was described by Longmire and Traverso. Both can be done by a minimally invasive approach such as laparoscopic surgery.

Operating Room Setup, Patient Positioning, and Surgical Team

Appropriate operating room may require a flexible table, cautery system, and energy system. Ideally, there are two monitors located at the head of the bed over both shoulders' side. One is for the surgeon and scrub nurse and another is for assistants. When lack of facility, given just one monitor, the placement should be on the left side of the patient.

Patient is placed in supine with slight head up. With head up, we can have better view resulting from gravity retraction. Patient's legs should be split to make space for cameraman. Arms are tucked to create free spaces for surgeon, assistants, and scrub nurse's activities.

The main surgeon and scrub nurse are positioned on the patient's right side. The first assistant's (cameraman) position is between patient's legs and second assistant stands on the left side. The back table is set up on the right side of patient, above the scrub nurse. The personnel is descried as in Fig. 1.

Technique

There are two main phases included in laparoscopic pancreaticoduodenectomy. They are resection and reconstruction.

Trocar Placement

First trocar is 12 mm in size which is placed at umbilicus' left side by Hasson technique.

One 12 mm trocar and three 5 mm trocars are placed as in Fig. 2.

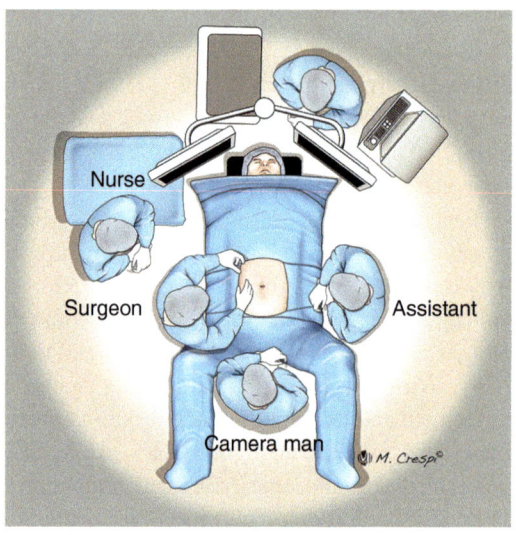

Fig. 1 OT setup

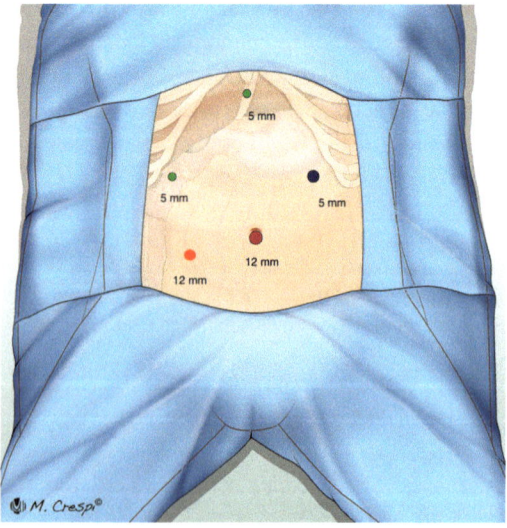

Fig. 2 Port placement

Inspection

Staging is very important in case of malignant or suspected malignant lesions. This is a mandatory step. Abdominal inspection is performed to assess liver, peritoneal, and mesenteric metastases. Beside this, we can assess resectability of tumor.

Dissection Phase

There are different approaches for LPD. We usually use clockwise approach for dissection phase. However, all patients were not applied the same kind of approach. It depended on proper situation. In case of a tumor located in uncinate process, we used superior mesenteric artery first approach. Clockwise approach includes below steps. Before these steps are described in detail, it is necessary to consider levels of lymphadenectomy in LPD. There are three levels of harvesting lymph nodes, but we only focus on standard lymphadenectomy which is recommended to perform routinely at present.

A consensus statement by the International Study Group on Pancreatic Surgery (ISGPS) was published in 2014 [3]. "After evaluating all the available literature and the expert opinions during the consensus meeting, a clear definition of a standard lymphadenectomy was reached: A standard lymphadenectomy should include Ln stations 5, 6, 8a, 12b1, 12b2, 12c, 13a, 13b, 14a right lateral side, 14b right lateral side, 17a, and 17b" (Fig. 3).

Infra-pancreatic Superior Mesenteric Vein Exposure

After abdomen is carefully explored and signs of advanced stage are not found, the lesser sac is entered by dividing gastrocolic ligament below the level of gastroepiploic vessels. Gastrocolic ligament should be divided from the left side to the duodenum to create enough space for working around head and body of pancreas. During this, transverse mesocolic vessels can be injured because of adhesion, especially at the site of pancreatic head. Avoiding these consequences, tips are following gastroepiploic vessels and duode-

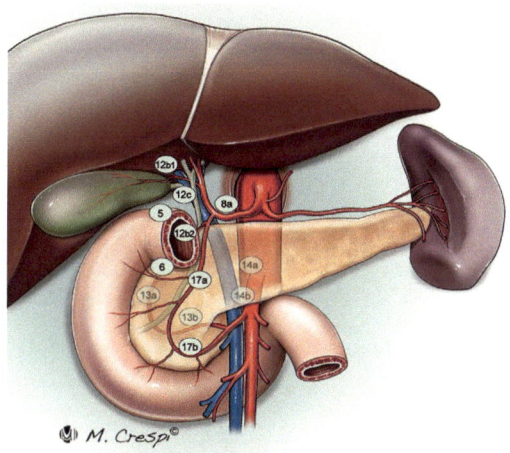

Fig. 3 Standard lymphadenectomy during PD

num. Moreover, meticulous dissecting is required. Greater omentum can become partly ischemic after dividing gastrocolic ligament but we do not need to resect it mostly.

Superior mesenteric vein (SMV) is dissected at inferior pancreatic border (Fig. 4). Right gastroepiploic and middle colic vein are important landmarks. SMV is covered by a thin layer called adventitial tissue and loose thin connective tissue outer. Dissector forceps can be useful to dissect and enter the loose thin connective tissue around SMV to expose SMV. Middle colic vein can drain separately or join with gastroepiploic vein to SMV. We prefer to leave middle colic vein unless it impedes such as in SMA first approach or some variations. Gastroepiploic vein must be ligated at the site draining to SMV as it drains separately. When gastroepiploic and superior right colic vein form gastrocolic trunk of Henle, the latter should be preserved.

SMV and portal vein (PV) exposures are slowly developed upward till superior border of pancreas. This work is recommended under viewing. Expanding our dissection to the left of SMV facilitates this work. During expanding dissection, we need to consider vessels nearby SMV.

Extended Kocher Maneuver

Right border of SMV is used to follow to push transverse mesocolon away from pancreatic head. Beside gastroepiploic and anterior pancreatico-

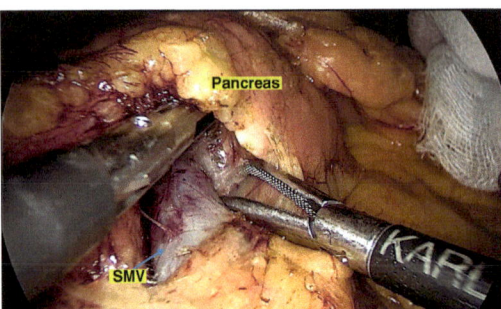

Fig. 4 Infra-pancreatic superior mesenteric vein (SMV) exposure

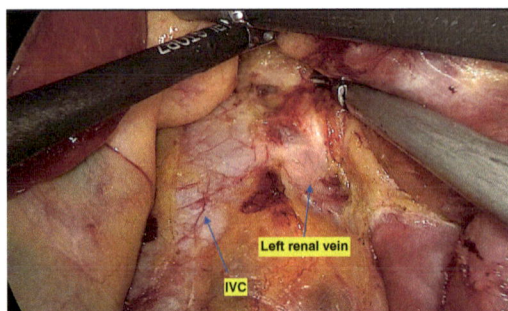

Fig. 6 Kocher maneuver

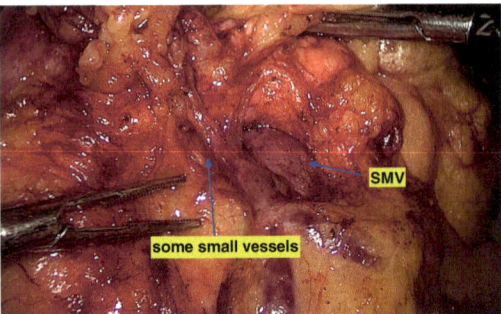

Fig. 5 Some small branches across dissecting plane

duodenal vein, there are some small vessels across this plane (Fig. 5). They usually cause bleeding during dissecting this plane that is difficult to control. Sharp dissection with energy devices shows effectively. Then duodenum part three and part four are separated from transverse mesocolon.

In laparoscopic surgery, it is easier for Kocher maneuver if this is dissected cephalad. Extended Kocher maneuver is completed when not only duodenum, pancreatic head, and uncinate are separated from retroperitoneum but inferior vena cava (IVC), left renal vein, and SMA are also exposed (Fig. 6).

Duodenal or Antral Transection
Pylorus preserving pancreaticoduodenectomy has been usually performed if signs of duodenal invasion have not appeared. It was preferred although delayed gastric empty was reported higher than classic PD.

It is similar to open surgery duodenum transected below pylorus 2–3 cm in LPPPD. Lymph

node group 5 and 6 will be left to remove en bloc with pancreatic head. For laparoscopic classic PD, antrectomy is performed at the level of third or fourth transverse vein on lesser curvature and at the confluence of the gastroepiploic veins on greater curvature. We use stapler for this step.

Upper Border of Pancreatic Neck Dissection and Gastroduodenal Artery Ligation
In laparoscopic PD, duodenal or antral transection (step 3) should be done prior this step and next step (dissection of porta hepatis) like outline in this chapter. In the condition of open PD, step 3 is usually performed when ability of radical tumor resection is ensured. This means step 3 has to follow step 4, 5, and 6. The explanation is because in LPD all laparoscopic instruments go upward from the ports and direction of dissection is in cephalad as well. Thus, surgical viewing becomes better after completing step 3 (Fig. 7). One more important tip to have good exposure to this area is liver retractor. We prefer liver retractor as in Fig. 8.

Anatomical variations may lead to inadvertent missing. Most of the major variations such as hepatic or gastroduodenal arterial anomalies, SMA, and bile duct variations are well identified on CT scan preoperatively. Among them, we need to care with accessory or replaced HA due to easily advertently missing (Fig. 9).

We usually started at upper border of pancreatic neck by incising the fascia and taking away large lymph nodes along common hepatic artery (CHA), lymph node group 8a. As a result, CHA was exposed. Follow CHA to extend lymphade-

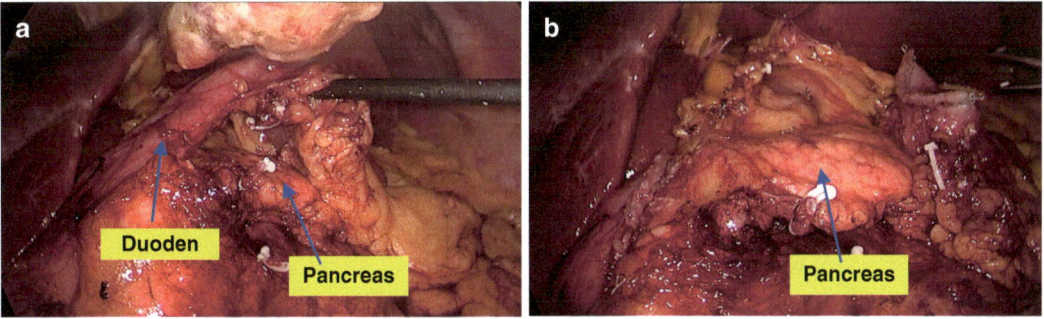

Fig. 7 Difference of surgical view between before (**a**) and after (**b**) duodenal or antral transection in laparoscopic PD

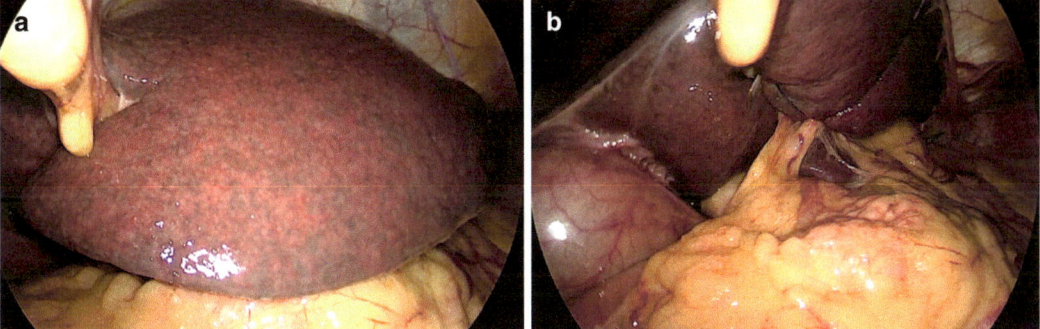

Fig. 8 Liver retractor: before (**a**) and after (**b**)

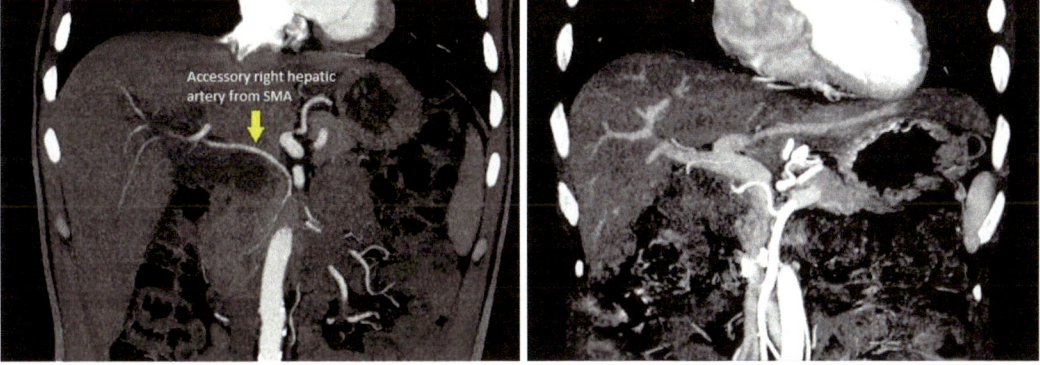

Fig. 9 Accessory or replaced right HA

nectomy bilaterally. According to standard lymph-adenectomy, lymph node dissection is extended to left gastric artery (LGA) at level of Celiac trunk in left direction. It is taken into consideration of preserving left gastric vein which drains to PV or PV–SMV junction or splenic vein. Continuing dissection toward right side, right gastric artery and GDA are exposed clearly and ligated. For GDA

ligation, we prefer to tie it with suture 2.0 as Vicryl or silk. Supra-duodenal branches should be divided to make a free space enough. Checking by bulldog before dividing GDA is necessary as in Fig. 10.

Dissection of Porta Hepatis

Dissection of porta hepatis is also one part of lymphadenectomy. First of this step is separation

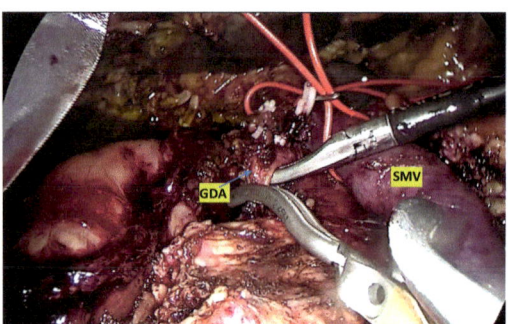

Fig. 10 Checking by using Bulldog before ligating GDA

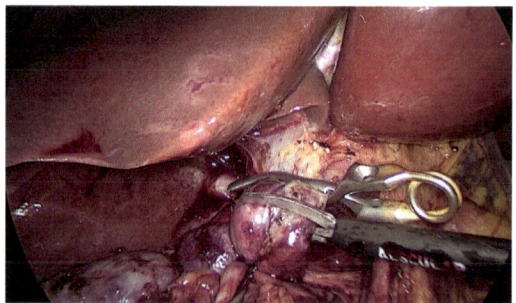

Fig. 11 Clamping bile duct before dividing

of fascia covering anterior porta hepatis to remove all fat and fascia around common hepatic duct (CHD), common bile duct (CBD), and cystic duct en bloc with CBD and gallbladder. These consist of lymph node groups namely 12b1, 12b2, and 12c belonging to the Japanese classification. After CBD, gallbladder and around tissue are taken down, PV is exposed. Despite not being included in standard lymphadenectomy definition, all fat and fascia surrounding HA and PV (group 12a and 12p) are practically taken away. These will be removed en bloc with lymph node group 8a, pancreatic head, bile duct, and duodenum at last dissecting step below. Although anatomical variations have been checked preoperatively, replaced or accessory right hepatic artery running right lateroposterior to CBD and CHD should be found during dissection of tissue surrounding PV and HA. Proximal stump of bile duct should be temporarily clamped by a bulldog and distal stump of bile duct should be ligation as well to prevent bile leakage as in Fig. 11. Biliary culture is recommended.

Pancreatic Neck Transection, Uncinate Dissection, and SMV, SMA Separation

Pancreatic neck transection is irreversible step on PD. Hence, it is usually completed when we believe that ability of doing PD is certain. This means SMA is able to separate from the tumor. We can check this by preoperative abdominal CT scan in most cases. However, we will get difficulty in suspicious cases. Actually, sureness is only achieved when we do arterial first approach. Arterial first approach is necessary in case of suspicious invasive SMA. This usually happens with tumors located in uncinate process. This is the reason why authors advise to perform uncinate dissection before pancreatic neck dissection, especially for open surgery.

For uncinate dissection, Treitz ligament is divided to give advantages for retractor duodenum and small bowel right laterally. Small venous branches draining to first jejunal vein and inferior pancreatoduodenal vein are ligation to free SMV. Clip and energic devices such as thunder beat and harmonic scalpel show effectively. First jejunal vein which curves posteromedially from the right side of SMV to course then posterior to SMA is usually protected. With our experience, if the ability of resection is almost certain, uncinate dissection will become easier and more advantageous after pancreatic neck transection.

Regarding pancreatic neck transection, tunnel under pancreatic neck which is created partly at the above steps is continued to complete. One tape is passed through this tunnel to lift pancreatic neck as transecting. After that pancreatic neck is transected at the level of SMV—PV.

Continue ligation of small branches draining to SMV and PV, usually from 3–5, to free completely SMV and PV as well. Then, SMV and PV are retracted left laterally to facilitate exposure of SMA wherein inferior pancreatic duodenal and first jejunal arteries are found. Inferior pancreatic duodenal artery (IPDA) may be divided in this step (Fig. 12) while first jejunal artery is usually protected. However, lymph nodes at origin of the latter should be harvested (Fig. 13) showing SMV and SMA separation.

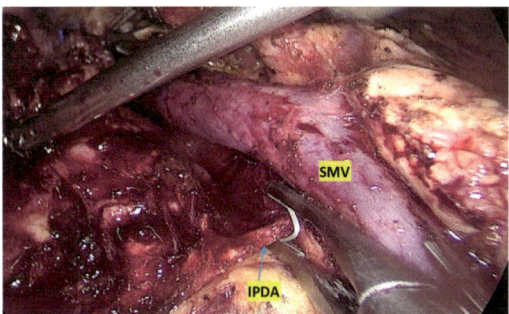

Fig. 12 Ligation of IPDA

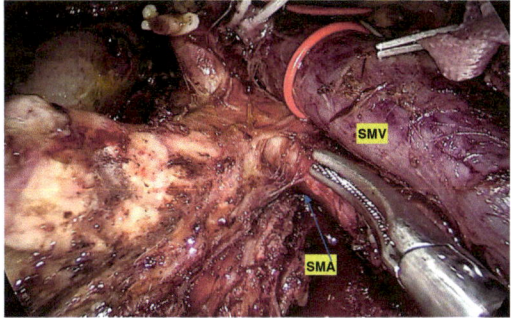

Fig. 13 SMV, SMA separation

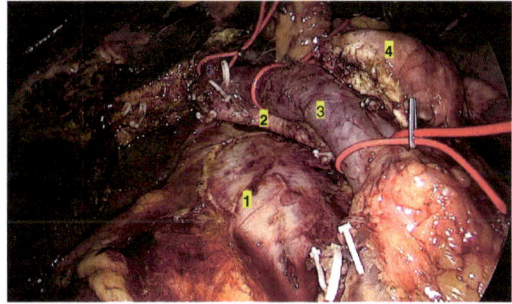

Fig. 14 After specimen removal in case of replaced RHA delivering from SMA (1: IV, 2: SMA, 3: SMV, 4: pancreas, 5: replaced RHA)

Jejunal Transection and Specimen Removal

Jejunum is transected by a stapler about 10 cm from Treitz flexure. Mesentery of proximal small bowel and connective tissue at the right side of SMA including lymph node group 14a and 14b are divided from SMA en bloc. Thus, the dissection phase is completed (Fig. 14).

Reconstruction Phase

Pancreatoenteric Reconstruction

At present, there is a range of procedures to do pancreatoenteric anastomosis. They are typically grouped into three main types with similar characteristics each. They are pancreaticogastrostomy, duct to mucosa pancreatojejunostomy (with or without parenchymal sutures), and invaginating pancreatojejunostomy. Although they are studied extensively, no kind is offered clearly superior to others in terms of improved outcomes [4–13]. Our team is in favor of end-to-side, two layers duct to mucosa pancreatojejunostomy.

Firstly, residual stump of jejunum is passed through transverse mesocolon where Treitz's ligament is divided. It is brought and placed close to pancreatic remnant. The latter is dissected to free approximately 1 cm from cut edge. Slowly absorbable suture monofilaments or bar sutures with 4.0 size are used for posterior parenchymal layer with continuous stitches. Next step is to open a hole at intestinal wall. Diameter of hole is equal to that of pancreatic duct. Then duct to mucosa suture is performed by interrupted stitches with absorbable suture (such as PDS) 4.0 or 5.0. We usually use an internal stent (Fig. 15) to ensure duct to mucosa pancreatojejunostomy working better and to prevent obstruction as well. Suturing to close anterior pancreatic parenchyma and jejunum is similar to posterior layer. Suction and irritation around pancreatic anastomosis are performed carefully. This will be repeated once after completing hepaticojejunostomy to prepare for collecting fluid around pancreatic anastomosis. This fluid will be exam-

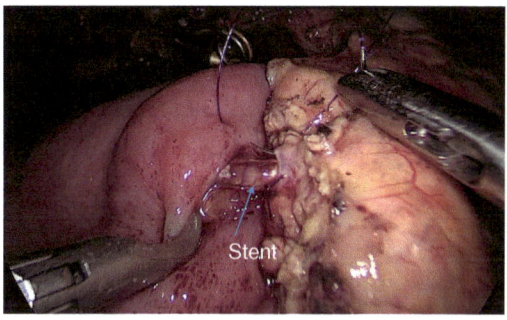

Fig. 15 Pancreaticojejunostomy with internal stent

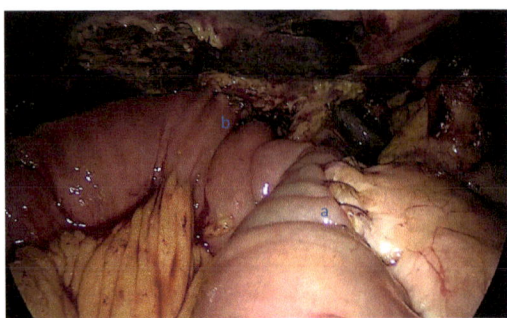

Fig. 16 Completed pancreaticojejunostomy (**a**) and hepaticojejunostomy (**b**)

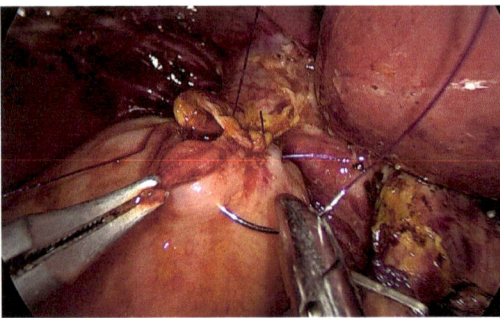

Fig. 17 End-to-side hepaticojejunostomy

ined for amylase concentration which can be used to evaluate the risk of postoperative pancreatic fistula. In the condition of unfound pancreatic duct due to very small size, we do pancreatojejunostomy like above procedure with only parenchymal layer and bigger opening on jejunum.

Hepaticojejunal Reconstruction

All three anastomoses including pancreatojejunostomy, hepaticojejunostomy, and enteroenteric anastomosis are performed with the same loop of jejunum (Fig. 17). End-to-side anastomosis is used for hepaticojejunostomy (Fig. 16). We prefer 4.0 or 5.0 absorbable sutures for this step. Continuous suture is used for both posterior and anterior half of hepatic duct's circumference if its diameter is upward of 5 mm. In contrast, if hepatic duct is less than 5 mm, we usually use interrupted suture. Important attention must be paid in this step to find the distance between pancreatic and hepatic duct anastomoses. This is not too long to avoid obstruction due to bending. Biliary stent is unnecessary. Authors routinely

stay jejunal limb to hilar plate to minimize tension of hepaticojejunostomy.

Enteroenteric Reconstruction

Duodenojejunostomy or gastrojejunostomy is technically easier than pancreatic and hepatic duct anastomoses. Hence, it is not difficult to do the former with totally laparoscopic surgery. However, expanding the incision of trocar to remove specimen (Fig. 18) is inevitable. Authors do it extracorporeally to save time instead.

Finally, checking for coagulation, bile leakage, gauze removal, and fluid clearance are completed. Drains are placed anterior pancreatic anastomosis and hepaticojejunostomy as well. Abdominal fascia defects and skin incisions are closed.

Complications and Management

Laparoscopic pancreaticoduodenectomy is a major surgery. When doing LPD, there will be common morbidities like other major surgery but the complication rate of LPD is higher. Moreover, there are complications only related to pancreatic resection. These can affect severely patients' health and lead to mortality [14]. Typically, there are three proper complications after doing PD such as pancreatic fistula (POPF), bleeding, and delayed gastric empty. Among them, POPF and bleeding have still been big problems [14, 15].

Postoperative Pancreatic Fistula

Postoperative pancreatic fistula (POPF) after LPD was reported at approximately 20% on average [14, 15]. POPF is defined and classified belong to the International Study Group for Pancreatic Surgery (ISGPS) 2016 [16]. There are different clinical conditions from asymptomatic to life-threatening patients. It may lead to further complications as inadequate management, for example, abdominal abscess, internal bleeding, wound infection, sepsis, and mortality.

The important key to treat POPF is to recognize this problem early and to prevent life-threatening sequela of this. An abdominal contrast-enhanced CT scan is necessary to assess

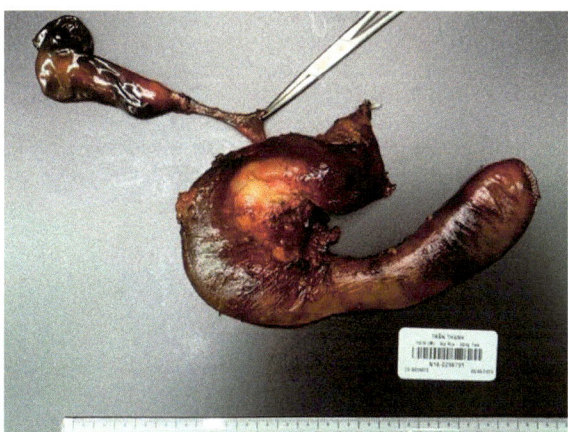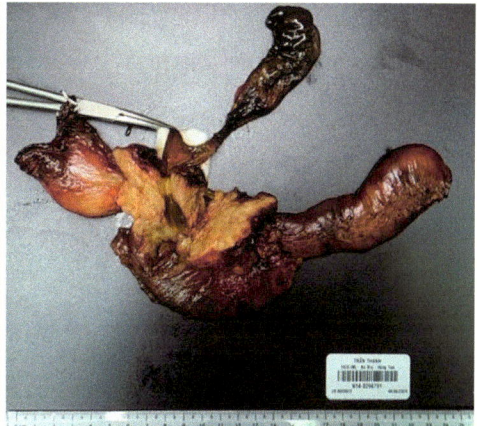

Fig. 18 Specimen

pancreatic anastomosis, fluid collections, signs of infected fluids, and intra-abdominal abscess.

Enteral nutrition is demonstrated to associate with higher rate of spontaneous fistula closure than parenteral nutrition in POPF patients. In pancreatojejunostomy where anastomosis is isolated from alimentary tract, oral diet is recommended although fistula is occurring.

Most POPF cases with stable clinical signs are treated by nonreoperation. The drains bringing well intra-abdominal fluids are remained and observed carefully. In case of fluid collection or intra-abdominal abscess, percutaneous or endoscopic ultrasonographic intervention is recommended.

Reoperation is indicated for sepsis shock, preventing sepsis or septic shock. Another indication of surgery is infected collection that requires lavage. Choice of open or laparoscopic surgery as reoperation depends on certain situation and surgeon's experience.

Bleeding

According to ISGPS [17], definition of hemorrhage after PD, called post-pancreatectomy hemorrhage (PPH), is based on three criteria: onset, location, and severity. Regard onset, hemorrhage is defined as early and late PPH happening in less or more than 24 h, respectively. Turning to location, PPH is defined intraluminal (intra-enteric) and extraluminal (extra-enteric). Finally, we have mild and severe PPH. Based on

these criteria, PPH is classified into grade A, grade B, and grade C.

Being similar to POPF, PPH in patients who remain clinically stable is treated by angiographic intervention. Reoperation is needed for catastrophic hemorrhage that requires rapid gaining of hemostasis.

Summary

PD can be done feasibly by totally laparoscopic surgery. It includes dissection phase and reconstruction phase. However, this is a technically difficult procedure. Both require surgeons with advanced laparoscopic skills and experience in pancreatic surgery. Although outcomes are significantly improved in recent years, the complication rate is still high and management is still difficult.

References

1. Whipple AO, Parsons WB, Mullins CR. TREATMENT OF CARCINOMA OF THE AMPULLA OF VATER. Ann Surg. 1935;102(4):763–79.
2. Gagner M, Pomp A. Laparoscopic pylorus-preserving pancreatoduodenectomy. Surg Endosc. 1994;8(5):408–10.
3. Tol JA, Gouma DJ, Bassi C, Dervenis C, Montorsi M, Adham M, et al. Definition of a standard lymphadenectomy in surgery for pancreatic ductal adenocarcinoma: a consensus statement by the international

study group on pancreatic surgery (ISGPS). Surgery. 2014;156(3):591–600.

4. Bassi C, Falconi M, Molinari E, Mantovani W, Butturini G, Gumbs AA, et al. Duct-to-mucosa versus end-to-side pancreaticojejunostomy reconstruction after pancreaticoduodenectomy: results of a prospective randomized trial. Surgery. 2003;134(5):766–71.

5. Berger AC, Howard TJ, Kennedy EP, Sauter PK, Bower-Cherry M, Dutkevitch S, et al. Does type of pancreaticojejunostomy after pancreaticoduodenectomy decrease rate of pancreatic fistula? A randomized, prospective, dual-institution trial. J Am Coll Surg. 2009;208(5):738–47. discussion 47–9

6. Clerveus M, Morandeira-Rivas A, Picazo-Yeste J, Moreno-Sanz C. Pancreaticogastrostomy versus pancreaticojejunostomy after pancreaticoduodenectomy: a systematic review and meta-analysis of randomized controlled trials. J Gastrointest Surg. 2014;18(9):1693–704.

7. El Nakeeb A, El Hemaly M, Askr W, Abd Ellatif M, Hamed H, Elghawalby A, et al. Comparative study between duct to mucosa and invagination pancreaticojejunostomy after pancreaticoduodenectomy: a prospective randomized study. Int J Surg (London, England). 2015;16(Pt A):1–6.

8. Hallet J, Zih FS, Deobald RG, Scheer AS, Law CH, Coburn NG, et al. The impact of pancreaticojejunostomy versus pancreaticogastrostomy reconstruction on pancreatic fistula after pancreaticoduodenectomy: meta-analysis of randomized controlled trials. HPB. 2015;17(2):113–22.

9. Hua J, He Z, Qian D, Meng H, Zhou B, Song Z. Duct-to-mucosa versus invagination Pancreaticojejunostomy following Pancreaticoduodenectomy: a systematic review and meta-analysis. J Gastrointest Surg. 2015;19(10):1900–9.

10. Keck T, Wellner UF, Bahra M, Klein F, Sick O, Niedergethmann M, et al. Pancreatogastrostomy versus pancreatojejunostomy for RECOnstruction after PANCreatoduodenectomy (RECOPANC, DRKS 00000767): perioperative and long-term results of a multicenter randomized controlled trial. Ann Surg. 2016;263(3):440–9.

11. Liu FB, Chen JM, Geng W, Xie SX, Zhao YJ, Yu LQ, et al. Pancreaticogastrostomy is associated with significantly less pancreatic fistula than pancreaticojejunostomy reconstruction after pancreaticoduodenectomy: a meta-analysis of seven randomized controlled trials. HP. 2015;17(2):123–30.

12. Menahem B, Guittet L, Mulliri A, Alves A, Lubrano J. Pancreaticogastrostomy is superior to pancreaticojejunostomy for prevention of pancreatic fistula after pancreaticoduodenectomy: an updated meta-analysis of randomized controlled trials. Ann Surg. 2015;261(5):882–7.

13. Xiong JJ, Tan CL, Szatmary P, Huang W, Ke NW, Hu WM, et al. Meta-analysis of pancreaticogastrostomy versus pancreaticojejunostomy after pancreaticoduodenectomy. Br J Surg. 2014;101(10):1196–208.

14. Liao CH, Wu YT, Liu YY, Wang SY, Kang SC, Yeh CN, et al. Systemic review of the feasibility and advantage of minimally invasive Pancreaticoduodenectomy. World J Surg. 2016;40(5):1218–25.

15. Chen K, Liu XL, Pan Y, Maher H, Wang XF. Expanding laparoscopic pancreaticoduodenectomy to pancreatic-head and periampullary malignancy: major findings based on systematic review and meta-analysis. BMC Gastroenterol. 2018;18(1):102.

16. Pulvirenti A, Ramera M, Bassi C. Modifications in the international study Group for Pancreatic Surgery (ISGPS) definition of postoperative pancreatic fistula. Trans Gastroenterol Hepatol. 2017;2(12):107.

17. Wente MN, Veit JA, Bassi C, Dervenis C, Fingerhut A, Gouma DJ, et al. Postpancreatectomy hemorrhage (PPH)–an international study Group of Pancreatic Surgery (ISGPS) definition. Surgery. 2007;142(1):20–5.

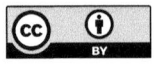

Laparoscopic Splenectomy

Marilou B. Fuentes and Davide Lomanto

Laparoscopic splenectomy has gained popularity as an option for patients having benign and malignant diseases as well as for trauma patients who are stable. Studies have shown that this procedure is prone to bleeding but with advanced technology and good anatomical knowledge of vasculature, the procedure is not only feasible but can be performed safely. Poulin who did the first laparoscopic partial splenectomy for ruptured spleen in 1995 proved it was possible. The inherent abundant blood supply and proximity of spleen to vital organs make it prone to 5–60% complication during its dissection, and hence utmost care and skills are needed during surgery [1].

Indications [2]

1. Benign hematologic diseases—mostly children.
2. Malignant hematologic diseases.
3. Splenic Cyst.
4. **Trauma**—a preoperative Computed Tomography (CT) scan is essential to assess the grade of splenic injury and to confirm that there is no multiple organ injury that would entail a need for laparotomy. Vital signs should be stable with a BP > 90/60 mmHg and HR <120 bpm [3]. Failure rate for conservative management of splenic injury ranges from 10 to 40% [4].

Contraindications [5, 6]

1. Portal hypertension secondary to liver cirrhosis.
2. Patient who cannot tolerate general anesthesia.
3. Coagulopathy.

Pre-OP Assessment and Management

1. CT scan with vascular reconstruction: Spleen size and volume (maximum diameter) [2, 5].
2. Triple Vaccination (Hemophilus influenza, Pneumococcus pneumonia, and Meningococcus): 15 days prior to scheduled surgery or 10 days after emergency surgery.
3. Prophylactic antibiotic upon induction of anesthesia and continued postoperatively for at least 24 hours.
4. Low-dose subcutaneous unfractionated heparin prophylaxis.

M. B. Fuentes (✉)
Department of Surgery, The Medical City, Pasig, Philippines

D. Lomanto
Department of Surgery, YLL School of Medicine, National University Singapore, Singapore, Singapore

© The Author(s) 2023
D. Lomanto et al. (eds.), *Mastering Endo-Laparoscopic and Thoracoscopic Surgery*,
https://doi.org/10.1007/978-981-19-3755-2_53

OT Setup

Instruments

Trocars: 12 mm, 10 mm, and two 5 mm
30° endoscope
Electrosurgical devices: electrothermal bipolar,
  advanced energy devices (ultrasonic shears,
  advanced bipolar)
Stapler or Clips
Specimen retrieval bag

Position

Patient in right lateral decubitus position.

Port Placement Fig. 1

Optical port:12 mm at umbilical area, 3–4 cm to
the left superiorly.

Second 10 mm at left anterior axillary line
below the costal margin or on or below the lower
edge of palpable spleen.

Working ports: Two 5 mm in the epigastric
(exposing hilum) and along midclavicular line
(retracting spleen) [7, 8].

Surgical Technique

It is best to do diagnostic laparoscopy to look for
an accessory spleen which is common in 10–30%
of the population. Failure to do so may lead to
recurrent or persistent thrombocytopenia. 75% of
accessory spleens are located at the splenic
hilum, 20% at the tail of the pancreas, and the
remaining 5% at the gastrosplenic, wall of the
stomach and intestines, greater omentum, mesentery, and pelvic area [9].

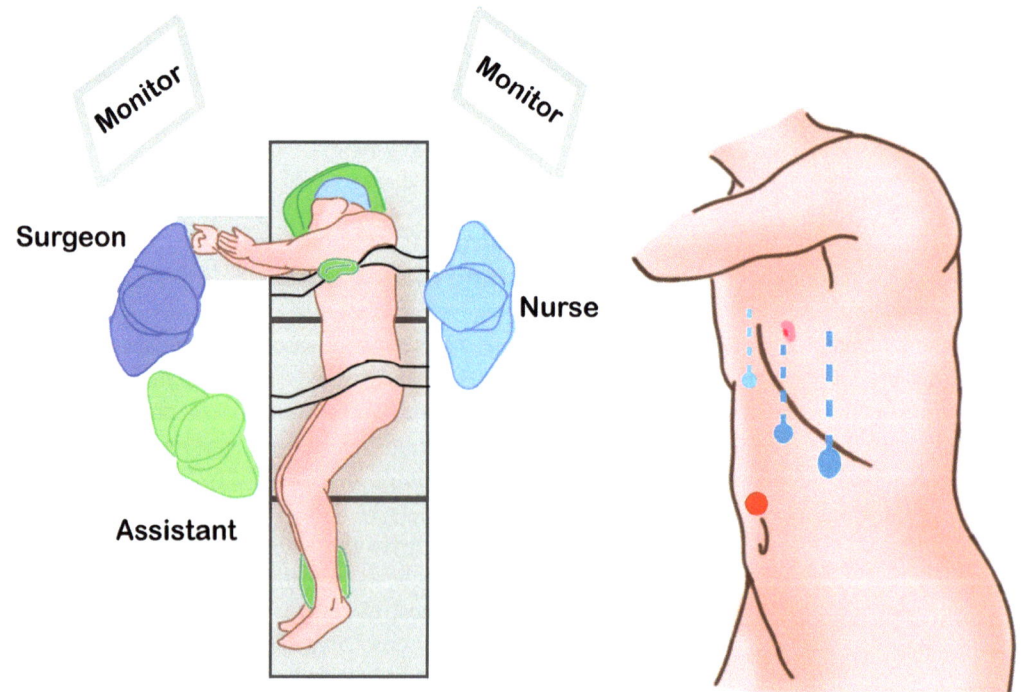

Fig. 1 Port placement: (1) umbilical area, (2) anterior axillary line, (3) midclavicular line, (4) epigastric

Approach

(a) *Anterior approach* has the advantage of having a direct view of the spleen just like what is seen in doing open splenectomy. The downside of this approach is poor visualization of hilum that may lead to vessel injury and bleeding [2, 6]. In this technique, spleen is exposed by downward traction of colon and medial retraction of the greater curvature of the stomach. The lesser sac is entered through the gastrocolic ligament (Fig. 2). The left gastroepiploic and short gastric vessels are divided to completely separate stomach and spleen and subsequent access and clipping of splenic vessels (Fig. 3) [6].

(b) *Posterolateral approach* has better visualization and access to vessels, the pancreas, and accessory spleen. This approach facilitates complete mobilization of the spleen by using gravity as a retractor [2, 6, 8]. The splenorenal and splenocolic ligaments are divided followed by dissection of the hilum, approaching it from the lower pole going to the upper pole (Fig. 4) [6].

Parenchymal Resection

(a) *Total Splenectomy* is indicated for centrally located, multifocal tumors and malignancy [7]. The drawback of infection and vascular

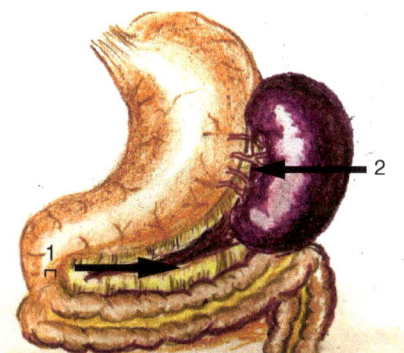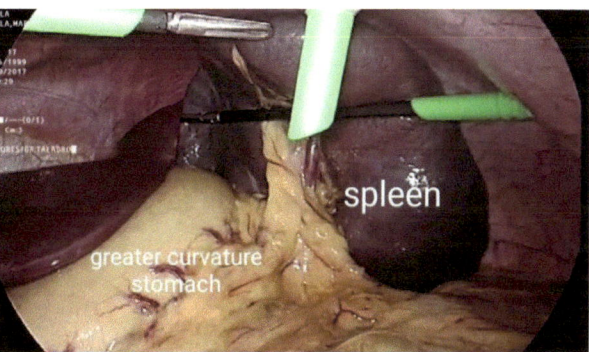

1.Open the lesser sac.
2.Short gastric vessels divided.

Fig. 2 (1) Open the lesser sac. (2) Short gastric vessels divided

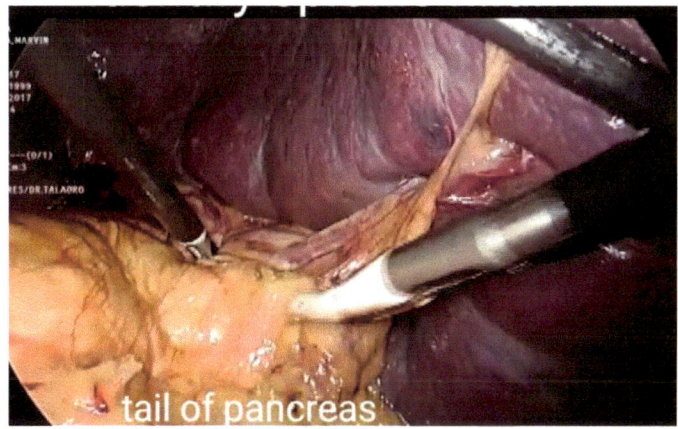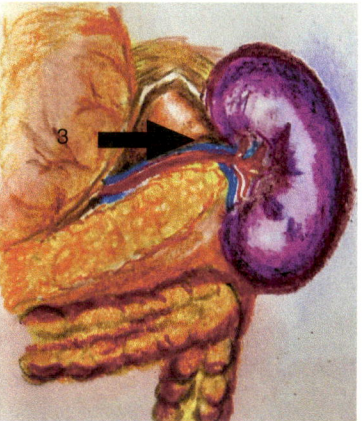

3.Access to splenic vessels

Fig. 3 (3) Access to splenic vessels

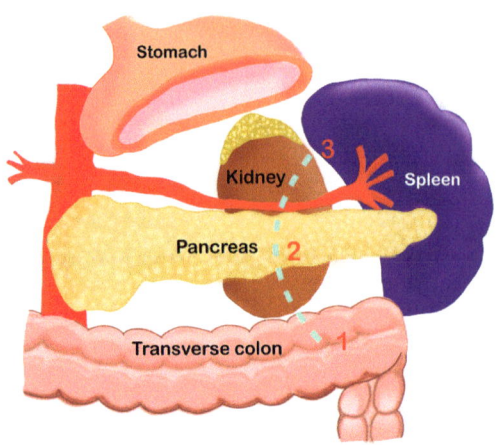

Fig. 4 Divide the *splenocolic* and *splenorenal* ligaments to expose the hilum. Dissection of the *hilum*. Free from lateral attachments

complications like thrombosis are noted in studies.

(b) *Partial splenectomy*: With the latest tools that are readily available and modifications of technique for improved visibility of structures, partial splenectomy with the removal of the lesion and preservation of function is now considered an option for treatment. The upper pole is often preserved for systemic disease because it is difficult to free from diaphragm as compared to dissecting the lower pole from splenic colon flexure.[20] This procedure makes use of selective devascularization of the splenic vessels and resection along or 1 cm inside the ischemic line to prevent bleeding [10, 11].

Spleen Remnant Size: 25–30% preserved spleen parenchyma allows good immunologic response [3, 5]. Studies done by Vasilescu et al. show that a mean volume of 41.4 cm³ is enough to preserve the spleen's immunologic function, while Stoher et al. noted it to be at 10 cm³ [10].

Vessel Dissection

(a) *Vessel first*: The main trunks of splenic artery and vein are identified at the pancreatic tail

and is the technique commonly used for large splenic vessels [12].

(b) *Hilar Transection*: The entire splenic hilum is transected as close as possible to the spleen and makes operative time shorter as compared to vessel first approach [12].

Complications, Prevention, and Management

Intraoperative Complications [2]

(a) *Bleeding* secondary to injury of the hilar vessels or splenic capsule. Studies showed that male sex and spleen measuring >19 cm by ultrasound are independent risk factors for intraoperative bleeding [13]. Importance of crucial exposure, knowledge of variations in anatomy, and careful dissection of structures are the initial step to prevention of bleeding. In the eventuality of bleeding from parenchyma, one can apply pressure/packing the area first, while bleeding from hilar vessels can be managed by clamping/grasping the vessel by a grasper and applying clips to bleeding vessel. When using stapler at the hilum, pedicle should be cleared and the stapler fired under direct vision. Splenic artery can be clipped to reduce the splenic size and make the spleen soft for easier extraction [1, 2].

(b) *Organ injury*: Chand et al. observed a 15% *pancreatic injury r*esulting in *pancreatic fistula*. Identification of pancreatic tail and dissecting it away from the hilum avoids this complication. *Bowel injury*, as well as *diaphragmatic injury*, can happen during mobilization of spleen, it is important that these complications are recognized and addressed intraoperatively [1, 2, 10].

Postoperative Complications

(a) *Postoperative hemorrhage* may occur at the splenic vessels at the tail of the pancreas, short gastric vessels, or trocar sites presenting as tachycardia, hypotension, decreasing hemoglobin with abdominal distension. Rapid resuscitation should be done for hemo-dynamically unstable patients followed by exploratory laparotomy for control of bleed-ers. If the patient is stable, may opt to do laparoscopy for control of bleeders [1].

(b) *Infection: Subphrenic abscess* is a known complication yet is difficult to diagnose resulting in a delay in management. Patients will usually present with intermittent fever, a chest X-ray may show pleural effusion, raised diaphragm, or basal atelectasis. An abdominal CT scan is essential for identifi-cation and as a guide to percutaneous drain-age. This complication can be avoided by meticulous hemostasis and suctioning of fluid prior to closure [1]. *Pancreatitis* is also a possibility when there is excessive manip-ulation or devascularization of the gland. *Overwhelming Post-Splenectomy Infection is seen in* 4.4% of cases with a 50–80% mor-tality rate, more common in children and more fatal after splenectomy for hemato-logic disorders. Immunization with pneu-mococcal vaccine 2 weeks before the scheduled surgery is the standard of care and for children younger than 5 year old who will undergo splenectomy, pediatricians advise a daily dose of penicillin until they reach the age of 10 [1, 14].

(c) *Vascular*: Splenic vein thrombosis can be encountered in 20% of patients who had splenectomy. his is associated with vague abdominal pain and can be documented using an ultrasound or CT scan. Routine postoperative ultrasound identifies 6.3–10% thrombosed portal vein (TPV). The risk of developing TPV is noted to be at 10–50% in patients who had laparoscopic splenectomy for myeloproliferative disorder, hemolytic anemia, and thalassemia. To prevent this complication, it is advised that splenic vein should be ligated as close as possible to the mesentery, routine postoperative ultrasound for high-risk patients. Once detected, the patient should receive systemic anticoagula-tion immediately as >90% will have recana-lization of the acutely thrombosed portal or mesentery vein.

(d) *Respiratory*: pneumonia and atelectasis.

(e) *Ileus*.

(f) *Hernia*: Port site hernias usually develop for incisions larger than 10 mm, which can be pre-vented by meticulous suturing of fascia [1].

Post-Op Care [7]

1. Splenic/Portal vein thrombosis—ultrasound screening on seventh postoperative day.

2. Antibiotic prophylaxis—oral Penicillin for 2 years after surgery but for a lifetime for immunosuppressed patients [15].

3. For ITP patients, platelet count evaluation is done 1 month after surgery as *Complete response* (platelet 100,000/mm^3 without sple-nectomy treatment), *Partial response* (platelet levels 30,000/mm^3, 100,000/mm^3 or at least twice the basal level), and *Complete unre-sponsiveness* (platelet below 30,000/mm^3 or twofold below basal level) [16].

4. Vaccination for patients who had emergency splenectomy is done 14 days after the proce-dure. However, for patients with poor follow-up, it is best to give the vaccination prior to discharge.

References

1. Bhandarkar D, Katara A, et al. Prevention and Management of Complications of laparoscopic sple-nectomy. Indian J Surg. 2011;73(5):324–30. https://doi.org/10.1007/s12262-011-0331-5.

2. Misiakos E, Bagias G, et al. Laparoscopic splenec-tomy: current concepts. World J Gastrointest Endosc. 2017;9(9):428–37. https://doi.org/10.4253/wjge.v9.i9.428.

3. Li H, Wei Y, et al. Feasibility and safety of emer-gency laparoscopic partial splenectomy. Medicine. 2017;96(16):e6450. https://doi.org/10.1097/MD.0000000000006450.

4. Prasad A, Agarwal N. Laparoscopic splenec-tomy in a case of blunt abdominal trauma. J Minim Access Surg. 2009;5(3):78–81. https://doi.org/10.4103/0972-9941.58503.

5. Somasundaram SK, Massey L, et al. Laparoscopic splenectomy is emerging 'gold standard' treatment even for massive spleens. Ann R Coll Surg Engl. 2015;97(5):345–8. https://doi.org/10.1308/0035884 14X14055925060479.

6. Garzi A, Ardimento G, et al. Laparoscopic splenectomy: Postero-lateral approach. Transl Med UniSa. 2019;20(3):9–12.

7. de la Villeon B, Le Bian A, et al. Laparoscopic partial splenectomy: a technical tip. Surg Endosc. 2014;29(1):94–9. https://doi.org/10.1007/s00464-014-3638-z.

8. Ji B, Wang Y, et al. Anterior versus posterolateral approach for Total laparoscopic splenectomy: comparative study. Int J. Med. Sci. 2013;10(3):222–9. https://doi.org/10.7150/ijms.5373.

9. Bajwa SA, Kasi A. Anatomy, abdomen and pelvis, accessory spleen. Treasure Island (FL): StatPearls Publishing; 2020.

10. Costi R, Ruiz C, et al. Partial splenectomy: who, when and how. A systematic review of the 2130 published cases. Journal of Pediatric Surgery. 2019;54(8):1527–38.

11. Esposito F, Noviello A, et al. Partial splenectomy: a case series and systematic review of literature. Ann Hepatobiliary Pancreat Surg. 2018;22(2):116–27.

12. Radkowiak D, Zychowicz A, et al. Quiet for optimal technique of laparoscopic splenectomy–vessel first or hilar transection? Videosurgery Miniinv. 2018;13(4):460–8. https://doi.org/10.5114/wiitm.2018.76071.

13. Wysocki M, Radkowiak D, et al. Prediction of technical difficulties in laparoscopic splenectomy and analysis of risk factors for postoperative complications in 468 cases. J. Clin. Med. 2018;7(12):547. https://doi.org/10.3390/jcm7120547.

14. Liu G, Fan Y. Feasibility and safety of laparoscopic partial splenectomy: a systematic review. World J Surg. 2019;43(6):1505–18. https://doi.org/10.1007/s00268-019-04946-8.

15. Leone G, Pizzigallo E. Bacterial infections following splenectomy for malignant and nonmalignant hematologic diseases. Mediterr J Hematol Infect Dis. 2015;7(1):e2015057. https://doi.org/10.4084/MJHID.2015.057.

16. Turkoglu A, Oguz A, et al. Laparoscopic splenectomy: clip ligation or en-bloc stapling? Turk J Surg. 2019;35(4):273–7.

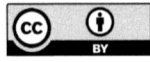

Intraoperative Splenic Injuries

Henry Chua and Vincent Matthew Roble II

Introduction

Intraoperative splenic injuries can occur in any abdominal surgical procedure. Reports range from vascular surgeons performing abdominal aortic aneurysm repairs to thoracic surgeons performing Nissen fundoplication to urologists performing radical nephrectomies [1]. Injury to the spleen during laparoscopic urological surgery has a reported incidence of 0.25% [2]. The reported incidence of splenic injury resulting in splenectomy during colonic surgery is 1.2–8%. The highest percentage of all incidental splenectomies are due to colonic surgeries, primarily to a large number of these operations and the close proximity between the colonic splenic flexure and the spleen [3]. Injuries to the spleen during laparoscopic adrenalectomy may be either access-related or caused by powerful retraction and handling of the organ [4].

Splenic injury may occur as a result of two etiologies. The first is due to traction injuries from excessive retraction of the spleen, resulting in a capsular tear or laceration. This is attributable to inadequate release of the ligamentous attachment of the spleen to surrounding structures. The second etiology is due to trauma from the instruments used during surgery.

Up to 40% of all splenectomies are performed for iatrogenic injury. The risk of splenic injury is highest during left hemicolectomy (1–8%), open antireflux procedures (3–20%), left nephrectomy (4–13%), and during exposure and reconstruction of the proximal abdominal aorta and its branches (21–60%). Splenic injury results in prolonged operating time, increased blood loss, and longer hospital stay. It is also associated with a two to tenfold increase in infection rate and up to a doubling of morbidity rates. Mortality rates are also reported to be higher in patients undergoing splenectomy for iatrogenic injury [5].

When splenic injury occurs intraoperatively, the surgeon is faced with the dilemma of whether to perform immediate splenectomy or treat the injury conservatively. The spleen is instrumental in immunity, especially with regards to encapsulated organisms. Splenectomy decreases resistance to certain infectious etiologies, necessitating prophylactic immunization. However, conservative treatment of a splenic laceration can be quite problematic owing to the friable and unforgiving nature of the splenic parenchyma, which may result in delayed hemorrhage and eventual splenectomy [2].

Management

The majority of splenic and liver injuries during laparoscopic surgery are minor capsular lesions which usually can be managed laparoscopically

H. Chua (✉) · V. M. Roble II
Advanced Minimally Invasive Surgery, Cebu
Doctors' University Hospital, Cebu, Philippines

© The Author(s) 2023
D. Lomanto et al. (eds.), *Mastering Endo-Laparoscopic and Thoracoscopic Surgery*,
https://doi.org/10.1007/978-981-19-3755-2_54

[6]. Splenic injuries that are dealt with conservatively will require multiple definitive hemostatic measures, and direct pressure alone is unlikely to provide durable success [2]. These injuries are typically sufficiently controlled with the combination of pressure and application of oxidized regenerated cellulose (Surgicel), absorbable gelatin sponges (Gelfoam), and fibrin glue (Tissucol) [4].

In a study by Coln et al., Gelfoam was the least effective in achieving hemostasis. It was also the least satisfactory agent studied from a convenience standpoint. Surgicel was much easier to use than Gelfoam and appeared to achieve faster hemostasis. Surgicel adhered well when applied to the lacerated surface and occasionally needed a second layer before hemostasis was achieved [7].

The use of fibrin sealants for rapid and definitive hemostasis for splenic injuries was described by Canby-Hagino et al. Fibrin sealant achieved adequate immediate hemostasis and each patient recovered without further splenic bleeding. It is simple to use in the open and laparoscopic approaches [8].

The use of gelatin thrombin granules (FloSeal), argon beam coagulator, and Surgicel was described by Chung et al. FloSeal consists of a gelatin matrix and a Thrombin component, which are mixed together before use. Cross-linked gelatin granules in the matrix swell approximately 20% on contact with blood or bodily fluids, slowing blood flow. The coagulation cascade is activated by the thrombin component to form a firm hemostatic plug. These two processes combine to effect hemostasis by tamponade [9]. Argon beam coagulator delivers radiofrequency electrical energy to tissue across a jet of argon gas, providing noncontact, monopolar, electrothermal hemostasis [10]. After evaluation of the extent of injury, Surgicel is initially placed on the injured area to provide hemostasis. If bleeding does not stop with the first application of Surgicel. Immediate coagulation of the area with the argon beam coagulator with application of FloSeal and additional Surgicel is done at the completion of every case, pneumoperitoneum is evacuated for 5 min and the site is reinspected to ensure perfect hemostasis. General surgery consultation is obtained if the bleeding does not stop with the application of argon beam, FloSeal, and Surgicel, or if the bleeding recurs after the 5 min pneumoperitoneum evacuation trial period. Laparoscopic splenectomy may be required in difficult situations (Fig. 1) [2]. More extensive lacerations to the spleen may warrant open conversion.

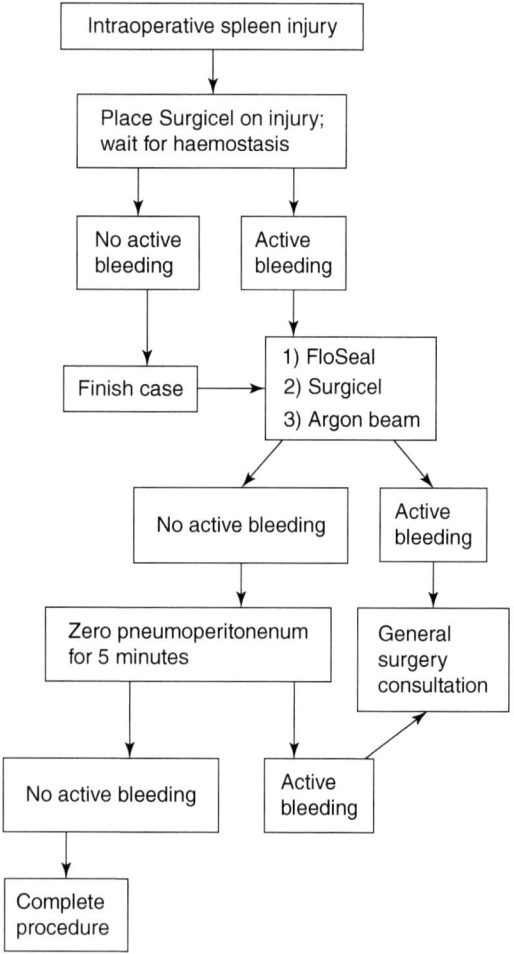

Fig. 1 Algorithm for optimal treatment of intraoperative splenic injury [2]

References

1. Holubar S. Splenic salvage after intraoperative splenic injury during colectomy. Arch Surg. 2009;144(11):1040–5.
2. Chung B, Desai MM, Gill IS. Management of intraoperative splenic injury during laparoscopic urological surgery. BJU Int. 2011;108(4):572–6.
3. Langevin J, Rothenberger D, Goldberg S. Accidental splenic injury during surgical treatment of the colon and rectum. Surg Gynecol Obstet. 1984;159(2):139–44.
4. Strebel R, Muntener M, Sulser T. Intraoperative complications of laparoscopic adrenalectomy. J Urol. 2008;26(6):555–60.
5. Cassar K, Munro A. Iatrogenic splenic injury. J R Collab Surg Edinb. 2002;47(6):731–41.
6. Hedican S. Complications of hand-assisted laparoscopic urologic surgery. J Endourol. 2004;18(4):387–96.
7. Coln D. Evaluation of hemostatic agents in experimental splenic lacerations. Am J Surg. 1983;145(2):145:256.
8. Canby-Hagino E, Morey A, Jatoi I, Perahia B, Bishoff J. Fibin sealant treatment of splenic injury during open and laparoscopic left radical nephrectomy. J Urol. 2000;164(6):2004–5.
9. Stacey MJ, Rampaul RS, et al. Use of FloSeal matrix hemostatic agent in partial splenectomy after penetrating trauma. J Trauma. 2008;64(2):507–8.
10. Go PM, Goodman GR, et al. The argon beam coagulator provides rapid hemostasis of experimental hepatic and splenic hemorrhage in anticoagulated dogs. J Trauma. 1991;31(9):1294–300.

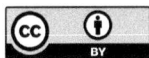

Transabdominal Pre-peritoneal Approach (TAPP)

Sajid Malik and Sujith Wijerathne

Introduction

History of inguinal hernia is as old as history of surgery itself. Bassini in 1887 published his original description of inguinal hernia repair with a later modification to Shouldice repair in 1945. Two real revolutions which have changed the hernia repair completely are the Lichtenstein "tensionless" mesh repair in 1989 and the introduction of laparoscopic surgery to hernia repair in the early 1990s [1].

Shortly afterward, surgeons have not only published their early experiences on laparoscopic intraperitoneal mesh (IPOM) (Fig. 1) repair of inguinal hernia but also described two major modifications to it—the transabdominal pre-peritoneal repair (TAPP) and the totally extra-peritoneal (TEP) repair. Such is the practice of modern science at a brisk pace [2].

Transabdominal Pre-Peritoneal (TAPP) repair, as compared to its counterpart TEP, provides easy learning in correlation to peritoneal and pre-peritoneal anatomy. This technique involves a diagnostic laparoscopy followed by an incision on peritoneum, careful blunt dissection to create

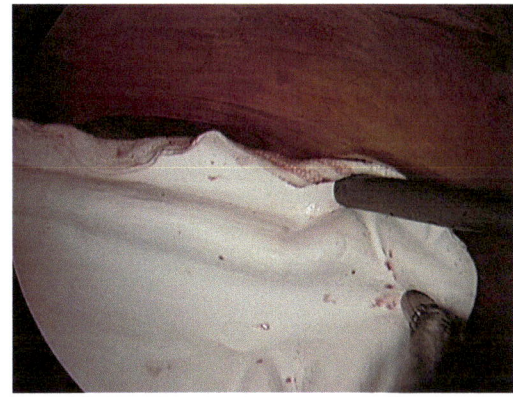

Fig. 1 Laparoscopic IPOM for inguinal hernia

peritoneal flap, reduction of hernia sac, placement of mesh, and closure of peritoneal flap again [3, 4].

Indications

- Reducible primary inguinal hernia (Figs. 2 and 3)
- Recurrent inguinal hernia after previous open repair
- Sliding inguinal hernia
- Hernia with adhesions at hernia orifices
- Alternative to difficult TEP

S. Malik (✉)
Department of Surgery, Allama Iqbal Medical College, Jinnah Hospital, Lahore, Pakistan

S. Wijerathne
Department of Surgery, National University Health System, Singapore, Singapore

© The Author(s) 2023
D. Lomanto et al. (eds.), *Mastering Endo-Laparoscopic and Thoracoscopic Surgery*,
https://doi.org/10.1007/978-981-19-3755-2_55

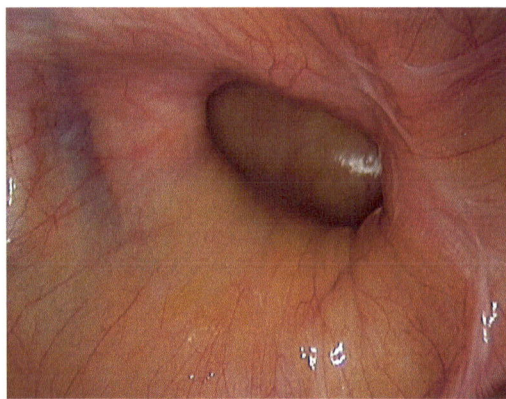

Fig. 2 Right direct inguinal hernia

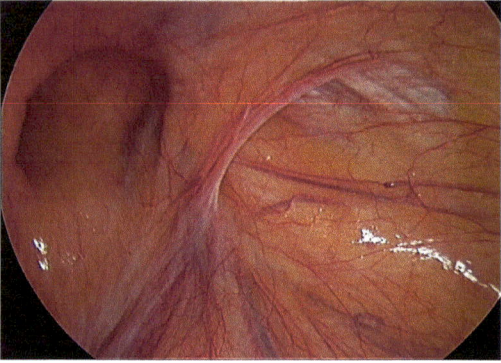

Fig. 3 Left direct inguinal hernia

Contraindications

- Inability to tolerate general anesthesia
- Clotting disorders
- Peritonitis
- Incarceration (relative)
- COPD
- Previous posterior mesh repair (relative)
- Prostatectomy (relative)
- Previous lower midline surgical incision (relative)
- Previous pelvic surgery for TAPP
- Ascites

Preoperative Preparation

- Antibiotic prophylaxis
- Empty bladder for primary unilateral inguinal hernia
- Foley's catheter for bilateral or recurrent inguinal hernia.

Operative Setup, Patient's Position, and Trocars Placement

- Monitor position: Position of monitor should be at patient's foot end, contralateral to surgeon's position. The Surgeon stand on the opposite side of the inguinal Hernia.
- **Instrumentation required**
  - Veress Needle or Hasson's Trocar for access
  - 30° telescope 10 mm
  - Atraumatic Graspers (2) 5 mm
  - Curved Scissors (1) 5 mm
  - Hook diathermy (1) 5 mm
  - Bowel Clamp (1) 5 mm
  - Suction/irrigation device
  - Endostaplers for mesh fixation 5 mm
  - Hemolock Clip applicator (1) 5 mm
  - Endoloop (1) (Optional)
- **Patient's position**
  - Patient should be in supine position with Trendelenburg position 15°
  - Surgeon stands on contralateral side of hernia and assistant stands behind or opposite to surgeon
  - Anesthetist should be reminding of endotracheal tubing positions due to the risk of collision of laparoscope cable with the tube.
- **Trocars size and position (Fig. 4)**
  - 10–12 mm periumbilical trocar
  - 2 × 5 mm cannula are inserted on the right and left flank for a good triangulation

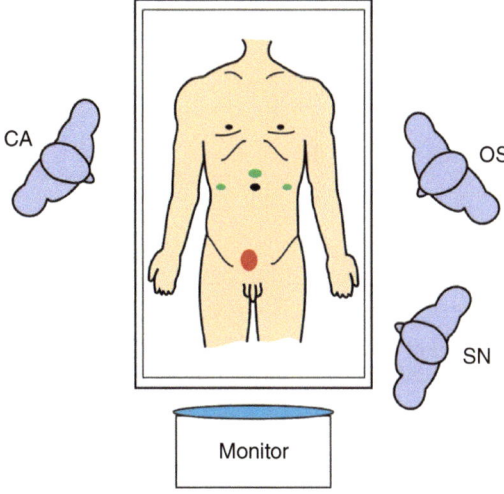

Fig. 4 Patient's and surgical team position; suggested trocars location

Surgical Technique

- General anesthesia with muscle relaxation is administered.
- 1–2 cm infraumbilical incision is made. Peritoneal cavity is entered either by creating the pneumoperitoneum with Veress needle or using open technique by Hasson' Trocar. Pneumoperitoneum is established with CO_2 pressures at 10–12 mmHg

- Two 5 mm trocars are inserted on either side of the camera port.
- The first step is to identify key anatomical landmarks (Figs. 5 and 6) such as [5]:
  - the pubic bone,
  - the medial umbilical ligament
  - the inferior epigastric vessels (IEV)
  - the anterior superior iliac spine (ASIS) by external palpation
- The definition of the type of hernia is in relation to the IEV (Fig. 7)
  - direct hernia: is medial to IEV
  - indirect hernia: is lateral to IEV
  - femoral hernia: is medial to the IEV and to the iliac vessels

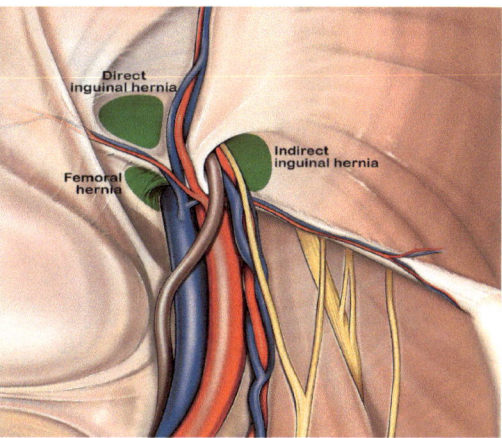

Fig. 5 The anatomy and landmarks of the myopectineal orifice (MPO) of Fruchaud

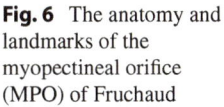

Fig. 6 The anatomy and landmarks of the myopectineal orifice (MPO) of Fruchaud

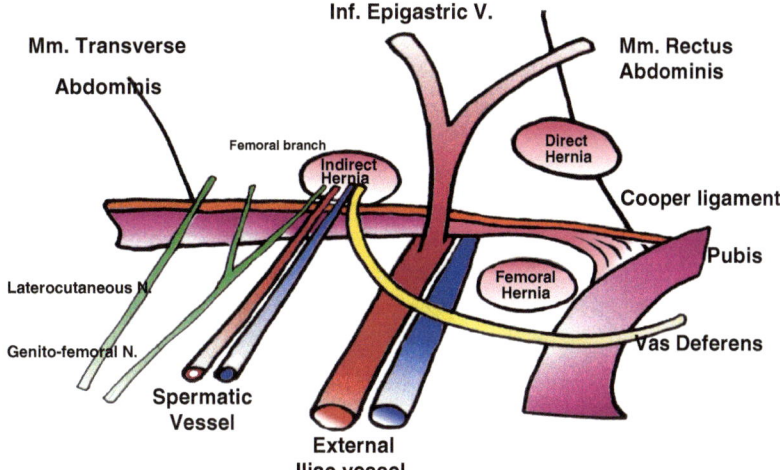

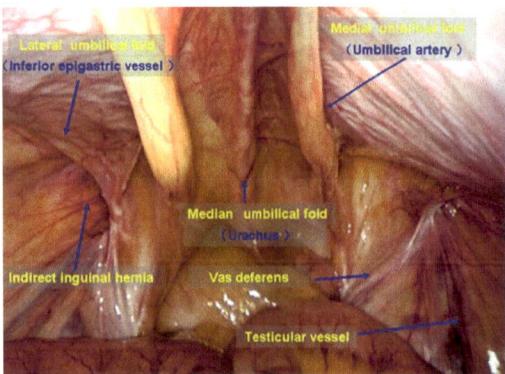

Fig. 7 Type of hernia in relation to IEV

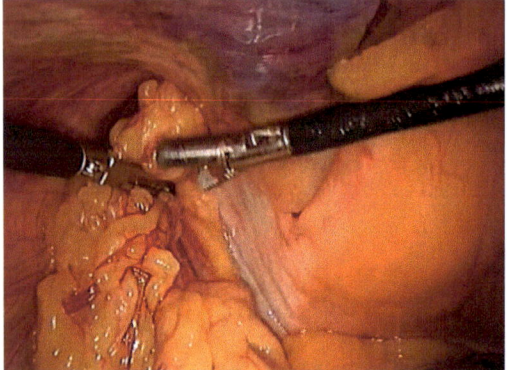

Fig. 8 Reduction of hernia content

- The next step is to reduce the hernia content into the abdominal cavity (Fig. 8). An atraumatic grasper or a bowel clamp is preferred to minimize any trauma to the contents of the hernia. It is advisable to avoid traction over the bowel and should attempt graded external compression.
- The peritoneal dissection starts laterally below the ASIS and about 5 cm above the upper limit of the hernia sac (Fig. 9a, b). The peritoneum is opened towards the midline by using diathermy hook or scissors and dissected inferiorly by blunt dissection. Peritoneal flap should be high enough to allow 2 cm overlap to avoid exposing the edge of the mesh. If incision is

too low, then the surgeon may try to push the mesh down which may crumple the mesh and ultimately suboptimal positioning.

- The indirect hernia sac is reduced and separated from the spermatic cord (Fig. 10).
- Occasionally, large indirect sacs cannot be completely reduced, and in such cases, the sac can be divided, and the proximal end should be ligated with a preformed laparoscopic loop ligature (Fig. 11). Alternatively, the sac can be ligated with a suture after ensuring it is empty and then can be divided distal to the ligated site.
- The final step is the mesh positioning and fixation. A rolled large pore polypropylene mesh (10 cm by 15 cm in size) is inserted through the 10 mm port, and with the use of graspers, the mesh is placed horizontally covering the myopectineal orifices from the midline of the pubis to lateral space of Bogros and inferiorly 2 cm below the pubic arch. The mesh is then anchored with laparoscopic absorbable tacks or staplers to Cooper's ligament and lateral to the IEV high at the abdominal wall to avoid the cutaneous nerves. This will help to prevent any mesh migration especially in case of large direct or indirect hernia. Mesh fixation is not necessary in smaller inguinal hernia [6]. A selective fixation for large hernia should be adopted (EHS classification; hernia defect > L2 and M2). Tacking should be avoided below the ileopubic tract and laterally below the ASIS where the risk of injury to the genitofemoral nerve and lateral femoral-cutaneous nerve of thigh [7] (Fig. 12).
- Mesh fixation is still a debatable topic. There is recommendation for fixation in patients with recurrent or large hernia (>3 cm). We suggest fixation in all large hernia during the early learning curve [8].
- Fibrin glue has been advocated as an alternative method of fixation, comparable to tacker and several studies have shown similar results between stapler fixation and fibrin

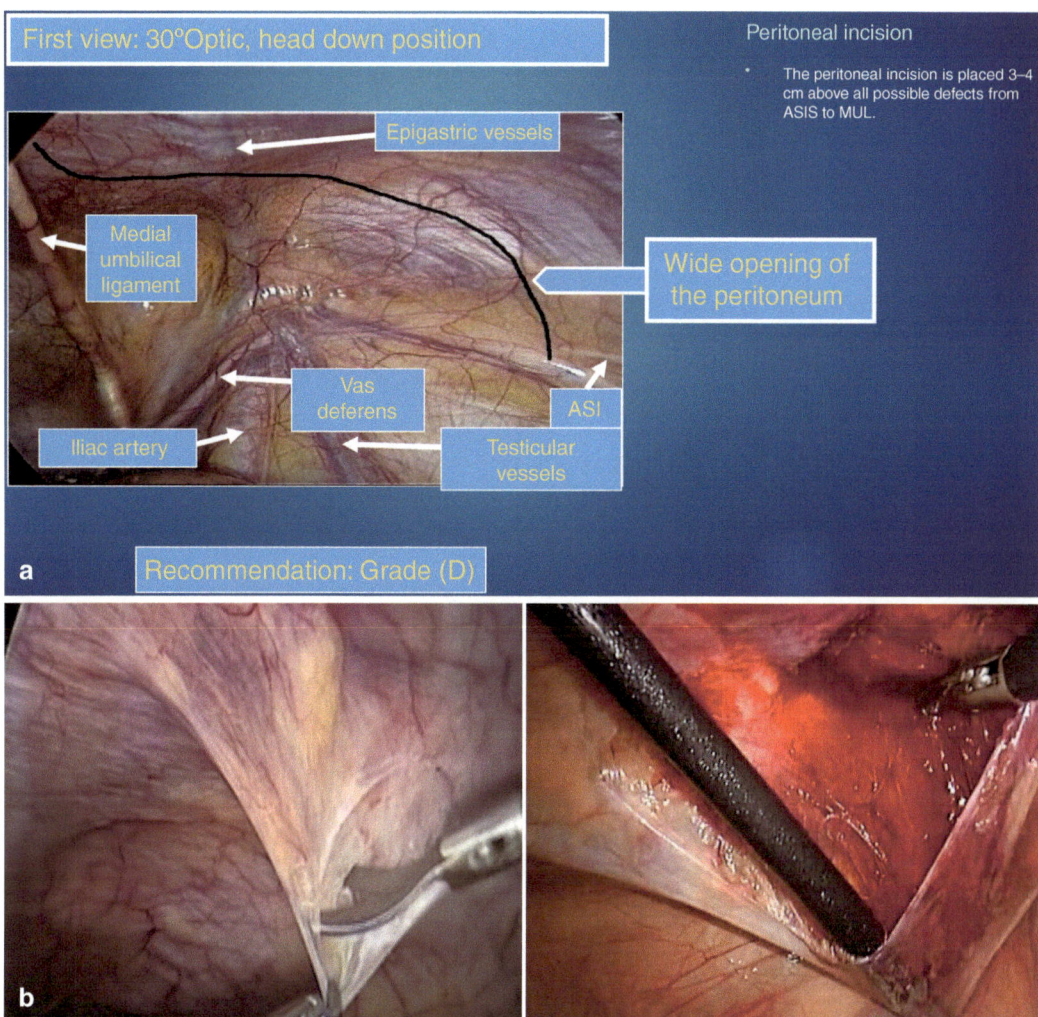

First view: 30°Optic, head down position

Peritoneal incision

* The peritoneal incision is placed 3–4 cm above all possible defects from ASIS to MUL.

Epigastric vessels

Medial umbilical ligament

Wide opening of the peritoneum

Vas deferens

ASI

Iliac artery

Testicular vessels

a

Recommendation: Grade (D)

b

Fig. 9 (**a**) Landmarks and incision of the peritoneal flap (black line). (**b**) Incision of the peritoneal flap using diathermy hook or scissor

glue with reduced risk of postoperative chronic pain [9, 10].

- Last step is adequate hemostasis and the closure of the peritoneum flap over the mesh by using:
  - Absorbable Tackers
  - Hemolocks
  - Continuous Absorbable suture (Fig. 13)
- It is advisable to close the peritoneal flap with continuous absorbable sutures under direct vision instead of tackers or staplers which can cause injury to the neurovascular structures located behind the peritoneum and the mesh. Care must be taken to avoid leaving gaps during the closure, as it may expose the mesh to the bowel which may lead to future adhesion formation or even fistulation.
- Fascia at the Infra umbilical 10 mm port site must be closed.
- Skin at the two 5 mm port site are closed with absorbable sutures or glue.

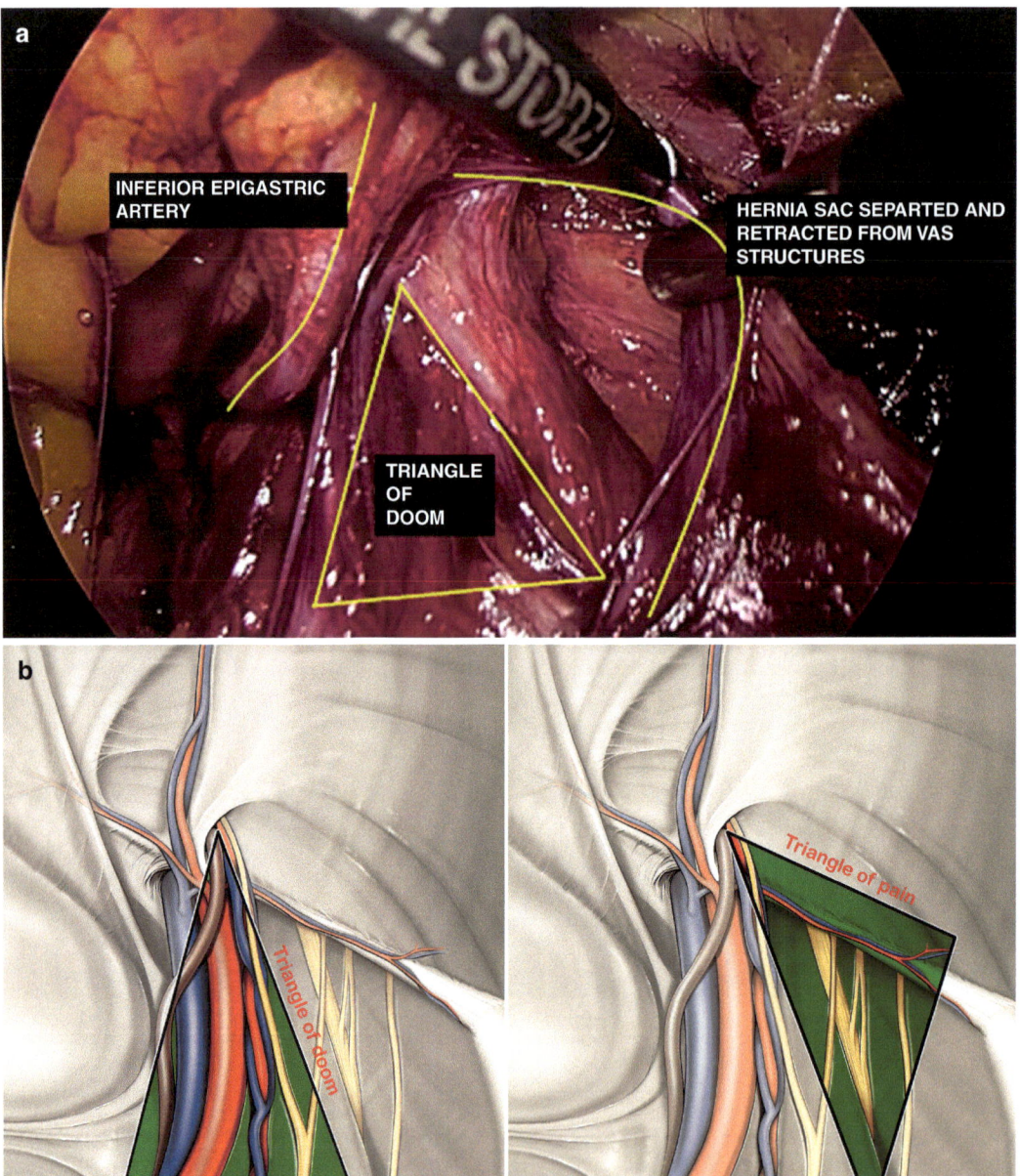

Fig. 10 (**a**) Indirect hernia sac is reduced and separated from the spermatic cord. (**b**) Indirect hernia sac is reduced and separated from the spermatic cord Figure

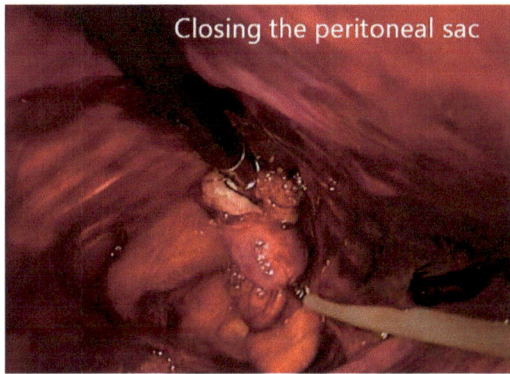

Fig. 11 The Indirect hernia sac is divided and ligated using an endoloop

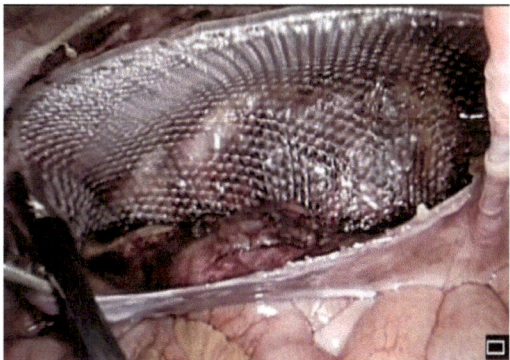

Fig. 12 Placement of an anatomical mesh in pre-peritoneal space with TAPP

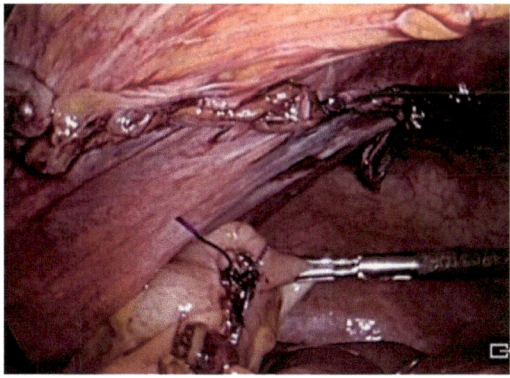

Fig. 13 Continuous absorbable suture is utilized to close the peritoneal flap

Postoperative Care

- Standard Analgesia
- Discharge the patient when the patient can ambulate and pass urine
- Avoid activities that require straining for up to 2–4 weeks

Postoperative Complications and Management [5]

- **Seroma**
  - Almost evident in majority
  - Size is important to determine the outcome
  - Avoid unnecessary dissection
  - Usually gets resolved spontaneously
- **Bleeding**
  - Injury to inferior epigastric vessels, spermatic vessels, and iliac vessels
  - Stop anticoagulation before surgery
  - Careful identification of vessels and dissection
  - Avoid rough dissection
  - Small hematoma would resolve in weeks, larger hematoma may require aspiration or surgical drainage but preferably done few weeks later to avoid mesh infection
- **Acute urinary retention**
  - Early mobilization
  - Preoperative counseling
  - Adequate analgesia
  - Foley's catheter may be inserted if patient is unable to pass urine after several attempts
- **Injury to surrounding structures**
  - Good knowledge of groin anatomy in the extraperitoneal plane is important
  - Injury to vas could be devastating, avoid holding vas and vessels
  - Care must be taken while parietalization of the peritoneum
  - Judicious use of surgical energy to avoid bladder and bowl injury

- **Postoperative pain**
  - Careful dissection in triangle of pain
  - Avoid injury to nerves
  - Absorbable tacking instead of metallic tackers and avoid any fixation over the triangle of pain
  - Prefer glue over tackers
- **Mesh infection**
  - Maintain sterility during the entire surgery
  - Non touch technique during handling the mesh
  - Prophylactic antibiotic
  - Careful inspection of surgical site after surgery
  - Early explanation of the mesh is advisable if mesh infection is suspected
- **Recurrence**
  - Look for contralateral orifice where possible
  - Adequate dissection
  - Appropriate mesh size
  - Proper orientation of mesh placement
  - Adequate medial coverage and overlap

Conclusion

Both techniques of endo-laparoscopic inguinal hernia repair (TEP and TAPP) are comparable in terms of the surgical outcomes [11]. Tailored approach in groin hernia repair by considering patient factors and surgeon's expertise is recommended.

References

1. Lichtenstein IL, Shulman AG, Amid PK, Montllor MM. The tension-free hernioplasty. Am J Surg. 1989;157:188–93.
2. Schultz LS, Graber JN, Pietrafitta J, Hickok DF. Early results with laparoscopic inguinal herniorrhaphy are promising. Clin Laser Mon. 1990;8:103–5.
3. Kavic MS, Roll S. Laparoscopic transabdominal Preperitoneal hernia repair (TAPP). In: Bendavid R, Abrahamson J, Arregui ME, Flament JB, Phillips EH, editors. Abdominal Wall hernias. New York, NY: Springer; 2001.
4. Bittner R, Arregui ME, Bisgaard T, et al. Guidelines for laparoscopic (TAPP) and endoscopic (TEP) treatment of inguinal hernia [international Endohernia society (IEHS)]. Surg Endosc. 2011;25(9):2773–843. https://doi.org/10.1007/s00464-011-1799-6.
5. Lovisetto F, Zonta S, Rota E, Bottero L, Faillace G, Turra G, Fantini A, Longoni M. Laparoscopic TAPP hernia repair: surgical phases and complications. Surg Endosc. 2007;21:646–52.
6. Khajanchee YS, Urbach DR, Swanstrom LL. Hansen PD outcomes of laparoscopic herniorrhaphy without fixation of mesh to the abdominal wall. Surg Endosc. 2001;15:1102–7.
7. Simons MP, Aufenacker B-NM, Bouillot JL, Campanelli G, Conze J, Lange D, Fortelny R, Heikkinen T, Kingsnorth A, Kukleta J, Morales-Conde S, Nordin P, Schumpelick V, Smedberg S, Smietanski M, Weber G, Miserez M. European hernia society guidelines on the treatment of inguinal hernia in adult patients. Hernia. 2009;13:343–403.
8. Saggar VR. Sarangi R laparoscopic totally extraperitoneal repair of inguinal hernia: a policy of selective mesh fixation over a 10-year period. J Laparoendosc Adv Surg Tech A. 2008;18:209–12.
9. Kathouda N, Mavor E, Friedlander MH, et al. Use of fibrin sealant for prosthetic mesh fixation laparoscopic extraperitoneal inguinal hernia repair. Ann Surg. 2001;233(1):18–25.
10. Olmi S, Scaini A, Erba L, et al. Quantification of pain in laparoscopic transabdominal preperitoneal (TAPP) inguinal hernioplasty identifies marked difference between prosthesis fixation system. Surgery. 2007;142(1):40–6.
11. McCormack K, Wake B, et al. Transabdominal preperitoneal (TAPP) versus totally extraperitoneal (TEP) laparoscopic techniques for inguinal hernia repair: a systematic review. Cochrane Database Syst Rev. 2005;25(1):CD004703.

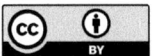

Totally Extraperitoneal Approach in Inguinal Hernia Repair

Davide Lomanto and Eva Lourdes Sta Clara

Introduction

Inguinal hernia can be repaired endoscopically via three methods namely total extraperitoneal (TEP), transabdominal pre-peritoneal (TAPP), and the less common intraperitoneal onlay mesh (IPOM) repair. The first two are widely utilized for the obvious advantages of lower recurrence and complication rates, and better outcome (less pain, less analgesic reqirement, less surgical site infection, reduced length of hospital stay, early return to daily activity, etc.) when compared to the open repair while covering all the potential hernia site in the myopectineal orifice with a large prosthesis [1, 2]. The TEP approach has a lower risk of intra-abdominal injury to organs and postoperative adhesions. On the other hand, in the TAPP approach, the contralateral side can be examined for occult or undiagnosed hernia and it can be useful as a diagnostic tool in an emergency hernia repair of irreducible cases.

Indications

- Patient with primary or recurrent reducible inguinal hernia
- Fit for general anesthesia

Contraindications

- Not fit for general anesthesia
- Acute abdomen with strangulated and infected bowel
- Respiratory distress
- Pediatric patients

Relative Contraindications

- Irreducible Hernia
- Sliding Hernia
- Inguino-scrotal Hernia
- Previous prostatectomy or pelvic surgery
- Previous TEP/TAPP Repair

Previous lower abdominal surgery is a relative contraindication. Adhesions can pose difficulty for the attending surgeon, and thus a surgeon who is

D. Lomanto
Department of Surgery, YLL School of Medicine, National University Singapore, Singapore, Singapore

E. L. Sta Clara (✉)
Department of Surgery, Asian Hospital Medical Center, Manila, Philippines

Training Officer (UMIST) and Training Committee Department of Surgery, Cardinal Santos Medical Center, Manila, Philippines

Deparment of Surgery, Rizal Medical Center, Manila, Philippines

Department of Surgery, University of Perpetual Help Dalta Medical Center, Las Pinas, Philippines

© The Author(s) 2023
D. Lomanto et al. (eds.), *Mastering Endo-Laparoscopic and Thoracoscopic Surgery*,
https://doi.org/10.1007/978-981-19-3755-2_56

attempting this should be skilled in doing both TEP and TAPP. But it should be explained to the patient that there is also a possibility that the operation can be converted to an open approach as deemed necessary by the surgeon. Previous open appendectomies are usually not a problem but requires one to be more careful during the lateral dissection.

Recurrent hernia from a previous TEP is a relative contraindication. This can still be done through TEP depending on the expertise of the surgeon.

Large inguinoscrotal hernia is also a relative contraindication depending on the experience of the surgeon since there would usually be a distorted anatomy and limited working space in this kind of inguinal hernias.

Preoperative Preparation

A thorough history and physical examination are necessary to assess the patient including the fitness for general anesthesia. If there is any doubt in the diagnosis of the inguinal hernia (large defect, sliding hernia, multiple recurrent, etc.) it may be prudent to do a preoperative imaging work-up by dynamic ultrasound or CT scan.

It should also be explained to the patient that there might be a risk of conversion to transabdominal pre-peritoneal (TAPP) inguinal hernia repair or open approach depending on the difficulty and safety of the procedure, which is based on the judgment of the operating surgeon. Risk for recurrence and complications should also be properly explained to the patient including vascular, nerve and vas injury, seroma, mesh infection, postoperative chronic pain, etc. [3].

Prophylactic antibiotic is recommended in the presence of risk factors for wound and mesh infection based on patient status (advanced age, recurrence corticosteroid use, immunosuppressive conditions, obesity, diabetes, and malignancy) or surgical factors (contamination, long operation duration, use of drains, urinary catheter) [4, 5].

Patient should also be advised to void prior to the procedure. However, in cases of complicated hernias (partially reducible, large defect, and/or the length of surgery more than 1.5 h) it is advisable to insert a urinary catheter, which can be removed at the end of the procedure.

Operating Theater Setup

Instruments

- 10 or 5 mm, 30° angled telescopes.
- Trocars
  - 10 mm Hasson's trocar
  - 5 mm trocar
- Balloon dissector
- Based on the IEHS guidelines, it is recommended to use a balloon dissector when creating the preperitoneal space to decrease operative time, especially during the learning period, when it is difficult to identify the correct preperitoneal plane and space [5]. Once the learning curve is overcomed, to reduce the cost of the procedure, a blind dissection can be achieved by swiping the telescope along the midline. A self-made dissector balloon can be arranged using finger gloves over an irrigation device.
- Graspers and atraumatic graspers
- Scissors, Hook
- Prosthetic mesh
- It is advisable to use a large pore polypropylene or multifilament polyester mesh with a size of at least 10 × 15 cm. Using a smaller mesh will increase the risk of recurrence. However, for larger defects of more than 3–4 cm (L > 3 according to EHS classification [4, 5] it is recommended to use a larger mesh (12 × 17 cm)
- Tackers and Fixation devices
- According to the IEHS Guidelines, fixation of the mesh is required only in particular cases like large hernia defect (>3–4 cm) especially in direct hernia to avoid translation of the mesh and to reduce the risk of recurrence [5]. Today either absorbable or permanent staplers/tackers are utilized to fix the mesh to the Cooper's ligament and to the rectus muscle. Sealants in the form of Fibrin Glue (Tisseel or Tissucol, Baxter USA) or synthetic glue (Liquiband, AMS UK; Histoacryl, BBraun, Germany; etc.) are also available and several studies have shown their efficacy and benefits.
- Endoloops
- Pre-made loop sutures are useful for closure of inadvertent tears in the peritoneum and ligation of the hernia sac. Based on the IEHS guidelines, it is recommended to close any peritoneal tears

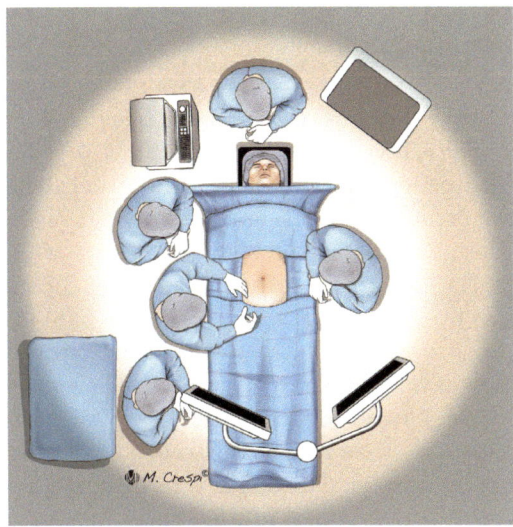

Fig. 1 Surgical team position

to decrease the risk of adhesions which may lead to bowel obstruction. If not available, the loop can be made using a 50–70 cm absorbable suture and an extracorporeal Roeder's knot.

Patient and Surgical Team Positioning

The patient is in a supine position under general anesthesia. The operating table is in a slight Trendelenberg position (10–15°) with both arms tucked at the sides. The attending surgeon stands at the opposite side of the hernia defect and the assistant stands beside the attending surgeon at the cephalad side of the patient (Fig. 1). The nurse then stands on the same side as the surgeon, near the feet of the patient. The monitor and video equipment are then placed at the caudal end of the operating table which can be midline or slightly ipsilateral to the defect. Monitors mounted on the boom arm will be helpful in improving visual space.

Surgical Technique

Entering and Creating the Preperitoneal Space

There are a few techniques to enter and create the preperitoneal space:

A 10 mm vertical/horizontal infraumbilical incision is first done. Subcutaneous tissue is bluntly dissected to expose the anterior rectus sheath using (2) S-retractors. The anterior rectus sheath is then incised, lateral from the midline, on the ipsilateral side of the hernia. This will avoid the linea alba and accidentally enter the peritoneal cavity. Then the rectus muscles are retracted laterally to expose the posterior rectus sheath.

Once the preperitoneal plane is entered, there are few techniques to create the space: (1) the optical balloon dissector; (2) the Veress' needle technique; and (3) the most common blunt dissection. Using the trocar with an optical balloon dissector, the space is created by inflating the balloon under vision (Fig. 2). This is the plane one should maintain and create up to the symphysis pubis using a gauze, finger, or a dissecting balloon depending on the preference and expertise of the surgeon. A Hasson's trocar is then inserted, and the plane is confirmed by inserting a 30° trocar. The rectus muscle should be visualized at the anterior area to be in the right plane. Insufflation is done with carbon dioxide at 8–12 mmHg.

Two 5 mm trocars are then inserted at the midline under direct vision to prevent any injury to the bladder, peritoneum, or bowels. The first 5 mm trocar is placed three fingerbreadths above the symphysis pubis. The second 5 mm trocar is then placed in between the Hasson's trocar and the first 5 mm trocar (Fig. 3).

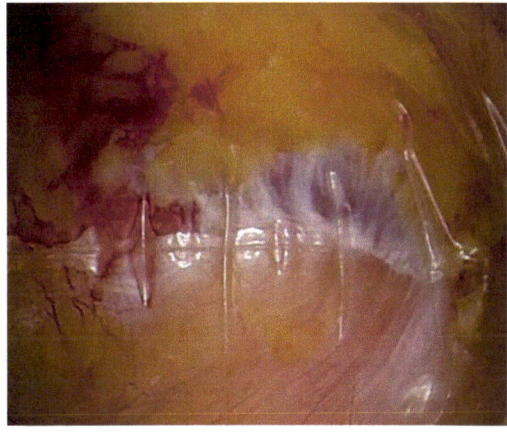

Fig. 2 Ballon dissector

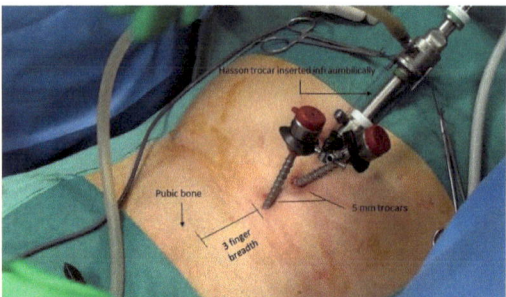

Fig. 3 Trocar placement

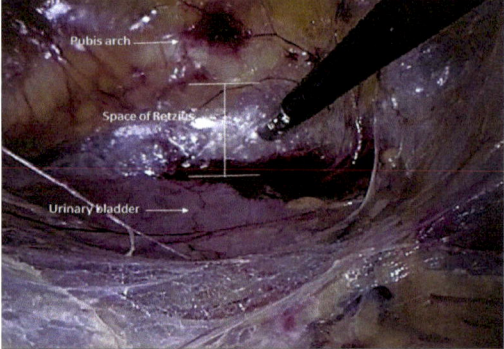

Fig. 4 Space of Retzius

Medial Dissection (Retzius or Pre-vesical Space)

Once all the working ports are inserted, using two atraumatic graspers, the dissection is conducted along the midline, below the rectus muscle and towards the pubis arch. The first landmark, cooper's ligament should be identified and is an excellent starting point for dissection. Dissection should follow the preperitoneal plane. Fatty tissue present in the preperitoneal space should be kept in contact with the inguinal floor and not with the peritoneum. The dissection should go 2 cm beyond the symphysis pubis till the obturator fossa to avoid missing any obturator hernia and to allow the medial lower corner of the mesh to be fixated once the space is deflated (Fig. 4). The limits of the dissection are medial, 1–2 cm beyond the midline and below the pubis arch; inferiorly till the peritoneal reflection is identified at the border with the retroperitoneal space.

Lateral Dissection (Lateral Space of Bogros)

Moving towards the anterior superior iliac spine (ASIS), in a surgical plane that is below the inferior epigastric vessels (IEV) and above the peritoneum, the lateral dissection is made. This plane is confined by the two layers of the fascia transversalis. The dissection is continued by pushing down the peritoneum until the psoas muscle can be seen. The lateral space of Bogros is delineated and cleaned all the way up to the anterior superior iliac spine. Attention should be made to avoid dissecting further laterally, beyond the lumbar fascia in the so-called lateral triangle of pain. This will prevent injury of the latero-cutaneous and genitofemoral nerves. The thin layer of fat covering the lateral fascia should be preserved and not skeletonized, similar energy and diathermy should not be used at this level (Figs. 5 and 6). Limits of the lateral dissection are inferiorly the psoas muscle, superiorly the ASIS, and cranially the arcuate line.

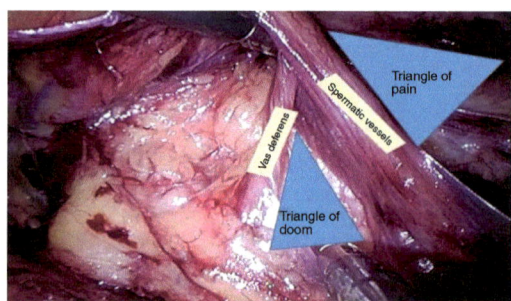

Fig. 5 Triangle of pain and triangle of doom

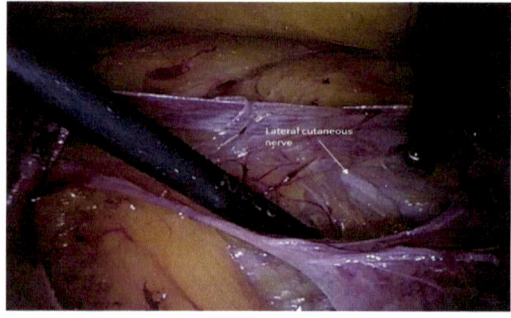

Fig. 6 Lateral cutaneous nerve at the Space of Bogros

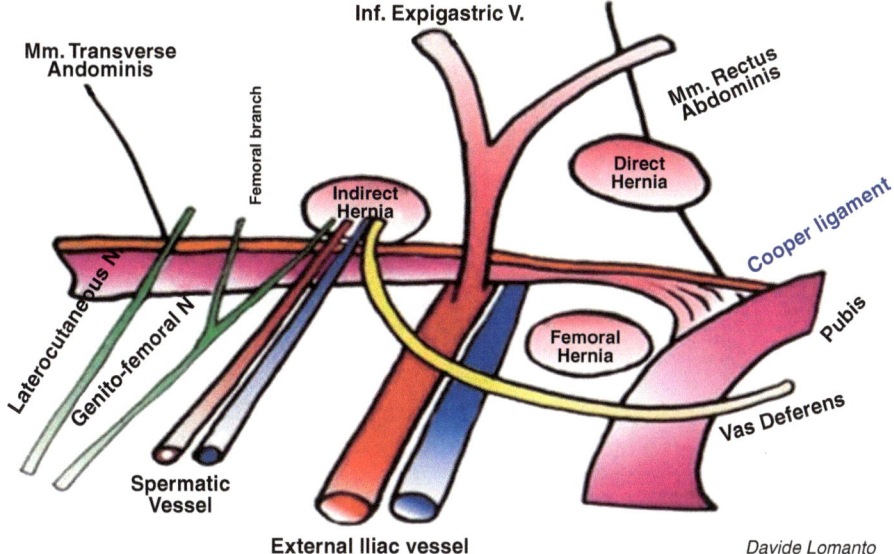

Fig. 7 Anatomic Landmarks in Endo-laparoscopic inguinal hernia repair

Hernia Sac Identification and Reduction

Once the medial and lateral dissections are completed (Fig. 7), we should be able to identify all the hernia defects followed by a proper hernia sac reduction and repair. This will allow the surgeon to visualize all the anatomical landmarks, lessen the risk of injuries, have a wider space for placing the prosthesis and in case of

inadvertent tear of the peritoneum to continue to work safely without being affected by the pneumoperitoneum.

The exposure of the whole Myopectineal Orifice should be made after a complete medial and lateral dissection followed by the hernia sac reduction (Fig. 8).

Hernia Reduction

Medial or Direct Hernia

In endo-laparoscopic approach, a defect medial to the inferior epigastric hernia and at the level of the

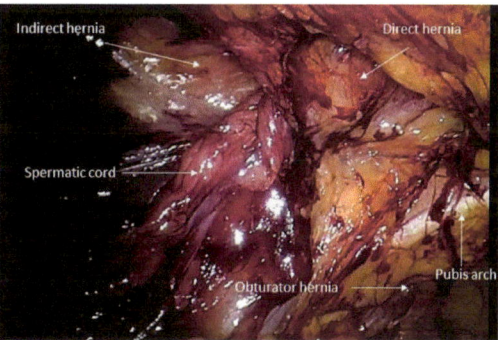

Fig. 8 Myopectineal orifice, left

Hesselblack triangle is a direct hernia. The reduction can be easily achieved by identifying and holding the hernia "pseudosac" and dividing it from the preperitoneal lipoma and peritoneum. When dissecting the direct hernia, the surgeon must remain in the correct plane in order to avoid injuring the bladder if it is part of the hernia. Careful dissection is done at the level of the pubis arch to avoid injury of the "corona mortis" and laterally of the iliac vessels and vas deferens. The pseudosac is grabbed, and the hernia contents are then reduced.

Femoral Hernia

The reduction of the hernia sac and content is achieved by gentle traction keeping in mind that the vessels hide behind the content (Fig. 9).

If the content is not reducible by traction due to the small size of the defect, it may be necessary to widen the femoral defect by using a hook diathermy ONLY on the medial-upper side (Fig. 10). This will facilitate the hernia sac reduction.

Obturator Hernia

In the same canal where the obturator vessels are, it is possible that preperitoneal fat and/or hernia sac is within. Gentle traction will allow the reduction of the hernia sac (Fig. 11).

Indirect Hernia

Lateral to the IEV, lies the deep ring and the indirect hernia. The standard approach to indirect hernia repair requires the spermatic structures to be separated from the hernia sac. This can be achieved

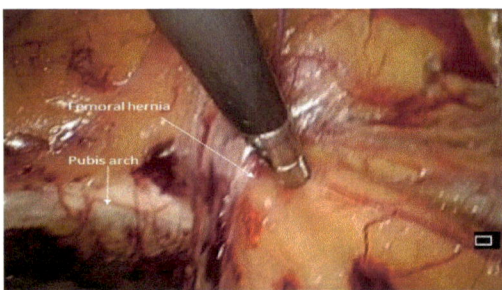

Fig. 9 Femoral hernia, right

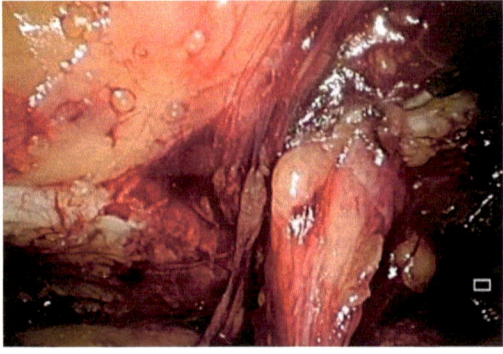

Fig. 10 Widening of the femoral ring using a hook diathermy at the medial-upper side

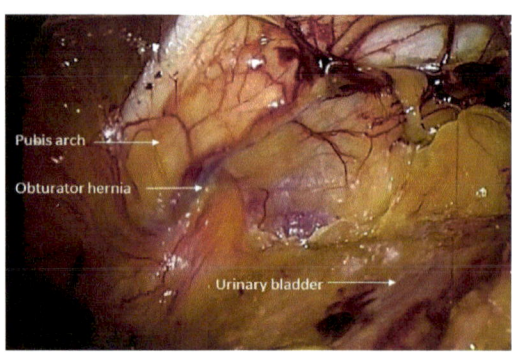

Fig. 11 Obturator hernia, left

using the medial approach and four simple steps: (1) Separate the whole sac and spermatic cord from the iliac vessels; (2) Slim the sac at the level of the deep ring with a partial reduction of both cord structures and sac; (3) Separate the cord structures from the sac on the inferior edge of the sac; and (4) Sac reduction by simple traction. Transection of the sac may be necessary in cases of long or complete sac to minimize injury to the testis by overtraction. It is suggested to divide the sac using diathermy to reduce the risk of hematoma and to ligate the proximal part using pre-made suture loop. Lipoma of the cord should be fully reduced.

Parietalization of the elements of the cord is considered sufficient when the peritoneum is dissected inferiorly until at least at the level at which the vas deferens crosses the external iliac vein and the iliopsoas muscle is identified.

In women, round ligament of the uterus is usually adherent to the peritoneum. Transection of the round ligament is then recommended, at least 1 cm proximal to the deep ring to avoid injury of the genital branch of the genitofemoral nerve at this location.

It is important to close all peritoneal holes/tears with absorbable suture loops or plastic clips (i.e., hem-o-lok, Teleflex Medical, USA) to prevent any internal herniation or adhesion formation with the mesh.

Mesh Repair

The final step is the hernia repair and it is achieved by covering all the myopectineal orifice with a synthetic large pore prosthesis of 10×15 cm. The mesh is rolled and inserted through the 10 mm trocar. A "no-touch technique" is mandatory to avoid mesh infection. The mesh is opened and inserted into the preperitoneal cavity avoiding any contact with the skin. The mesh is then placed horizontally and unrolled over the myopectineal orifice making sure to cover all the hernia sites. One-third of the mesh should be below the symphysis pubis, the upper margin reaching the lower trocar medially and laterally lining over the psoas muscle. In bilateral hernias, there should be a 1–2 cm overlap of the meshes at the midline. It is important to make sure that no part of the peritoneum is under the mesh to prevent any recurrence. The mesh should be placed without wrinkles or folds and should not be split to avoid chronic pain or recurrence.

The mesh is then anchored using tackers or sealant to prevent mesh migration and possible recurrence. Two to three point fixations are necessary: the Cooper's ligament, medial to the inferior epigastric vessels at the rectus muscle and if necessary lateral to the inferior epigastric vessels. Avoid tackers or stapler fixations below the iliopubic tract and too laterally considering a 15–20% of abnormalities in the nerves path. This will help prevent any nerve injuries and consequent postoperative chronic pain.

An accurate hemostasis should be guaranteed if the correct surgical plane is identified. The carbon dioxide is then released while visualizing that the mesh is not rolled, and the peritoneum stays in front of the mesh to prevent any recurrence. The lateral inferior edge of the mesh can be held with a grasper, if necessary. The ports are then removed and the anterior rectus sheath incision at the 10 mm trocar site is sutured. The skin incisions are then closed with absorbable sutures or glue.

Postoperative Care

- Diet, as tolerated, is resumed
- Analgesia is given (etoricoxib 90 mg daily for 3 days)
- Patient is discharged on the same day once voiding freely
- Follow-up is at 1 week, 1, and 3 months

Complications

Complications can be categorized into intraoperative and postoperative complications. Intraoperative complications specific to TEP occur in about 4–6% of the cases and can be due to vascular, visceral, nerve, and spermatic cord structures injury [6–8]. Vascular injuries would include injury to the external iliac vessels, inferior epigastric vessels, spermatic vessels, or the vessels over the pubic arch including the corona mortis veins. The most common is the injury of the IEV and this can be avoided by using the midline approach and by inserting all the ports under direct vision. Injury to the major vessels are catastrophic, a correct lateral traction of the sac and spermatic structure with a medial approach may be helpful in avoiding it. Visceral injuries including but not limited to the bowels and urinary tract can be reduced by careful dissection and limiting the use of diathermy. Transmitted energy through the thin peritoneal layer may result in injury of the bowel underlying. Patients with previous pelvis surgery, sliding hernia, or large inguinoscrotal are at risk for bladder injury, in this case a urinary catheter may be necessary. In case of injuries, they can be managed by an endolaparoscopoic suture repair. Nerve injuries can be prevented by accurate lateral dissection, limiting the number of staplers/tackers if fixation is needed, and the use of absorbable tackers or sealant. Spermatic cord injuries can be lessened by properly identifying the anatomy and avoiding too much traction of the cord. Tears in the peritoneum can also occur especially during the early stage of the learning curve. All peritoneal tears should be closed by using suture loops or hem-o-loks.

Postoperative complication like seroma commonly occur in patients with large direct and indirect hernia, the seroma usuall appear after 7–10 days and do not require any treatment. It may be mistaken for an early recurrence. In principle, it should be treated conservatively and will be reabsorbed spontaneously within 4–6 weeks. However, if it is symptomatic and persists after 2 months it is advisable to drain by aspiration and in sterile condition. In cases of complex serohematoma, an excision after 4–5 months should be considered.

Early recurrence is usually due to inadequate surgical technique and can be due to wrong case selection for beginners, inadequate fixation of the mesh, inadequate mesh size, inadequate dissection of the myopectineal orifice, and failure to cover unidentified hernia defects [9].

References

1. Memon MA, Cooper NJ, et al. Meta-analysis of randomized clinical trials comparing open and laparoscopic inguinal hernia repair. Br J Surg. 2003;90(12):1479–92.
2. Feliu X, Claveria R, Besora P, et al. Bilateral inguinal hernia repair: laparoscopic or open approach? Hernia. 2011;15(1):15–8.
3. Lomanto D. Katara Avinash. Managing intraoperative complications during totally extraperitoneal repair of inguinal hernia. Minim Access Surg Sep. 2006;2(3):165–70.
4. Simons MP, Aufenacaker T, Bay-Nielsen M, et al. European Hernia Society guidelines on the treatment of inguinal hernia in adult patients. Hernia. 2009;13(4):343–403.
5. Bittner R, Arregui ME, Bisgaard T, et al. Guidelines for laparoscopic (TAPP) and endoscopic (TEP) treatment of inguinal hernia [international EndoHernia society (IEHS)]. Surg Endosc. 2011;25:2773–843.
6. Tetik C, Arregui ME, Dulucq JL, et al. Complications and recurrences with laparoscopic repair of groin hernias: a multi-institutional retrospective analysis. Surg Endosc. 1994;8:1316–23.
7. Kraus MA. Nerve injury during laparoscopic inguinal hernia repair. Surg Laparosc Endosc. 1993;3:342–5.
8. Felix E, Habertson N, Varteian S. Laparoscopic hernioplasty: surgical complications. Surg Endosc. 1999;13:328–31.
9. Pablo RM, Reusch M, et al. Laparoscopic hernia repair–complications. JSLS. 1998;2(1):35–40.

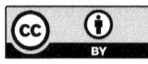

Laparoscopic Management of Recurrent and Re-recurrent Hernia

Sajid Malik, James Lee Wai Kit, Sujith Wijerathne, and Davide Lomanto

Introduction

Despite the best surgical techniques and measures, we still see recurrence rates between 0.5 and 15% in the current literature, following primary hernia repair and this depends on the hernia site, method of repair as well as circumstances of the timing of surgery [1]. With such a growing number of patients presenting with hernia recurrence, it is imperative that general surgeons are familiar and comfortable with various modalities of repair [2].

Re-recurrent inguinal hernia is defined as a recurrence of a hernia which has been repaired at least twice before at the same site [3] (Fig. 1).

According to the EHS, IEHS Guidelines, and HerniaSurge Group (2018), endo-laparoscopic posterior approach is preferred for recurrences after anterior repair and open anterior approach can be used for recurrence after posterior approach [4].

As the population is aging, the number of cases done laparoscopically has increased and

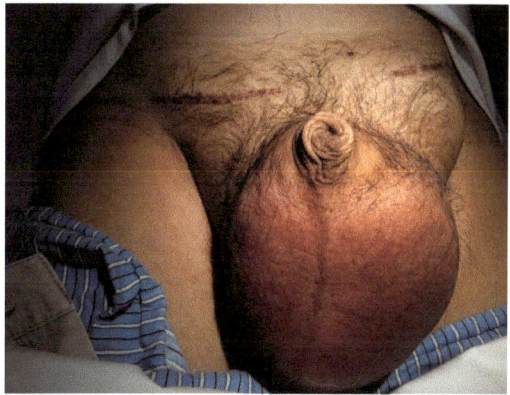

Fig. 1 Patient with recurrent hernia after bilateral open repair

with other challenging factors like robotic prostatectomy, we presume that in the future we are going to experience more cases of either multiple recurrences and recurrence after both anterior and posterior repairs in which there is a lack of data and guidelines to guide surgeons on the choice of treatment [1].

We would stress that these cases can be extremely challenging in which the failure of a previous treatment not only leads to a difficult surgery but also to an outcome that can be suboptimal and poor for the patients. In our modest opinion, these cases for the best of the patients should be referred and treated by Hernia Centers of Excellence where expertise and high volume will make the difference [5].

S. Malik (✉)
Department of General Surgery, Allama Iqbal Medical College, Jinnah Hospital, Lahore, Pakistan

J. L. W. Kit
Minimally Invasive Surgery Centre, National University Hospital, Singapore, Singapore

S. Wijerathne
Department of Surgery, National University Health System, Singapore, Singapore

D. Lomanto
Department of Surgery, YLL School of Medicine, National University Singapore, Singapore, Singapore

© The Author(s) 2023
D. Lomanto et al. (eds.), *Mastering Endo-Laparoscopic and Thoracoscopic Surgery*,
https://doi.org/10.1007/978-981-19-3755-2_57

In this chapter, we aim to outline the key points in the use of endo-laparoscopic techniques for the repair of recurrent and re-recurrent inguinal hernias, based on our experience at a high-volume hernia center.

Indications

Indication for repair of hernia recurrences are similar to primary hernia repair. In patients who have an asymptomatic recurrence, there is a role for watchful waiting as the risk of complications remain low even in the recurrent hernia group [1, 6]. In patients who are symptomatic, repair should be undertaken after evaluation of the recurrence with a balanced discussion considering the patient's underlying comorbidities and quality of life. Urgent repair should be undertaken in patients who present with complications related to the hernia such as perforation, strangulation, or obstruction [6].

Recurrences are usually classified according to the timing of the recurrence—immediate, early, and late. Although there is no consensus with regards to the actual definitions of the timing and some authors have used a period of 5 years to differentiate between early and late recurrences. Immediate recurrences are usually due to technical issues such as excessive intra-abdominal pressure or trauma to the repair site, as well as the presence of occult hernia which was missed during the initial repair. Early recurrences are generally related to surgeon factors with regards to surgical technique, tissue handling, and the choice of tissue versus mesh repair. Late recurrences are generally due to hernia biology from patient factors such as age-related weakening of the anterior abdominal wall, obesity, smoking as well as the presence of new risk factors such as chronic constipation and retention of urine that can lead to chronic increased abdominal pressure resulting in recurrences [7].

For Re-recurrences, multiple factors will influence the decision on repair: type of previous repair, age, comorbidities (DM, obesity, Diverticular diseases, etc.), concomitant pelvic surgery. An accurate analysis of all risk factors should be balanced with the benefits, patient's expectations and expected outcome, and ultimately with the surgeon's experience [8].

Contraindications

In the repair of hernias, contraindications can be divided into general contraindications for surgery due to the risk of anesthesia, specific contraindications to hernia repair as well as contraindications in the consideration of the modality of hernia repair.

Hernia repair in general can be considered as mild to moderate risk procedure. Therefore, generally, most patients would be fit for the procedure. Furthermore, with the advent of options of general, spinal, and even local anesthesia in the course of the repair, the technique can be tailored to minimize the risk of anesthesia, especially in patients with very poor underlying comorbidities (e.g., Poor heart function, poorly controlled cardiovascular risk factors, etc.). However, the surgeon needs to also take into consideration the extent of surgery for these cases and marry the type of anesthesia with the extent of surgery indicated to ensure a good outcome.

Contraindications related to the repair of hernias would include those who would not benefit from the hernia repair (poor quality of life prior to surgery to begin with and are unaffected by the hernia recurrence), lifestyle risk factors for hernia development that the patients are unwilling to modify which would result in further hernia recurrence in the future and futility of the current repair [9].

A specific relative contraindication would be the repair of hernias in pregnant patients soon after delivery. In these patients often the abdominal wall is lax due to the pregnancy. Most guidelines recommend delaying elective hernia repair in pregnant patients until at least 4 weeks postpartum to allow for sufficient time for the abdominal wall to regain sufficient normality prior to repair to allow for a meaningful repair [4, 10].

Pre-Op Assessment

All patients undergoing hernia repair should undergo appropriate preoperative assessment for surgery. Evaluation of underlying comorbidities and preoperative optimization should be performed with a referral to anesthesia as required [4].

Specific assessment of the hernia should also be performed. In patients with recurrent hernia with complex anatomy or possible complications, cross-sectional imaging should be performed to further delineate the anatomy as required in order to assist with planning of the hernia repair. A dedicated Informed Consent should be taken highlighting the risk for bladder injury, bowel injury, and injury to the cord structures including vas deferens transection.

A dynamic Ultrasound by an expert radiographer in hernia may be helpful together with a CT Scan for more complex or complicated situations like inguinoscrotal hernia which are not reducible, previous pelvic surgery or radiotherapy, etc. [11].

OT Setup

- See setup for inguinal hernias in TAPP or TEP chapters
- Urinary Catheter for complex recurrent and re-recurrent cases

Instrumentations

- Standard endo-laparoscopic set for Inguinal hernia (see chapter on TEP and TAPP)

Surgical Technique

At present, surgery is the mainstay approach for all recurrent and re-recurrent inguinal hernias. The surgical approach is determined by the nature of the previous repair (mesh vs nonmesh) as well as previous approach (anterior vs posterior). The main principle is the choice of approach should avoid the route of previous approach with a preference for entry through virgin planes to mini-mize trauma and injury to both cutaneous nerves as well as the cord structures. Previous tissue repair offers more flexibility in view of the absence of a mesh which can potentially complicate the surgical repair of the recurrent hernia due to adhesions to the mesh [2, 4, 10].

Principles of Recurrent Repair

1. Approach through virgin tissue planes
2. Anticipate scarring and distortion of normal tissue planes
3. Reinforcement of the inguinal floor
4. Dissection from normal tissue to scarred tissue and avoiding the use of scarred tissue for repair
5. Tension-free technique for suture lines
6. Leave previous mesh in place and incorporate the edge of the previous mesh into the new repair where possible
7. Dissection to expose and evaluate all hernia orifices to avoid missing an occult hernia
8. Adequate mesh size for coverage of all hernia orifices and to prevent rerecurrence

Challenges and Strategies

In case of post open anterior repair, repair of recurrent hernias can be similar to primary repair through the posterior approach. In some cases, it is difficult to reduce the direct or indirect sac if the prior anterior repair had utilized stitches to plicate the transversalis fascia, inadequate isolation of the sac or if a mesh plug was utilized in the previous anterior repair to fix a direct hernia. Adhesions are the main challenge in the repair of recurrent hernias. Initiating dissection at a more anterior location would ensure safer dissection and a reduction in injury to the vas deferens, corona mortis, or bladder. TEP repair is preferred if the necessary expertise is present; however, TAPP is a good alternative option as well in such recurrent repairs [10, 11].

In cases of re-recurrent hernias, the surgical technique and related repair can be even more tricky should there have been prior anterior and posterior repairs during the first two surgeries. In such cases, one needs to ask what is the best approach? If you attempt endo-laparoscopic repair which approach is the best? Is it even worth the challenges to attempt an endo-laparoscopic repair for re-recurrent hernias?

Treatment of re-recurrent hernias needs to be individualized to the patient. Risk and benefit of the procedure would need to be considered by the attending surgeon after a thorough discussion with the patient [12, 13].

In cases where the patient is elderly (e.g., more than 80 years old) with multiple comorbidities who presents with an asymptomatic re-recurrent hernia, it is prudent to consider that conservative management is a viable alternative given the risk benefit of performing a complex repair for an asymptomatic patient.

In cases whereby the patient is young, fit, and healthy with evidence of a re-recurrent hernia after both an anterior and posterior repair failure, our recommendation is to perform a transabdominal posterior approach (TAPP). Using this approach we are able to make a clear diagnosis of the hernia type, size, and location of the recurrence. Using this method we can also understand the reason for failure having a clear view of the myopectineal orifices during the procedure. We recommend using a urinary catheter during the intraoperative period to keep the urinary bladder decompressed and to prevent bladder injuries during both recurrent and re-recurrent inguinal hernia repairs [14].

In our experience, majority of the recurrences after multiple previous open anterior repairs are usually medial recurrences (70–75%) [1] (Fig. 2).

Re-recurrences after both anterior and posterior repairs are usually because of improper previous mesh placement, which could be placement of the mesh too high or the repair of a large direct hernia (15–20% of the time), resulting in either medial or lateral recurrences (Figs. 3, 4, 5, 6, and 7).

Our recommended approach for such cases can be outlined below

- Initiation of the dissection where the posterior myopectineal orifice of Fruchaud (MPO) is not covered by mesh.
- Attempt to reduce the hernia sac or excise it.

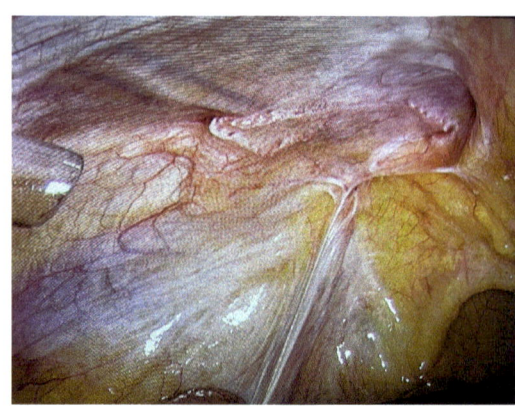

Fig. 2 Medial recurrence after open mesh repair and TEP mesh repair

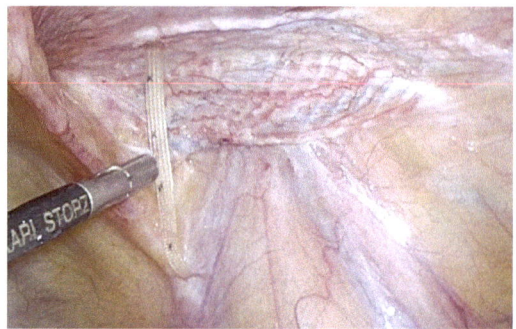

Fig. 3 Recurrence with mesh shrinkage

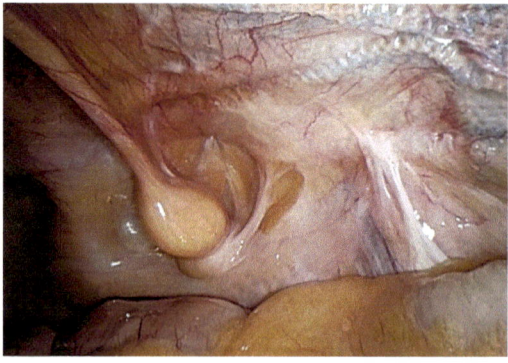

Fig. 4 Recurrence due to mesh placed higher on the myopectineal orifice

- Attempt to get a strong medial fixation point for the next mesh, and if you cannot dissect up to the Cooper's ligament because of high risk for bladder injury, then consider overlapping the new mesh to the old and use titanium fixa-

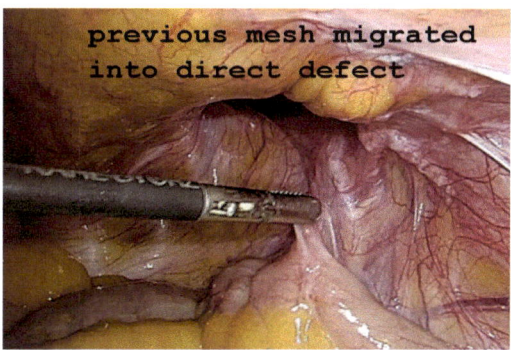

Fig. 5 Medial recurrence after large direct hernia repair and mesh displaced inside the hernia

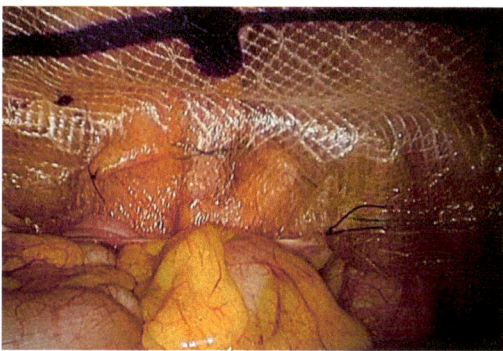

Fig. 8 After laparoscopic IPOM Plus repair for re-recurrent inguinal hernia

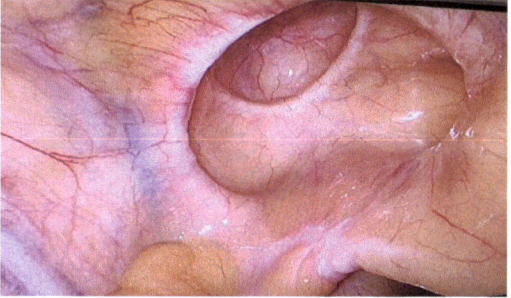

Fig. 6 Rerecurrence after previous TEP mesh repair

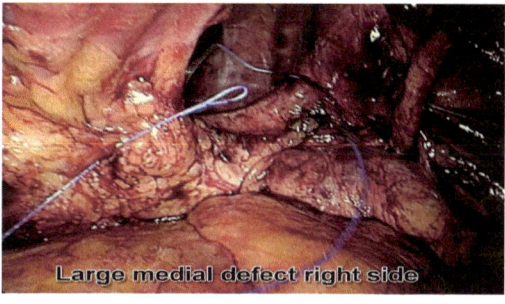

Fig. 9 Direct Defect Closure as a measure to prevent recurrence and reduce seroma

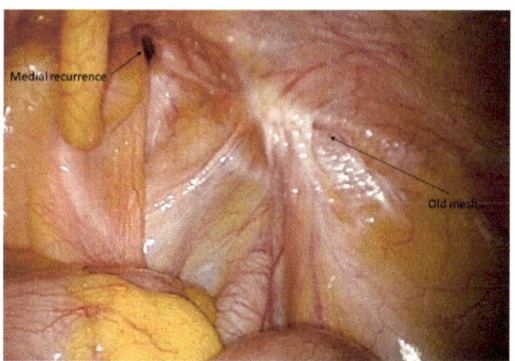

Fig. 7 Medial recurrence after previous TEP

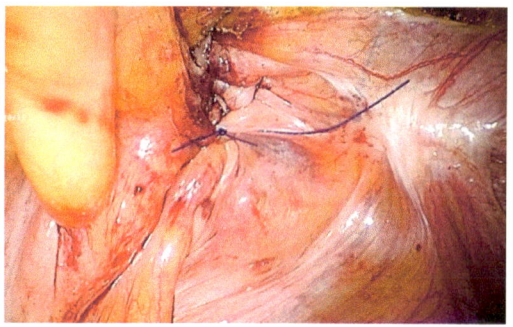

Fig. 10 After the closure of medial defect

tion above the pubis arch [15]. Consider an Intraperitoneal onlay (IPOM) or transabdominal partial extraperitoneal mesh placement (TAPE) and fix it using staplers on top and the upper medial side of the old mesh (Fig. 8).

• Fixing the mesh medially to the Cooper's ligament using tackers in both approaches is important and during IPOM repair the lower

edge of the mesh needs to be sutured to the peritoneum to prevent further recurrences. Close the direct defect using nonabsorbable sutures (Figs. 9 and 10. Usmani et al. have described primary closure of direct inguinal hernia defects with a barbed suture (TEP/ TAPP plus technique) which is also supported and recommended by the International

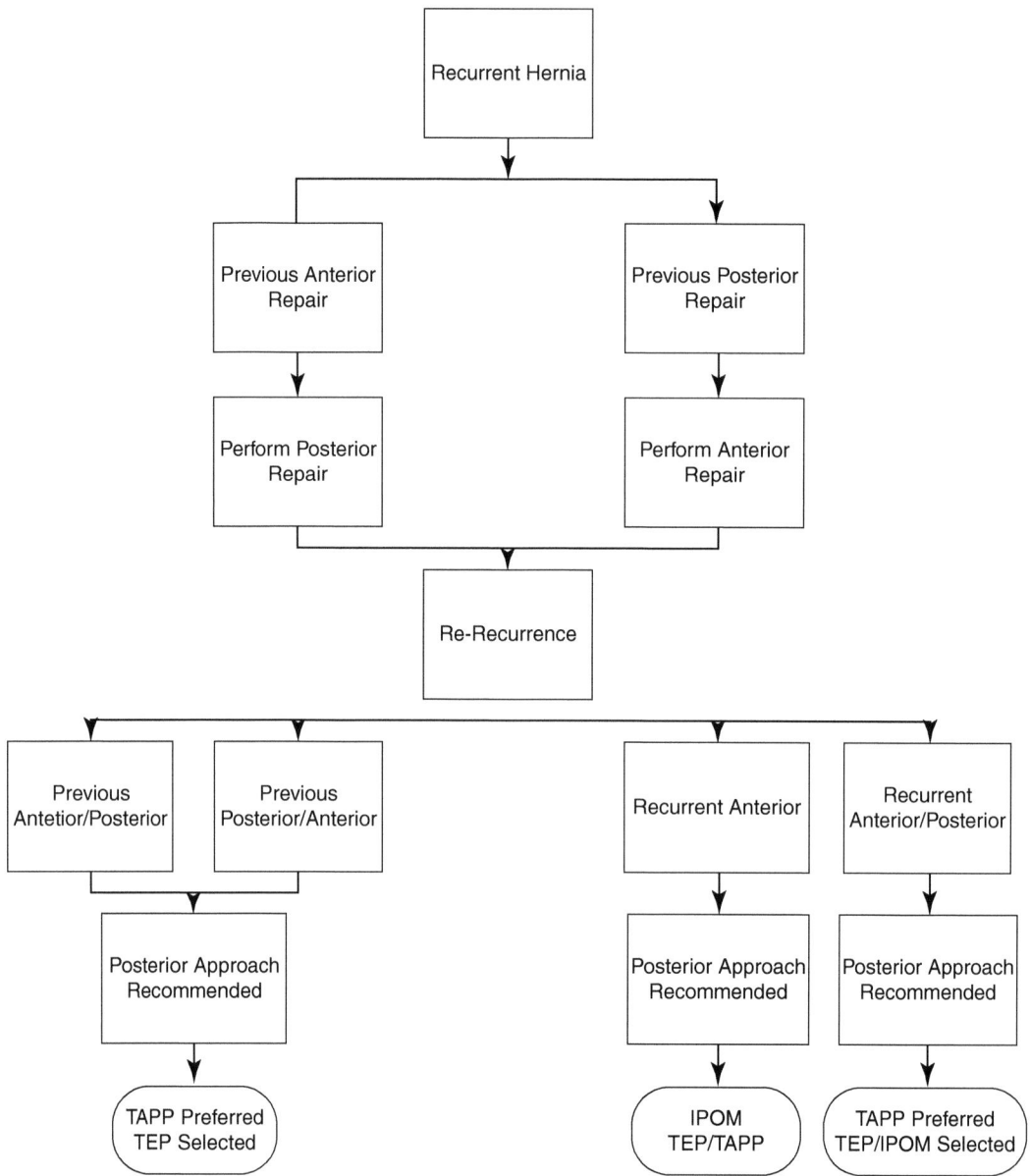

Fig. 11 Algorithm for repair of recurrent and re-recurrent groin hernias

Endohernia Society's Update of Guidelines in 2015 [16]. This technique is known to reduce the incidence of seroma and recurrence rates in large direct inguinal hernia repairs.

- In some patients, a thin layer of fat may allow you a good dissection plan between the mesh and the MPO. The surgeon needs to be extra cautious in the lower area where the Vas defer-

ens, spermatic artery and veins, and iliac vessels are located.

- Consider distorted anatomy always in the repair of re-recurrent hernias.
- Authors have devised this algorithm which can be used to decide on a tailored approach to manage cases of recurrent and re-recurrent inguinal hernia (Fig. 11).

Complications and Management

Complications related to the repair of recurrent hernias are similar to the complications of repair of primary hernias. However, specific to the repair of recurrent hernias, the surgeon should be mindful that distorted anatomy, nonvirgin planes, and the presence of possible previous meshes do increase the risk of postoperative pain. Dissection through previous plans also increases the risk of bowel, bladder, and vessel injury especially through the posterior approach for recurrent and re-recurrent hernias as adhesions would have developed from the previous surgery.

Postoperative Care

See chapter on hernia postoperative care.

Conclusion

Recurrent hernias will become a predictably bigger problem in the future with the increasing number of hernia cases being done worldwide. Although challenging, it is imperative that general surgeons are knowledgeable in various approaches of repair to arm themselves with the skills in dealing with these cases based on the initial repair approach. Re-recurrences which are even more challenging should be referred to specialist hernia centers where possible as their repair might require further advanced techniques.

References

1. Schmidt L, Öberg S, Andresen K, Rosenberg J. Recurrence rates after repair of inguinal hernia in women–a systematic review. JAMA Surg. 2018;153:1135–42. https://doi.org/10.1001/jamasurg.2018.3102.
2. Bullen NL, Massey LH, Antoniou SA, Smart NJ, Fortelny RH. Open versus laparoscopic mesh repair of primary unilateral uncomplicated inguinal hernia: a systematic review with metaanalysis and trial sequential analysis. Hernia. 2019;23:461–72. https://doi.org/10.1007/s10029-019-01989-7.
3. Burcharth J, Andresen K, Pommergaard HC, et al. Recurrence patterns of direct and indirect inguinal hernias in a nationwide population in Denmark. Surgery. 2014;155:173–7.
4. HerniaSurge group. International guideline for groin hernia management. Hernia. 2018;22:1–165. https://doi.org/10.1007/s10029-017-1668-x.
5. Bisgaard T, Bay-Nielsen M. Kehlet H re-recurrence after operation for recurrent inguinal hernia. A nationwide 8-year follow-up study on the role of type or repair. Ann Surg. 2008;247:707–11. https://doi.org/10.1097/SLA.0b013e31816b18e3.
6. van den Heuvel BJ, Wijsmuller AR, Fitzgibbons RJ. Indications–treatment options for symptomatic and asymptomatic patients. In: International guidelines for groin hernia management. Hernia. 2018;22:1–165. https://doi.org/10.1007/s10029-017-1668-x.
7. Siddaiah-Subramanya M, Ashrafi D, Memon B, Memon MA. Causes of recurrence in laparoscopic inguinal hernia repair. Hernia. 2018;22:975–86. https://doi.org/10.1007/s10029-018-1817-x.
8. Burcharth J. The epidemiology and risk factors for recurrence after inguinal hernia surgery. Dan Med J. 2014;61:B4846.
9. Murphy BL, Zhang J, Ubl DS, Habermann EB, Farley DR, Paley K. Surgical trends of groin hernia repairs performed for recurrence in medicare patients. Hernia. 2018;23:677–83. https://doi.org/10.1007/s10029-018-1852-7.
10. Bittner R, Arregui ME, Bisgaard T, et al. Guidelines for laparoscopic (TAPP) and endoscopic (TEP) treatment of inguinal hernia [international Endohernia society (IEHS)]. Surg Endosc. 2011;25:2773–843.
11. Niebuhr H, Pawlak M, Śmietański M. Diagnostic testing modalities. In: International guidelines for groin hernia management. Hernia. 2018;22:1–165. https://doi.org/10.1007/s10029-017-1668-x.
12. Köckerling F, Schug-Pass C. Diagnostic laparoscopy as decision tool for re-recurrent inguinal hernia treatment following open anterior and laparo-endoscopic posterior repair. Front Surg. 2017;4:22. https://doi.org/10.3389/fsurg.2017.00022.
13. Karthikesalingam A, Markar SR, Holt PJE, Praseedom RK. Meta-analysis of randomized controlled trials comparing laparoscopic with open mesh repair of recurrent inguinal hernia. Br J Surg. 2010;97:4–11. https://doi.org/10.1002/bjs.6902.
14. Tran H, Weyhe D, Berrevoet F, Recurre Weyhe D, Klinge U. Meshes. In: International guidelines for groin hernia management. Hernia. 2018;22:1–165. https://doi.org/10.1007/s10029-017-1668-x.
15. Fortelny RH, Sanders DL, Montgomery A. Mesh fixation. In: International guidelines for groin hernia management. Hernia. 2018;22:1–165. https://doi.org/10.1007/s10029-017-1668-x.
16. Usmani F, Wijerathne S, Malik S, et al. Effect of direct defect closure during laparoscopic inguinal hernia repair ("TEP/TAPP plus" technique) on postoperative outcomes. Hernia. 2020;24:167–71. https://doi.org/10.1007/s10029-019-02036-1.

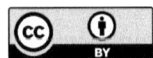

Laparo-Endoscopic Approach to Complex Inguinal Hernia [Inguinoscrotal Hernias: Sliding Hernias]

Rakesh Kumar Gupta and Davide Lomanto

Abbreviations

CSTs	Component separation techniques
PPP	Preoperative progressive pneumoperitoneum
SSIs	Surgical site infections
TAPP	Trans abdominal preperitoneal repair
TEP	Totally extraperitoneal repair

Background

Very few surgical entities have fascinated surgeons over centuries than the complexity of inguinal hernia repair. Despite being one of the commonest procedures performed, the surgical fraternity all over the world is still in the quest for the final word on the best type of repair. Similarly, treatment of complex groin hernia remains the same [1]. Complex groin hernia can be defined as those with large size, e.g., inguinoscrotal hernia, sliding hernia, multiple recurrences, infected mesh and strangulation, etc. The approach to these hernias involves a great deal of preoperative preparations and decision-making that is carried through the operation and postoperative period. The laparoscopic approach in these cases is feasible and with good outcomes provided that the surgeon adheres to three M's; mastery of the anatomy, meticulous dissection, and modus operandi [2]. No wonder hundreds of procedures have been described for the treatment of complex groin hernia. There has been always a concern about whether complex groin hernia can be treated with laparoscopy or not but more favorable outcomes have been found with laparoscopy than in open surgery [1].

The laparoscopic exploration allows for the treatment of incarcerated/strangulated hernias and the intraoperative diagnosis of occult hernias.

TAPP appeared to be superior in terms of learning curve, diagnosis of occult hernia, and the feasibility for incarcerated or strangulated hernia [3].

Complex Inguinoscrotal Hernias

Any hernia that passes beyond the inguinal ligament and extends to the scrotum is termed as inguinoscrotal hernia [4, 5]. Scrotal hernia has been defined subjectively in the past as scrotal, big scrotal, giant scrotal hernia, etc. Decision to

R. K. Gupta (✉)
GS & MIS Unit, Department of Surgery, B.P. Koirala Institute of Health Sciences, Dharan, Nepal

D. Lomanto
Department of Surgery, YLL School of Medicine, National University Singapore, Singapore, Singapore
e-mail: surdl@nus.edu.sg

© The Author(s) 2023
D. Lomanto et al. (eds.), *Mastering Endo-Laparoscopic and Thoracoscopic Surgery*,
https://doi.org/10.1007/978-981-19-3755-2_58

choose the best approach to treat such a hernia is not unanimous and is different to treating surgeons. This may be attributed to absence of uniformity in classification of such type of hernias. In this scenario, Ertem M et al. have proposed a volumetric classification and based on this, the surgical procedure [4] (Table 1 and Fig. 1).

The clinical external measurement will provide almost exact volume. Normally the CECT for decision-making for scrotal hernia is not required, except in giant hernias and hernia with loss of domain.

Those inguinoscrotal hernias that are hanging below the midpoint of the inner thigh when the patient is standing is called as giant inguinal hernias [6] (Fig. 2). The term giant scrotal hernia should be used if the hernia volume is greater than 1000 ml [4].

Table 1 Choice of surgery in relation to scrotal volume

Textile	Volume (ml)	Surgical procedure
S	0 - 500	
M	500 - 1000	
L	1000-2000	
XL	2000-3000	
XXL	3000 <	

* depends on surgeon's experience and preference

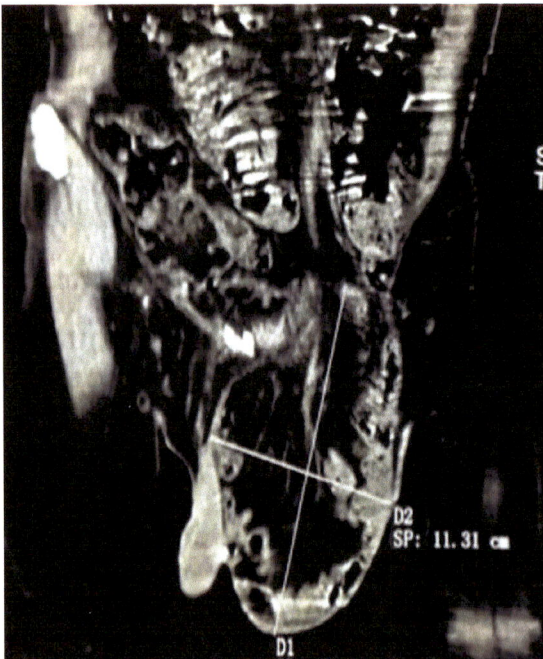
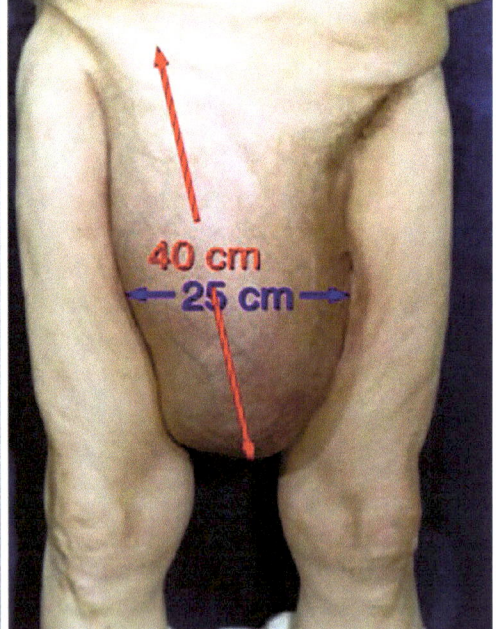

Fig. 1 Measurement of scrotum volume in giant hernia Scrotal volume can be calculated with the following formula [4]

Scrotal volume = length * width * depth * 0.52

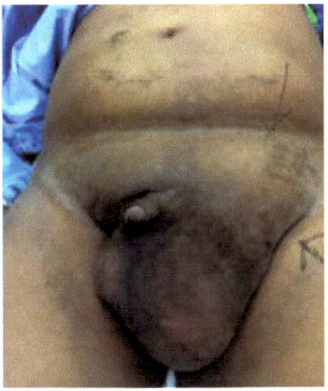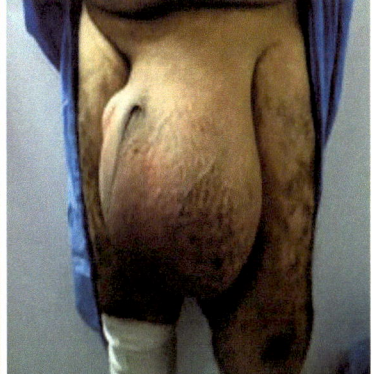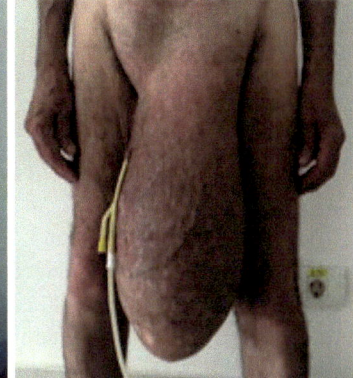

Fig. 2 Showing giant scrotal hernias Type I, II, and III

Challenges with Complex Inguinoscrotal Hernia

1. Large abdominal wall defects [EHS:M/L $\geq$ 3].
2. Difficulty in dissecting large hernia sac.
3. Increased risk of injury to inferior epigastric artery, testicular vessels, urinary bladder, sigmoid colon, etc.
4. Chronic bacterial and fungal skin infections.
5. Loss of domain.
6. Scrotal reconstruction.

Laparoscopy vs. Open

1. Comparison of laparoscopic and Lichtenstein repair in recurrent hernia by Z. Demetreshavili showed similar operative time ($p = 0.068$) and postoperative outcomes (infection, seroma, hematoma) ($p = 0.19$), less postoperative pain ($p = 0.002$) and few sicker days leave in TAPP ($p < 0.001$) [7].
2. Laparoscopic repair in cases of sliding hernia is safe and feasible with safe outcome. TAPP is the preferable method [1].

We will here be discussing about the laparoscopic management of the same. Complex groin hernia is much more difficult to repair through the anterior approach, not only because of the large volume to be reduced but also due to the retroperitoneal sliding component that usually occurs [8].

Indications for Laparoscopic Approach

All complex groin hernia cases are fit for surgery.

Contraindications for Laparoscopic Approach

1. Prior groin irradiation.
2. Prior pelvic lymph node.
3. Poor candidate for general anesthesia.
4. Giant inguinal hernia type II and III.

Relative Contraindications

1. Prior laparoscopic herniorrhaphies [9].

Preoperative Assessment

1. Select those patients who give consent for laparoscopic surgery.
2. Conditions predisposing hernia such as constipation, prostatism, pulmonary conditions asthma, COPD) should be addressed.
3. Adoption of lifestyle modifications such as cessation of smoking, exercise, and weight loss should be encouraged.
4. Hernia characteristics such as size, recurrent, bilateral, incarcerated, and strangulation should be assessed.

5. Consent should be taken and should be explained about the increased risk of complications such as seroma, SSI, vascular injury, injury to vas deferens, injury to bowel and urinary bladder, chronic groin pain, and recurrence.

As techniques of TEP and TAPP has been already discussed in the previous chapter, in this chapter an overview of special consideration that must be kept in mind while approaching laparoscopically will be discussed.

Special Considerations in Dealing Inguinoscrotal Hernias

1. Insertion of an additional fourth 5 mm trocar may be needed to facilitate the exposure (Fig. 3).
2. Wider preperitoneal space creation is required.
3. In the case of large and incarcerated hernias, *releasing incision* on transversalis sling is given with hook cautery at the 10 o'clock position (if necessary division of the epigastric vessels may be done) to allow *remote hernial access* and *increases working space* and complete reduction of the sac (Fig. 4).

4. Inferior epigastric vessels may be divided which allow access to the deep internal ring without injury and also allows the smooth placement of mesh without wrapping.
5. If hernia is not reducible, ring can be enlarged with anteromedial incision in case of direct hernia whereas antero-lateral incision in case of indirect hernia.
6. As sac is quite large in these patients, if complete reduction is not possible, it can be divided as distal as possible.
7. In order to check the viability of bowel in case of TEP, umbilical port is transferred from preperitoneal position to intraperitoneal position. If there is a need for resection of nonviable segment it can be done intraperitoneally once the repair of hernia is completed preperitoneally.
8. Hybrid approach: Combined laparoscopic approaches and open extraperitoneal approach when the content of the sac cannot be reduced (Fig. 5).
9. As defect is large, a standard weight mesh with wider covering (at least 4–5 cm) is preferable. The fixation must be favored in such cases.
10. A closed suction drain is inserted to prevent the inevitable incidence of postoperative seroma (optional).

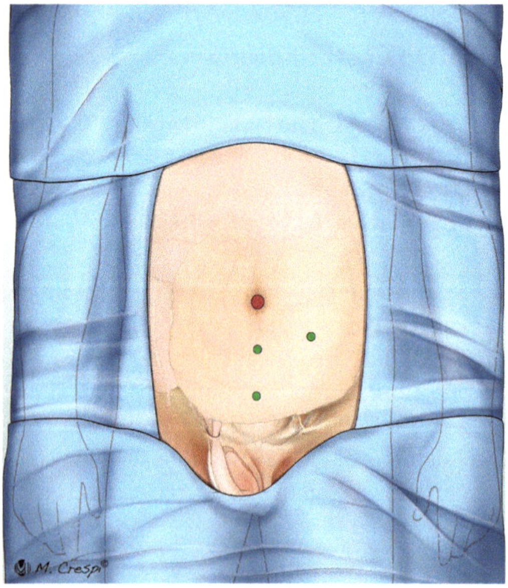

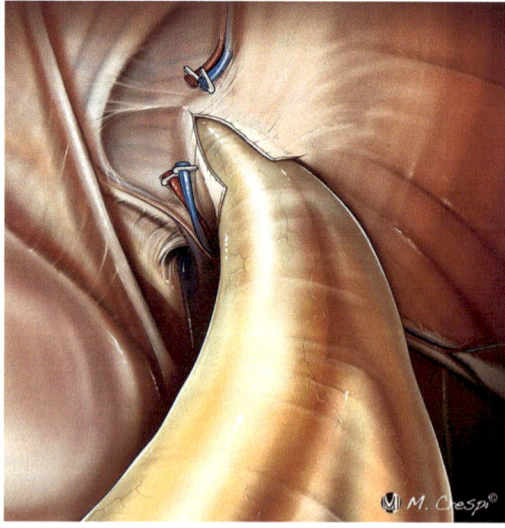

Fig. 3 Creation of extra port in TEPP

Fig. 4 Showing division of transverse sling

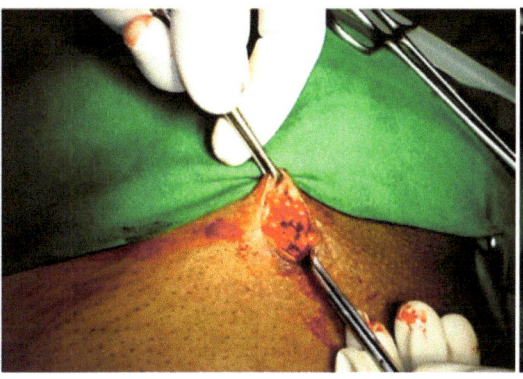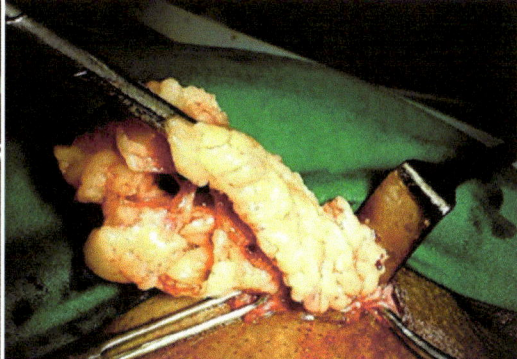

Fig. 5 Hybrid approach: combined laparoscopy and open

11. In patients with loss of domain: various adjuncts to increase intra-abdominal space is required (i.e., preoperative progressive pneumoperitoneum, Botulinum toxins, component separation, musculocutaneous flaps, etc.) [6].

Sliding Inguinal Hernia

Sliding hernia is very uncommon of all hernia and contributes 6–8% of all hernia cases [10, 11]. It is a type of hernia in which the posterior wall of the sac is not only formed by the parietal peritoneum but also formed by the sigmoid colon with its mesentery on its left side, caecum on the right side, and often with the portion of bladder in both sides [10, 12]. Sliding hernia is also called as "longstanding hernia" and usually developed in old age patients with a history of long duration [10, 11].

Bendavid defines a sliding hernia as a "protrusion through an abdominal wall opening of a retroperitoneal organ, with or without its mesentery, with or without an adjacent peritoneal sac" [1, 10].

He describes three types of sliding hernia [1, 10, 11] (Fig. 5).

1. Type 1: most common and contributes 95% of sliding hernias
     : when a part of the peritoneal sac is made up by the wall of a viscus,
2. Type 2: contributes 5% of sliding hernias

     : when the mesentery of a retroperitoneal viscus forms part of the wall of the peritoneal sac
3. Type 3: very rare
     : when the viscus itself protrudes without a peritoneal sac.

Challenges with Sliding Hernia

1. Diagnosis of this hernia is not possible preoperatively and is usually an intraoperative finding [11] (Figs. 6 and 7).
2. This hernia continues to test the surgeon's understanding of the inguinal canal's anatomy and technical expertise with a significant rate of complications and a higher rate of recurrence [1, 10].

The surgeon's *experience* and *comfort level* should dictate the choice of the *safest* repair for the patient. The common techniques and consideration of laparoscopic approach [TEP/TAPP] to inguinoscrotal hernias is already discussed in earlier chapter. We will here be discussing about the common pitfalls and the techniques/precautions to deal with it. Laparoscopic repair of sliding inguinal hernias is feasible and safe with impressive results. TAPP approach is preferred over TEP approach as it allows better identification of these hernias and offers easier method of sac reduction [1].

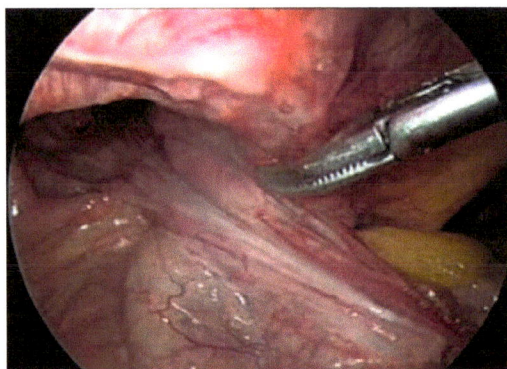

Fig. 6 Transabdominal view of sliding hernia

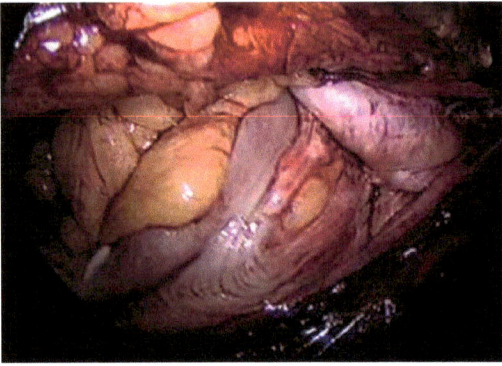

Fig. 7 Totally extraperitoneal view of sliding hernia

Special Considerations [1]

1. Foleys's catheter needs to be inserted after induction of anesthesia-risk of urinary bladder injury is minimized by doing this.
2. After induction of general anesthesia attempt to reduce hernia content should be made. For irreducible hernias, TAPP should be done whereas reducible hernia needs to be operated by TEP.
3. Insertion of an additional fourth 5 mm trocar may be needed to facilitate the exposure.
4. As diagnosis of sliding hernia is intraoperative we should see whether the content of the sac is forming the wall of the sac or adhered to it. moreover sliding hernia may be missed during TEP repair as diagnosis is made only after opening of peritoneal sac which is not routinely opened in TEP repair.

5. Usually sliding hernia presents with irreducibility and also poses difficulty in reduction of sac, most surgeons prefer TAPP repair. Moreover, due to the high incidence of recurrence, retroperitonealization of the organ is also recommended which is possible with TAPP repair.
6. Attempt to separate the sac from the sliding component should never be made. In case of difficulty in reduction of sac, it may be divided beyond the level of the content. The deep inguinal ring may be cut on superolateral aspect to facilitate reduction of hernia contents.
7. The technique of a combined approach to these difficult cases can simply be another useful tool in the hernia surgeons' armamentarium.
8. Do not hesitate to convert laparoscopic approach to open approach in cases where there is difficulty in reduction of sac and high risk of injuries to hernia contents. Stoppa or Lichtenstein repair may be preferable in some situations.

To ensure the proper safe landing of both patients and surgeons while approaching complex inguinoscrotal hernias laparoscopically, we strongly advised to follow the 10 golden rules for a safe MIS inguinal hernia repair [3] (summarized below) along with the abovementioned special considerations.

Summary of the Ten Golden Rules [3]

1. Beginning of surgery.
   Creation of peritoneal flaps in TAPP.
   Dissection of preperitoneal space in TEP.
2. Dissection should always follow the peritoneal plane.
3. Dissection must be creating enough space to accommodate an adequately sized mesh.
4. External iliac vein must be visible so that there is no chance of missed femoral hernias.
5. Parietalization of the elements of the cord must be sufficient.

6. If needed the distal hernia sac can be transected or abandoned in case of complex inguinoscrotal hernias.
7. The deep inguinal canal should be explored in search of lipoma of cord.
8. Mesh should properly cover the myopectineal orifice with overlap of atleast 3–4 cm.
9. Surgeon can decide intraoperatively if the mesh needs fixation.
10. Deflation should be done under direct visualization.

Complications

Intraoperative

1. Pneumoperitoneum.
2. Injury to inferior epigastric artery.
3. Injury to major vessels.
4. Bowel/Urinary bladder injury.
5. Inability to reduce hernia contents.

Postoperative

1. Acute urinary retention.
2. Seroma: The risk of seroma formation is higher for endoscopic techniques than for open repairs [9].
3. Hematoma: The incidence of hematomas is lower for endoscopic (4.2–13.1%) techniques than for open repair (5.6–16%) [9].
4. Chronic pain.
5. Ischemic orchitis.
6. Testicular atrophy.
7. Early recurrence.

Postoperative Care

1. Acute urinary retention: single shot rubber catheter drainage/Foley's catheterization.
2. Day care surgery: can be discharged on the same day.

3. Analgesics: injectables/orals,
   To improve postoperative pain, infiltration of trocar site with local anesthesia is recommended.
4. Thromboprophylaxis: It is recommended that thromboembolic prophylaxis is given according to usual routines in patients with risk factors [9].

Conclusion

There has been little evidence about laparoscopic approach to complex inguinoscrotal hernias and sliding inguinal hernias. Before making a bold claim which technique is the best, more research should be conducted on this. Laparoscopic approach to these hernias is possible with a meticulous selection of patients and taking special considerations into account. The choice of techniques whether TAPP/TEPP depends upon the surgeon's choice with which he/she is comfortable.

References

1. Patle NM, Tantia O, Prasad P, Khanna S, Sen B. Sliding inguinal hernias: scope of laparoscopic repair. J Laparoendosc Adv Surg Tech. 2011;21(3):227–31. https://doi.org/10.1089/lap.2010.0473.
2. Simons MP, Smietanski M, Bonjer HJ, et al. International guidelines for groin hernia management. Hernia. 2018;22(1):1–165. https://doi.org/10.1007/s10029-017-1668-x.
3. Claus C, Furtado M, Malcher F, Cavazzola LT, Felix E. Ten golden rules for a safe MIS inguinal hernia repair using a new anatomical concept as a guide. Surg Endosc. 2020;34(4):1458–64.
4. Ertem M, Gök H, Özben V, Hatipoğlu E, Yildiz E. Can volumetric measurement be used in the selection of treatment for inguinoscrotal hernias? Turkish J Surg. 2018;34(1):13–6. https://doi.org/10.5152/turkjsurg.2017.3710.
5. Siow SL, Mahendran HA, Hardin M, Chea CH, Nik Azim NA. Laparoscopic transabdominal approach and its modified technique for incarcerated scrotal hernias. Asian J Surg. 2013;36(2):64–8. https://doi.org/10.1016/j.asjsur.2012.11.004.

6. Hodgkinson DJ, McIlrath DC. Scrotal reconstruction for giant inguinal hernias. Surg Clin North Am. 1984;64(2):307–13. https://doi.org/10.1016/S0039-6109(16)43287-1.

7. Demetrashvili Z, Qerqadze V, Kamkamidze G, et al. Comparison of lichtenstein and laparoscopic transabdominal preperitoneal repair of recurrent inguinal hernias. Int Surg. 2011;96(3):233–8. https://doi.org/10.9738/CC53.1.

8. Beitler JC, Gomes SM, Coelho ACJ, Manso JEF. Complex inguinal hernia repairs. Hernia. 2009;13(1):61–6. https://doi.org/10.1007/s10029-008-0432-7.

9. Bittner R, Köckerling F, Fitzgibbons RJ, LeBlanc KA, Mittal SK, Chowbey P. Laparo-endoscopic hernia surgery: evidence based clinical practice; 2018. p. 1–483. https://doi.org/10.1007/978-3-662-55493-7.

10. Adams RA, Wysocki AP. Outcome of sliding inguinal hernia repair. Hernia. 2010;14(1):47–9. https://doi.org/10.1007/s10029-009-0563-5.

11. Shoba Rani B, Lokesh K, Sudha MG, Babu YM. A clinical study on sliding inguinal hernias. J Evid Based Med Healthc. 2015;2(39):6327–43. https://doi.org/10.18410/jebmh/2015/870.

12. Wang P, Huang Y, Ye J, Gao G, Zhang F, Wu H. Large sliding inguino-scrotal hernia of the urinary bladder. Med (United States). 2018;97(13):e9998. https://doi.org/10.1097/MD.0000000000009998.

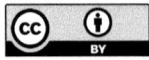

Part XVII

Incisional/Ventral Hernia Repair

Laparoscopic Intraperitoneal Onlay Mesh (IPOM) and IPOM Plus

Sajid Malik and Sujith Wijerathne

Introduction

The field of minimally invasive surgery has revolutionized the surgical practice by imparting its ability to avoid major abdominal wall incisions [1]. It is expected that laparoscopic surgery might reduce the burden of incisional hernias which is the most common complication after abdominal surgery and despite ongoing research in wound closure and reparative techniques, abdominal incisional hernia remains an unresolved problem [1]. The outcome of incisional hernia may have major social and economic implications and worldwide 10–30% of patients undergoing laparotomy will develop an incisional hernia and subsequent conventional open repair often fails to adequately address this substantial problem [2]. The recurrence rate for primary tissue repairs may approach the 35% range, which is higher than the primary occurrence rate; when repaired for recurrence, rates have been reported greater than 50%. Although the advent of prosthetic repair has significantly reduced the recurrence rate compared with that of primary suture repair, it remains in the ranges of 10–24% [3].

Gradual decreases in recurrence rates have been realized over the last decade as minimally invasive techniques have been increasingly utilized. For example, in some series, the recurrence rate of initial incisional hernias has been reduced to 2–9% [4–6].

Moreover, multiple studies demonstrate that laparoscopic repair of ventral hernia results in a short length of stay and a quick return to normal activities [6]. The recurrence rate after laparoscopic repair of a recurrent hernia ranges between 9% and 12%, which is an improvement when compared with recurrence rates of 20% after conventional repair with prosthetic material [6, 7]. Clearly, the laparoscopic approach to repair ventral hernia has significantly improved the management of this problem. This technique involves either an intraperitoneal onlay mesh (IPOM) with or without defect closure (IPOM+) or preperitoneal mesh-placement (PPOM) as in the open sublay repair [8, 9].

This chapter will review the risk factors, indications, contraindications, preoperative preparation, and postoperative care after laparoscopic ventral hernia repair. Additionally, it will discuss the complications and steps to avoid these complications for safe practice.

S. Malik (✉)
Department of General Surgery, Allama Iqbal Medical College, Jinnah Hospital, Lahore, Pakistan

S. Wijerathne
General Surgery and Minimally Invasive Surgery, Department of Surgery, National University Health System, Singapore, Singapore

Department of General Surgery, Alexendra Hospita, Singapore, Singapore

© The Author(s) 2023
D. Lomanto et al. (eds.), *Mastering Endo-Laparoscopic and Thoracoscopic Surgery*,
https://doi.org/10.1007/978-981-19-3755-2_59

Risk Factors for Primary and Recurrent Ventral Hernia

Risk factors for the development of incisional hernia formation are not well defined and prevention strategies are still a long way to know. Some well-established systemic and local factors being reported in many studies are enlisted as follows [10, 11].

Systemic Factors

- obesity
- diabetes
- steroid use
- benign prostatic hypertrophy
- pulmonary disease
- advancwed age
- Male gender
- Chronic coughing
- Pregnancy
- Weight lifting

Local Factors

- size of fascial defect
- type of incision
- method of fascial closure
- postoperative hematoma
- postoperative wound infection

Indications

- symptomatic ventral/incisional hernia larger than 3 cm
- recurrent hernia

Contraindications

- Loss of domain (ventral larger 20 cm)
- Strangulated hernia
- Gangrenous bowel
- Peritonitis
- Intra-abdominal Sepsis
- Infection

- Eventration
- Systemic condition like cirrhosis with caput medusae

Preoperative Preparation

- Routine blood investigations
- Bowel Preparation (optional)
- Antibiotic prophylaxis
- CT-Scan (selected cases: recurrent, incarcerated, etc.) (Fig. 1)
- Pulmonary function (obese)
- Informed Consent (risk for enterotomy, conversion, seroma, etc.)
- DVT prophylaxis

OT Setup, Patient's Position, and Trocars Placement

- Monitor position (Fig. 2)
  - Position of the monitor should be opposite to the trocars
  - Height and distance should follow standard principles
- Instrumentation required (Fig. 3)
  - Veress Needle (Optional)
  - Trocars
  - Laparoscopic camera unit with 30° telescope 10 mm and 5 mm
  - Atraumatic Graspers (2) 5 mm
  - Curved Scissors (1) 5 mm

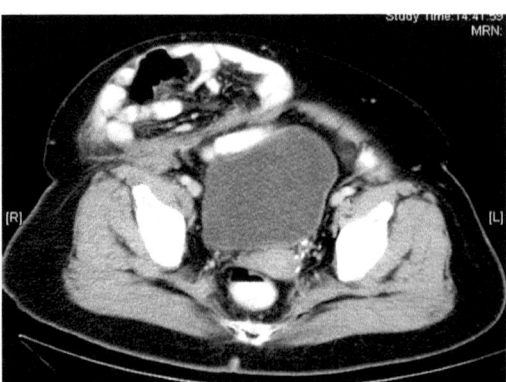

Fig. 1 Axial contrast-enhanced reformatted CT image of the abdomen shows herniation of gut and omental fat through a large abdominal defect

- Bowel Clamp (2) 5 mm
- Suction/irrigation device
- Energy source preferably LigaSure (1) 5 mm
- Suture passer/14 G IV Cannula and nonabsorbable suture
- Tackers; absorbable or nonabsorbable (for mesh fixation)
- Clip applier (1) 5 mm (optional)
- Hook diathermy (1) 5 mm (optional)
• Patient Position and preparation
  - Standard supine position with both arms tucked at the side or on the arm board depending on the size and site of hernia
  - Surgeon and Assistant stand on the side of the patient

- Foleys catheter for large, recurrent, incisional, or partially or irreducible hernia
• Trocars size and position
  - 12 mm Optical trocar (1)
  - 5 mm trocars (2)
  - 12 mm port inserted laterally between the costal margin and the Anterior superior iliac spine (ASIS)
  - 5 mm ports (2) inserted on either side of the optical trocar
  - an additional 5 mm port may be required in an approachable position for the mesh fixation.

Surgical Technique

The hernia defect should be marked before the abdominal cavity is entered (Fig. 4).

First Trocar Insertion

Pneumoperitoneum can be established using either a Veress needle or a Hasson trocar. The "open technique" using Hasson's trocar should be preferred. In our experience, we establish the pneumoperitoneum using open Hasson's technique which is quite safe entry. Optical trocar entry should be preferred in obese male with thick anterior abdominal wall where open technique would be difficult to achieve (i.e., Opti-View) (Fig. 5a, b).

The direct view trocar with 0° scope is very useful to avoid bowel injury accessing the abdo-

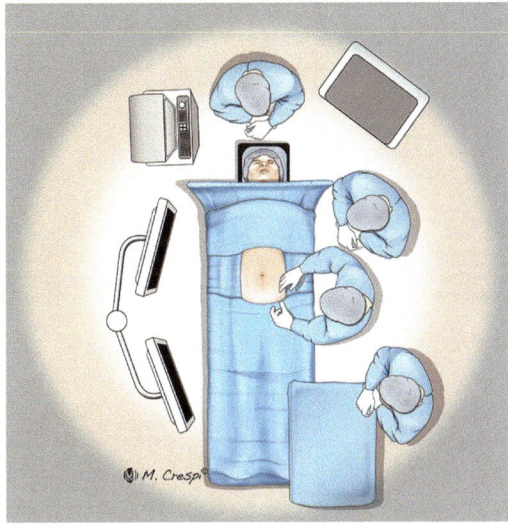

Fig. 2 OT setup

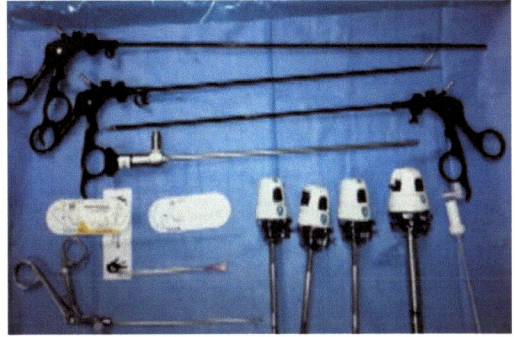

Fig. 3 Common instruments for IPOM/IPOM+ repair

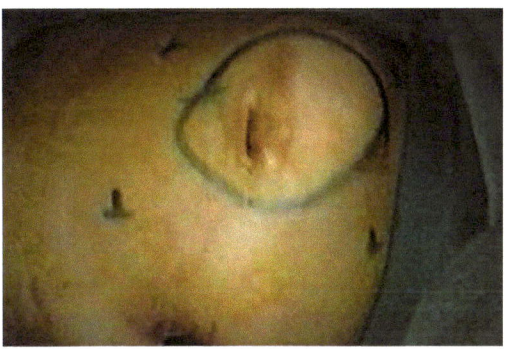

Fig. 4 Marking of defect

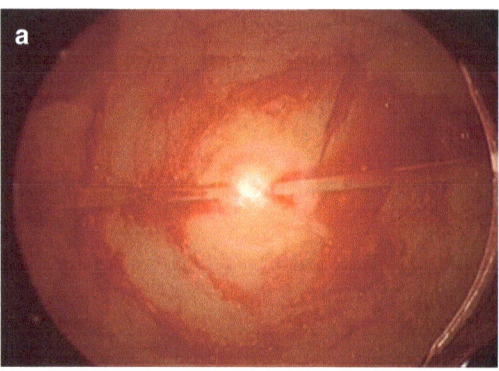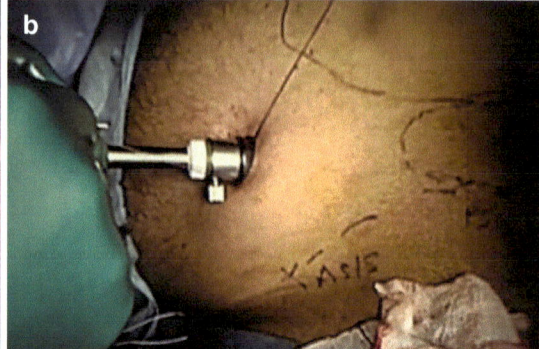

Fig. 5 (**a**) Endoscopic view of Opti-view. (**b**) Hasson's technique

men. The first trocar is inserted laterally between the anterior iliac spine and the subcostal margin (anterior axillary line). An angled [30° or 45°] laparoscope, inserted through the 10–12 mm trocar, must be utilized to facilitate the visualization of the anterior abdominal wall.

Working Trocars

Working Trocars placed too close to the edge of the defect may not allow adequate working space. Trocars placed too laterally may limit the downward displacement of the instrument handle. Once the first trocar is inserted, usually two, 5 mm trocars are placed under vision and well lateral to the defect, on either side of the 10–12 mm port.

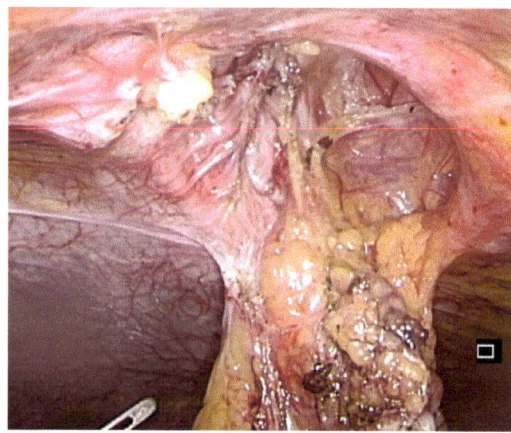

Fig. 6 Abdominal wall defect with adhesions

Preparing the Defect: Adhesiolysis

If necessary, adhesiolysis is first performed to clear the margins of the defect and to avoid bowel injury, the use of diathermy or the ultrasonic dissector should be very careful. Any thermal injury to intestine could result in catastrophic peritonitis and result in delayed repair. Despite the fact that there are plenty of video material available on social media for using Ultrascission®, LigaSure®, or Thunderbeat®, authors are confident in using these devices, but with caution, being aware of the inherent risk. After adhesiolysis is performed a reduction of hernia contents is started with the steady hand-over-hand withdrawal of the sac contents (Figs. 6 and 7).

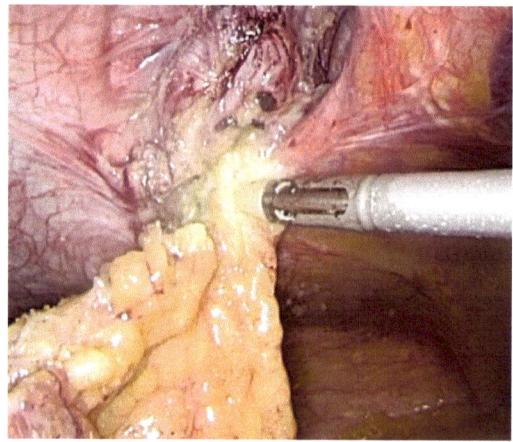

Fig. 7 Adhesiolysis to delineate defect margins

External countertraction applied by the assistant may facilitate the reduction of the hernia sac contents and can lower the abdominal "ceiling" to provide better working space. Care must be taken to avoid excessive tension with grasper to minimize the risk of intestinal injury at this step. In rare cases, when incarceration is not possible to reduce then sharp dissection of the fascial edge of the defect will facilitate the reduction.

Measurement of Defect Size

Once the margins of the hernia are well delineated and cleared, the defect can be measured by external palpation or with an intra-abdominal ruler/suture, or even with a laparoscopic instrument. It is best practice to reduce intra-abdominal pressure to 6 mmHg in order to get accurate size. Mesh overlap to defect according to mesh type should be selected appropriately.

Mesh Size and Choice of Mesh

At the moment, plenty of different types of mesh are available in the market: Gore-Tex and PTFE (dual mesh or dual mesh plus), polyester, or polypropylene coated with different antiadhesive agents. All the mesh comes in different sizes and dimensions. A prosthetic mesh is then tailored to ensure at least 5 cm overlap of all defect margins. Distinct "orienting" marks are placed on the mesh and on the skin (Fig. 6), respectively, to assist with intra-abdominal orientation. Individual needs and properties should be kept in mind for appropriate mesh size and choice.

Mesh Fixation

Suture, tacking devices, and glue fixation methods are common in practice while authors believe to use a tailor approach for devising a final method of mesh fixation based on previous repair, site, size, and other factors. Main idea of fixation is to keep the mesh in contact with the anterior abdominal wall in order to achieve fibrosis and to avoid landing of mesh in the peritoneal cavity to prevent complications. Authors recommend to practice absorbable spiral tack fixation over

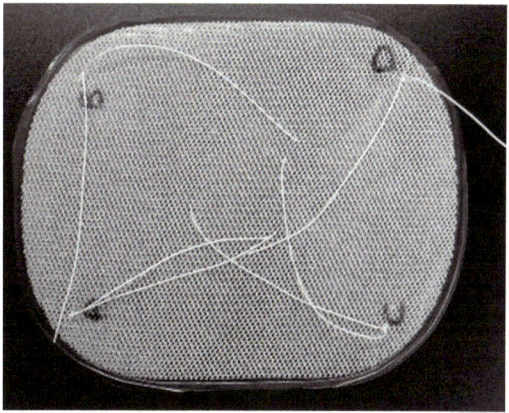

Fig. 8 Four cardinal sutures for mesh anchoring

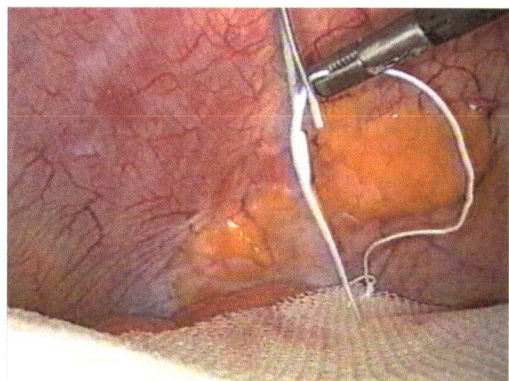

Fig. 9 Transabdominal suture

suture repair but a tailored approach should always be practiced before making any decision.

If suture fixation is decided then sutures should be placed at four cardinal points of the mesh (Fig. 8).

For larger prosthesis, additional sutures may be placed between these four sutures. The mesh is then wrapped around a laparoscopic grasper and inserted through the 12 mm trocar. Once inserted, the mesh is unfurled and oriented correctly; the preplaced sutures are pulled transabdominally using a suture passer through the previously marked locations (Fig. 9).

Sutures should not be tied until all sutures are pulled, so that the mesh must be adjusted. If we need to readjust the mesh to better cover the hernia defect, the sutures can simply be pulled back into the abdomen and replaced.

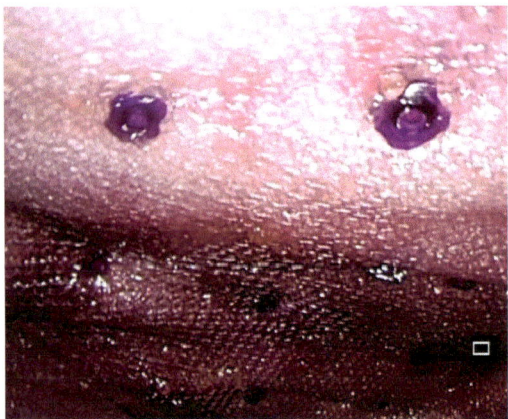

Fig. 10 Spiral AbsorbaTack with safe distance and with one closest to trocar

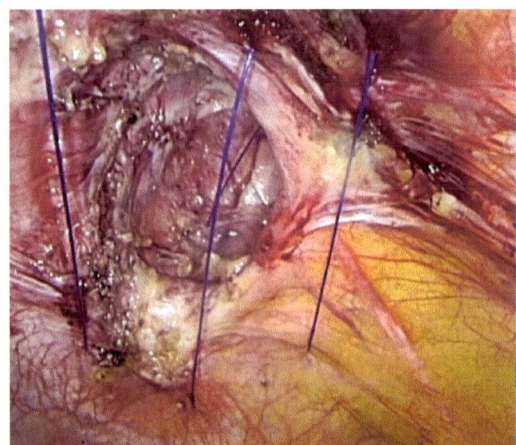

Fig. 11 Placement of Tranfascial suture with suture passer to close the defect before mesh placement

Metallic or Absorbable tacks can be used for fixation but the latter is preferred for less pain, less seroma, and to prevent other long-term post complications. Larger meshes require more number of tacks but it is recommended to keep a safe distance of 1–1.5 cm between two tacks aiming for no gaps in between in order to prevent small bowel obstruction. Selection of length of tack depends on individual factors like abdominal wall fats, distance of solid layer (fascial layers) from mesh, and also type of mesh (prosthetic vs biological). Spiral tack is 3.9 mm long, AbsorbaTack® 4.1 mm (functionally), Sorbafix® 6.4 mm, and Securestrap® 7.1 mm. These lengths are aimed for solid layers like fascia and not just peritoneal or preperitoneal fat. The most difficult part of tack fixation is the one which is the closest to the trocars. In order to fix properly, it is recommended to place a contralateral trocar or use different angels with a combination of camera and working ports to achieve solid fixation (Fig. 10).

IPOM+

In IPOM + additional transfascial sutures should be placed transabdominally to ensure defect closure after sutures passed every 3–5 cm. Suture passer or 14 G IV Cannula should be used in

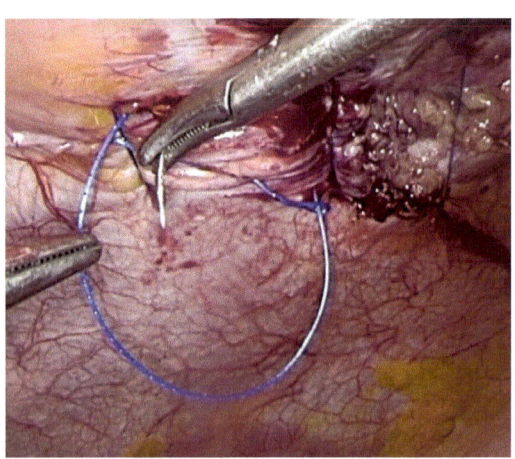

Fig. 12 Intracorporeal continuous repair of defect and divarication as IPOM + repair

order to pass nonabsorbable sutures for this technique. One length of suture should not be used for more than two passes. Care must be taken to avoid underlying visceral injury (Fig. 11).

Intracorporeal continuous repair of defect site or divarication of recti repair by this technique gives an additional benefit to restore anatomy but at the cost of increased post-op complications like pain, seroma, and prolonged immobility (Fig. 12).

Closure

Once mesh fixation is done, abdominal cavity should be explored to look for any bleeding or injury. All CO_2 should allow to exit from the cavity, and 10 mm trocar site should be closed with either nonabsorbable suture or PDS. Care must be taken to avoid any injury or taking abdominal content in sutures. Finger inspection before closure ensures safety.

When to Convert

- dense bowel adhesion
- adhesion between the bowel and previous mesh repair
- Enterotomy with important spillage for enteric fluid
- Unidentified bleeding

Postoperative Care

- Standard Analgesia
- Compressive bandage for 5 post-op days
- Abdominal binder for 4–6 weeks
- Antibiotic therapy if needed
- Conservative management of the seroma, treat by aspiration only if symptomatic (pain) (Fig. 13)

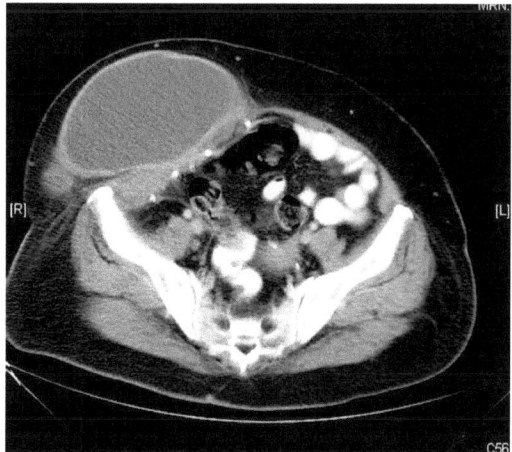

Fig. 13 Postoperative large seroma after mesh repair

Difficult Hernia Location

- *For lateral/flank hernias:* mobilize the colon to get adequate space to place the mesh laterally.
- *For hernia near the costal margin:* sutures may be passed around the rib/costal cartilage to anchor.
- *For Suprapubic hernia*: it is a quite common defect and it is the most difficult and challenging location to repair either in open or laparoscopic repair. Actual experience shows that the best solution is to fix the mesh extraperitoneally at the Cooper's ligament using a TAPP-like technique.

Complications and Management

- Trocar injury
  - Open Hasson's technique
  - Direct visualization
  - Care in scarred abdomen
  - Check for injury
- Adhesiolysis leading to injury
  - Patience in adhesiolysis
  - Careful dissection
  - Use scissors instead of cautery
  - Bipolar hemostasis instead of monopolar
- Post-op ileus or intestinal obstruction
  - Larger mesh with more sutures
  - Composite mesh instead of simple polypropylene meshes
  - Tackering at periphery of mesh
  - Bring omentum at top of bowl after mesh placement
- Mesh infection
  - Consider for first case on list
  - Achieve complete sterilization
  - Antibiotic prophylaxis
  - Change gloves before putting in mesh
  - Minimum handling of mesh
  - Nontouch technique for mesh placement
  - New fixation device (absorbable)
  - Mesh with larger pore size
- Seroma/Bleeding
  - Avoid extensive adhesiolysis

- Safe entry into the abdomen with injury to epigastric vessels
- Invert sac before closing the defect
- Less cautery—less infection
- Compression dressing
- Recurrence
  - Pre-op optimization for systemic conditions as well as for defects
  - Apply appropriate technique
  - Transfascial sutures
  - Use larger mesh to overlap 5 cm from defect
  - Centralization of mesh
  - No gaps at mesh edges
- Suture site pain
  - Liberal but judicious use of local analgesia
  - Adequate post-op analgesia
  - Use glue where preferable to close skin
  - Adequate IV analgesia
  - Abdominal binder
- Missed or delayed bowel injury
  - Use atraumatic graspers
  - Careful inspection of bowel and other structures
  - Gentle manipulation of bowel, if needed then hold mesentery instead of bowel itself
  - Avoid energy devices in the vicinity of bowel
  - Careful inspection at end of the procedure
  - Re-laparoscope if in doubt

Clinical Results

Since its introduction in 1992, the laparoscopic approach has achieved better outcomes than the historical conventional open approach. Patients have also the benefits associated with MIS approach such as less pain, shorter length of hospital stay, and less blood loss [12, 13].

In several series, for laparoscopic ventral hernia repair the length of stay in the hospital ranges between 1 and 3 days, the operating time for laparoscopic repair is less than the conventional repair by as much as 30–40 min and the recurrence rate is significantly reduced around 2–8% [13, 14]. Intraoperative complications like enterotomies should be managed by immediate repair

of the enterotomy and if there is important enteral spillage the mesh repair should be delayed for 1–2 months. Extensive adhesiolysis increases the risk of prolonged ileus, another possible complication that may lengthen the hospital stay.

Lastly, the laparoscopic approach provides additional benefit as a complete exploration of the abdominal cavity, the possibility to add another procedure if needed, an easier adhesiolysis due to the magnification of the view, and a lower chronic postoperative abdominal pain because no wide dissection is performed.

References

1. Wright BE, Niskanen BD, Peterson DJ, Ney AL, Odland MD, Vancamp J, Zera RT, Rodriguez JL. Laparoscopic ventral hernia: are there competitive advantages over traditional methods of repair? Annals Surg. 2002;68:291–5.
2. Söderbäck H, Gunnarsson U, Hellman P, Sandblom G. Incisional hernia after surgery for colorectal cancer: a population-based register study. Int J Color Dis. 2018;33(10):1411–7.
3. Misiakos EP, Patapis P, Zavras N, Tzanetis P, Machairas A. Current trends in laparoscopic ventral hernia repair. JSLS. 2015;19(3):e2015.00048. https://doi.org/10.4293/JSLS.2015.00048.
4. Luijendijk RW, Hop WC, van den Tol MP, de Lange DC, Braaksma MM, JN IJ, et al. A comparison of suture repair with mesh repair for incisional hernia. N Engl J Med. 2000;343:392–8.
5. Mudge M, Hughes LE. Incisional hernia: a 10-year prospective study of incidence and attitudes. Br J Surg. 1985;72:70–1.
6. Köckerling F. Recurrent Incisional hernia repair-an overview. Front Surg. 2019;6:26. https://doi.org/10.3389/fsurg.2019.00026.
7. LeBlanc KA. Booth WV laparoscopic repair of incisional abdominal hernias using expanded polytetrauoroethylene: preliminary findings. Surg Laparosc Endosc. 1993;3:39–41.
8. Heniford BT, Park A, Ramshaw BJ, Voeller G. Laparoscopic repair of ventral hernias: nine years' experience with 850 consecutive hernias. Ann Surg. 2003;238(3):391–9. discussion 399–400
9. Bittner R, et al. Guidelines for laparoscopic treatment of ventral and incisional abdominal wall hernias (international Endohernia society (IEHS))-part 1. Surg Endosc. 2014;28(1):2–29. https://doi.org/10.1007/s00464-013-3170-6.
10. Hoer J, Lawong G, Klinge U, Schumpelick V. Factors influencing the development of incisional hernia. A retrospective study of 2983 laparotomy patients over a period of 10 years. Der Chirurg; Zeitschrift fur alle

Gebiete der operativen Medizen. 2002;73(5):474–80. https://doi.org/10.1007/s00104-002-0425-5.

11. Kokotovic D, Bisgaard T, Helgstrand F. Long-term recurrence and complications associated with elective incisional hernia repair. JAMA. 2016;316(15):1575–82. https://doi.org/10.1001/jama.2016.15217.

12. Pradeep CK, Sharma A, Mehrotra M, Khullar R, Soni V, Baijal M. Laparoscopic repair of ventral/incisional hernias. J Minimal Access Surg. 2006;2:192–8.

13. Lomanto D, Iyer SG, Shabbir A, Cheah WK. C laparoscopic versus open ventral hernia mesh repair: a prospective study. Surg Endosc. 2006;20(7):1030–5.

14. Pierce RA, Spitler JA, Frisella MA, et al. Pooled data analysis of laparoscopic vs open ventral hernia repair: 14 years of patient data accrual. Surg Endosc. 2007;21:378–86.

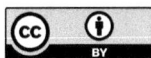

Extraperitoneal Ventral Hernia Repair

Kiyotaka Imamura and Victor Gheorghe Radu

Introduction

"Bridged-IPOM" of Leblanc has been introduced in the 1990s [1]. IPOM is still the mainstay of the repair of ventral hernia, but it has not been without limitation. Adhesive bowel obstruction, mesh erosion, enterocutaneous fistula, and chronic pain are due to tight mesh fixations [2]. Extraperitoneal mesh placement offer advantages: the retromuscular positioning of the mesh permits the integration of both sides, providing the repair with superior tensile strength and costly coated mesh is unnecessary. Nevertheless, the laparoscopic extraperitoneal approach continues to pose limitation in available degree of freedom and significant ergonomic challenge to the operating surgeons.

To overcome these technical difficulties, two approaches were developed, the enhanced-view totally extraperitoneal (eTEP) technique and the mini or less open sublay (MILOS) repair. eTEP has initial approach for the inguinal hernia repair [3], but combined with other retromuscular and preperitoneal repair of ventral hernia repairs such as Rives-Stoppa or Transversus Abdominis Release (TAR), it enables us to put the mesh preperitoneal space and restore the midline defect

[4]. MILOS permits insertion of a large mesh in the retromuscular or preperitoneal space and anatomical reconstruction of the abdominal wall via a small transhernial incision [5].

Indications

Ventral hernias (primary, incisional, and also complex ventral hernias—multiple sites hernias)

Contraindications

- Mesh infection and/or fistula
- Loss of domain
- Dystrophic or ulcerated skin (relative)
- Incarcerated (relative)
- Previous retromuscular ventral hernia repair (relative)
- Previous incision from xiphoid process to the pubic bone (relative)

Preoperative Assessment

- Detailed history (review of prior medical and surgical records of previous interventions, anatomy, and the presence of any mesh or fixation devices)
- Physical examination
- Biochemical studies to assess their baseline health

K. Imamura (✉)
Minimally Invasive Surgery Center,
Yotsuya Medical Cube, Tokyo, Japan
e-mail: k-imamura@mcube.jp

V. G. Radu
Medlife, Bucharest, Romania

© The Author(s) 2023
D. Lomanto et al. (eds.), *Mastering Endo-Laparoscopic and Thoracoscopic Surgery*,
https://doi.org/10.1007/978-981-19-3755-2_60

427

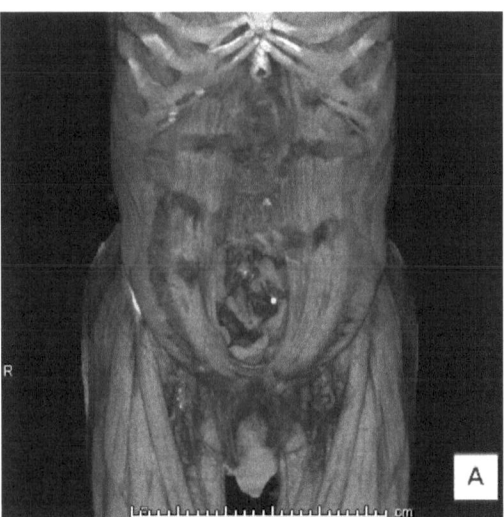

Fig. 1 3D reconstructed CT images are useful to know the relationship between the location of the hernia orifice and anatomy of the abdominal muscle wall

- Defect location and size: up-to-date computed tomography (CT) study of abdomen and pelvis is recommended (Fig. 1)
- Prior or current wound complication
- Presence of ostomy
- Excess skin
- Screening colonoscopy for patients over the age of 50 years (optional)

Enhanced-View Totally Extraperitoneal (eTEP) Technique

OT Setup and Patient's Position

- Supine position with arms tacked by the side; the table is flexed, putting the patient in hyperextension
- After induction of general anesthesia and intubation, a Foley catheter is routinely placed
- Instrumentation required: 0 or 30° telescope 10 mm
- 30° telescope 5 mm
- Atraumatic Graspers [2] 5 mm
- Curved Scissors [1] 5 mm
- Suction/irrigation device
- Needle driver
- Hook electrocautery

- Energy device (optional)
- Trocars size and position (see below)

Surgical Technique

1. Development of the retrorectus space and port placement

   - General rule for the port placement: Trocars to be placed at the opposite part of the abdomen from the location of the hernia defect (Fig. 2).
     - Lower midline defects: cranial approach (Fig. 2 top left).
     - Upper midline defects: caudal approach (Fig. 2 top right).
     - Lateral defects: contralateral lateral approach (Fig. 2 bottom).
   - Dissecting the retrorectus space using a balloon trocar or an optic trocar (Fig. 3).

     Caution: To avoid pneumoperitoneum, trocar should be held horizontally along the anterior layer of the posterior sheath. Figure 4 indicates the tip of the optic trocar mistakenly breaks the posterior sheath.

     Caution: When using a balloon dissector, it is critical to avoid overinflation which may rupture the linea semilunaris and consequently injure the neuromuscular bundles passing through posterior sheath to the rectus muscle.
   - The retromuscular space is insufflated with CO_2 to a pressure of 10–15 mmHg (Fig. 5).

2. Crossover of the midline

   - "Crossover" refers to the surgical dissection that joins one retrorectus space to its contralateral counterpart without violating the intra-abdominal cavity.
   - Accomplished by remaining superficial to the falciform or umbilical ligaments—depending on where the crossing-over of linea alba is performed (Fig. 6).
   - Crossover should ideally be performed at a level of the midline which has not been previously violated.

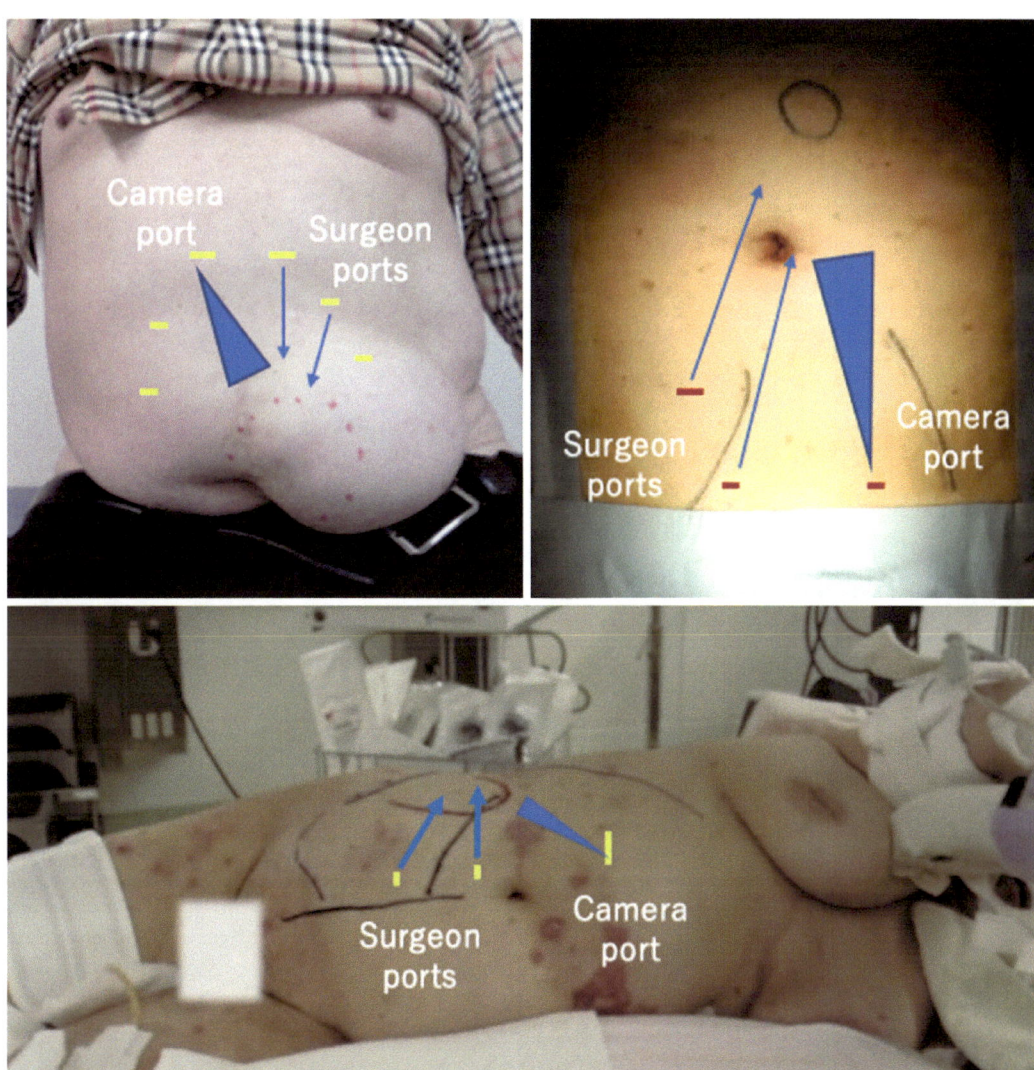

Fig. 2 Ports placement and patient's position in three different situations. Upper left: Cranial approach. Upper right: Caudal approach for an epigastric hernia, inferior epigastric arteries were marked by using preoperative ultrasound. Bottom: Lateral approach for an incisional hernia located just cephalic of the right iliac crest

3. Connection of both retrorectus spaces, left and right

- Both retrorectus spaces are linked by the preperitoneal bridge represented by the falciform ligament and/or umbilical ligament (Fig. 7).
- The retrorectus dissection is limited laterally by the semilunaris lines, where neurovascular bundles pass through the posterior sheath to the rectus muscles.

4. TAR (when needed)

- Indication of TAR: additional TAR may be necessary if maximal defect width closely approximates or exceeds 2× rectus width (Dr. Alfredo Carbonell-ninth Annual AWR Summit, Montana, Feb 2018), tension on the posterior layer, narrow unilateral retrorectus space(<5 cm), poor compliant abdominal wall.

Fig. 3 Dissecting the retrorectus space using an optic trocar

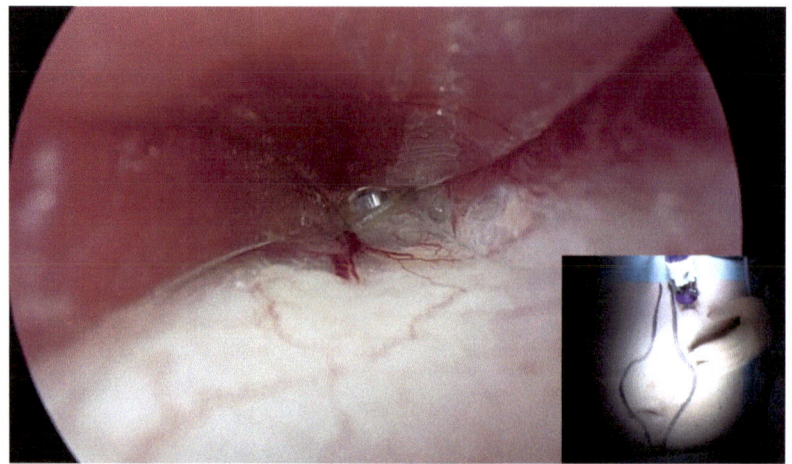

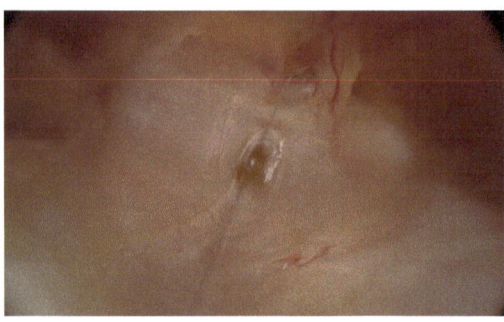

Fig. 4 Tip of the optic trocar entered the extraperitoneal fat

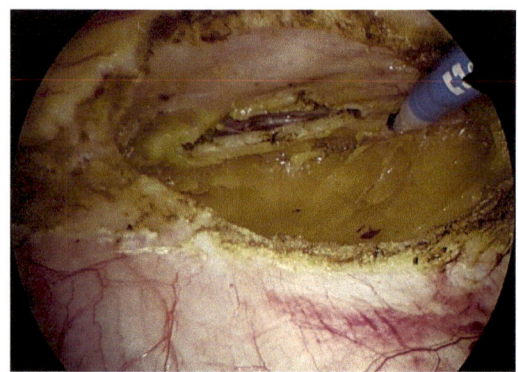

Fig. 6 Crossing the midline anteriorly to the falciform ligament

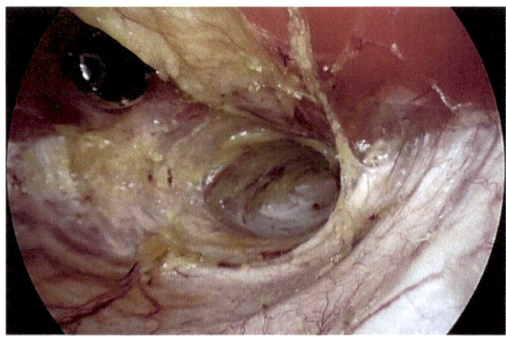

Fig. 5 Retrorectus dissection

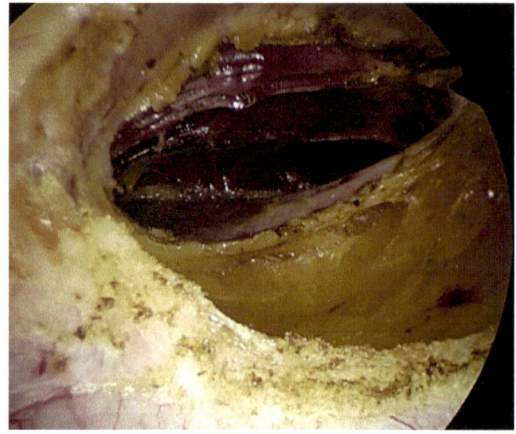

Fig. 7 Connecting the both retrorectus spaces

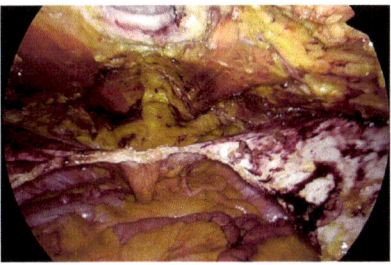 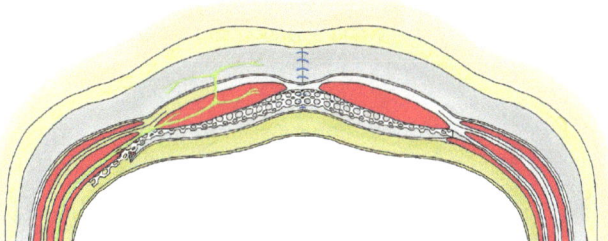

Fig. 8 Hemi-TAR

- Incision of the posterior lamella of the internal oblique fascia 1 cm medially to the semilunaris line to protect the neurovascular bundles (the last 6 pairs of intercostal nerves).
- "Bottom to top" or "top to bottom" depending on comfort of the surgeon.
- Transection of transversus abdominis muscle (TA) and posterior component separation should be done as laterally as possible, to the psoas muscle, and as cranial (behind the diaphragm) as it is needed, depending on hernia location.

5. Closure of the posterior fascial layer defect

- Closure of the posterior layer is necessary to keep a barrier between the mesh and viscera.
- This posterior layer is not a layer of resistance, so it is recommended to preserve the peritoneum (the falciform ligament) as a bridge between the rectus sheaths.
- It is strongly recommended to avoid any tension in the suture line on the posterior layer. To reduce tension between the posterior sheath, hemi-TAR (unilateral) or TAR could be necessary (Fig. 8).

Compared with the anterior hernia orifice, the gap between the posterior layers became larger. In this case, right hemi-TAR was useful to close the posterior layer without tension.

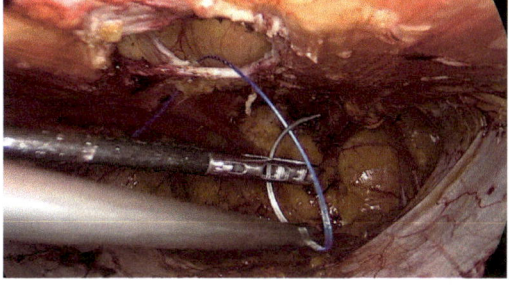

Fig. 9 Closure of anterior sheath by nonabsorbable suture

6. Closure of the anterior fascia (Restoration of linea alba)

- Restoration of the linea alba is done by suturing the anterior rectus sheaths on the midline. Nonabsorbable barbed 0 (zero) sutures in running fashion (Fig. 9)
- When we pull the stitch, reduce the pressure of insufflation to 5–6 mmHg

7. Mesh placement

- Appropriate mesh size selection: entire dissected area should be covered
- Medium weight macroporous mesh (polypropylene or polyester) (Fig. 10)
- Deployed through 12 mm trocar
- Mesh fixation is not necessary, except in the situation of suprapubic defect.

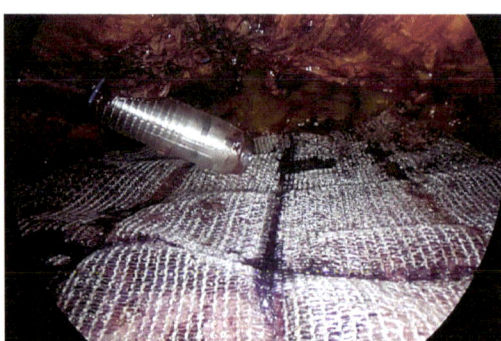

Fig. 10 Mesh placement

8. Drain placement (optional)
9. Exsufflation
   - Slow exsufflation under direct vision to ensure the mesh remains in the correct position.

Mini or less Open Sublay (MILOS) Repair

MILOS is a minimally invasive transhernial approach. It is an open procedure, using endoscopic dissection instruments. eMILOS is an endoscopic MILOS variation and divided into single-port and multiple port.

OT Setup and Patient's Position

Supine position with arms tacked by the side or in lithotomy position

Instrumentation required
- Standard laparoscopic instruments
- 30° telescope 10 mm
- Atraumatic Graspers (2) 5 mm
- Curved Scissors (1) 5 mm
- Rectangular retractors
- Light-armed laparoscopic instruments: EndoTorch ™ (Wolf TM, Knittlingen, Germany) (optional)
- Flexible single ports (optional)
- Suction/irrigation device

- Needle driver
- Hook electrocautery

Surgical Technique

1. Small incision directory above the center of the hernia defect (Fig. 11)
   - skin incision of 2–5 cm = mini-open, 6–12 cm = less-open
2. Hernia sac preparation (Fig. 12)
3. Small incision of the peritoneum for diagnostic laparoscopy (Fig. 13)
4. Resection of abundant peritoneum of the hernia sac (Fig. 14)

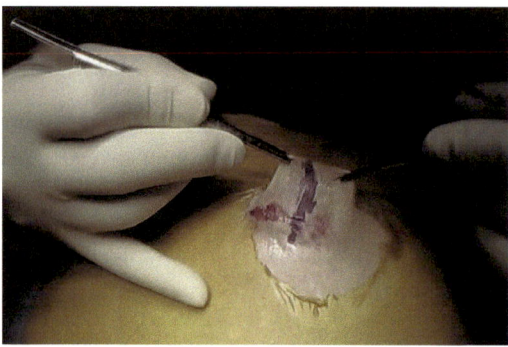

Fig. 11 Skin incision (4 cm) over the hernia sack. (Courtesy of Dr. Taketo Matsubara at St. Luke's International Hospital, Tokyo, Japan)

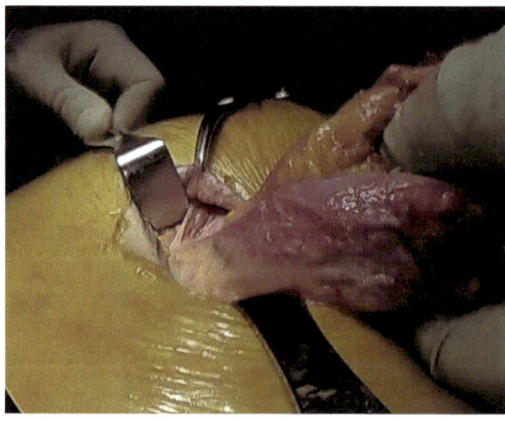

Fig. 12 Dissection of the hernia sac and clear exposition of the hernia ring. (Courtesy of Dr. Taketo Matsubara at St. Luke's International Hospital, Tokyo, Japan)

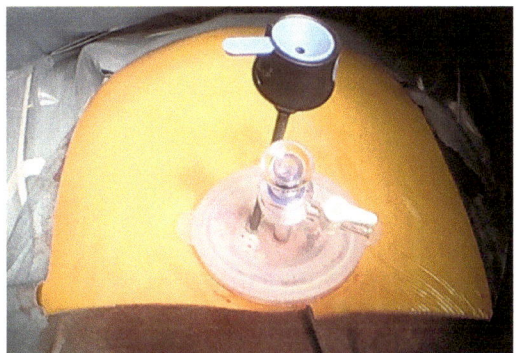

Fig. 13 Dissection of the hernia sac and clear exposition of the hernia ring. (Courtesy of Dr. Taketo Matsubara at St. Luke's International Hospital, Tokyo, Japan)

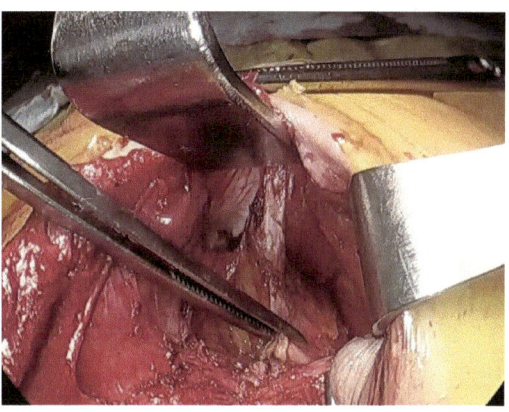

Fig. 15 Resection of abundant peritoneum of the hernia sac. (Courtesy of Dr. Taketo Matsubara at St. Luke's International Hospital, Tokyo, Japan)

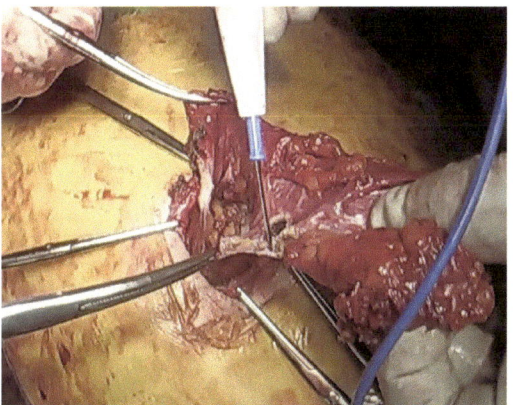

Fig. 14 Transhernial laparoscopy. (Courtesy of Dr. Taketo Matsubara at St. Luke's International Hospital, Tokyo, Japan)

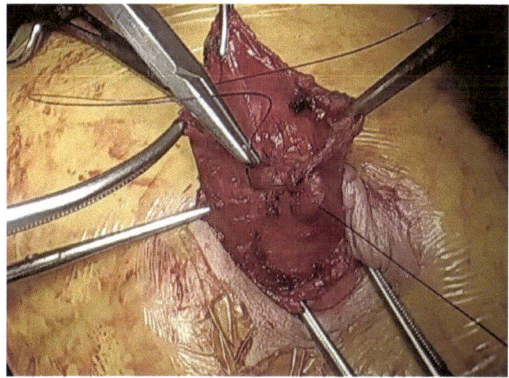

Fig. 16 Closure of peritoneum. (Courtesy of Dr. Taketo Matsubara at St. Luke's International Hospital, Tokyo, Japan)

5. Complete and precise exposure of the fascial edge of the hernia orifice
6. Transhernial extraperitoneal dissection around the hernia gap

   - Rectangular retractors are used to lift the abdominal wall.
   - EndoTorch™ (laparoscopic instruments armed with a light tube) is a specially designed instrument for this dissection (optional).
   - It is important to clearly expose the posterior sheath to enable safe opening of the retromuscular space (Fig. 15).

   - With large ventral hernias, MILOS and eMILOS operation can be combined with TAR.

7. Closure of the abdominal cavity (Figs. 16 and 17)
8. Transhernial extraperitoneal mesh implantation
   - The mesh should posteriorly overlap the hernia defect by at least 5 cm (Fig. 18).
9. Mesh fixation (optional)
10. Hernia defect closure (Fig. 19)

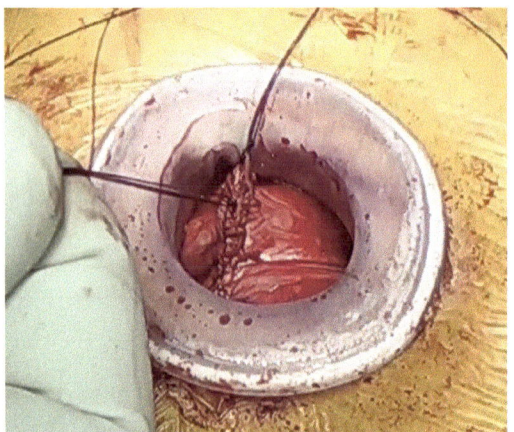

Fig. 17 Closure of posterior rectus sheath. (Courtesy of Dr. Taketo Matsubara at St. Luke's International Hospital, Tokyo, Japan)

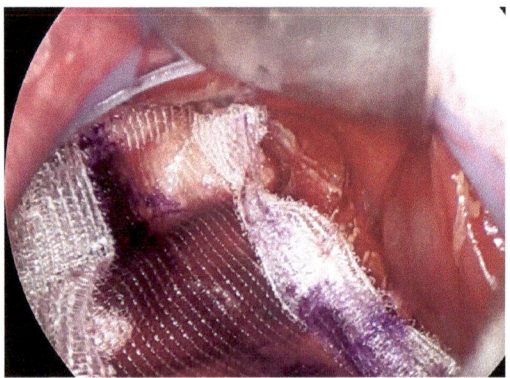

Fig. 18 Mesh with at least 5 cm overlap. (Courtesy of Dr. Taketo Matsubara at St. Luke's International Hospital, Tokyo, Japan)

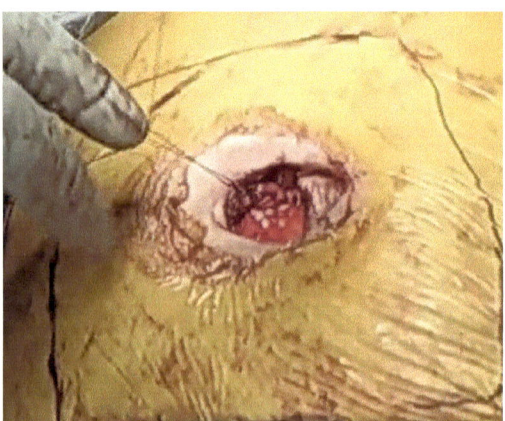

Fig. 19 Anterior rectus sheath closure. (Courtesy of Dr. Taketo Matsubara at St. Luke's International Hospital, Tokyo, Japan)

Complications and Management

- Injury to the bowel
- Hematoma
- Recurrence
- Intraparietal hernia: Dehiscence of the posterior sheath closure results in an intraparietal hernia in which the viscera may become incarcerated between mesh anteriorly and the posterior sheath (Fig. 20). To avoid any tension on the suture line, change the direction of suturing to close the posterior fascia.

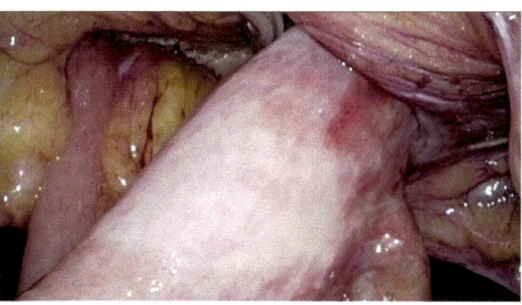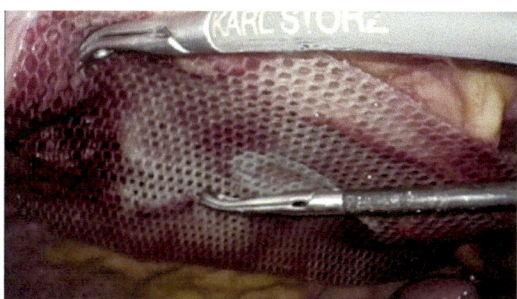

Fig. 20 Intraparietal hernia developed 19 days after the index operation. Treated by using IPOM

Postoperative Care

- Standard Analgesia
- Discharge the patient when the patient is able to ambulate
- Reduce sports activities and carrying heavy weight for 2 weeks

References

1. LeBlanc KA, et al. Laparoscopic repair of incisional abdominal hernias using expanded polytetrafluoroethylene: preliminary findings. Surg Laparosc Endosc. 1993;3:39–41.

2. Robinson TN, et al. Major mesh-related complications following hernia repair. Surg Endosc Other Interv Tech. 2005;19:1556–60.
3. Daes J. The enhanced view-totally extraperitoneal technique for repair of inguinal hernia. Surg Endosc. 2012;26:1187–9.
4. Belyansky I, et al. A novel approach using the enhanced-view totally extraperitoneal (eTEP) technique for laparoscopic retromuscular hernia repair. Surg Endosc. 2018;32:1525–32.
5. Reinpold W, et al. Mini-or less-open sublay operation (MILOS): a new minimally invasive technique for the extraperitoneal mesh repair of incisional hernias. Ann Surg. 2019;269:748–55.

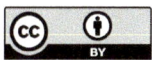

Endoscopic Anterior Component Separation Technique (eACS)

Kiyotaka Imamura and Victor Gheorghe Radu

Component separation technique (CST) provides a substantial amount of medial advancement of myofascial components of the abdominal wall and is useful in addressing large and complex hernia defects during open ventral hernia repair. Classic anterior CST is associated with high rates of surgical site occurrences and infection [1]. To reduce wound complications, endoscopic approach was developed [2]. Although endoscopic anterior CS (eACS) has lost popularity due to recent trend toward TAR for complex abdominal wall reconstruction cases [3], eACS result in a similar wound morbidity and recurrence rate as TAR [4]. eACS could be another option in the armamentarium to deal with complex ventral hernias.

Indications

- Large ventral hernias (primary, incisional)
- To close the abdominal wall primarily without mesh in contaminated fields.

- *Caution! CST without mesh reinforcement has high rates of hernia recurrence [5].

K. Imamura (✉)
Minimally Invasive Surgery Center,
Yotsuya Medical Cube, Tokyo, Japan
e-mail: k-imamura@mcube.jp

V. G. Radu
Medlife, Bucharest, Romania

Contraindications

- Noncompliant abdominal wall from previous repair/mesh
- Concomitant TAR
- Defects are disproportionally wider than longer (relative)

Preoperative Assessment

- Same as previous chapter: "extraperitoneal ventral hernia repair."

OT Setup and Patient's Position

- Supine position with both arms tacked in alongside the trunk of the patient.
- Using ultrasound imaging, semilunar line lateral to the rectus abdominis muscle is identified and marked on the skin bilaterally.

Instrumentation Required

- 0° telescope 10 mm
- 30° telescope 5 mm
- A cylindrical dissection balloon dissector—Spacemaker™ Pro Blunt Tip Trocar (Medtronic, New Haven, CT)
- Atraumatic Graspers (2) 5 mm

© The Author(s) 2023

D. Lomanto et al. (eds.), *Mastering Endo-Laparoscopic and Thoracoscopic Surgery*,
https://doi.org/10.1007/978-981-19-3755-2_61

- Curved Scissors (1)] 5 mm
- Suction/irrigation device
- Hook electrocautery

Surgical Technique

Three options should be considered.

1. eACS first or median laparotomy first?
   - Some surgeons prefer to do eACS first to avoid contamination of lateral abdominal space from the midline wound [3] but others perform median laparotomy first to titrate the need for eACS [6]. The latter avoids overtreatment, for hernia width cannot be the only determinant; patient's height, visceral fat amount, and abdominal wall compliance should be considered.
2. Depending on the place where the first port is placed; precostal [6] or inguinal approach [7].
   - Precostal approach: 13–15 cm away from the xiphoid depending on the patient's height, and 4 cm above the costal arch.
   - Inguinal approach (Fig. 1): lower lateral quadrant of the abdomen, lateral to the previously marked semilunar line.
3. Depending on the location of the "endoscopic pocket"; subfascial [6] and subcutaneous [3] approach.

A Case of eACS for Large Midline Defect (Width 10 cm × Length 21 cm): eACS First, Inguinal and Subfascial Approach

1. Identify and mark the bilateral semilunar line (Fig. 2) under ultrasound guidance.
2. Create the lateral endoscopic pockets.
   - 12 mm incision is made in the lower quadrant of the abdomen, lateral to the semilunar line (Fig. 3)
   - Balloon dissector is introduced and advances below the aponeurosis of exter-

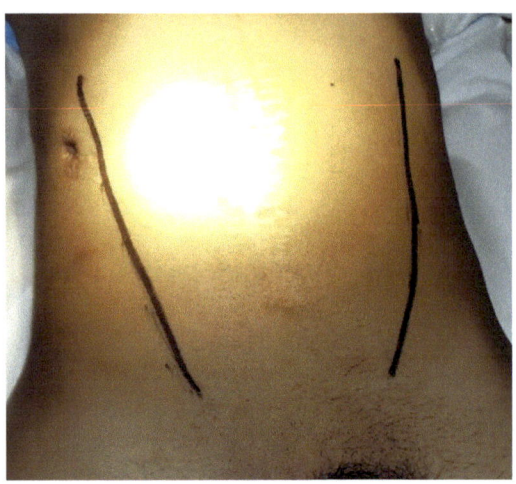

Fig. 2 Bilateral semilunar line is identified and marked

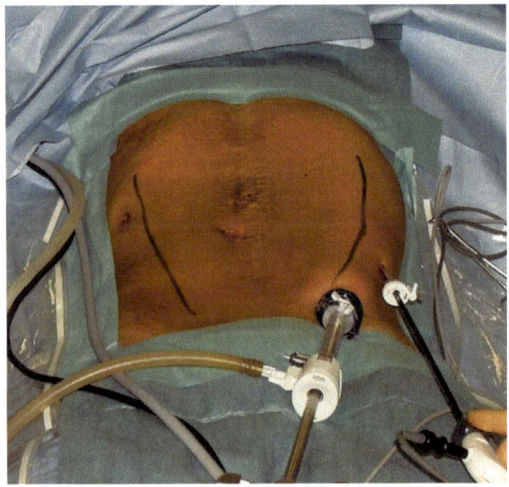

Fig. 1 Inguinal approach of eACS

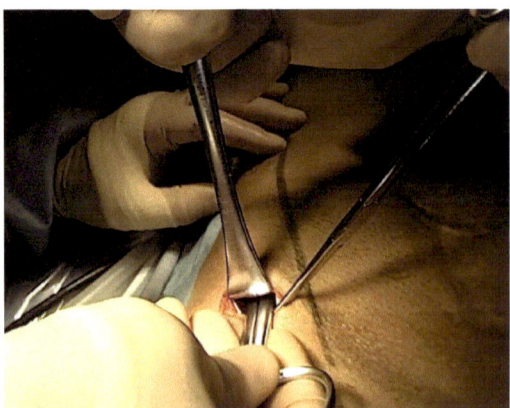

Fig. 3 As in a standard inguinal hernia repair, the external oblique aponeurosis is incised and the space between external and internal oblique muscle was identified

nal oblique muscle then the balloon is inflated (Fig. 4).

- The space is insufflated with CO_2 and maintained at a pressure of 10 mmHg (Fig. 5).

3. Transection of the external oblique muscle (Fig. 6).
   - Additional 5 mm port is introduced at a position lateral and superior to the camera port.
   - The external oblique aponeurosis is incised laterally to the right semilunar line.
   - The external oblique aponeurosis is incised from inguinal ligament to 4–6 cm above the costal margin (Fig. 7).

4. Adhesiolysis and restoration of the linea alba (Fig. 8). the linea alba is reconstructed using continuous endo-laparoscopic intracorporeal suturing

5. Upon the restoration of the linea alba, a synthetic mesh is rolled and inserted in the surgical space and apposed to reinforce the abdominal wall (Fig. 9)

Here, below is a CT scan reconstruction of the abdominal wall before and after 1 year follow-up showing the excellent reconstruction and repair of the abdominal wall midline defect (Fig. 10).

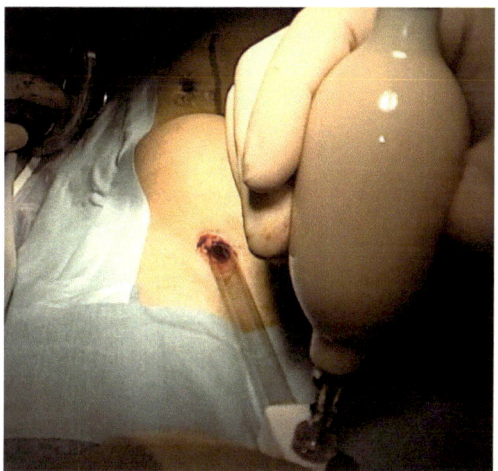 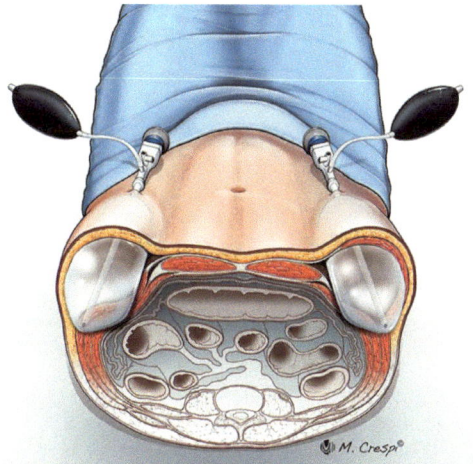

Fig. 4 *Left*: the Balloon dilatation is inserted in the subfascial space; *Right*: schematic of the balloon dilation within the lateral muscles

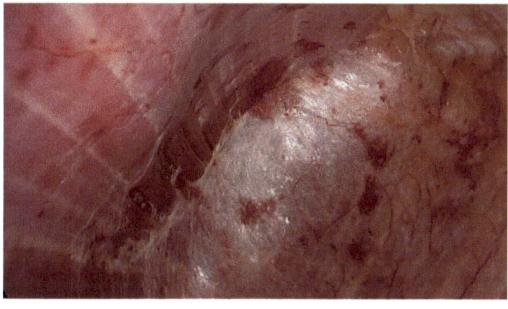

Fig. 5 Overview of the space between the right external and internal oblique muscle after removal of the balloon and gas insufflation

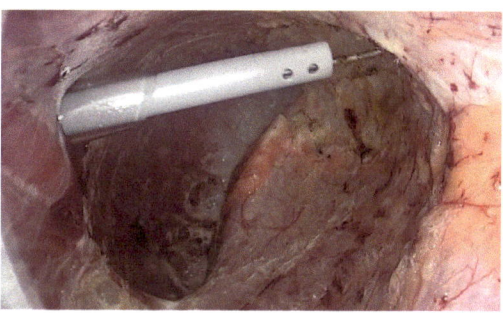

Fig. 6 Incise the elevated external oblique aponeurosis

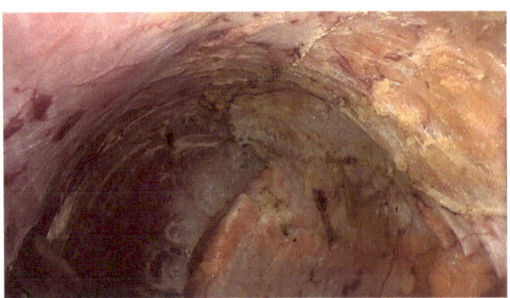

Fig. 7 Endoscopic view after release of external oblique muscle

Complications and Management

- Small bowel injury during adhesiolysis
- Mesh infection
- Seroma
- Recurrence
  - same as the previous chapter: "laparo-scopic IPOM and IPOM+."
- Lateral hernia
  - resulting from full-thickness injury to the linea semilunaris,
  - repair using TAR [8].

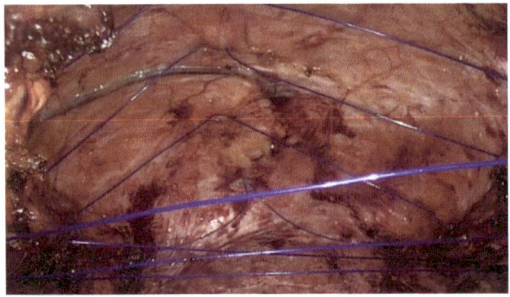

Fig. 8 The extracorporeal interrupted suture technique is used to close the fascial defect

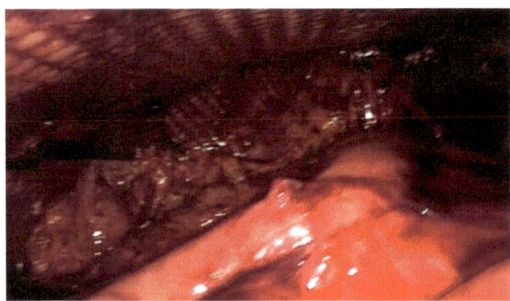

Fig. 9 IPOM reinforcement

Peroperativ 3D-CT   1 year postop 3D-CT

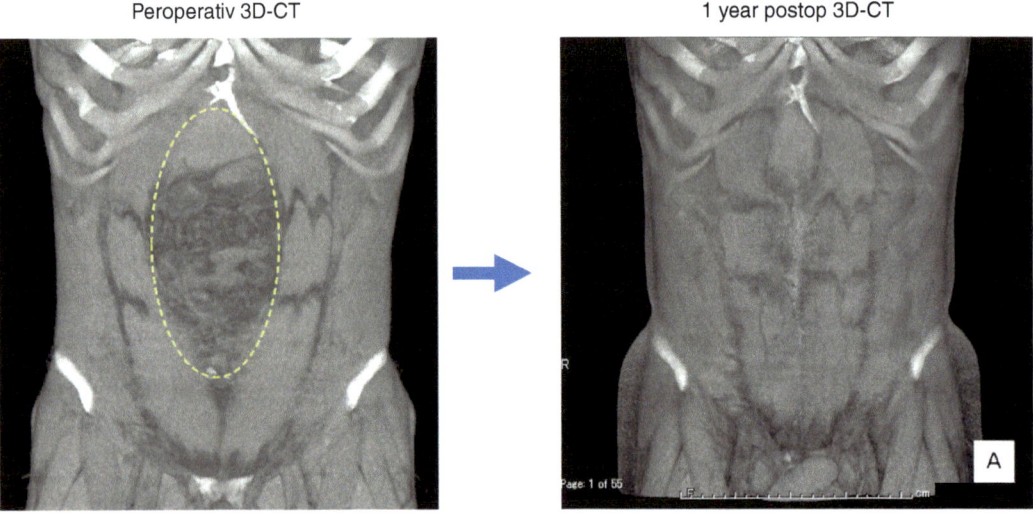

Fig. 10 Left: preoperative 3D-CT image, yellow circle means hernia orifice. Right: 1-year postoperative 3D-CT image

Postoperative Care

- Standard Analgesia
- Discharge the patient when the patient is able to ambulate
- Reduce sports activities and carrying heavy weight for 2 weeks

References

1. Ramirez OZ, et al. "Components separation" method for closure of abdominal-wall defects: an anatomic and clinical study. Plast Reconstr Surg. 1990;86:519–26.
2. Rosen MJ, et al. Laparoscopic versus open-component separation: a comparative analysis in a porcine model. Am J Surg. 2007;194:385–9.
3. Daes J, et al. Endoscopic subcutaneous component separation as an adjunct to abdominal wall reconstruction. Surg Endosc. 2017;31:872–6.
4. Bittner R, et al. Update guidelines for laparoscopic treatment of ventral and incisional abdominal wall hernias (International Endohernia Society (IEHS)): part B. Surg Endosc. 2019;33:3511–49.
5. Liang MK, et al. Ventral hernia management: expert consensus guided by systematic review. Ann Surg. 2017;265:80–9.
6. Köhler G, et al. Evolution of endoscopic anterior component separation to a precostal access with a new cylindrical balloon trocar. J Laparoendosc Adv Sug Tech A. 2017;28:730–5.
7. Clarke JM. Incisional hernia repair by fascial component separation: results in 128 cases and evolution of technique. Am J Surg. 2010;200:2–8.
8. Pauli EM, et al. Posterior component separation with transversus abdominis release successfully addresses recurrent ventral hernias following anterior component separation. Hernia. 2015;19:285–91.

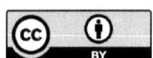

Role of Botulinum Toxin-A in Chemical Component Separation Technique

Sajid Malik and Davide Lomanto

Introduction

Ventral incisional hernia is one of the most common log-term surgical complications after open midline surgeries and accounts for almost 20–30% of the cases [1, 2]. Repair of this incisional hernia is always challenging for general surgeons, especially for complex abdominal wall hernia (CAWH) which also have a major physical, social, and mental repercussions on patients [3]. Ramirez et al. devised a component separation technique (CST) which aims medicalization of rectus abdominis muscles by complete division of bilateral external oblique aponeurosis [4].

CAWH is the one with large hernia defects with size >10 cm; re-recurrence; loss-of-domain; large abdominal wall/soft tissue defect and or enterocutaneous fistula; hernias in anatomically peripheral locations; and close-to-bone or local recurrent infection [4].

Recently, Surgeon's technological armamentarium has been widened for CAWH with introduction of preoperative injection of botulinum toxin A (BTA). It is a protein with neurotoxin activity and is produced by *Clostridium botulinum* and has an inhibitory effect on presynaptic

cholinergic nerve endings [5]. This technique was first reported by Ibarra-Hurtado et al. in 2009, where he used BTA to facilitate fascial closure in 12 patients [6]. Lateral muscle paralysis was successfully achieved for tension-free hernia defect closure. BTA gives an additional advantage of narcotic analgesia with due action blocking the acetylcholine and also by preventing the release of substance P from presynaptic motor nerve endings [7]. Although BTA is a dangerous chemical, small well-calculated doses at specific points on abdominal wall, and also by avoiding vital muscles and viscera have good safety profile [7, 8].

Botulinum Toxin

Types, Mechanism, Effects, and Duration of Action

Commercially available brands of BTA are Botox® (Fig. 1) and Dysport®. This protein blocks the release of acetylcholine in nerve terminals and paralyzes the muscles.

BTA is injected into ventral abdominal wall muscles to achieve functional denervation with paralyzing effect that starts in 3–4 days and reaches maximum effect in 2 weeks [8]. This flaccid paralysis of muscles leads to an increase in abdominal cavity volume. This helps abdominal wall reconstruction without tension. Working in close collaboration with interventional radiologists provides very promising results.

S. Malik (✉)
Department of Surgery, Allama Iqbal Medical College, Jinnah Hospital Lahore, Lahore, Pakistan

D. Lomanto
Department of Surgery, YLL School of Medicine, National University Singapore, Singapore, Singapore

© The Author(s) 2023
D. Lomanto et al. (eds.), *Mastering Endo-Laparoscopic and Thoracoscopic Surgery*,
https://doi.org/10.1007/978-981-19-3755-2_62

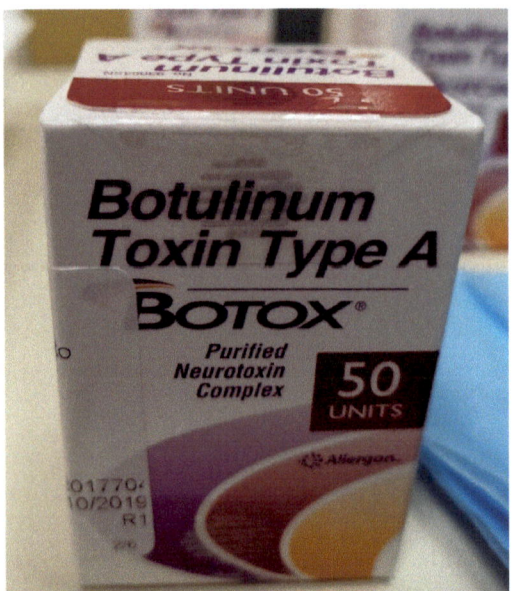

Fig. 1 One of the commercially available brand in author's own practice

Practical Applications

Selection of Patient

Initially, we have to make certain selection criteria on the basis of which we can provide benefits to the patients. There is no consensus but little evidence on certain criteria which are published in the literature, the most important of which is the complex abdominal wall hernia repair (CAWR) according to the size and site. The average length of frontal abdominal musculature from the linea alba to midaxillary line is about 15–20 cm; and the length gained by BTA administration is 3–4 cm on each side; and 6–8 cm in total. This suggests that a defect of 6–8 cm size would likely get benefit from the best results without component separation technique and the repair would be tension free as well [9]. The author has performed a limited number of cases and more randomized trials are needed to establish the facts.

Injections and Interventional Radiological Kit

Author recommends six injections of 50 IU Botox® (Botulinum Toxin A), Sterile water for dilution, and six sets of 25G spinal needles. Ultrasound kit should include minimum of linear transducer (4–12 MHz) in sterile housing; chlorhexidine can additionally be used as a coupling agent (Fig. 2).

Selection of Site

The site of BTA is crucial and needs to be defined very accurately. Elstner, Ibarra-Hurtado, Zielinski, and Zandejas have described four different techniques but with one end result. They concluded that BTA administration between midclavicular and midaxillary line pattern could be of a straight line or triangular from costal margin to superior iliac fossa [6, 10, 11]. According to Ibarra-Hurtado technique, patient is placed in left or right lateral position and five sites are identified. Two on midaxillary line at equal distance, three more on anterior axillary and midclavicular lines, and reciprocal is produced for other side as well. These techniques give advantage of increased length and decreased thickness of lateral ventral abdominal muscles (Fig. 3).

Consenting, Selection of Dose, and Procedure

Standard precautions for any interventional radiological procedure should be practiced as per national guidelines. Counseling and consenting regarding steps, and risks vs benefits should be explained in a surgical clinical visit by the surgeon first and later by interventional radiologists. Back ache once paralyzing effects of toxin on muscles should be addressed and abdominal binder therefore should be prescribed before-

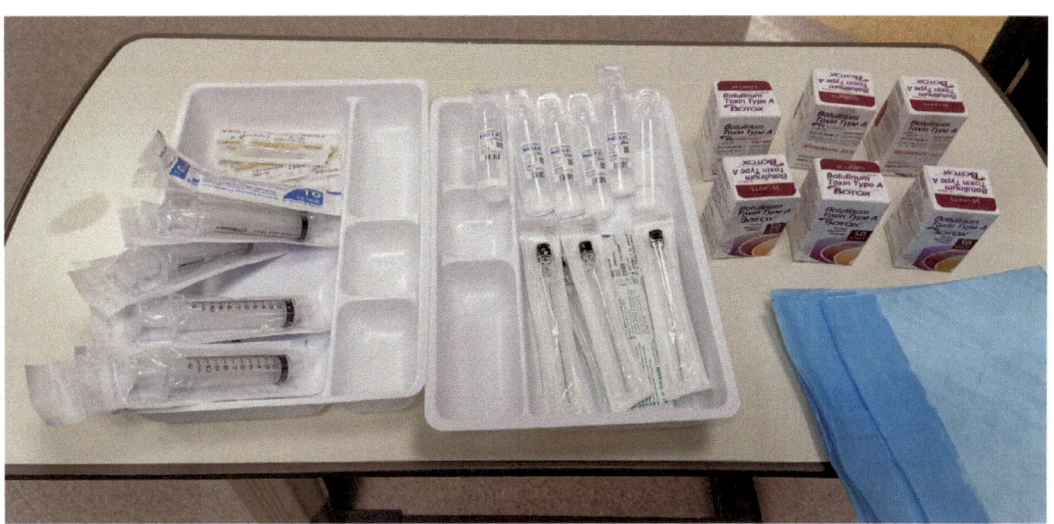

Fig. 2 Equipment required in procedure room under ultrasound guidance

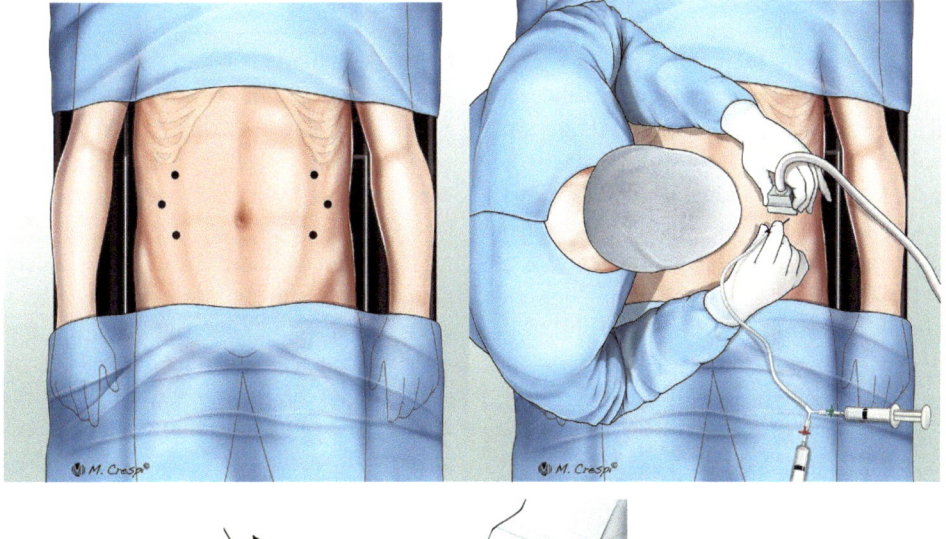

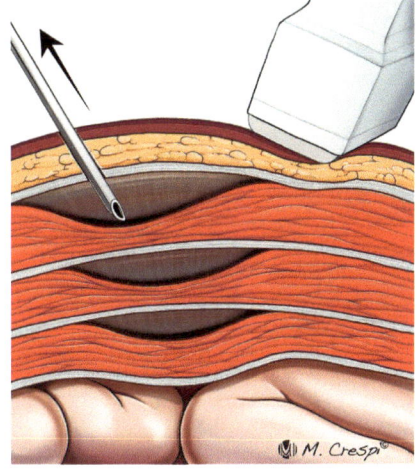

Fig. 3 Various sites of injections and positioning of probe and needle

hand. Always explain to patient that respiration may be labored especially if undertaking heavy activity.

During the procedure, inform the patient that injections would be at various sites and not to cough or take any sudden deep breath during the procedure to avoid any injury to underlying structures. Identify three muscles [*External Oblique Muscle (Ex Ob M.); Internal Oblique Muscle (In. Ob M.); and Transversus Abdominus (Tr. Ab M.)* (Figs. 3 and 4)].

There is a great personal bias in the selection of dose for BTA. Doses are varying in different studies but all are aiming to decide "good effective" amount with "best" dilution at "appropriate" time at "the best" site. Some believe a larger amount (400 IU) of BTA is safe but the author suggests 150 IU on each side with a total and maximum amount of 300 IU (six injections total as mentioned above).

Recently, we have proposed even a more conservative approach to reduce the dosing amount to 100 IU on each side to a total of 200 IU for up to 10 cm defect. Equal amount of six doses at six sites (three on each side) should be administered under ultrasound guidance by an expert hand to avoid complications [9, 10]. Although the surgeons are also expert in doing this procedure; radiologists are more helpful to perform this procedure [12].

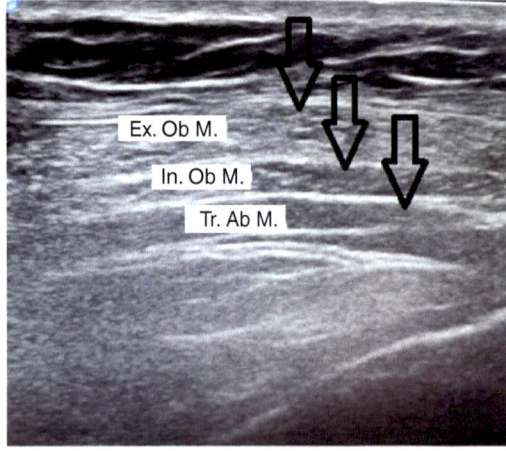

Fig. 4 Identify three muscles shown with black arrow [External Oblique Muscle (Ex Ob M.); Internal Oblique Muscle (In. Ob M.); and Transversus Abdominus (Tr. Ab M.)]

Aftermath

The author's routine is to request interventional radiologist, master in this technique and familiar with the results and outcome, of his hospital to perform the BTA injection to the bilateral anterior abdominal wall muscles (external oblique, internal oblique, and transversus abdominis) 3 weeks before the operation. Ideal time for surgery is in third or fourth week after injections. Either laparoscopic (preferably) or lap-assisted surgery is performed when BTA provides its peak effect at 4 weeks resulting in flaccid paralysis, and then declined gradually in the next 3–4 months. During this whole time, the patient is advised to wear an abdominal binder to avoid complications which might be a result of this flaccid muscle paralysis.

Complications

A study by Nielsen et al. reported one patient who had pain related to BTA injections which was managed by narcotic pain medications and resolved prior to surgery [13].

Three more studies [11, 14, 15] reported patients reporting with weak cough or sneeze after BTA injections but their condition improved after wearing an abdominal binder [14]. In addition to this weak coughing, few patients reported with a sense of bloating that resolved after hernia repair while some others reported with backache and dyspnea which improved with abdominal binder [15]. Based on these complications, the author devised a way to reduce the amount from 300 IU to 200 IU with a rationale of sparing the transverses abdominis muscle which may allow to increase core stability and ultimately will reduce the side effects.

Conclusion

Initial results have shown BTA as a very good alternative to CST for CAWH with minor side effects. Dual advantages of tension-free hernia repair and analgesic effect have raised the interest of researchers. Additionally, flaccid relaxation of abdominal muscles decreases the intra-abdominal pressure thus improving ventilation complications and ultimately reducing the need for and duration of invasive ventilation support. These advantages further facilitate the postoperative healing process as well. All these discussions are from initial results and large randomized control studies on the dosage, techniques, and timing of BTA would be needed to reach a consensus.

References

1. Jairam AP, Timmermans L, Eker HH, Pierik REGJM, van Klaveren D, et al. Prevention of incisional hernia with prophylactic onlay and sublay mesh reinforcement versus primary suture only in midline laparotomies (PRIMA): 2-year follow-up of a multicentre, double-blind, randomised controlled trial. Lancet. 2017;390:567–76.
2. Bikhchandani J, Fitzgibbons RJ Jr. Repair of giant ventral hernias. Adv Surg. 2013;47:1–27.
3. Deerenberg EB, Harlaar JJ, Steyerberg EW, Lont HE, van Doorn HC, et al. Small bites versus large bites for closure of abdominal midline incisions (STITCH): a double-blind, multicentre, randomised controlled trial. Lancet. 2015;386:1254–60.
4. Ramirez OM, Ruas E, Dellon AL. "Components separation" method for closure of abdominal-wall defects: an anatomic and clinical study. Plast Reconstr Surg. 1990;86:519–26.
5. Jankovic J, Brin MF. Therapeutic uses of botulinum toxin. N Engl J Med. 1991;324:1186–94.
6. Ibarra-Hurtado TR, Nuño-Guzmán CM, Echeagaray-Herrera JE, Robles-Vélez E, De Jesús G-JJ. Use of botulinum toxin type A before abdominal wall hernia reconstruction. World J Surg. 2009;33:2553–6.
7. Jankovic J, Albanese A, Atassi MZ, Dolly JO, Hallet M, Mayer NH. Botulinum toxin: therapeutic clinical practice and science. Philadelphia: Saunders Elsevier; 2009. p. 512.
8. Dressler D. Clinical applications of botulinum toxin. Curr Opin Microbiol. 2012;15:325–36. https://doi.org/10.1016/j.mib.2012.05.012.
9. Lien SC, Hu Y, Wollstein A, Franz MG, Patel SP, Kuzon WM, Urbanchek MG. Contraction of abdominal wall muscles influences size and occurrence of incisional hernia. Surgery. 2015;158:278–88. https://doi.org/10.1016/j.surg.2015.01.023.
10. Weissler JM, Lanni MA, Tecce MG, Carney MJ, Shubinets V, Fischer JP. Chemical component separation: a systematic review and meta-analysis of botulinum toxin for management of ventral hernia. J Plast Surg Hand Surg. 2017;51:366–74. https://doi.org/10.1080/2000656X.2017.1285783.
11. Elstner KE, Read JW, Rodriguez-Acevedo O, Ho-Shon K, Magnussen J, Ibrahim N. Preoperative progressive pneumoperitoneum complementing chemical component relaxation in complex ventral hernia repair. Surg Endosc. 2017;31:1914–22. https://doi.org/10.1007/s00464-016-5194-1.
12. Bueno-Lledó J, Torregrosa A, Ballester N, Carreño O, Carbonell F, Pastor PG, et al. Preoperative progressive pneumoperitoneum and botulinum toxin type A in patients with large incisional hernia. Hernia. 2017;21:233–43.
13. Nielsen M, Bjerg J, Dorfelt A, Jørgensen LN, Jensen KK. Short-term safety of preoperative administration of botulinum toxin A for the treatment of large ventral hernia with loss of domain. Hernia. 2020;24:295–9.
14. Farooque F, Jacombs AS, Roussos E, Read JW, Dardano AN, et al. Preoperative abdominal muscle elongation with botulinum toxin A for complex incisional ventral hernia repair. ANZ J Surg. 2016;86:79–83.
15. Rodriguez-Acevedo O, Elstner KE, Jacombs ASW, Read JW, Martins RT, et al. Preoperative botulinum toxin A enabling defect closure and laparoscopic repair of complex ventral hernia. Surg Endosc. 2018;32:831–9.

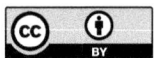

Endo-laparoscopic Repair of Lateral Ventral Hernia

James Lee Wai Kit, Sajid Malik, Sujith Wijerathne, and Davide Lomanto

Introduction

Lateral ventral hernia (LVH) repair is a challenging procedure for surgeons because of the difficult anatomy, the difficult location, the little knowledge on treatment as compared to midline defects, and the scarcity of cases and experience. Till now the poor outcomes including the potential risks of postoperative pain, infection, and higher risk of recurrence have compromised the success of several approaches [1–5].

Briefly, as LVH is described as a primary or secondary defect located at the subcostal, flank, iliac, or lumbar regions. According to the European Hernia Society (EHS) classification [6–8], these defects are classified from L1 to L4, respectively (Table 1). Different types of secondary hernias include defect or wide laxity that can also occur due to denervation of the muscles as a result of previous spine surgery, lobectomy incision, injury, or rupture of the muscles due to blunt trauma [9]. The abdominal wall musculature is innervated in segments by the T7–T12 spinal roots and any disturbance to these nerves can lead to a weakening of the lateral wall muscles resulting in bulges or hernias [10].

Most surgeons opt for open repair of these hernias because of their familiarity with the approach and its accompanying greater ease of tissue manipulation [2]. Conversely, Minimally Invasive Surgery (MIS) approaches in abdominal wall hernia repair have evolved significantly with the advent of several reported techniques which include classical Intraperitoneal Onlay Mesh repair (IPOM) or IPOM with defect closure (IPOM plus/IPOM+), extended Totally Extraperitoneal (e-TEP) repair, endoscopic retro-muscular repair, and Transabdominal Preperitoneal (TAPP) approach. These described techniques combine the advantages of retromuscular or preperitoneal mesh placement with the well-known benefits of MIS approaches [2, 11, 12].

Recent guidelines acknowledge with Grade C (Oxford Classification) the laparoscopic lateral ventral hernia mesh repair of LVHR. This approach seems to be associated with fewer surgical site infections but equal rates of hernia recurrence and chronic pain when compared to open mesh repair, but in conclusion they recommend both open and laparoscopic mesh repair equally [2, 6, 13]. Outcomes of LVH repair are

J. L. W. Kit
Minimally Invasive Surgery Centre, National University Hospital, Singapore, Singapore

Department of Surgery, YLL School of Medicine, National University Singapore, Singapore, Singapore

S. Malik
Allama Iqbal Medical College, Jinnah Hospital, Lahore, Pakistan

S. Wijerathne (✉) · D. Lomanto
Minimally Invasive Surgery Centre, National University Hospital, Singapore, Singapore

General Surgery and Minimally Invasive Surgery, Department of Surgery, National University Health System, Singapore, Singapore

Department of Surgery, YLL School of Medicine, National University Singapore, Singapore, Singapore

© The Author(s) 2023
D. Lomanto et al. (eds.), *Mastering Endo-Laparoscopic and Thoracoscopic Surgery*,
https://doi.org/10.1007/978-981-19-3755-2_63

Table 1 EHS classification of ventral hernia based on location [8]

Zones	Region	Description
L1	Subcostal	Between the costal margin and a horizontal line 3 cm above the umbilicus
L2	Flank	Lateral to the rectal sheath in the area 3 cm above and below the umbilicus
L3	Iliac	Between a horizontal line 3 cm below the umbilicus and the inguinal region
L4	Lumbar	Latero-dorsal of the anterior axillary line

affected by both, patient factors and operative technique and especially by the large size of hernia defects [11–14]. The complexity of the surgical approach, with its limited dissection plane, the limitations placed on the overlapping of the prosthesis by structures like the iliac crest, ribs, and spine, combined with the lack of proper fixation makes this repair vulnerable to higher rates of surgical complications and hernia recurrence.

Thus, a successful repair of LVH repair necessitates careful patient optimization, a thorough understanding of the anatomy of the hernia including its size, location, and etiology, together with a tailored surgical approach to ensure optimal outcomes [2, 12, 15].

This chapter aims to provide guidance on the management of these complex hernias.

Indications

Patients with asymptomatic ventral hernias can be considered for surgery. However, in patients who decline elective surgical intervention, they should be counseled on the risks of a watchful waiting approach with early recognition of symptoms of hernia complications.

Patients with symptomatic ventral hernias should undergo surgical repair as the mainstay of treatment.

Patients with hernia-related complications such as strangulation, obstruction, or incarceration should aim to undergo early or emergent repair depending on their clinical condition. Concerns during the repair for such hernias include the risk of a contaminated field from bowel perforation or the necessity of bowel resection, which may affect the decision for mesh versus tissue repair in such cases.

Patients with symptomatic but uncomplicated lateral ventral hernias should undergo surgical repair barring the absence of contraindications.

Absolute contraindications to elective repair include severe comorbidities unsuitable for general anesthesia, uncontrollable coagulopathy, giant hernia with major loss of domain, major abdominal sepsis, giant hernia with loss of abdominal domain as well as poor quality of life that would preclude meaningful outcome postsurgical repair.

Relative contraindications that are modifiable prior to surgery include smoking, obesity, and diabetic control. Smoking increases the risk of surgical site infection and should ideally be stopped 6–8 weeks prior to elective ventral hernia surgery. Obesity increases the risk of surgical site infection, hernia recurrences as well as prolongs hospital stay post elective surgery. Patients prior to elective lateral ventral hernia repair should aim for a BMI less than 30 kg/m^2. Diabetic patients should also aim for adequate glucose control of Hba1c less than 8% prior to surgery.

As with all surgical cases, patients should be assessed prior to surgery for fitness for anesthesia. Management of underlying comorbidities especially that of diabetes, smoking, and obesity are important as they pose risks to ventral hernia repair.

Specific for lateral ventral hernias, it is important that these patients undergo cross-sectional preoperative imaging in order to delineate the location of the defect and its contents. Evaluation of the defect size is important as we recommend the use of Botox injections for defects larger than 8 cm 4–6 weeks prior to surgery to increase abdominal domain to assist with the surgical repair process.

OT Setup

- Please refer to OT setup chapter for laparoscopic hernia repair
- Mesh preparation preoperatively is important to ensure all necessary equipment are on site and sized appropriately for the defect
- The choice of operative technique (Open vs Lap vs Robotic) should be individualized to the patient

Surgical Technique

We advocate a tailored MIS approach for patients undergoing repair of lateral ventral hernias.

All patients undergoing surgical repair with MIS approaches should be done under general anesthesia. The repair techniques available are as follows:

Repair Techniques

- Laparoscopic Intraperitoneal Onlay Mesh Repair Plus (IPOM+)
- Laparoscopic/Robotic Transabdominal Preperitoneal Repair (TAPP/rTAPP)
- Extended Totally Extraperitoneal Repair (e-TEP)
- Laparoscopic Transabdominal Partial Extraperitoneal Repair (TAPE)

The repair of lateral ventral hernias via the MIS approach can be divided into the following categorical steps:

General Steps

- Positioning
- Diagnostic Laparoscopy (except in e-TEP)
- Adhesiolysis (as required)
- Closure of fascia defect
- Mesh placement with at least 5 cm overlap from original defect size
- Tacking of mesh with double-crown fixation technique

Patient positioning is supine for most L1, L2, and L3 cases with slight variations. L1, L2, and L3 cases required tiling the table with the hernia side up towards the surgeon. L1 cases require a further reverse Trendelenburg positioning of about 15–30°. L3 cases require a further Trendelenburg position of 15–30°. L4 cases being lateral require a lateral decubitus (Figs. 1 and 2) with the hernia side tilted away from the surgeon.

Diagnostic laparoscopy should be performed after gaining access to the peritoneal cavity for IPOM+, TAPP, and TAPE cases. Adhesiolysis should be carefully performed if

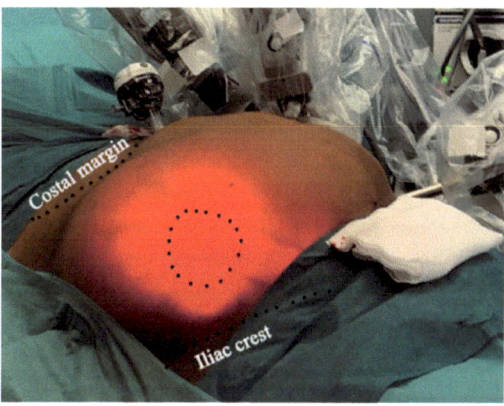

Fig. 1 Performing robotic TAPP (rTAPP) in lateral decubitus position for a hernia in L4 region that resulted after bone harvesting from the iliac crest

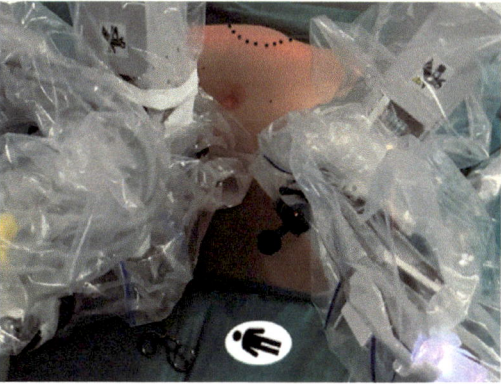

Fig. 2 Performing robotic TAPP in lateral decubitus position for a hernia in L4 region that resulted from likely traumatic rupture of muscle

required for incisional hernia cases to clearly delineate the fascia defect as well as ensure adequate exposure for mesh placement. Closure or approximation of defect followed by mesh placement is thereafter performed for all cases of lateral ventral hernia repair via the MIS technique.

Choice of mesh is determined by the location of the mesh placement, surgical technique utilized as well as the presence of contamination during the surgery process. In extraperitoneal mesh placement like TAPP (lap or robotic) and e-TEP, standard macroporous polypropylene or polyester meshes are utilized; in some cases, self-gripping meshes may be useful to avoid challenges in mesh placement and fixation. Composite meshes are used for IPOM+ and TAPE approaches. A minimum 5 cm overlap of the original defect prior to closure is required. For lateral hernia closer to bone structures like the iliac crest, mesh should be fixed to it using permanent metal tackers while absorbable tackers can be used for fixation to soft tissue in a classical "double-crown" technique.

IPOM+ Approach

We recommend a standard IPOM technique for the IPOM+ approach with the addition of closing the fascia defect using either transfacial nonabsorbable sutures or intra-corporeal nonabsorbable barbed sutures or both. Access is done using a 10–12 mm port on the contralateral abdominal wall to the hernia away from the defect with adequate space for mesh overlap after defect closure. Two 5 mm working ports should be placed on either side of the 10–12 mm port about 6–8 cm away. A composite mesh posterior to the peritoneum should be placed in an underlay position. IPOM+ approach should be considered in cases where intra-abdominal adhesions are expected and where peritoneum damage secondary to adhesiolysis is expected. We also recommend this technique for L1 hernias (Fig. 3) at the subcostal region where extraperitoneal dissection beyond the costal margin can be technically challenging.

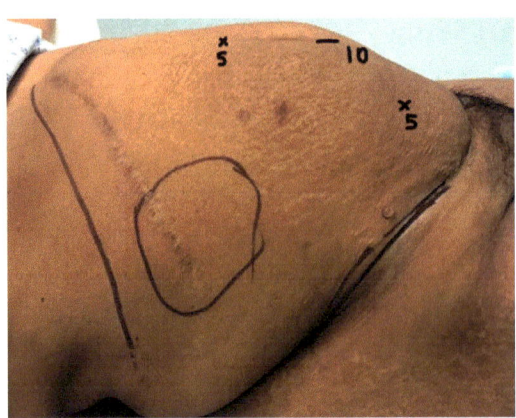

Fig. 3 Planned port placement for laparoscopic IPOM+ repair of an incisional hernia in L1 region

TAPP/rTAPP Approach

Both endo-laparoscopic or robotic technique can be used for the TAPP approach and they are similar in technique. Access is like the IPOM+ technique with care to ensure adequate space between the ports and defect to allow room for creation of the peritoneal flap. Surgeons should be mindful that more space is needed for bigger defects. The peritoneal flap should be created at least 8 cm away from the edge of the defect and for defects larger than 3–4 cm, this distance should be revised to be greater than 8 cm. This is to ensure sufficient ergonomics for operating, mesh placement, and closure of the peritoneal flap. For the robotic approach, we recommend an additional 10–12 mm port to facilitate insertion and removal of sutures as well as for suctioning where required. We recommend laparoscopic TAPP for L2 cases with defects no larger than 4–5 cm and robotic TAPP for cases with larger defects, especially in the L4 region where ergonomics of laparoscopic repair are not favorable, especially during laparoscopic closure of the defect requiring plication.

e-TEP Approach

Access for the e-TEP approach (see Chapter on e-TEP) is like groin hernias with the 10–12 mm port placed through an infraumbilical incision medial to the semilunar line on the opposite side of the hernia after entering the preperitoneal retrorectus plane. The plane should subsequently be developed using the camera as well as insufflation of gas through the port to aid dissection. Two 5 mm working ports can thereafter be placed inferior to the camera port after creating adequate space at the space of Bogros and Retzius (Fig. 4). We recommend the e-TEP approach for primary hernias in the L2 region for defects no larger than 4–5 cm in size. This technique is also applicable for selected hernias in L3 region.

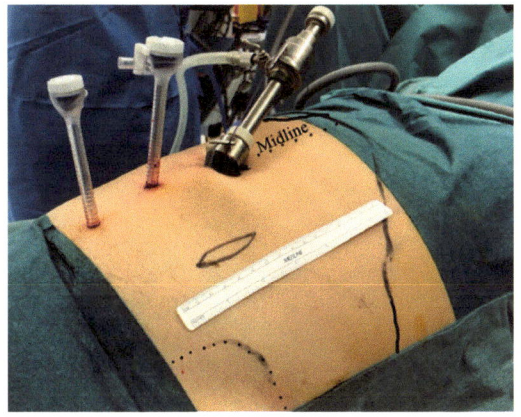

Fig. 4 Port placement for e-TEP repair of a Spigelian hernia

TAPE Approach

Access and port placement for the Transabdominal Partial Extraperitoneal approach (TAPE) is similar to the TAPP technique. We recommend a dissection of the peritoneal flap-like TAPP for groin hernias to be undertaken until the clear identification of the pectineal ligament of Cooper and the landmark myopectineal structures is performed. A composite mesh is used in the TAPE technique as part of the mesh will be exposed beyond the free edge of the peritoneal flap. We recommend this technique in cases where the peritoneal coverage of the defect and mesh is not adequate due to prior extensive adhesiolysis. After placement of the mesh, the free edges of the remaining peritoneum should be tacked over the mesh and abdominal wall using absorbable tackers. This approach is mostly utilized for midline and lateral flank hernia.

Suggested Diagram for a Tailored Endo-Laparoscopic Lateral Ventral Hernias Repair (Fig. 5).

In a nutshell, lateral ventral hernia which is actually a quite challenging condition can be

Fig. 5 Tailored approach for lateral ventral hernia

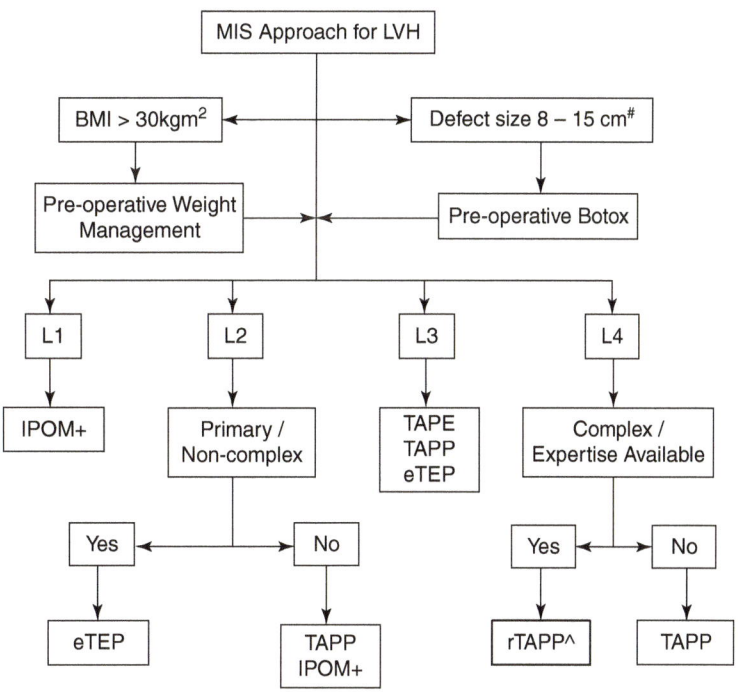

Open approach should be considered for defects larger than 15cm

^ Robotic approach can be used to repair hernia in all 4 regions if expertise is available

Table 2 Summary of procedure techniques

	IPOM+	TAPP	e-TEP	TAPE
Access	10–12 mm port opposite hernia with 2 × 5 mm working ports approximately 6–8 cm away from the camera port	10–12 mm port opposite hernia with 2 × 5 mm working ports approximately 6–8 cm away from the camera port. Consider additional 10–12 mm port for rTAPP	10–12 mm port opposite hernia with 2 × 5 mm working ports approximately 6–8 cm inferior from the camera port	10–12 mm port opposite hernia with 2 × 5 mm working ports approximately 6–8 cm away from the camera port
Mesh choice	Composite mesh	Synthetic mesh—Consider self-gripping	Synthetic mesh—Consider self-gripping	Composite mesh
Mesh location	Underlay	Sublay	Sublay	Sublay/underlay
Useful situations	Expected intra-abdominal adhesions, near costal margin			Inadequate peritoneal coverage
Appropriate defect size	Large defects	4–5 cm defects	4–5 cm defects	4–5 cm defects
Hernia sites	L1/L2	L2/L3/L4	L2/L3	L2/3/4
Flap entry	N.A	8 cm from edge of defect	10–12 mm Portsite	8 cm from edge of defect

managed by endo-laparoscopic method using TAPP, TAPE, e-TEP, and rTAPP with each having individualized selection criteria (Table 2).

Complications and Management

General postoperative complications apply to lateral ventral hernia repairs as well such as mesh-related infections, seroma formation, and recurrence.

Post-Op Care

The use of prophylactic antibiotics is essentially in view of mesh implantation. There is no role for continuation of antibiotics postsurgery. Patients should receive a standardized analgesia package for pain control. They should also be counseled on the use of an abdominal binder, especially in the presence of large hernias. Return advice looking out for symptoms of fever, worsening abdominal pain, and erythema over the hernia site should be done routinely to both patients and relatives.

Patients should be followed up in the clinic at routine intervals initially 2 weeks after surgery and thereafter at the 1 month, 3 month, 6 month, and 1 year mark.

Discussion

Lateral ventral hernia is a challenging condition to treat. Our approach via an endo-laparoscopic method using TAPP, TAPE, e-TEP, and rTAPP has also been described by other authors [16]. They also conclude that extraperitoneal or pre-peritoneal mesh placement allows adequate abdominal wall reinforcement and reduces the need for extensive surgical fixation and related complications.

Authors such as Cavalli et al. [3] and Katkhouda et al. [4] have also published their approaches to lateral ventral hernia repair through an open method. Cavalli et al. describe a four-step technique with an open extraperitoneal approach for complex LVH in particular for large hernia size white Katkhouda et al. recommended an open technique with mesh fixation to bony structures to reduce recurrences.

We advocate a tailored approach for lateral ventral hernias. No technique is superior to the other for MIS LVH repair and a tailored approach based on patient and hernia characteristics and also taking the facilities and expertise in complex hernia techniques into consideration can provide the best results and the value of open surgical approach should not be taken lightly in a large and complex hernia.

References

1. Cobb WS, Kercher KW, Heniford BT. Laparoscopic repair of incisional hernias. Surg Clin North Am. 2005;85(1):91–103, ix. https://doi.org/10.1016/j.suc.2004.09.006.
2. Regner JL, Mrdutt MM, Munoz-Maldonado Y. Tailoring surgical approach for elective ventral hernia repair based on obesity and National Surgical Quality Improvement Program outcomes. Am J Surg. 2015;210(6):1024–9; discussion 1029–30. https://doi.org/10.1016/j.amjsurg.2015.08.001.
3. Cavalli M, Aiolfi A, Morlacchi A, et al. An extraperitoneal approach for complex flank, iliac, and lumbar hernia. Hernia. 2020;25(2):535–44. https://doi.org/10.1007/s10029-020-02214-6.
4. Katkhouda N, Alicuben ET, Pham V, et al. Management of lateral abdominal hernias. Hernia. 2020;24(2):353–8. https://doi.org/10.1007/s10029-020-02126-5.
5. Webber V, Low C, Skipworth RJE, Kumar S, de Beaux AC, Tulloh B. Contemporary thoughts on the management of Spigelian hernia. Hernia. 2017;21(3):355–61. https://doi.org/10.1007/s10029-017-1579-x.
6. Bittner R, Bain K, Bansal VK, et al. Update of guidelines for laparoscopic treatment of ventral and incisional abdominal wall hernias (international Endohernia society (IEHS))—part a. Surg Endosc. 2019;33(10):3069–139. https://doi.org/10.1007/s00464-019-06907-7l.
7. Bittner R, Bain K, Bansal VK, et al. Update of guidelines for laparoscopic treatment of ventral and incisional abdominal wall hernias (international Endohernia society (IEHS)): part B. Surg Endosc. 2019;33(10):3069–139. https://doi.org/10.1007/s00464-019-06908-6.
8. Muysoms FE, Miserez M, Berrevoet F, et al. Classification of primary and incisional abdominal wall hernias. Hernia. 2009;13(4):407–14. https://doi.org/10.1007/s10029-009-0518-x.
9. Dakwar E, Le TV, Baaj AA, et al. Abdominal wall paresis as a complication of minimally invasive lateral transpsoas interbody fusion. Neurosurg Focus. 2011;31(4):E18. https://doi.org/10.3171/2011.7.FOCUS11164.
10. Pulikkottil BJ, Pezeshk RA, Daniali LN, Bailey SH, Mapula S, Hoxworth RE. Lateral abdominal wall defects: the importance of anatomy and technique for a successful repair. Plast Reconstr Surg Glob Open. 2015;3(8):e481. https://doi.org/10.1097/GOX.0000000000000439.
11. Van Ramshorst GH, Eker HH, Hop WCJ, Jeekel J, Lange JF. Impact of incisional hernia on health-related quality of life and body image: a prospective cohort study. Am J Surg. 2012;204(2):144–50. https://doi.org/10.1016/j.amjsurg.2012.01.012.
12. Holihan JL, Alawadi Z, Martindale RG, et al. Adverse events after ventral hernia repair: the vicious cycle of complications. J Am Coll Surg. 2015;221(2):478–85. https://doi.org/10.1016/j.jamcollsurg.2015.04.026.
13. Belyansky I, Daes J, Radu VG, et al. A novel approach using the enhanced-view totally extraperitoneal (eTEP) technique for laparoscopic retromuscular hernia repair. Surg Endosc. 2018;32(3):1525–32. https://doi.org/10.1007/s00464-017-5840-2.
14. Stoppa RE. The treatment of complicated groin and incisional hernias. World J Surg. 1989;13(5):545–54. https://doi.org/10.1007/BF01658869.
15. Hesselink VJ, Luijendijk RW, De Wilt JHW, Heide R, Jeekel J. An evaluation of risk factors in incisional hernia recurrence. Surg Gynecol Obstet. 1993;176(3):228–34.
16. Shahdhar M, Sharma A. Laparoscopic ventral hernia repair: extraperitoneal repair. Ann Laparosc Endosc Surg. 2018. https://doi.org/10.21037/ales.2018.09.07.

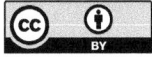

Posterior Plication or Combined Plication of the Recti Diastasis

Davide Lomanto, Raquel Maia, and Enrico Lauro

The anterior abdominal wall consists of the abdominal rectus muscles separated by the linea alba, which is the fusion of the aponeuroses of external and internal oblique muscles and transversus abdominis.

Rectus abdominis diastasis (RAD) is a clinical condition where the inter-rectus distance is abnormally wide with a consequent bulging on the midline, due to a weaker and thinner linea alba (Fig. 1).

Even though there is not an agreement about the average inter-rectus distance (IRD) to be considered abnormal, many authors describe a separation wider than 2 cm as RAD [1].

The measurements may differ based on the location along the linea alba above or below the umbilicus.

Beer et al. examined 150 nulliparous women between 20 and 45 years of age by ultrasound at three reference points to evaluate the normal IRD.

The survey revealed a broad range of widths, and the data collection allowed the authors to consider "normal" up to a width of 15 mm at the xiphoid, up to 22 mm at the reference point 3 cm above the umbilicus, and up to 16 mm at the reference point 2 cm below the umbilicus [2].

Mota et al. studied the IRD during and after pregnancy in primiparous women considering as "normal" the measurements between the 20 and 80th percentiles. During pregnancy, the IRD measured 49–79 mm at 2 cm below the umbilicus, 54–86 mm at 2 cm above the umbilicus, and 44–79 mm at 5 cm above the umbilicus, while in the postpartum period 6 months after birth, the IRD decreased to 9–21 mm, 17–28 mm, and 12–24 mm at 2 cm below, 2 cm above and 5 cm above the umbilicus, respectively [3].

The authors concluded that in primiparous women, the IRD may be considered "normal" up to values wider than in nulliparous.

As shown in an anatomical study by Rath et al. the normal inter-rectus width is age-related: below 45 years of age diastasis is considered as a separation of the two rectus muscles exceeding 10 mm above the umbilicus, 27 mm at the umbilical ring, and 9 mm below the umbilicus, while above 45 years of age these values increase up to 15 mm, 27 mm, and 14 mm, respectively [4].

D. Lomanto (✉)
Department of Surgery, Yong Loo Lin School of Medicine, National University Singapore, Singapore, Singapore
e-mail: surdl@nus.edu.sg

R. Maia
Brazilian College of Gastric Surgeons, Sao Paulo, Brazil

E. Lauro
General Surgery Division, St. Maria del Carmine Hospital, Rovereto, Italy

© The Author(s) 2023
D. Lomanto et al. (eds.), *Mastering Endo-Laparoscopic and Thoracoscopic Surgery*,
https://doi.org/10.1007/978-981-19-3755-2_64

459

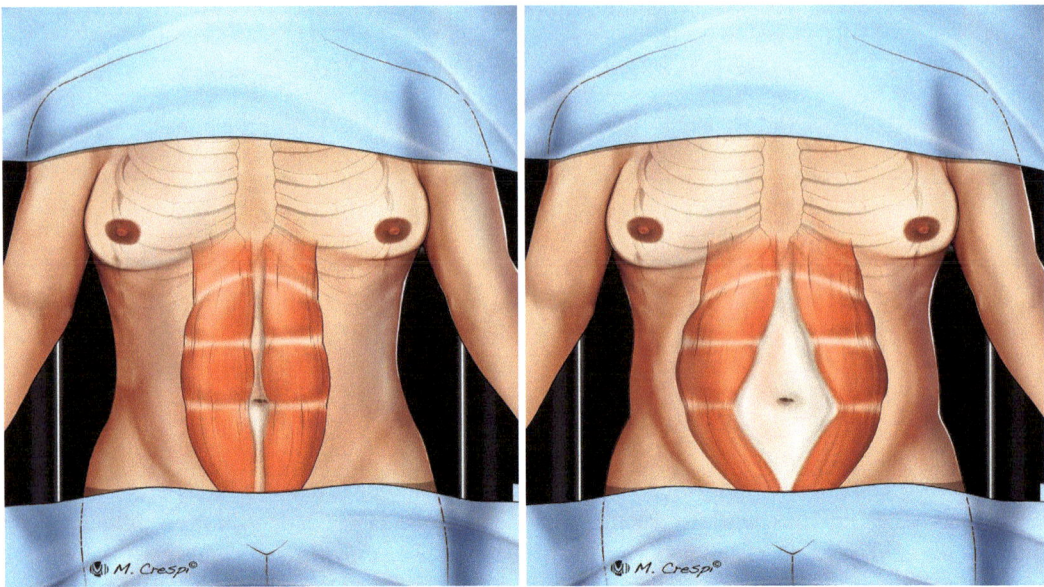

Fig. 1 Schematic of normal linea alba and Recti muscle diastasis

Risk Factors

Rectus abdominis diastasis can be congenital or acquired.

Several *congenital anomalies* are associated either with defects of the anterior abdominal wall, involving malformation of the somatic and visceral layers (i.e., the Cantrell pentalogy or *thoracoabdominal syndrome*, Beckwith-Wiedemann syndrome, Opitz syndrome, midline defect syndrome, and prune belly syndrome), or with an autosomal dominant transmission as an abdominal wall development failure [5, 6].

In the *acquired RAD*, the weakening and laxity of the abdominal wall tissues result in an abnormal inter-rectus distance and often in a typical abdominal protrusion.

The fascia can become thin due to stretching, which can be caused by an elevated intra-abdominal pressure, such as in pregnant and obese patients, or due to prior abdominal surgery. An association of RAD with other disorders affecting connective tissue suggests an underlying tissue weakness.

Risk factors for acquired RAD are:

- **Pregnancy**—Pregnancy increases the risk of developing RAD; however, not all pregnant women develop diastasis. The amount of the

separation can increase, decrease, or stay the same during the postpartum period [7, 8].

Exercise significantly reduced the risk of developing RAD [9].

Obesity—Weight gain with an increase in the intra-abdominal pressure can lead to a gradual rectus muscle separation [10].

Collagen disease—As in patients with hernias or aortic aneurysm, patients with diastasis recti present decreased levels of type I and III collagen [11, 12].

Aneurysm—Some, but not all studies, support such an association as a result of a collagen tissue disorders [13].

Classification

Ranney proposed a classification of RAD based on the width of the IRD: width < 3 cm, between 3 and 5 cm, or > 5 cm are classified as mild, moderate, or severe, respectively [14].

Recently, the German Hernia Society and the International Endo Hernia Society proposed a more specific classification based on the diastasis length and location (subxiphoidal M1, epigastric M2, umbilical M3, infraumbilical M4, and suprapubic

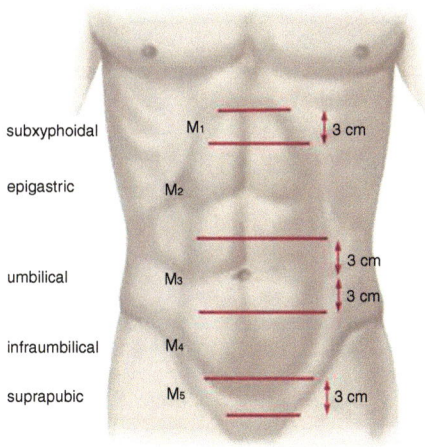

Rectus Diastasis Classification			
Midline	M1 subxiphoidal		
	M2 epigastric		
	M3 umbilical		
	M4 infraumbilical		
	M5 suprapubic		
Length: cm		Width: cm	
Width cm	W1 < 3 cm	W2 3 - ≤ 5 cm	W3 > 5 cm

subxyphoidal — M1 — 3 cm
epigastric — M2
umbilical — M3 — 3 cm / 3 cm
infraumbilical — M4
suprapubic — M5 — 3 cm

Fig. 2 Classification of RAD based on length and width of the IRD

M5), diastasis width (W1 < 3 cm, W2 = 3 ≤ 5 cm, and W3 > 5 cm), concomitant hernias, previous operations, number of pregnancies/births, skin laxity, and pain assessment [15] (Fig. 2).

Clinical Features

Rectus abdominis diastasis may be symptomatic or asymptomatic. An abnormally wide abdominal muscle distance results in a modification of the inner abdominal pressure and can affect the stability of the abdominal "box," having an impact on the vertebral column, the diaphragm, and the pelvic floor.

Symptoms include abdominal pain or discomfort, lumbar back pain, and pelvic instability, with urogynecological symptoms, such as urinary incontinence, fecal incontinence, and pelvic organ prolapse.

In addition, patients affected by RAD often report a lower acceptance of their body image and a lower quality of life compared with the general population.

Patients with acquired RAD typically are middle-aged and older men with central obesity, or small, fit women with previous multiple or large fetus births.

RAD does not consist of a proper abdominal wall defect, and therefore there is no risk of incarceration or strangulation, although ventral (umbilical, epigastric) or incisional hernias can coexist with RAD.

Diagnosis

The physical examination can detect a RAD as a bulged linea alba by a head lift maneuver in most patients.

This protrusion normally extends from the xiphoid to the umbilicus and possibly more caudally to the pubis.

The width between the two rectus abdominis muscles can be easily taken at rest and during contraction at several levels along the linea alba but, if a surgical treatment is required, an imaging investigation is mandatory.

Ventral and incisional hernias are obviously associated with a fascial defect, while RAD does not present any fascial interruption.

Imaging

Ultrasound (US) is a useful noninvasive method that can confirm diastasis and at the same time exclude other causes of bulging.

Measurements are usually taken at rest and during abdominal muscle activation (i.e., during a head lift maneuver) at different reference points above and below the umbilicus.

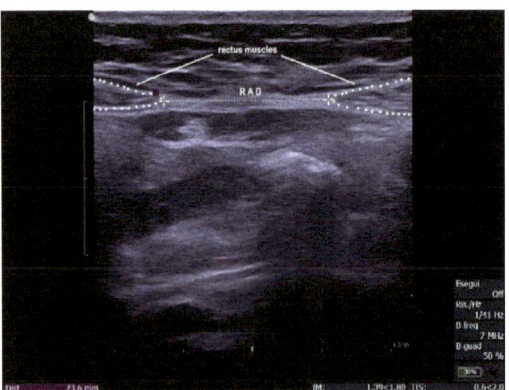

Fig. 3 Ultrasound findings

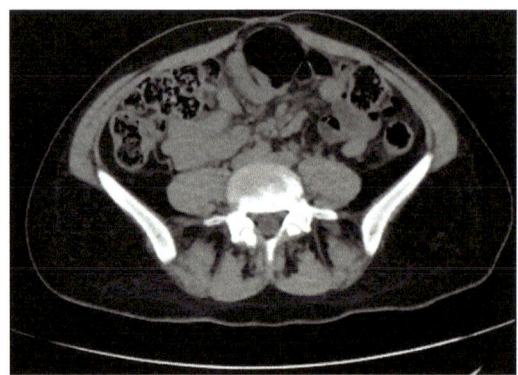

Fig. 5 CT SCAN imaging showing RAD at the umbilicus

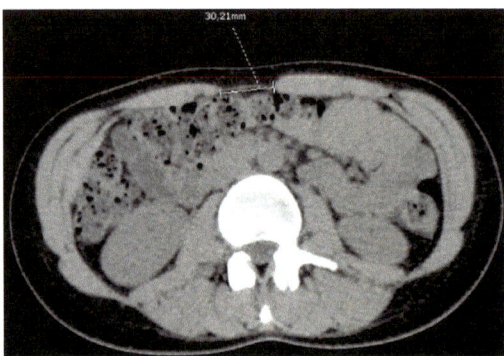

Fig. 4 CT SCAN imaging showing RAD above the umbilicus

US intersession reliability has been shoved to be high in the supraumbilical region, but poor when measuring IRD below the umbilicus [16] (Fig. 3).

Computed tomography (CT) without contrast medium at rest and during Valsalva maneuver offers an accurate investigation of the inter-rectus distance and of the whole abdominal wall anatomy, including the possible association with ventral or incisional hernias.

In addition, CT Scan allows a useful three-dimensional reconstruction for better anatomical preoperative assessment (Figs. 4 and 5).

Indications and Management

RAD alone does not require surgical repair: conservative management with weight loss and exercise are the suggested treatment [17–19].

In case of RAD associated with abdominal hernias, rectus abdominis plication with mesh reinforcement is recommended [19, 20].

Indications for mini-invasive (MIS) surgical repair include the presence of a midline/umbilical hernias, medium size RAD (measuring up to 5 cm, but no consensus reached in the current literature), no prior hernia repair or laparotomy (relative contraindication), and no need for abdominoplasty. Repair of the RAD with concomitant midline hernia is critical as may lead to a so-called pseudo-recurrence where the presence of a midline bulge may affect patient satisfaction.

Surgical Repair

Different surgical approaches have been reported from open to endo-laparoscopic or robotic. Similarly, several different techniques have been described for the RAD repair like anterior or pos-

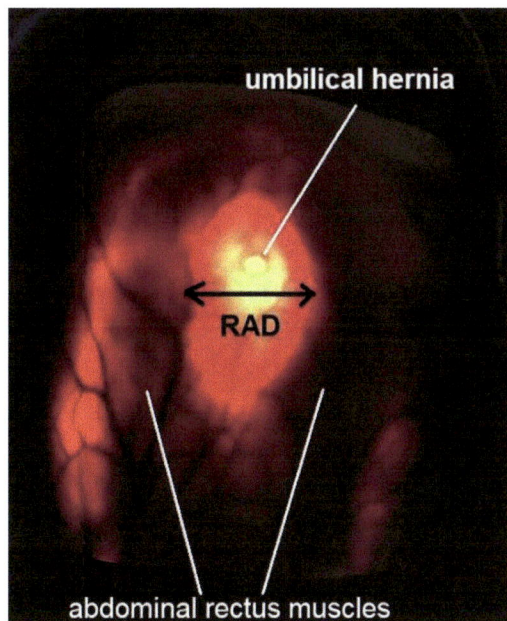

Fig. 6 Intraoperative view of the abnormal inter-rectus distance in a patient with RAD

terior rectus sheath plications and mesh repair (Fig. 6).

If we classify the different techniques, we have:

For the MIS approaches:
- Laparoscopic with Intraperitoneal Onlay Mesh (IPOM) reinforcement
- Endo-laparoscopic in which the mesh is positioned extraperitoneal sublay or onlay
- Robotic-assisted for all above

Plication

Suture plication of the anterior, posterior, or both rectus aponeurosis can be performed using a single or double-layer suture technique or a triangular "mattress" running suture technique. Slowly absorbable or nonabsorbable 2–0 sutures can be

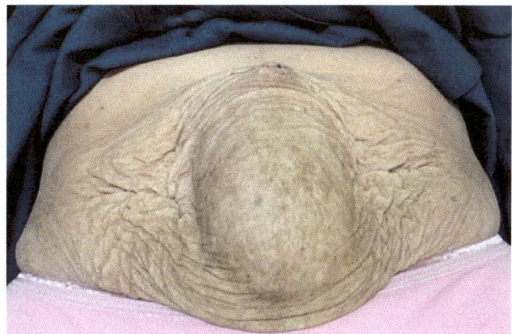

Fig. 7 Large W3 Rectus Diastasis

utilized for the plication. The plication can be completed by using a mesh for reinforcement.

If an anterior plication is performed, the mesh can be placed either in onlay position or in the retrorectus space (sublay). In case of laparoscopic posterior plication, the mesh is placed intraperitoneal (IPOM). Absorbable or nonabsorbable can be utilized.

In this chapter, we will focus on the Combined or Posterior plication of the RAD with mesh reinforcement. Our Indication for this technique is ONLY for a RAD associated with primary midline hernia in which an only hernia repair may lead to failure due to the lack of midline support. In fact, in the long term, the hernia repair is going to fail if not treated concurrently with RAD [21, 22] (Fig. 7).

Our technique is derived from the classical IPOM Plus in which the defect closure is added to the simple IPOM repair (see related Chapter).

Preoperative Preparation

- Routine blood investigations
- Bowel Preparation (optional)
- Antibiotic-prophylaxis
- CT Scan (in selected cases: recurrent, incarcerated, etc.)
- Weight Loss if BMI >30

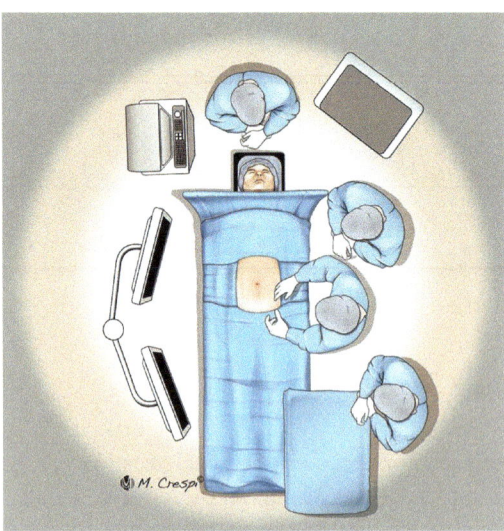

Fig. 8 OR Setup for Ventral Hernia and RD Repair

OT Setup, Patient's Position and Trocars Placement (Fig. 8)

- Monitor position
  - Position of the monitor should be opposite to the Surgeon Operator.
- Patient Position and preparation
  - Standard supine position with both arms tucked at the side or on the arm board depending on the size and site of hernia (Fig. 3)
  - Surgeon and Assistant stand on the side of the patient
- Instrumentation required
  - Hasson or Optical Trocar or Veress Needle
  - Trocars: One 10–12 mm and two 5 mm
  - Laparoscopic camera unit with 30 telescope 10 mm and 5 mm
  - Atraumatic Graspers (×2) 5 mm
  - Curved Scissors (×1) 5 mm
  - Bowel Clamp (×1) 5 mm
  - Suction/irrigation device
  - Advance Energy Device (Thunderbeat, Olympus, Japan)
  - Suture passer
  - Nonabsorbable suture (Polypropilene 0 or 1)

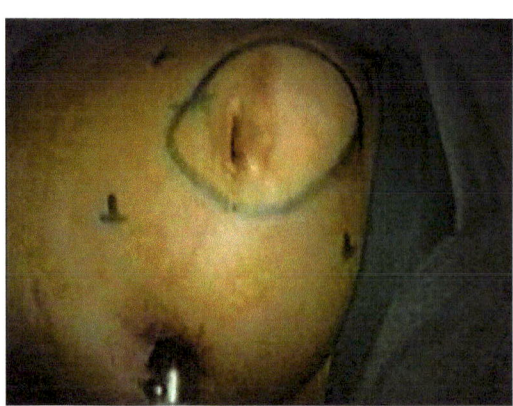

Fig. 9 Port placement

- V-Lock suture, nonabsorbable 0 (Medtronic, USA)
- Composite Mesh with anti-adhesive barrier
- Tackers; absorbable (for mesh fixation)
- Trocars size and position (Fig. 9)
  - *12 mm port inserted laterally between the costal margin and the Anterior superior iliac spine (ASIS)*
  - *5 mm ports (2) inserted on either side of the optical trocar*
  - *An additional 5 mm port may be required in an approachable position for the mesh fixation*

Surgical Technique

The hernia defect and RAD should be marked preoperatively. Pneumoperitoneum can be established using either a Veress needle and Optical Trocar or a Hasson trocar.

The first 12 mm trocar is inserted on the anterior axillary line between the anterior iliac spine and the subcostal margin. A 30° laparoscope is inserted and diagnostic laparoscopy is carried out. Two 5 mm trocars are inserted under vision on both sides of the 12 mm trocar. Trocars should be at least 8 cm away from the lateral edge of RAD.

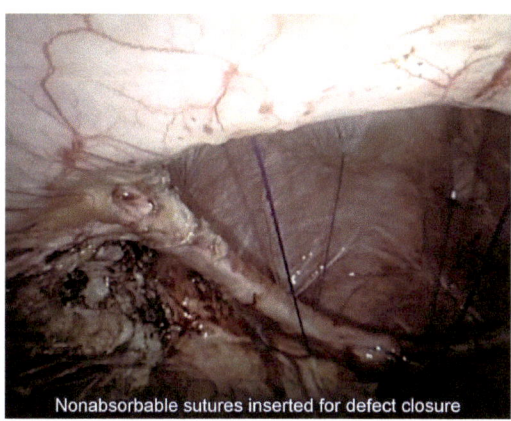

Nonabsorbable sutures inserted for defect closure

Fig. 10 Nonabsorbable transfascial suture utilized to approximate large RD

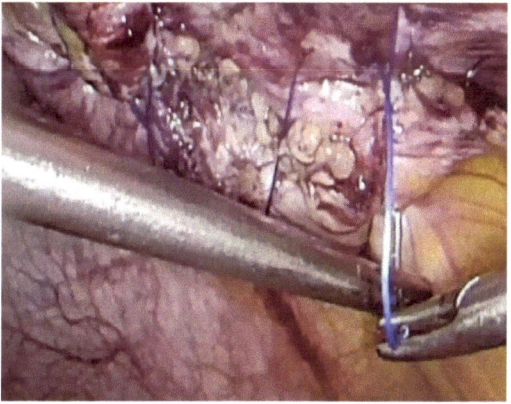

Fig. 11 An intracorporeal continuous suture with nonabsorbable material is utilized to approximate the edges of the recti mm

Hernia defect and diastasis are identified and adhesiolysis is performed if needed.

Our alternative for the RAD closure involves either the use of nonabsorbable transfascial suture (Fig. 10) or the closure of the posterior rectus muscle aponeurosis by a continuous nonabsorbable suture (Fig. 11). Suture plication of posterior can be performed using a single- or double-layer suture technique or a triangular "mattress" running suture technique.

For large RAD, we prefer the use of transfascial suture approximation (Laparoscopic-Assisted Rectus Diastasis Approximation: LARDA) this can be utilized alone or with the posterior endosuturing plication (Fig. 12).

After the recti mm approximation, an intraperitoneal mesh is positioned for reinforcement to repair the concomitant ventral hernia that follows the same surgical technique of the Laparoscopic IPOM technique, similar to the complications and postoperative care we refer to in the laparoscopic IPOM Chapter.

Since we do not have at this time randomized clinical trials to support and clinical evidence, we will summarize our clinical experience to validate our approach. RD is present in about 18–20% of our primary midline hernia. Since 2013, we have started to consider the repair of the RD as mandatory and we have collected data from 89 patients (78 F; 11 M) with a mean age of 37 years old. Among the Female patients: all had at least two deliveries and 85% had a cesarian section. Mean defect size was (W2: 3.8 cm) with a mean length of 13 cm. we performed a posterior plication with endosuturing in 33 pts. and in 56 we used transfascial suture (LARDA Technique). Mesh was utilized in all cases (65 pts. had 10 × 15 cm; 24 pts has a 15 × 20 cm); Mean VAS score was 2 (range 0–7) at 24 h and 1 at movement at 48 h. No complications were recorded and the recurrence rate was 0 at 22 months follow-up. Satisfaction rate using Carolinas Comfort Scale score was very good in 96% of the patients.

In conclusion, the posterior approach either with LARDA or posterior endosuturing plication allows to correct umbilical hernia and rectus diastasis concurrently. Patient with normal BMI with minimal skin excess and rectus diastasis are the best candidates. The minimal dissection and the use of MIS improve the cosmetic results. Without dissection of the supra-aponeurotic space, we can reduce the incidence of seroma and skin infection and necrosis. Both techniques are feasible, safe with acceptable clinical outcome, and with a shorter learning curve.

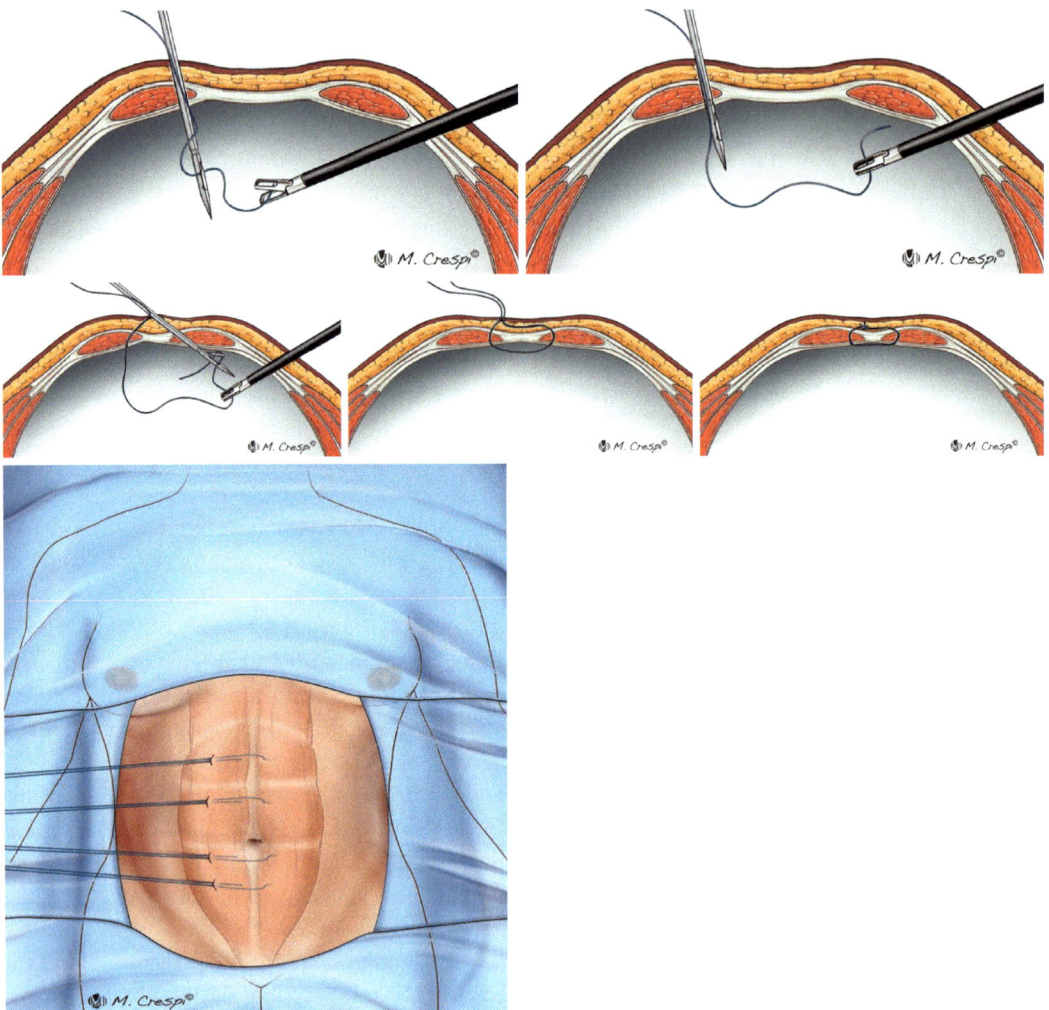

Fig. 12 Showing the use of transfascial suture for the closure of the defect (photo above) and the final results

Complications

Complications following surgery are mainly represented by seromas, hematomas, or wound complications, such as skin or flap ischemia, surgical site infections, or hypertrophic scarring. Dissection and suturing may be responsible. Complications may be more frequent when mesh is used.

Postoperative Care, Follow-Up, and Outcomes

Suction drains can be used and should be removed when serosal output is less than 30–40 mL/24 h. There is no evidence suggesting the benefit of an abdominal binder, but it can be considered to provide compression and increase patient comfort postoperatively. Patients should avoid heavy lifting for at least 4 weeks. Follow-up is indicated in the first 3 months postoperative to rule out seroma, collections, and recurrences, then as planned. Patient satisfaction after surgery is often high and recurrence rate low but further long-term RCTs are needed.

References

1. Brooks DC. Overview of Abdominal Wall hernias in adults. 2015.
2. Beer GM, Schuster A, Seifert B, et al. The normal width of the linea alba in nulliparous women. Clin Anat. 2009;22:706.
3. Mota P, Pascoal AG, Carita AI, Bo K. Normal width of the inter-recti distance in pregnant and postpartum primiparous women. Musculoskelet Sci Pract. 2018;35:34–7.
4. Rath AM, Attali P, Dumal JL, Goldlust D, Zhang J, Chevrel JP. The abdominal linea alba: an anatomo-radiologic and biomechanical study. Surg Radiol Anat. 1996;18:281–8.
5. Digilio MC, Capolino R, Dallapiccola B. Autosomal dominant transmission of nonsyndromic diastasis recti and weakness of the linea alba. Am J Med Genet A. 2008;146A:254.
6. Okayasu I, Kajita A, Shimizu K. A variant form of median defect syndrome. Syndrome of combined congenital defects involving the supraumbilical abdominal wall, sternum, diaphragm, pericardium, and heart. Acta Pathol Jpn. 1978;28:287.
7. Hsia M, Jones S. Natural resolution of rectus abdominis diastasis. Two single case studies. Aust J Physiother. 2000;46:301.
8. Fernandes da Mota PG, Pascoal AG, Carita AI, Bø K. Prevalence and risk factors of diastasis recti abdominis from late pregnancy to 6 months postpartum, and relationship with lumbo-pelvic pain. Man Ther. 2015;20:200.
9. Benjamin DR, van de Water AT, Peiris CL. Effects of exercise on diastasis of the rectus abdominis muscle in the antenatal and postnatal periods: a systematic review. Physiotherapy. 2014;100:1.
10. Lockwood T. Rectus muscle diastasis in males: primary indication for endoscopically assisted abdominoplasty. Plast Reconstr Surg. 1998;101:1685.
11. van Keulen CJ, et al. The role of type III collagen in family members of patients with abdominal aortic aneurysms. Eur J Vasc Endovasc Surg. 2000;20(4):379–85.
12. Blotta RM, et al. Collagen I and III in women with diastasis recti. Clinics (Sao Paulo). 2018;73:e319.
13. McPhail I. Abdominal aortic aneurysm and diastasis recti. Angiology. 2008;59:736.
14. Ranney B. Diastasis recti and umbilical hernia causes, recognition and repair. SDJ Med. 1990;43:5–8.
15. Reinpold W, Köckerling F, Bittner R, Conze J, Fortelny R, Koch A, Kukleta J, Kuthe A, Lorenz R, Stechemesser B. Classification of rectus diastasis—a proposal by the German hernia society (DHG) and the international Endohernia society (IEHS). Front Surg. 2019;28:6.
16. Keshwani N, McLean L. Ultrasound imaging in postpartum women with diastasis recti: inter-rater between-session reliability. J Orthop Sports Phys Ther. 2015;45(9):713–8.
17. Akram J, Matzen SH. Rectus abdominis diastasis. J Plast Surg Hand Surg. 2014;48:163.
18. Nahas FX, Augusto SM, Ghelfond C. Should diastasis recti be corrected? Aesthetic Plast Surg. 1997;21:285.
19. Köhler G, Kuketina RR, Emmanuel K. Sutured repair of primary small umbilical and epigastric hernias: concomitant rectus diastasis is a significant risk factor for recurrence. World J Surg. 2015;39:121–6.
20. Bellido Luque J, et al. Totally endoscopic surgery on diastasis recti associated with midline hernias. The advantages of a minimally invasive approach. Prospective cohort study. Hernia. 2014;19:493–501.
21. Köhler G, Kuketina RR, Emmanuel K. Sutured repair of primary small umbilical and epigastric hernias: concomitant rectus diastasis is a significant risk factor for recurrence. World J Surg. 2015;39:121–6. https://doi.org/10.1007/s00268-014-2765-y.
22. Costa TN, Abdalla RZ, Santo MA, Tavares RRFM, Abdalla BMZ, Cecconello I. Transabdominal midline reconstruction by minimally invasive surgery: technique and results. Hernia. 2016;20:257–65. https://doi.org/10.1007/s10029-016-1457-y.

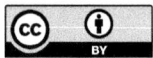

Endo-laparoscopic Retromuscular Repair

Enrico Lauro, Giovanni Scudo, and Salvatore Rizzo

Introduction

Although few data exist to guide the management of rectus abdominis diastasis (RAD), during past decades many articles were published to describe techniques to correct RAD and concomitant abdominal midline defects [1–4]. Among these, stapled techniques are acquiring an increasing interest [5–8].

Main common points of these techniques are:

- Respect of Rives-Stoppa principles
- Use of staplers to repair the widened linea alba and keep together the rectus muscles at the same time
- Sublay mesh reinforcement

Retromuscular space can be accessed from the Retzius space, as during TEP procedure, using a space maker balloon or directly by blind dissection.

An infra-umbilical incision is an effective alternative to gain the same retromuscular space.

The space between rectus muscles and posterior sheath is then dissected endoscopically.

The widened midline is cut and sutured by stapling, bringing the two rectus muscles closer together and repairing the diastasis at the same time.

Section of the linea alba creates a retromuscular box where to place the mesh in a sublay position.

Indications

Endo-laparoscopic stapled repair must be considered for:

- Small, single, and multiple midline or incisional hernias (W1, according to EHS classification) associated with RAD up to 5 cm width
- Patients fit for general anesthesia
- Absence of contraindications to laparoscopy

Contraindications

- Large midline defects > W2, in accord to EHS classification (relative)
- Previous retromuscular mesh repair for abdominal hernias
- Skin excess or need for abdominoplasty
- Major loss of abdominal domain
- Pediatrics patients
- Cancer patients
- Pregnancy or desire for future pregnancy
- Portal hypertension

E. Lauro (✉) · G. Scudo
General Surgery Division, St. Maria del Carmine Hospital, Rovereto, Italy
e-mail: enrico.lauro@apss.tn.it

S. Rizzo
General Surgery Division, Cavalese Hospital, Cavalese, Italy

© The Author(s) 2023   469
D. Lomanto et al. (eds.), *Mastering Endo-Laparoscopic and Thoracoscopic Surgery*,
https://doi.org/10.1007/978-981-19-3755-2_65

- Previous placement of a peritoneal dialysis catheter (relative)
- Emergency setting (relative)

Preoperative Assessment

- Careful clinical history and physical examination
- CT scan without contrast, at rest and during Valsalva's maneuver
- Routine investigations according to hospital protocols
- Prophylactic antibiotics according to hospital protocols
- Previous stop of any anticoagulant according to its wash-out time
- Administration of Low-molecular-weight heparin (LMWH) if indicated
- Gastric and Bladder decompression

OT Setup

- Patient in standard supine position (split legs optional)
- Monitor is on the patient's head side
- Laparoscopic Instrumentation required:
  - 30° scope 5 mm
  - 1 Trocar 5 mm
  - 1 monoport
  - 2 atraumatic graspers 5 mm
  - 1 Veress needle (optional)
  - 1 curved Maryland dissector 5 mm
  - 1 curved scissor
  - 1 bipolar forceps
  - 1 hook diathermy (optional)
  - Suction/irrigation device

Surgical Technique: How We Do It

Laparoscopic Phase

Pneumoperitoneum is induced by the closed technique.

We prefer to use the Veress needle at Palmer's point. A 5 mm port is placed on the left flank lateral to the semilunar arcuate line, and laparoscopic exploration of the abdomen is then performed to assess the real defect to treat. If needed, other 5 mm ports can be positioned to reduce all hernial contents. At the end of this phase, the intra-abdominal pressure is reduced to a lower value of 6–8 mmHg.

Endoscopic Phase

It starts by obtaining access to the retromuscular space (according to the chosen technique). We prefer to perform an infra-umbilical 4 cm incision, reducing eventual umbilical hernias if present. Access to the retromuscular space is gained bilaterally by small incisions on the anterior rectus muscles fascia.

The two branches of a linear stapler are inserted respectively beneath the right and the left rectus muscles (Fig. 1).

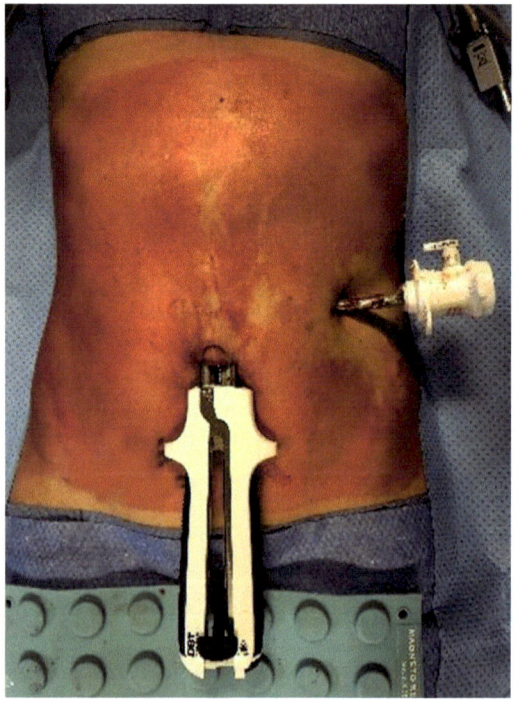

Fig. 1 Insertion of Stapler beneath the rectus muscle

The Stapler, placed in the retromuscular space, is then fired cranially and, after been reloaded, caudally towards the pubis (Fig. 2).

A monoport is placed through the infra-umbilical incision to proceed with the endoscopic retromuscular dissection (Fig. 3).

The neurovascular bundles must be identified and preserved (Fig. 4).

Using endoscopic staplers, the widened linea alba is cut and sutured bringing the rectus muscles closer together (Fig. 5).

The retromuscular space is prepared to obtain a single chamber from the xiphoid to the suprapubic region or exceeding the defect for at least 4 cm (Fig. 6); it is highly recommended for a laparoscopic check before stapling, to avoid bowel injuries.

In case of large defects, an oversewn suture of the anterior plication is performed in order to reinforce the stapled suture and reduce the gap between the two rectus muscles (Fig. 7).

Once the retromuscular space is prepared, measurements are taken to choose the mesh size.

We usually do not fix the mesh, but fibrin glue or a self-gripping mesh is an option (Fig. 8).

Finally, a laparoscopic check is performed to exclude breaches in the peritoneum.

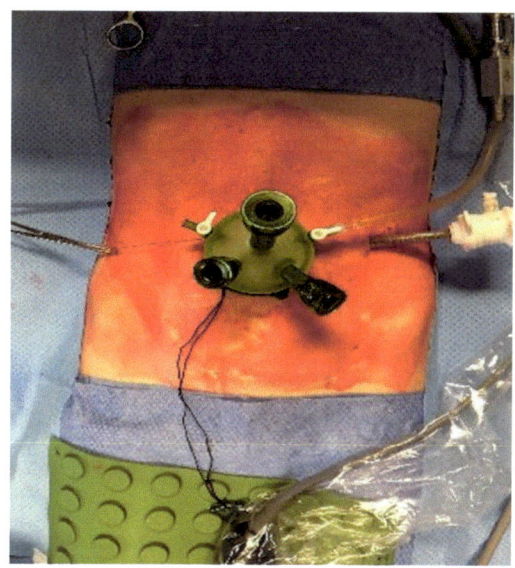

Fig. 3 Monoport at infra-umbilical incision

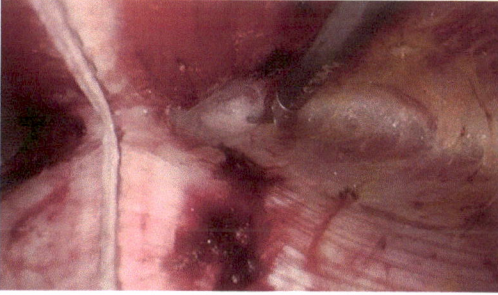

Fig. 4 Retromuscular space dissection

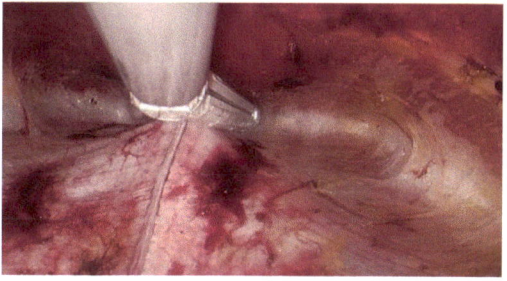

Fig. 5 Stapled midline plication

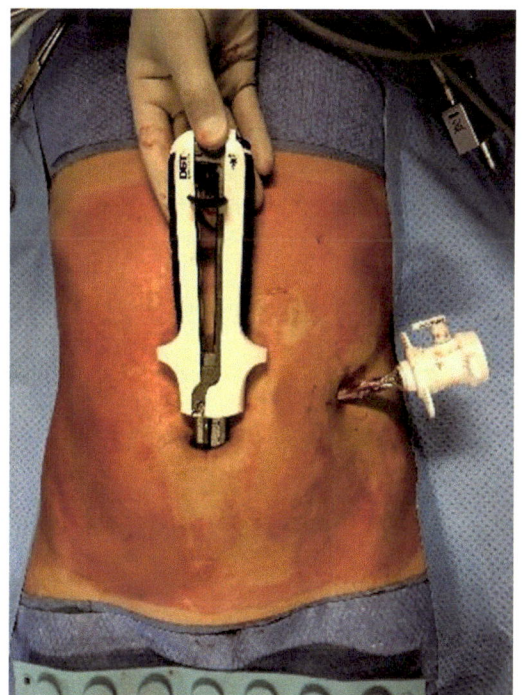

Fig. 2 Firing of stapler in the retromuscular space

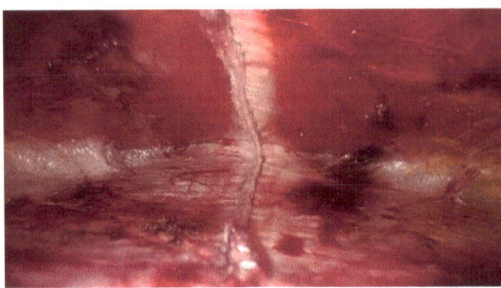

Fig. 6 Final view of the retromuscular space

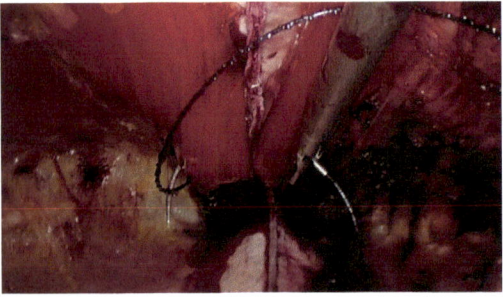

Fig. 7 Ower-sewn suture of the anterior stapled plication with a 2/0 barbed wire

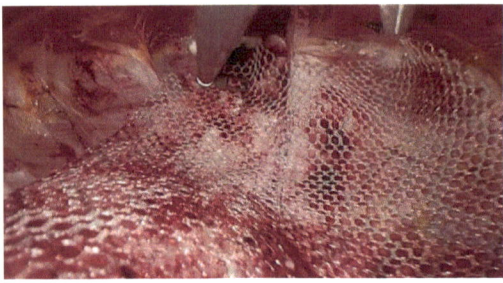

Fig. 8 Retromuscular mesh placement

At the end of the procedure, the intraperitoneal port is removed from the peritoneum into the retromuscular space, to place a closed-suction drain.

The monoport is now retracted, and a suture of the anterior rectus sheath is done with small bites technique through the infra-umbilical incision. Skin closure completes the operation.

Complications and Management

- *Intraoperative complications:*
- In case of posterior fascia breaches, repair can be attempted by endoscopic approach to avoid intraperitoneal mesh exposure.
- Bowel injuries need immediate treatment by suture or bowel resection.
- Muscular bleeding is a rare complication and can be approached endoscopically or, in case of massive bleeding, converting to open technique.
- *Postoperative complications:*
- Small retromuscular hematomas can be treated conservatively. In case of deep epigastric vessel bleeding, we suggest an urgent angiographic treatment.
- Seromas can be managed conservatively, while chronic or symptomatic seromas can be aspirated in an aseptic setting.
- Chronic pain can require further investigations and specialistic management.

Postoperative Care

- Diet and mobilization are resumed starting on the first postoperative day
- Analgesia is prescribed according to hospital protocol
- Discharge is feasible as soon as possible, according to diet tolerance, pain control, and adequate mobilization of the patient
- If closed-suction drainage is present, it can be removed when output is less than 50 cc/24 h
- All patients are advised to wear an abdominal binder for a period of at least 1 month after operation and avoid weight lifting for at least 2 months

References

1. Palanivelu C, Rangarajan M, Jategaonkar PA, et al. Laparoscopic repair of diastasis recti using the 'Venetian blinds' technique of plication with prosthetic reinforcement: a retrospective study. Hernia. 2009;13(3):287–92.
2. Muas DMJ, Palmisano E, Poa Santoja G, et al. Preaponeurotic endoscopic repair (REPA) as treatment of the diastasis of the recti associated or not to hernias of the middle line. Multicenter study. Rev Hispanoam Hernia. 2019;7(2):59–65. https://doi.org/10.20960/rhh.194.
3. Köckerling F, Botsinis MD, Rohde C, Reinpold W, Schug-Pass C. Endoscopic-assisted linea alba reconstruction: new technique for treatment of symptomatic umbilical, trocar, and/or epigastric hernias with concomitant rectus abdominis diastasis. Eur Surg. 2017;49(2):71–5. https://doi.org/10.1007/s10353-017-0473-1.
4. Bellido Luque J, Bellido Luque A, Valdivia J, et al. Totally endoscopic surgery on diastasis recti associated with midline hernias. The advantages of a minimally invasive approach. Prospective cohort study. Hernia. 2015;19(3):493–501. https://doi.org/10.1007/s10029-014-1300-2.
5. Abdalla RZ, Garcia RB, da Costa RID, Abdalla BMZ. Treatment of mid-line abdominal wall hernias with the use of endo-stapler for mid-line closure. Arq Bras Cir Dig. 2013;26(4):335–7.
6. Carrara A, Lauro E, Fabris L, Frisini M, Rizzo S. Endo-laparoscopic reconstruction of the abdominal wall midline with linear stapler, the THT technique. Early results of the first case series. Ann Med Surg. 2019;38:1–7.
7. Costa TN, Abdalla RZ, Santo MA, Tavares RRFM, Abdalla BMZ, Cecconello I. Transabdominal midline reconstruction by minimally invasive surgery: technique and results. Hernia. 2016;20(2):257–65.
8. Moore AM, Anderson LN, Chen DC. Laparoscopic stapled sublay repair with self-gripping mesh: a simplified technique for minimally invasive Extraperitoneal ventral hernia repair. Surg Technol Int. 2016;29:131–9.

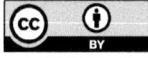

Endoscopic Subcutaneous Onlay Laparoscopic Approach

Andreuccetti Jacopo, Di Leo Alberto, and Enrico Lauro

Introduction

In recent years, abdominal wall surgery has shown a clear interest in reproducing traditional open techniques and avoiding intraperitoneal mesh placement. The endoscopic Subcutaneous Onlay Laparoscopic Approach (SCOLA) is very popular in South American countries, especially for small umbilical and epigastric hernias with concomitant rectus muscles diastasis. In these cases, a full midline reconstruction should be scheduled, because hernia repair alone is affected by a higher recurrences rate compared to simultaneous hernia and diastasis repair [1–5]. Through an endoscopic dissection of the preaponeurotic subcutaneous space is possible to reconstruct the abdominal wall by placing an onlay prosthesis in those patients without excess skin or subcutaneous tissue. Although SCOLA repair is safe and feasible to correct diastasis recti and symptomatic midline hernias with excellent cosmetic results, seroma and abdominal numbness are frequent complications.

A. Jacopo (✉)
General Surgery 2, ASST Spedali Civili of Brescia, Brescia, Italy
e-mail: jacopo.andreuccetti@asst-spedalicivili.it

D. L. Alberto
U.O. di Chirurgia Generale, Ospedale San Camillo, Trento, Italy

E. Lauro
General Surgery Division, St. Maria del Carmine Hospital, Rovereto, Italy

Indications

- Small/medium (≤4 cm) primitive hernias or multiple defects of the abdominal wall midline (umbilicus and/or epigastric hernia) associated with rectus muscles diastasis >2 cm
- Patients fit for general anesthesia

Contraindications

- Midline defects ≥5 cm
- Excess of skin and/or subcutaneous tissue
- BMI >30 kg/m^2
- Complex hernias
- Loss of abdominal domain
- Desire for pregnancy

Preoperative Assessment

- Careful history and physical examination
- Routine investigations according to hospital protocols
- Prophylactic antibiotics according to hospital protocols
- Suspension of any anticoagulant according to its wash-out time
- Ultrasound or CT scan (without contrast at rest and during Valsalva's maneuver)
- Preoperative antiseptic shower
- Prophylactic antibiotics

© The Author(s) 2023
D. Lomanto et al. (eds.), *Mastering Endo-Laparoscopic and Thoracoscopic Surgery*,
https://doi.org/10.1007/978-981-19-3755-2_66

OT Setup (Fig. 1)

- *Laparoscopic (Lps) Instrumentations*
  - Lps camera (10 mm, 30°)
  - 1 × 11 mm trocar (or balloon tip trocar)
  - 2 × 5 mm trocars
  - Lps bipolar forceps
  - Lps curved scissor
  - 2 × Johann forceps
  - Lps needle holder
  - Suture for linea alba plication (2–0 or 0 absorbable barbed suture)
  - Prosthesis (lightweight and large porous mesh)
  - Fibrin glue
- *Patient's Position (Figs. 2 and 3)*
  - The patient is positioned supine on the surgical table with the legs lower than the hip's level in order to avoid the fighting between surgeon's hands and patient's limbs.

- The surgeon places himself between the patient's legs.
- The endoscopic equipment is positioned to the right of the patient.
- *Essential Steps in Synthesis*
  - Trocars setup (Figs. 2 and 3).
  - Creation of a pyramid-shaped preaponeurotic work chamber (Fig. 4).
  - Reduction of the ventral hernia (Fig. 5).
  - Plication of the linea alba (Fig. 6).
  - Mesh positioning and fixation (Figs. 7, 8, and 9).

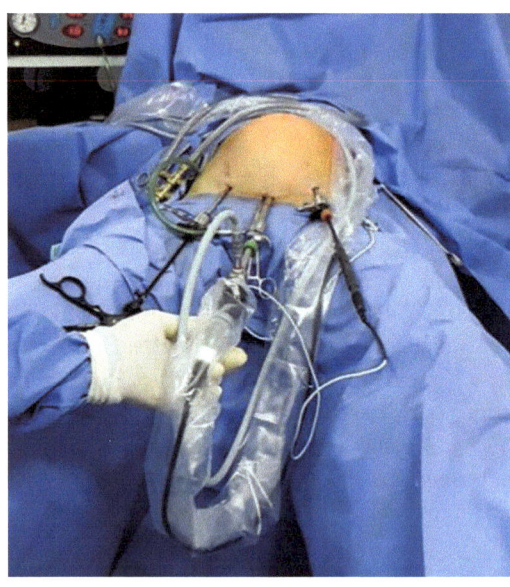

Fig. 3 Patient's position

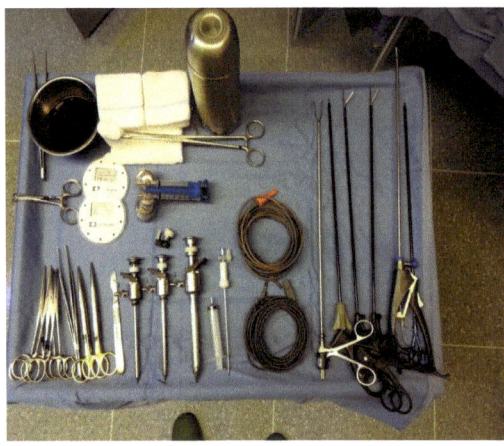

Fig. 1 OT Setup

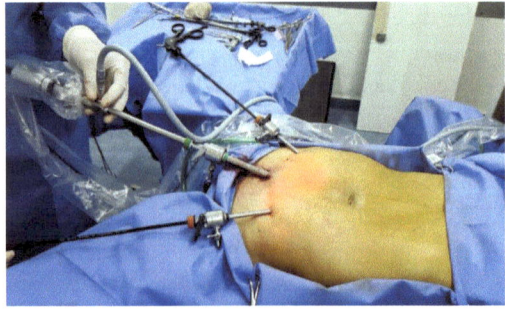

Fig. 2 Patient's position

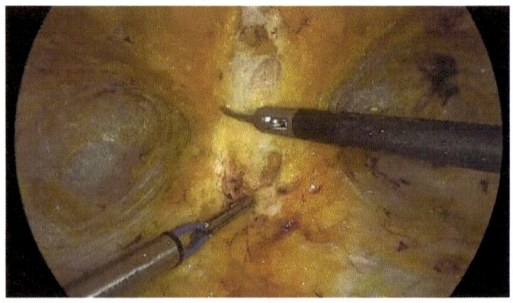

Fig. 4 Creation of a pyramid-shaped preaponeurotic work chamber

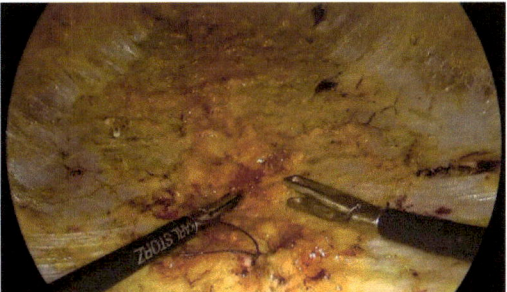

Fig. 5 Reduction of the ventral hernia in abdomen

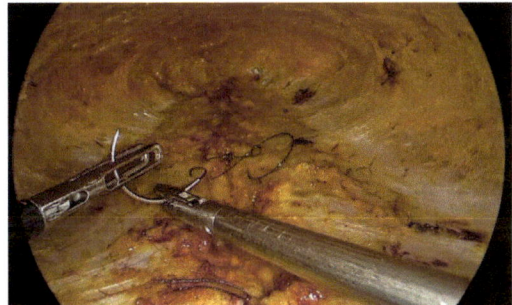

Fig. 6 Plication of the linea alba

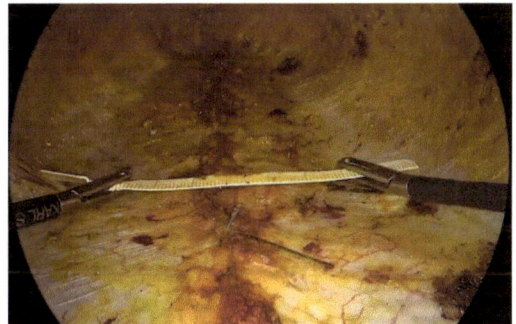

Fig. 7 Final aspect after midline plication and defect closure. Measuring the prosthesis width

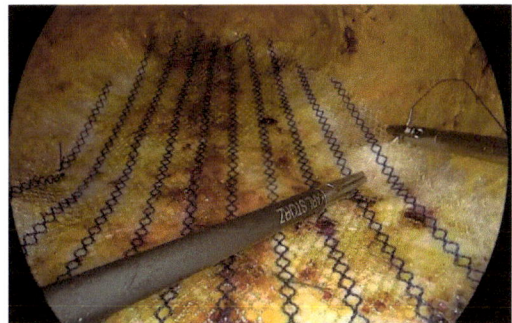

Fig. 8 Mesh positioning

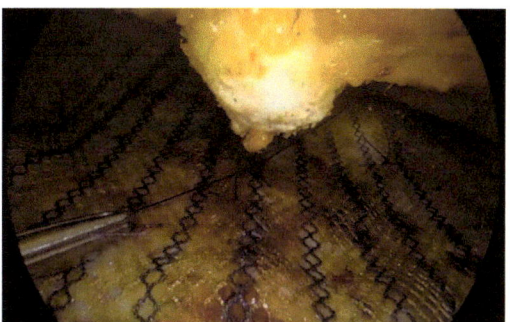

Fig. 9 Anchoring the umbilicus

- *Description of the technique*

A surgical incision is made in the suprapubic region on the midline. After identifying the aponeurotic fascia, a small workspace is created with finger dissection and the first 11 mm trocar is there positioned (a balloon tip Trocar is an option). A subcutaneous chamber is created throughout blunt dissection using the camera, to the right and then to the left towards the anterior superior iliac spines. The other two 5 mm trocars are now positioned obtaining an optimal triangulation. The dissection proceeds in the preaponeurotic space separating the anterior rectus sheath and subcutaneous tissue, preserving the perforating vessels (Fig. 4). During the subcutaneous space dissection hernias, defects are identified, and their content is reduced (Fig. 5). The dissection extends up to the xiphoid. The linea alba plication is performed by suturing the medial margins of the anterior fascia of the rectus muscles with a barbed running suture (Fig. 6). A fixed macroporous lightweight mesh is placed onlay according to the dimension of the plane (Figs. 7 and 8). The last step of the intervention involves anchoring the umbilicus on the fascial plane (Fig. 9). If a suction drain is used it is held in place until the output is less than 30 cc/24 h.

Postoperative Care

- All patients are prescribed an abdominal binder to wear for about 2 months
- Analgesia is required
- Discharge is possible even after 24 h
- Advised against lifting weight for 3 months

References

1. Reinpold W, Köckerling F, Bittner R, et al. Classification of rectus diastasis-a proposal by the German hernia society (DHG) and the international Endohernia society (IEHS). Front Surg. 2019;6:1. https://doi.org/10.3389/fsurg.2019.00001.
2. Muas DMJ, Palmisano E, Poa Santoja G, et al. Preaponeurotic endoscopic repair (REPA) as treatment of the diastasis of the recti associated or not to hernias of the middle line. Multicenter study. Rev Hispanoam Hernia. 2019;7(2):59–65. https://doi.org/10.20960/rhh.194.
3. Juárez Muas DM. Preaponeurotic endoscopic repair (REPA) of diastasis recti associated or not to midline hernias. Surg Endosc. 2019;33(6):1777–82. https://doi.org/10.1007/s00464-018-6450-3.
4. Claus CMP, Malcher F, Cavazzola LT, et al. Subcutaneous onlay laparoscopic approach (SCOLA) for ventral hernia and rectus abdominis diastasis repair: technical description and initial results. Arq Bras Cir Dig. 2018;31(4):e1399. https://doi.org/10.1590/0102-672020180001e1399.
5. Bellido Luque J, Bellido Luque A, Valdivia J, et al. Totally endoscopic surgery on diastasis recti associated with midline hernias. The advantages of a minimally invasive approach. Prospective cohort study. Hernia. 2015;19(3):493–501. https://doi.org/10.1007/s10029-014-1300-2.

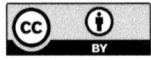

Minimally Invasive Surgery for Diaphragmatic Hernia

Hrishikesh Salgaonkar, Kanagaraj Marimuthu, Alistair Sharples, Vittal Rao, and Nagammapudur Balaji

Diaphragmatic hernia (DH) is a rare entity, more commonly seen in children as compared to adults. It is classified as congenital or acquired. Most common cause of acquired hernia is following trauma. Management of DH is primarily surgical repair which can be performed by laparotomy, laparoscopy, thoracotomy, or thoracoscopy. Due to the rarity of the disease, there is a paucity of data in the literature regarding the best approach for the repair. With the advent of laparoscopy or thoracoscopy, these are the preferred options as it offers us all the known benefits associated with minimally invasive surgery (MIS). For the scope of this chapter, our focus will be on the role of thoracoscopy and laparoscopy in the management of adult DH, the technical details, and its associated complications.

Introduction

An important muscle of respiration, the diaphragm forms a physical wall which separates the contents of the chest from the abdomen. In diaphragmatic hernia (DH), there is herniation of abdominal viscera into the pleural space through a weakness or defect in the diaphragm.

The single most important factor is due to the pressure gradient between the abdominal and thoracic cavities. During respiratory cycle, this may reach up to 100 mm of Hg and contributes to herniation of abdominal contents into the thoracic cavity [1]. DH can be classified as congenital or acquired [2]. Congenital DH is seen mainly in pediatric population and occurs due to failure of the fusion of foraminas of diaphragm. In Bochdalek hernia, there is an incomplete fusion of posterolateral foramina and in Morgagni hernia, it is at the anterior midline through the sterno-coastal region. Acquired DH is most commonly traumatic in origin, mainly due to penetrating or blunt trauma to the abdomen or thorax. Spontaneous DH is a rarity where the patient denies any history of trauma or symptoms and accounts for less than 1% of cases [3, 4]. But a possibility of a previously forgotten trauma cannot be ruled out completely. The presentation of DH can be acute or chronic. For chronic DH, the classification criteria concerns the temporal parameter of its development and diagnosis. As per Carter's Scheme [5].

1. Acute phase (time between the original trauma and the patient's recovery)
2. Latent phase (time post-recovery during which patient may or may not be symptomatic and obstructive phase)
3. Obstructive phase (when contents become incarcerated with potential risk of ischemia, necrosis, and perforation)

H. Salgaonkar (✉) · K. Marimuthu · A. Sharples · V. Rao · N. Balaji
Department of Bariatric and Upper GI Surgery, University Hospitals North Midlands, Stoke-on-Trent, UK

© The Author(s) 2023
D. Lomanto et al. (eds.), *Mastering Endo-Laparoscopic and Thoracoscopic Surgery*, https://doi.org/10.1007/978-981-19-3755-2_67

The diagnosis of traumatic DH is often delayed as at the time of the accident or trauma it is difficult to detect a small defect or rent in the diaphragm [6]. Most symptoms are masked due to the associated symptoms from the traumatic injury [5, 7]. It only raises suspicion when complications of DH occur, e.g., gastrointestinal obstruction, strangulation of contents, or cardiopulmonary compromise. Traumatic DH is more common on left side (80%) and can be bilateral in 1–3% of cases. The left preponderance is thought to be due to the protective effect of the bare area of liver dissipating the force of the injury. The incidence of DH post penetrating trauma is almost double after a gunshot injury (20–59%) as compared to stab wounds (15–32%) [8]. Classically a chronic DH is a sequelae of an undiagnosed and untreated diaphragmatic injury while managing an acute traumatic event. Both penetrating and blunt thoracoabdominal injuries may cause a DH.

The clinical features of DH differ based on the location of the hernia and the organs herniating through it. Most common organs involved are the liver and gallbladder on the right side and the stomach, colon, and small bowel on the left side. In large hernia, solid organs like liver and spleen may also herniate. DH is often asymptomatic or produces very mild symptoms, till serious complications like obstruction or strangulation manifest. It is not unusual for the patient to present months to years after the index injury. Symptomatology may be related to respiratory tract, gastrointestinal organs, or a nonspecific general pain. When complications occur, patient may have severe respiratory, gastrointestinal, or cardiovascular symptoms which may mimic a tension pneumothorax also.

In some cases, a DH may be discovered incidentally on a radiological examination performed for unrelated reasons. A high index of suspicion is necessarily combined with a detailed history, thorough clinical examination, proper interpretation of the radiological images namely chest radiograph which is a preliminary investigation ordered in most outpatient or emergency setup. Usual findings are loss of diaphragmatic integrity with bowel haustrations or gas shadows within thorax, mediastinal shift to normal side, atelecta-

sis, pleural effusion, or hydro-pneumothorax. If a nasogastric tube is inserted, very commonly this may be seen in the chest in defect on the left side if stomach has herniated through. A CT scan of chest and abdomen or MRI may be helpful when diagnosis is uncertain.

Once diagnosed, irrespective of symptoms it is advisable to offer surgery if the patient is fit. This can be via laparotomy, thoracotomy, laparoscopy, or thoracoscopy or a combined approach based on the surgeon's preference, anatomic location of defect, degree of infra-diaphragmatic adhesions, and previous abdominal repair [9]. It is not advisable to delay the surgery as this may lead to complications, e.g., volvulus, incarceration, strangulation, etc. The goal is to reduce the contents back into the abdominal cavity and repairing the defect in the diaphragm. Minimal invasive surgery in the form of laparoscopy or thoracoscopy offers us all the benefits in terms of lesser pain, shorter hospitalization, reduced respiratory complications, and early return to work [3, 9]. Although data from randomized control trials is lacking results of both thoracoscopy or laparoscopy have been found to be comparable [9]. Laparoscopy in particular by delineating clear anatomy, better working space is increasingly thought to be a safe and feasible option to repair DH [10].

Acute DH with obstruction/strangulation or Acute traumatic DH: In an acute scenario, surgical approach should be immediate without any delay. Traditionally this would involve a laparotomy or thoracotomy. Use of prosthesis when contaminated field is present is debatable. Use of biological mesh may be considered. For the scope of this chapter, we would keep our focus on minimal invasive modalities.

Preoperative Work-Up

A thorough preoperative assessment is required to assess fitness to withstand the surgery, nutritional assessment, and optimization of medical comorbidities. This includes routine blood, urinalysis, chest radiograph, barium swallow if needed, or a CT scan. If a history of smoking is present it is advisable to abstain immediately.

Acute presentation of DH is a true surgical emergency and we may need to proceed to surgery immediately. Correction of dehydration and electrolyte abnormalities if any should be done. In left side hernias, it is advisable to decompress the stomach with nasogastric tube. Counsel the patient regarding the risk of complications with particular emphasis on recurrence.

Operative Technique: Laparoscopy

Theater layout and patient position: The patient is placed in supine position with split legs. Secure the patient safely to the operative table with straps at mid-thigh levels, to both legs separately and foot support if patient is morbidly obese. The stability should be tested preoperatively by placing patient in anti-Trendelenburg position before starting the surgery. The arms are tucked by the patient side. Compression stockings and pneumatic compression devices are applied to both legs until unless contraindicated. The surgeon stands in between the legs, camera operator on the right side, and another assistant on the left in left side DH. On right side DH, the camera operator and assistant change their positions. It is ideal to have two monitors one on either side of the patient's head. If only one monitor is present place it above the affected side shoulder.

Abdominal access and techniques: Creation of pneumoperitoneum can be done using a Veress needle, by direct trocar entry (Optical entry) or open Hasson's technique. Insufflating the abdomen to 12–14 mmHg. The table is then placed in anti-Trendelenburg position 25–30⁰. This allows better visualization of the upper abdominal cavity and tissue spaces that need to be dissected. Rest trocars are placed under vision. A liver retraction device is placed through one of these port sites, usually substernal to retract the liver if it is not herniating. The port position and numbers vary slightly depending upon the side of the hernia. Total 4–5 trocars technique is used based upon the side of DH, the contents herniating through. On the right side DH, a 10/12 mm port just above the umbilicus for scope, two additional ports laterally on the right side one in the midclavicular line and another along the anterior axil-

lary line, one additional 5 mm port in the midline epigastric region for assistant. For left side DH, five ports are generally used. A 10/12 mm port just above the umbilicus, two working lateral ports on either side in the midclavicular line at the level of umbilicus, 5 mm substernal port for liver retraction, and additional port left side laterally along the anterior axillary line for assistant.

Always start by performing a general examination of the peritoneal cavity to exclude any other pathology, e.g., other abdominal wall hernia, adhesions, or what organs are herniating to the defect (Fig. 1). Visualize the entire diaphragm on both sides and assess for contents of the DH.

Reducing the contents and delineating the defect: Use nontraumatic graspers to retract bowels caudally away from the operative field. Contents of the hernia are gently reduced using nontraumatic graspers (Fig. 2).

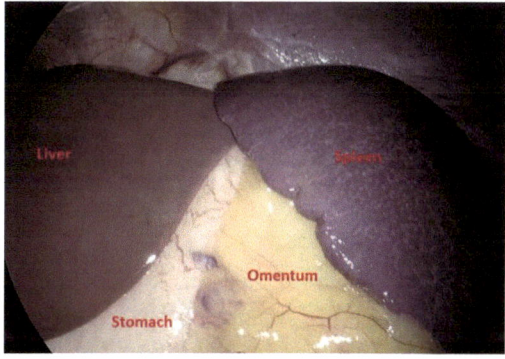

Fig. 1 Diaphragmatic hernia with stomach, liver, and spleen pulled up into the defect

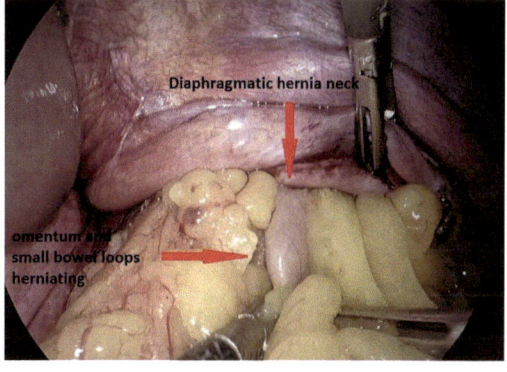

Fig. 2 Gentle traction with nontraumatic graspers to reduce the contents

In acute cases the contents especially stomach, small bowel, or colon may be edematous and can be easily damaged with serosal tears or enterotomies. Special care is taken while handling and reducing solid organs, e.g., spleen if seen herniating to avoid hemorrhage. Any adhesions between the herniated organs and sac which are continuous with the pleural lining should be meticulously separated using an energy device as per surgeon preference. It is not uncommon to end up making multiple openings in the pleural lining. Any openings in the pleural lining can be sutured using 3–0 absorbable sutures. In difficult cases, a thoracoscopy may be performed additionally to aid the release of adhesions of herniated abdominal contents from the thoracic cavity. In longstanding DH, the lung on the affected side is hypoplastic in many cases. Once the defect is delineated, clear out any adhesions around the edges so as to gain space for suturing the edges and mesh placement/fixation. At this stage, if required one can pass an intercoastal drain under vision into the pleural cavity. In large defects this may involve mobilizing the splenic flexure on the left side, Gerota's fascia or the triangular ligaments of the liver. In cases of large and redundant hernial sacs, excess sacs can be excised to facilitate proper closure. If eventration of diaphragm is present, we can plicate the diaphragm with polypropylene or ethibond sutures. The plication helps to bring the diaphragm to the desired level which will help us during defect closure.

Defect closure: With regards to defect closure, some surgeons prefer simple suturing of the defect, whereas others prefer to additionally reinforce the defect with prosthetic material. However, it is generally agreed that defects which are larger than 20–30 cm² do require the use of prosthesis [11]. The author prefers the use of barbed suture or ethibond to close the defect. Meticulous defect closure is attempted in all cases (Fig. 3).

If required peritoneal flaps or muscular flaps can be utilized. In addition to providing a flat surface for prosthesis placement, it prevents mesh extrusion through the defect [12]. Once the defect is closed, different types of prosthesis can be used for reinforcement. In the literature review, polypropylene, composite mesh, and biological meshes have been used. In the authors opinion, composite or biological mesh should be used. Although more expensive, they are preferred due to lower infection rates and less risk of erosion into hollow viscus [13]. Like any hernial repair, the mesh should overlap the defect by at least 5 cm all around to reduce risk of recurrence. Until and unless contraindicated, we always reinforce the closed defect with a prosthesis to reduce the risk of recurrence. Also, placing the mesh on the peritoneal surface of diaphragm by physiology of intra-abdominal pressure keeps the mesh opposed to the defect (Laplace's law). The mesh is then fixed using sutures, tackers, or glue

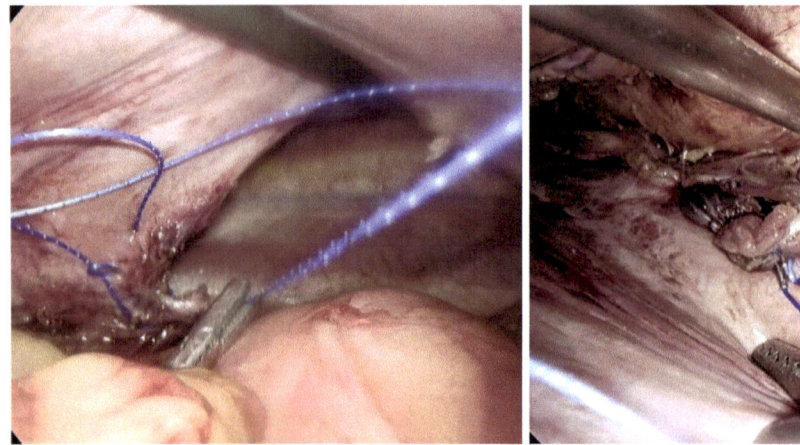

Fig. 3 Completely delineate and close the defect of diaphragmatic hernia

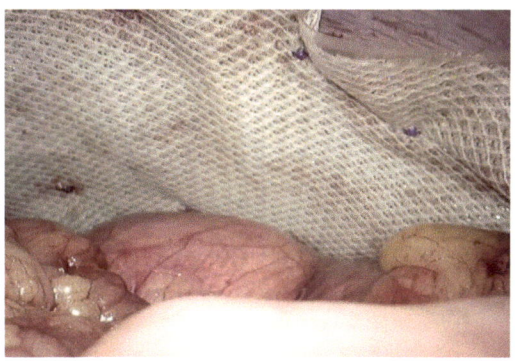

Fig. 4 Mesh reinforcement and fixation over the defect

(Fig. 4). While tackers are the most commonly used modality, it is advisable to use them carefully so as to avoid injury to vital structures in the vicinity.

Thoracoscopy: A thoracic approach may be preferred to treat recurrent diaphragmatic hernia, following a previous abdominal repair. It can also be used in combination with laparoscopy, especially in presence of dense adhesions between the contents and the thoracic cavity inner lining [14]. It is also easier to plicate diaphragmatic eventration thoracoscopically as compared to laparoscopically. If a thoracoscopic or laparo-thoracoscopic approach is planned it is advisable to perform general anesthesia with a double-lumen tube to achieve single-lung ventilation.

Postoperative Care

Patient who has preoperative respiratory distress (emergency scenarios) or a severely hypoplastic lung on affected side, recovery from anesthesia may be difficult and may need ventilatory support postoperatively. Similarly, in patients where bowel resection is performed, e.g., strangulation of contents, etc., may need nutritional support in the form of TPN or enteric feeding.

In elective setup, as per ERAS protocol (Early recovery after surgery) adequate analgesia and anti-emetics are prescribed. Early mobilization and feeds are encouraged. Postoperative anti-thrombotic prophylaxis based upon hospital recommendations should be followed. Anti-microbial

cover is decided on a case-to-case basis. All patients should undergo a postoperative chest radiograph. Intercoastal drain is removed based upon the quantity of draining fluid from the pleural cavity, resolution of pneumothorax, and lung expansion. Regular follow up is needed, ideally after 1 week, every 3 months in the first year, and then annually for 4–5 years after surgery. A detailed clinical examination and chest radiograph should be performed.

Complications

Fatal intraoperative complications such as failure to return viscera to the abdominal cavity, irreparable bowel abnormalities, e.g., ischemia, gangrene, etc., failure to repair large defects, and difficulty maintaining ventilation and oxygenation ultimately leading to mortality are not uncommon particularly in emergency scenarios. Routine complications of any thoracoscopic or gastrointestinal surgery such as chest infection, wound infections, bleeding, incisional hernia, adhesions, and postoperative ileus are reported. While performing adhesiolysis, bleeding and visceral injuries can occur. Pneumothorax and pleural effusion are common complication. Longstanding DH predisposes patients to pulmonary hypertension. Although there is a paucity of evidence from randomized control trials, minimal invasive modalities of managing DH offer us all the benefits namely reduced pain, shorter hospitalization, early return to work, respiratory, and wound-related complications.

Recurrence: The incidence of recurrence is debatable. In congenital DH this ranges from 3 to 50% in various studies. It is advisable to repair a recurrent DH after a laparotomy or laparoscopy with thoracoscopic approach [15].

Bowel obstruction: Handling of intra-abdominal viscera invariably leads to adhesions, which may progress to bowel obstruction. These are more common after laparotomy as compared to laparoscopic DH repair [16, 17].

Long-term morbidity: Significant proportions of patients with longstanding DH suffer from long-term complications even after surgical repair. These are chronic respiratory disease, pulmonary hypertension, gastroesophageal reflux disease, and musculoskeletal deformities (more common after thoracotomy).

Conclusion

Minimally invasive surgery for DH repair offers us all the routine benefits such as magnified vision, shorter hospitalization, and reduced wound and pulmonary complications as compared to open methods. Laparoscopic or thoracoscopic repair of DH is a safe and effective method for managing adult diaphragmatic hernias, especially in experienced hands.

Practical Tips

- Having a trained and regular team assisting during the surgery cannot be over-emphasised.
- Combining laparoscopy and thoracoscopy is a good option especially when adhesions are present between the contents and the thoracic cavity.
- Insertion of additional trocars and conversion to open technique in difficult scenarios should not be considered as failure of surgery.
- For defects closed under tension or defects larger than 10 cm use a prosthetic reinforcement.
- In cases where the defect cannot be closed, local muscle flaps (intercostals, latissimus dorsi) or Intraperitoneal fascial flaps (Toldt's) are performed to cover the defect with help of plastic surgeons.
- Diaphragmatic hernia is a rare diagnosis. Surgical results are best in experienced hands. These are to be borne in mind before offering surgery to patients, especially in an elective setting.

Acknowledgments Kind regards to Dr. Sunil Kumar Nayak, Department of Minimal invasive surgery, GEM Hospital and Research Centre, Coimbatore for providing all the intraoperative images.

References

1. İçme F, Vural S, Tanrıverdi F, Balkan E, Kozacı N, Kurtoğlu GÇ. Spontaneous diaphragmatic hernia: a case report. Eurasian J Emerg Med. 2014;13:209–11.
2. de Meijer VE, Vles WJ, Kats E, den Hoed PT. Iatrogenic diaphragmatic hernia complicating nephrectomy: top-down or bottom-up? Hernia. 2008;12(6):655–8.
3. Gupta S, Bali RK, Das K, Sisodia A, Dewan RK, Singla R. Rare presentation of spontaneous acquired diaphragmatic hernia. Indian J Chest Dis Allied Sci. 2011;53(2):117–9.
4. Gupta V, Singhal R, Ansari MZ. Spontaneous rupture of the diaphragm. Eur J Emerg Med. 2005;12(1):43–4.
5. Carter BN, Giuseffi J, Felson B. Traumatic diaphragmatic hernia. Am J Roentgenol Radium Ther. 1951;65(1):56–72.
6. Bani Hani MN. A combined laparoscopic and endoscopic approach to acute gastric volvulus associated with traumatic diaphragmatic hernia. Surg Laparosc Endosc Percutan Tech. 2008;18(2):151–4.
7. Dwari AK, Mandal A, Das SK, Sakar S. Delayed presentation of traumatic diaphragmatic rupture with herniation of the left kidney and bowel loops. Case Rep Pulmonol. 2013;2013:814632.
8. Ahmed N, Jones D. Video-assisted thoracic surgery: state of the art in trauma care. Injury. 2004;35(5):479–89.
9. Saroj SK, Kumar S, Afaque Y, Bhartia AK, Bhartia VK. Laparoscopic repair of congenital diaphragmatic hernia in adults. Minimal Invas Surg. 2016;2016:1–5.
10. Thoman DS, Hui T, Phillips EH. Laparoscopic diaphragmatic hernia repair. Surg Endosc. 2002;16(9):1345–9.
11. Jee Y. Laparoscopic diaphragmatic hernia repair using expanded polytetrafluoroethylene (ePTFE) for delayed traumatic diaphragmatic hernia. Wideochir Inne Tech Maloinwazyjne. 2017;12(2):189–93.
12. Palanivelu C, Jani KV, Senthilnathan P, Parthasarathi R, Madhankumar MV, Malladi VK. Laparoscopic sutured closure with mesh reinforcement of incisional hernias. Hernia. 2002;11(3):223–8.
13. Esposito F, Lim C, Salloum C, Osseis M, Lahat E, Compagnon P, et al. Diaphragmatic hernia following liver resection: case series and review of the literature. Ann Hepatobiliary Pancreat Surg. 2017;21(3):114–21.
14. Chauhan SS, Mishra A, Dave S, Naqvi J, Tamaskar S, Sharma V, et al. Thoracolaparoscopic management of diaphragmatic hernia of adults: a case series. Int Surg J. 2020;7(5):1627–33.
15. Keijzer R, van de Ven C, Vlot J, et al. Thoracoscopic repair in congenital diaphragmatic hernia: patching is safe and reduces the recurrence rate. J Pediatr Surg. 2010;45(05):953–7.

16. Putnam LR, Tsao K, Lally KP, et al. Congenital diaphragmatic hernia study group and the pediatric surgery research collaborative. Minimally invasive vs open congenital diaphragmatic hernia repair: is there a superior approach? J Am Coll Surg. 2017;224(04):416–22.

17. Davenport M, Rothenberg SS, Crabbe DCG, Wulkan ML. The great debate: open or thoracoscopic repair for oesophageal atresia or diaphragmatic hernia. J Pediatr Surg. 2015;50(02):240–6.

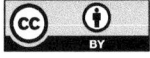

Laparoscopic Parastomal Hernia Repair

Isaac Seow-En, Yuan-Yao Tsai, and William Tzu-Liang Chen

Introduction

Parastomal hernia is an incisional hernia resulting from an abdominal wall stoma creation [1]. The published incidence of parastomal hernia varies widely, with 2–28% and 4–48% affecting end ileostomies and end colostomies, respectively, depending on the severity of the hernia, method of diagnosis, and the duration of follow-up [2]. Loop stomas have a much lower incidence of parastomal herniation, as these tend to be reversed before a hernia can develop. The risk of herniation is cumulative with time but appears to be highest within 2 years of ostomy formation. Most patients are asymptomatic or have mild complaints such as intermittent discomfort or sporadic obstructive symptoms, but many eventually have symptoms significant enough to warrant surgical intervention, including incarceration, strangulation, and perforation. The bulging around the stoma can also cause result in difficulty applying the stoma appliance, resulting in leakage and skin irritation [2].

As with other types of incisional hernia, risk factors associated with parastomal hernia development can be categorized into patient- or technique-related. Patient factors include underlying comorbid conditions which raise intra-abdominal pressure, adversely affect wound healing and nutrition, or predispose to wound infection. Obesity with a BMI ≥ 25 kg/m^2 has also been found to be an independent risk factor [3].

Surgery-related or technical factors include the site of stoma creation, the size of the trephine, intraperitoneal versus extraperitoneal route, and the prophylactic use of a mesh. It is a common belief that stomas formed through the rectus abdominis muscle have lower hernia rates than those formed lateral to the muscle. However, a 2003 review [2] observed that only one study [4] out of six comparing the two approaches found any significant benefit in the transrectus positioning. A 2019 Cochrane review similarly could not demonstrate a lower rate of hernia if the stoma were placed through versus lateral to the rectus muscle [5]. It is noteworthy that another recent meta-analysis showed a significantly reduced incidence of

I. Seow-En
Department of Colorectal Surgery, Singapore General Hospital, Singapore, Singapore

Division of Colorectal Surgery, China Medical University Hospital, Taichung, Taiwan

Y.-Y. Tsai
Division of Colorectal Surgery, China Medical University Hospital, Taichung, Taiwan

W. T.-L. Chen (✉)
Division of Colorectal Surgery, Department of Surgery, China Medical University Hsinchu Hospital, Zhubei City, Hsinchu County, Taiwan
e-mail: wtchen@mail.cmuh.org.tw

parastomal herniation with preoperative stoma site marking, which the authors suggested was a result of transrectus ostomy creation [6]. The ideal trephine size is not yet established, although an increased risk of herniation has been associated with a defect of 3 cm and above [7, 8].

The extraperitoneal technique of end stoma creation, described by Goligher in 1958, was devised to reduce small bowel internal herniation into the lateral peritoneal space [9]. This method was also found in a 2016 meta-analysis to have a significantly lower rate of parastomal herniation compared to the transperitoneal approach (6% vs 18%) as well as stomal prolapse rate (1% vs 7%) [10]. Similar benefits were reported with the "Goligher method" following a laparoscopic approach to bowel resection and stoma formation [11]. Many recent studies have also evaluated the utility of prophylactic mesh placement, either biologic or synthetic, at the time of permanent ostomy creation. A 2018 Cochrane meta-analysis of 10 randomized controlled trials with 944 patients looked at mesh placement for prevention of parastomal herniation [12]. Seven of these trials described an open sublay and three a laparoscopic intraperitoneal onlay method, of which the most recent [13] employed a laparoscopic modified Sugarbaker technique. The authors found that using a prophylactic mesh halved the incidence of hernia (41% vs. 22%) without increasing stoma-related infection rates, although the overall quality of evidence was low due to a high degree of clinical heterogeneity [12]. The 2018 European Hernia Society guidelines strongly recommend the use of a prophylactic nonabsorbable mesh upon the construction of an end colostomy [14].

The transrectus, transperitoneal route without the use of mesh prophylaxis is still a popular approach for end ostomy creation, and parastomal herniation remains a common complication. There are several different approaches to surgical repair of parastomal hernias. In this chapter, we evaluate the various methods with a focus on laparoscopic repair.

Indications

The best remedy for parastomal hernia is to reverse the stoma and restore intestinal continuity. This option may not be always possible, as in the case of an abdominoperineal resection. In our practice, end colostomies following abdominoperineal resections complicated by symptomatic parastomal hernias is the most common indication for surgery. Patients with bothersome symptoms, cosmetic concerns, or emergency indications should undergo surgical intervention. Based on current evidence no recommendation can be made for operative repair over regular observation for asymptomatic patients or those with mild complaints [14]. Support garments may improve some symptoms.

Surgical Approach

Options for surgical repair of parastomal hernias include local suture repair, stoma relocation, and various forms of mesh repair. Suture repair is the easiest method and avoids a repeat laparotomy or laparoscopy. After parastomal incision and hernia sac reduction, the fascial opening is narrowed using absorbable or nonabsorbable sutures. Of all methods, direct suture repair has the highest rate of hernia recurrence ranging from 46 to 100% [2], with an overall morbidity and infection rate of 23% and 12%, respectively [15]. Despite this, direct repair may have a role in selected emergency cases or frail patients who are unable to tolerate more major surgery. Stoma relocation involves resiting the stoma to a new position on the abdominal wall. While this has a lower recurrence rate (0–76%) than direct tissue repair [2], it is inferior to mesh repair and should only be used if the existing stoma site is unsatisfactory.

Mesh repair can be onlay (fixation onto the fascia of the anterior rectus sheath and aponeurosis of the external oblique muscle), retromuscular sublay (dorsal to the rectus muscle and anterior to the posterior rectus sheath), or intraperitoneal (intra-abdominal fixation onto the peritoneum) [14]. Two common methods are used for intraperitoneal prosthesis placement, the Sugarbaker technique, first described in 1985 [16], and the keyhole technique. A third method, the sandwich technique, involves a combination of both methods and uses two meshes. In a 2012 review, recurrence rates for mesh repair ranged from 7 to 17% and did not differ significantly between the different methods when open surgery was performed [15]. Overall morbidity and mesh infection rates were low and comparable for each type of mesh repair.

Perhaps the success of laparoscopy for ventral hernia repair has led to an increased uptake of the laparoscopic modality for parastomal hernia repair [17], with both having similar short-term outcomes [18]. A 2013 retrospective review of more than 2000 patients, of which 10% were performed by laparoscopy, showed that the minimally invasive approach was associated with a shorter operating time, decreased length of hospital stay, lower risk of morbidity, and lower risk of surgical site infection, following adjustment for all potential confounders including age, gender, ASA score, emergency or elective surgery, hernia type, and wound class [19]. Interestingly, while the intraperitoneal mesh techniques have similar recurrence rates when performed via open surgery, using laparoscopy the same meta-analysis reported the modified Sugarbaker approach having a significantly lower recurrence rate than the keyhole method [15]. Moreover, the laparoscopic sandwich method showed promising initial results [20] but requires further evaluation before routine use can be recommended [14].

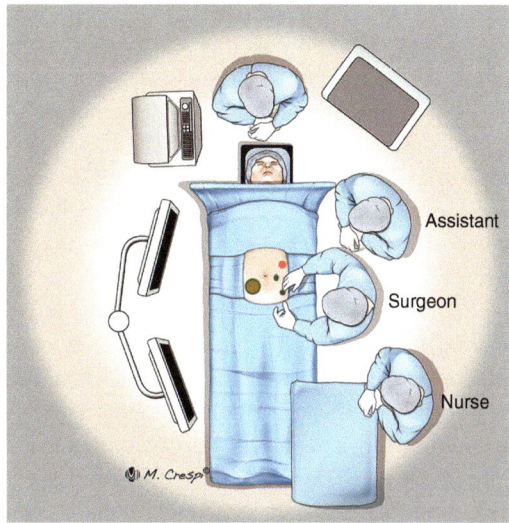

Fig. 1 Schematic of the operating setup and port placement for repair of a right lower quadrant parastomal hernia. The 12 mm camera port can be placed at either of the two superior "x" markings with 5 mm ports placed at the other two

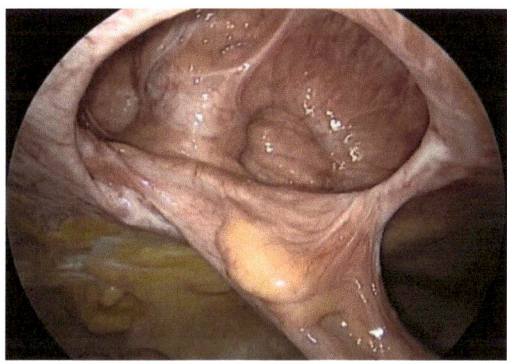

Fig. 2 Fascial defect and proximal bowel limb clearly seen following reduction of hernia sac and adequate adhesiolysis

OT Setup

Schematic of the operating setup and port positioning for repair of parastomal herniation of an end colostomy following abdominoperineal resection is shown in Fig. 1. The patient is placed supine. A 12 mm camera trocar is placed under direct vision at the right flank to avoid adhesions from previous midline surgery. Two 5 mm working trocars are placed at the right abdomen. Prophylactic intravenous antibiotics are given at anesthetic induction.

Surgical Technique

Essential steps and technique
1. Adhesiolysis
2. Reduction of the hernia sac contents
3. Placement and fixation of the prosthesis

Following laparoscopic entry, adequate adhesiolysis and careful reduction of hernia sac contents are performed as per usual. The fascial defect should be clearly seen by the end of this process (Fig. 2). The keyhole technique uses a slit mesh with a 2–3 cm "keyhole" cut-out to allow passage of the bowel while covering the entire fascial defect. There is a risk of bowel obstruction if too small a keyhole is made and risk of hernia recurrence if the keyhole is too large. The Sugarbaker technique is more easily accomplished by securing a piece of non-slit mesh over the entire fascial defect. We favor the latter technique, for its relative simplicity and lower recurrence rates.

In the Modified Sugarbaker method, the proximal bowel is anchored using Ethibond 2–0 to the peritoneum lateral to the hernial defect at two points (Fig. 3). The fascial defect can be accurately measured using a ruler (Fig. 4) to assist in preparation of the mesh. We use a Bard™ Composix™ E/X mesh, which is comprised of a synthetic layer of polypropylene, combined with a permanent barrier layer of expanded polytetrafluoroethylene (ePTFE) [21]. The mesh is first prepared exter-

nally. Appropriate mesh size is selected such that the fascial defect can be overlapped by 4–5 cm circumferentially after fixation [22]. A larger mesh can be chosen and trimmed if necessary. A length of Prolene 2–0 suture with a straight needle is anchored to the anticipated cranial end and another similar length anchored to the lateral aspect of the mesh, both on the synthetic side. The mesh is then tightly rolled up along with the attached straight needles and introduced into the abdomen through the 12 mm trocar.

Within the peritoneal cavity, the mesh can be unfurled and positioned with the synthetic surface facing up. The straight needles are passed through the anterior abdominal wall at the corresponding superior and lateral positions adjacent to the hernia defect (Fig. 5). The sutures are held with clamps and held taut; this two-point temporary fixation to the abdominal wall spreads the

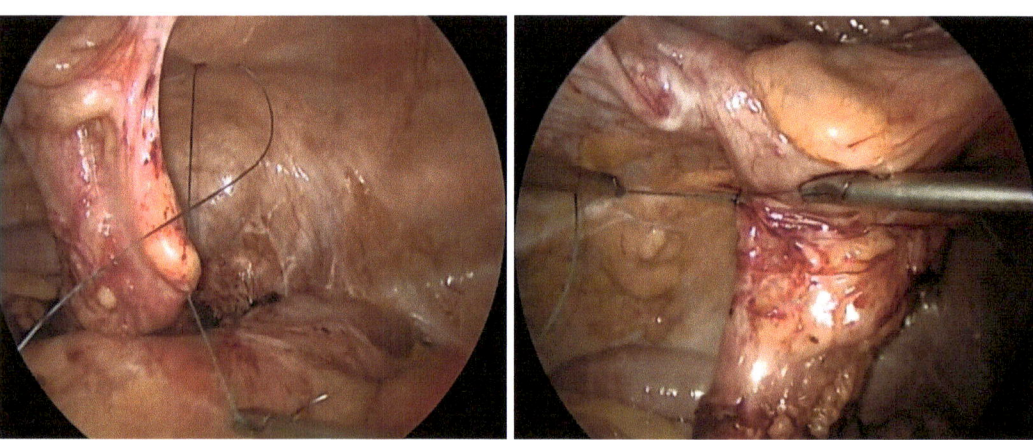

Fig. 3 The bowel limb is secured on either side to the peritoneum just lateral to the fascia defect

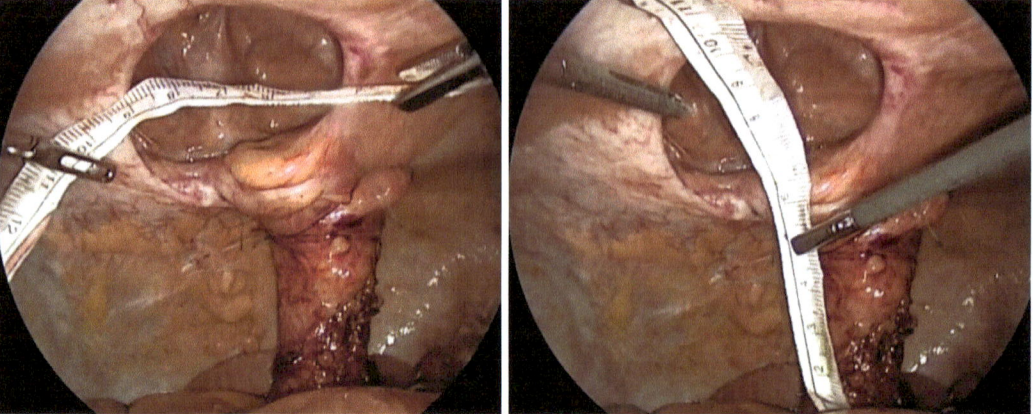

Fig. 4 The fascia defect is accurately measured to assist in mesh preparation

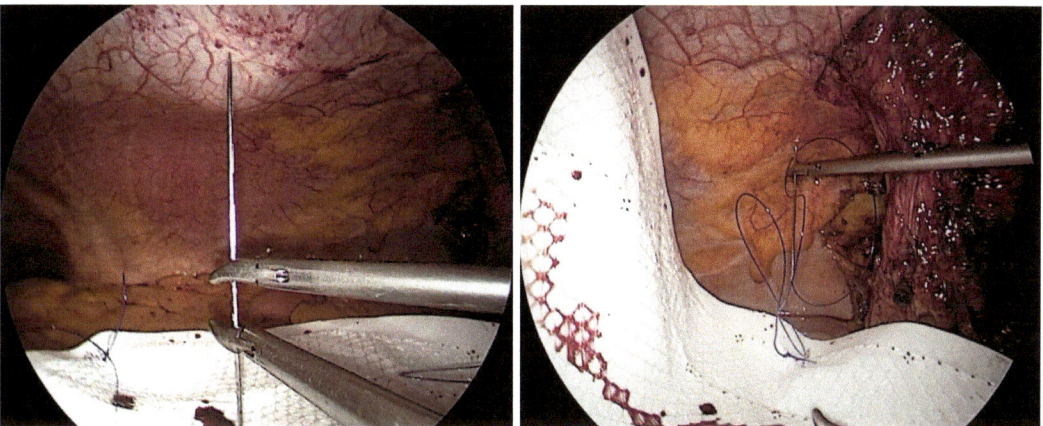

Fig. 5 Prolene 2/0 with straight needles are anchored to the mesh and passed through the anterior abdominal wall at the 12 and 3 o'clock positions

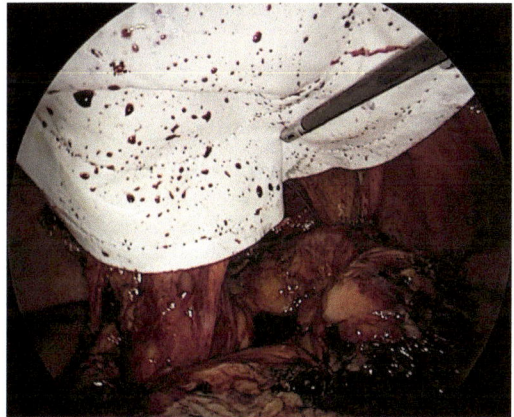

Fig. 6 Once the trans-fascial sutures are held taut, the mesh can be appropriately positioned to facilitate subsequent fixation

mesh out over its intended position to facilitate tacking (Fig. 6). Next, the mesh is secured using a ProTack™ Fixation Device in a double crown fashion (Fig. 7) just beyond the fascial defect and a second layer at the outer periphery of the mesh. While applying the tacks laterally it is important not to injure the bowel. A reasonable amount of space is left to accommodate passage of stool through the lateralized bowel "mesh flap valve." The trans-fascial Prolene 2–0 sutures can be cut externally, and the surgery is concluded.

The choice of mesh is an important consideration. Synthetic uncoated meshes, such as polypropylene, should not be used for intraperitoneal repair as they are associated with a significant risk of adhesions and mesh erosion [15, 23]. Biologic meshes have been shown to have high recurrence rates of 16–90% [24]. Composite prostheses are the ideal design for intraperitoneal hernia repair as these meshes comprise of a permanent synthetic material for the parietal side to encourage adhesion formation and an adhesion barrier layer for contact with the visceral side [21]. The adhesion barriers can either be absorbable or permanent. Thus far, ePTFE mesh has been the popular choice for laparoscopic Sugarbaker repair [17]. The advantage of ePTFE is the microporous structure which prevents tissue ingrowth into the prosthesis, with a low tendency for developing adhesions [25].

Surgeons should also be aware of mesh shrinkage over time. Shrinkage of the mesh and enlargement of the central hole is likely the greatest contributing factor to the higher reported recurrence rate of the keyhole method compared to the Sugarbaker technique [15]. It is therefore essential to achieve good mesh positioning and adequate fascial overlap of the mesh circumferentially.

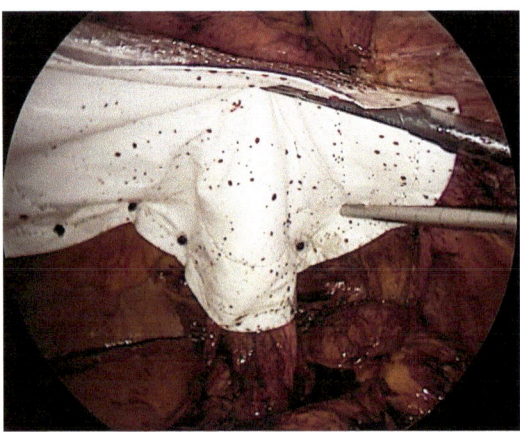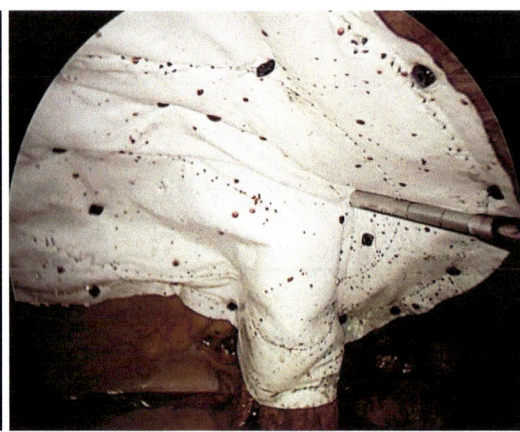

Fig. 7 The mesh is secured using the double crown method. (*left*) The outer layer of tacks is applied leaving adequate space for the lateralized bowel. (*right*) The inner layer of tacks applied just beyond the fascial defect

Complications and Management

A 2015 meta-analysis of laparoscopic parastomal hernia repair studied 15 articles with 469 patients [17]. The overall postoperative morbidity rate was 1.8%, with no differences between techniques. The most common complication was surgical site infection in 3.8%, with mesh infection occurring in 1.7% and obstruction requiring reoperation in 1.7%. The overall recurrence rate using laparoscopy for hernia repair was 17%, with the laparoscopic modified Sugarbaker technique showing superior recurrence rates at almost one-third that of the keyhole approach (10% vs. 28%).

Postoperative Care

The postoperative management of patients following parastomal hernia repair is similar to that of any incisional hernia repair. In general, no further antibiotics are given beyond the induction dose unless significant bowel manipulation and adhesiolysis were performed. The patient is advised to avoid heavy lifting and strenuous activity for 4–6 weeks and modifiable risk factors which can contribute to hernia recurrences are controlled.

References

1. Pearl RK. Parastomal hernias. World J Surg. 1989;13(5):569–72.
2. Carne PWG, Robertson GM, Frizelle FA. Parastomal hernia. Br J Surg. 2003;90(7):784–93.
3. Kojima K, Nakamura T, Sato T, Matsubara Y, Naito M, Yamashita K, Watanabe M. Risk factors for parastomal hernia after abdominoperineal resection for rectal cancer. Asian J Endosc Surg. 2017;10(3):276–81.
4. Sjödahl R, Anderberg B, Bolin T. Parastomal hernia in relation to site of the abdominal stoma. Br J Surg. 1988;75(4):339–41.
5. Hardt J, Meerpohl JJ, Metzendorf MI, Kienle P, Post S, Herrle F. Lateral pararectal versus transrectal stoma placement for prevention of parastomal herniation. Cochrane Database Syst Rev. 2019;4(4):CD009487.
6. Hsu MY, Lin JP, Hsu HH, Lai HL, Wu YL. Preoperative Stoma Site Marking Decreases Stoma and Peristomal Complications: A Meta-analysis. J Wound Ostomy Continence Nurs. 2020;47(3):249–56.
7. Pilgrim CHC, McIntyre R, Bailey M. Prospective audit of parastomal hernia: prevalence and associated comorbidities. Dis Colon Rectum. 2010;53(1):71–6.
8. Hotouras A, Murphy J, Thaha M, Chan CL. The persistent challenge of parastomal herniation: a review of the literature and future developments. Color Dis. 2013;15(5):e202–14.
9. Goligher JC. Extraperitoneal colostomy or ileostomy. Br J Surg. 1958;46(196):97–103.
10. Kroese LF, de Smet GHJ, Jeekel J, Kleinrensink GJ, Lange JF. Systematic Review and Meta-Analysis of Extraperitoneal Versus Transperitoneal Colostomy

for Preventing Parastomal Hernia. Dis Colon Rectum. 2016;59(7):688–95.

11. Hino H, Yamaguchi T, Kinugasa Y, Shiomi A, Kagawa H, Yamakawa Y, Numata M, Furutani A, Suzuki T, Torii K. Relationship between stoma creation route for end colostomy and parastomal hernia development after laparoscopic surgery. Surg Endosc. 2017;31(4):1966–73.

12. Jones HG, Rees M, Aboumarzouk OM, Brown J, Cragg J, Billings P, Carter B, Chandran P. Prosthetic mesh placement for the prevention of parastomal herniation. Cochrane Database Syst Rev. 2018;7(7):CD008905.

13. López-Cano M, Serra-Aracil X, Mora L, Sánchez-García JL, Jiménez-Gómez LM, Martí M, Vallribera F, Fraccalvieri D, Serracant A, Kreisler E, Biondo S, Espín E, Navarro-Soto S, Armengol-Carrasco M. Preventing Parastomal Hernia Using a Modified Sugarbaker Technique With Composite Mesh During Laparoscopic Abdominoperineal Resection: A Randomized Controlled Trial. Ann Surg. 2016;264(6):923–8.

14. Antoniou SA, Agresta F, Alamino JMG, Berger D, Berrevoet F, Brandsma HT, Bury K, Conze J, Cuccurullo D, Dietz UA, Fortelny RH, Frei-Lanter C, Hansson B, Helgstrand F, Hotouras A, Jänes A, Kroese LF, Lambrecht JR, Kyle-Leinhase I, López-Cano M, Maggiori L, Mandalà V, Miserez M, Montgomery A, Morales-Conde S, Prudhomme M, Rautio T, Smart N, Śmietański M, Szczepkowski M, Stabilini C, Muysoms FE. European Hernia Society guidelines on prevention and treatment of parastomal hernias. Hernia. 2018;22(1):183–98. https://doi.org/10.1007/s10029-017-1697-5.

15. Hansson BME, Slater NJ, van der Velden AS, Groenewoud HMM, Buyne OR, de Hingh IHJT, Bleichrodt RP. Surgical techniques for parastomal hernia repair: a systematic review of the literature. Ann Surg. 2012;255(4):685–95.

16. Sugarbaker PH. Peritoneal approach to prosthetic mesh repair of paraostomy hernias. Ann Surg. 1985;201(3):344–6.

17. DeAsis FJ, Lapin B, Gitelis ME, Ujiki MB. Current state of laparoscopic parastomal hernia repair: A meta-analysis. World J Gastroenterol. 2015;21(28):8670–7.

18. Levy S, Plymale MA, Miller MT, Davenport DL, Roth JS. Laparoscopic parastomal hernia repair: No different than a laparoscopic ventral hernia repair? Surg Endosc. 2016;30(4):1542–6.

19. Halabi WJ, Jafari MD, Carmichael JC, Nguyen VQ, Mills S, Phelan M, Stamos MJ, Pigazzi A. Laparoscopic versus open repair of parastomal hernias: an ACS-NSQIP analysis of short-term outcomes. Surg Endosc. 2013;27(11):4067–72.

20. Berger D, Bientzle M. Polyvinylidene fluoride: a suitable mesh material for laparoscopic incisional and parastomal hernia repair! A prospective, observational study with 344 patients. Hernia. 2009;13(2):167–72.

21. Deeken CR, Faucher KM, Matthews BD. A review of the composition, characteristics, and effectiveness of barrier mesh prostheses utilized for laparoscopic ventral hernia repair. Surg Endosc. 2012;26(2):566–75.

22. Hansson BME, Morales-Conde S, Mussack T, Valdes J, Muysoms FE, Bleichrodt RP. The laparoscopic modified Sugarbaker technique is safe and has a low recurrence rate: a multicenter cohort study. Surg Endosc. 2013;27(2):494–500. https://doi.org/10.1007/s00464-012-2464-4.

23. Halm JA, de Wall LL, Steyerberg EW, Jeekel J, Lange JF. Intraperitoneal polypropylene mesh hernia repair complicates subsequent abdominal surgery. World J Surg. 2007;31(2):423–9. discussion 430.

24. Slater NJ, Hansson BME, Buyne OR, Hendriks T, Bleichrodt RP. Repair of parastomal hernias with biologic grafts: a systematic review. J Gastrointest Surg. 2011;15(7):1252–8.

25. Koehler RH, Begos D, Berger D, Carey S, LeBlanc K, Park A, Bruce R, Smoot R, Voeller G. Minimal adhesions to ePTFE mesh after laparoscopic ventral incisional hernia repair: reoperative findings in 65 cases. JSLS. 2003;7(4):335–40.

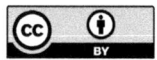

Part XX

Colorectal Surgery

Laparoscopic Right Hemicolectomy with Complete Mesocolic Excision and Central Vascular Ligation (CME/CVL) for Right Sided Colon Cancer

Ming Li Leonard Ho and William Tzu-Liang Chen

Introduction (with Clinical Data)

Hohenberger et al. [1] advocated CME/CVL for resection of right-sided colon cancers. CME involves sharp dissection along Toldt's fascia with the goal of removing the primary tumor, its mesentery, and an undisrupted envelope of mesocolic fascia. The specimen would contain adjacent blood vessels, draining lymphatics, and neural tissue, which are potential pathways through which the tumor may spread. The second component is CVL whereby the tumor-supplying vessels are ligated at their origin. This ensures the maximal harvest of all regional lymph nodes.

CME/CVL for right-sided colon cancer has been shown to result in reduced local recurrence [1], higher lymph node yield [2], and improved disease–free survival [3].

Indications

Adenocarcinoma is located from the cecum to the mid-transverse colon with pre-op staging of cT3–4 or N1–2.

Contraindications

Patients with distant metastases should not be considered for this operation. Cancers related to hereditary syndromes such as familial adenomatous polyposis (FAP) or Lynch syndrome are contraindicated as well. Other contraindications to the operation include obstructed or perforated tumors, previous abdominal surgery, or comorbidities (such as severe heart or lung disease) that render the patient unfit for laparoscopic surgery.

Preoperative Assessment

A colonoscopy is done to biopsy the tumor as well as to confirm its location. The tumor is tattooed routinely. Computed tomography (CT) of the thorax, abdomen, and pelvis is performed to assess for metastatic disease. Bowel preparation is not routinely ordered. A routine anesthetic assessment is performed prior to the surgery.

OT Setup

The patient is placed in a modified Lloyd Davis position with both arms tucked in. The surgeon stands between the patient's legs while the camera assistant is positioned on the right of the surgeon. If a surgical assistant is available, he/she will stand on the surgeons' left. Refer to Fig. 1 for OT setup.

M. L. L. Ho · W. T.-L. Chen (✉)
Division of Colorectal Surgery, Department of Surgery, China Medical University Hsinchu Hospital, Zhubei City, Hsinchu County, Taiwan
e-mail: wtchen@mail.cmuh.org.tw

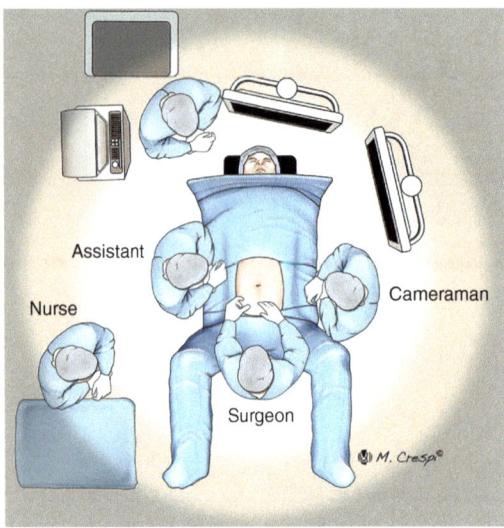

Fig. 1 OT setup

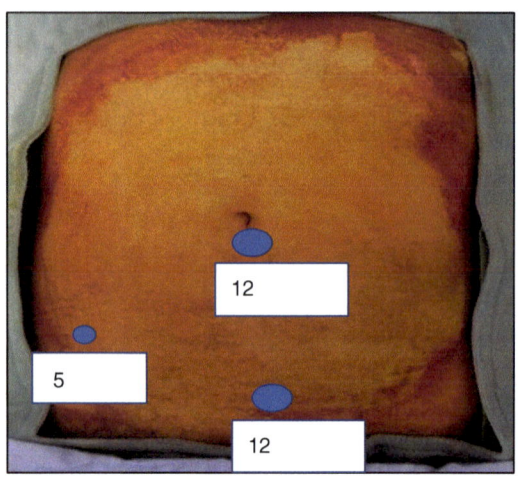

Fig. 2 Port placement

Surgical Technique

Port Placement: The camera port is usually inserted supra or infra umbilically. A 12 mm port is inserted 2 cm superior to the pubic symphysis at the midline while a 5 mm port is inserted at the right iliac fossa. An additional 5 mm port may be inserted at the right hypochondrial region for the assistant. Refer to Fig. 2.

Colon mobilization: Pneumoperitoneum is created at 10–15 mm Hg. The abdominal cavity is inspected for metastases. Once the patient is positioned in a Trendelenburg position with the left side down, the omentum, small bowel, and transverse colon are swept to a cephalad direction. The terminal ileum is lifted anteriorly towards the abdominal wall (refer to Fig. 3), exposing the cleavage plane between ileal mesentery and retroperitoneum. Peritoneum overlying this plane is scored with either monopolar diathermy or an advanced energy device. As dissection proceeds along Toldt's fascia, the ileal mesentery, and posterior aspect of the right colon are mobilized off the retroperitoneum. The authors routinely leave the lateral attachments of the colon untouched, as this helps to provide additional counter traction.

During dissection in the superior direction, it is important to look out for the duodenum and

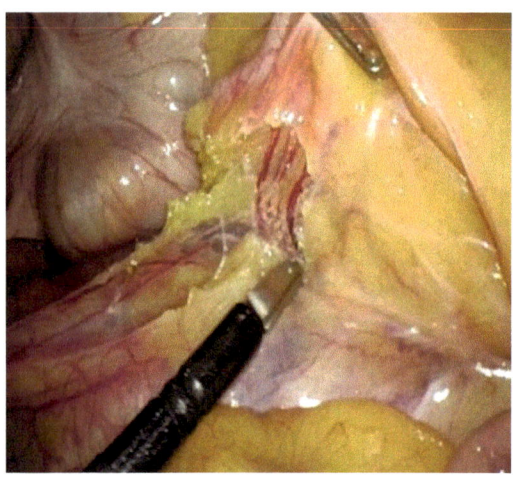

Fig. 3 Tenting the terminal ileum mesentery and mobilization of the retroperitoneum using monopolar cautery

subsequently dissect anterior to it. In the author's practice, the medial extent of dissection is reached when the duodenum and pancreatic head are exposed (refer to Fig. 4). Further mobilization is performed in towards the direction of Morrisons' pouch until the dissection plane is separated from Morrisons' pouch by a layer of peritoneum. A gauze is placed at the dissected area to demarcate the dissected plane.

CVL: Prior to commencing the CVL, the mesentery of the ascending and transverse colon is spread out to visualize the location of the ileocolic (IC), middle colic (MC), and superior

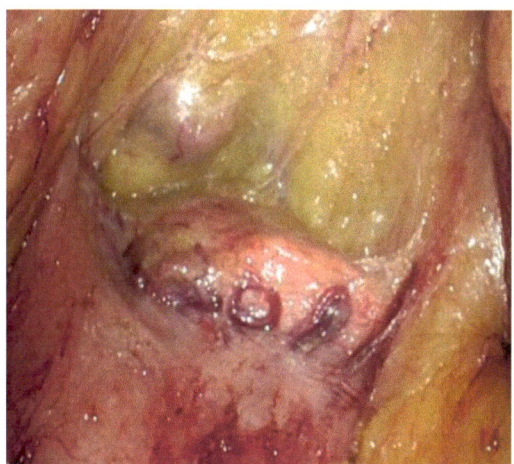

Fig. 4 At the medial extent of mobilization, the duodenum and pancreatic head are exposed

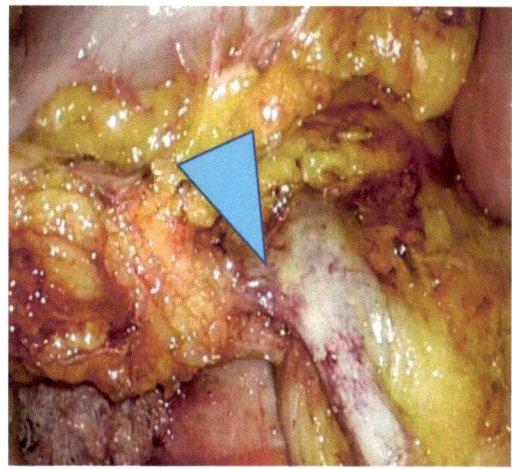

Fig. 5 Ileocolic artery and vein (arrowed) take-off from SM pedicle

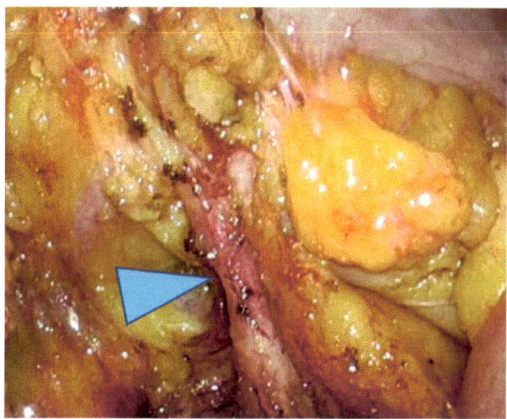

Fig. 6 Middle colic artery (arrowed) branching off from SMA

mesenteric (SM) pedicles. The peritoneum overlying the pedicles is scored. Next, the terminal ileum is located and the proximal transection point is decided. Using an energy device, a mesenteric window is created adjacent to the proximal transection point. A laparoscopic stapler is introduced through this window to transect the ileum. The ileal mesentery is divided using energy device in the direction of the SMA pedicle.

At the junction of the IC and SM pedicles, fine dissection is performed to skeletonize the vessels and demonstrate the take-off of the IC from the SM vessels (refer to Figs. 5 and 6). Failure to demonstrate this could lead to inadvertent ligation of the SM vessels, resulting in excessive small bowel ischemia. In the event that initial vessel identification is in question, it is advised that dissection continues along the SM pedicle in the cephalad direction; dissected vessels subsequently arising from the SM pedicle will provide more information on vascular anatomy.

After ligation of the IC pedicle, the next vessel to be ligated is the right colic artery should it be present. Approximate location of the middle colic (MC) pedicle can be located via inspection of the transverse colonic mesentery. For tumors located between the cecum and the proximal transverse colon, the right branch of MC vessels is ligated. The main MC vessels are dissected free and

ligated for mid-transverse colon tumors. The gastrocolic trunk is usually identified and preserved. Once this is done, the CVL is completed. A laparoscopic stapler is used to transect the transverse colon at the intended distal transection point. (Fig. 7).

Anastomosis: This can be performed in the iso or antiperistaltic fashion. Using diathermy, an opening is made in the ileum/colon immediately beyond the staple line at the anti-mesenteric surface. A 60 mm laparoscopic stapler is inserted into the bowel lumen to form the anastomosis. The anastomosis is subsequently closed using sutures (either vicryl 3/0 or V—lock) or stapler.

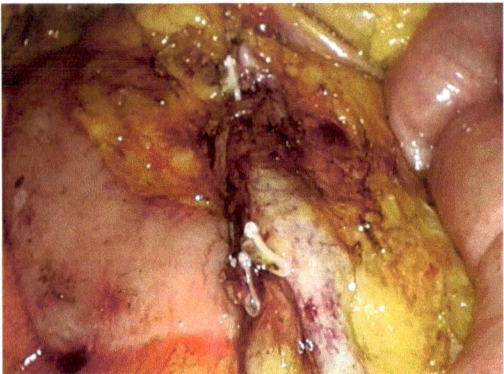

Fig. 7 Post CVL, the SMV is exposed. The SMA is not dissected free as lymph node metastasis tends not to spread beyond the SMV. Leaving the SMA undissected also results in better function

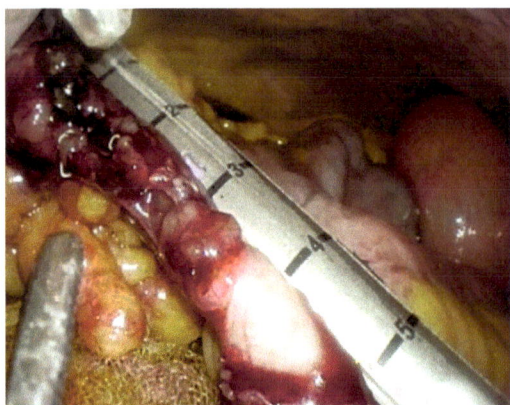

Fig. 9 Closure of the anastomosis using stapler

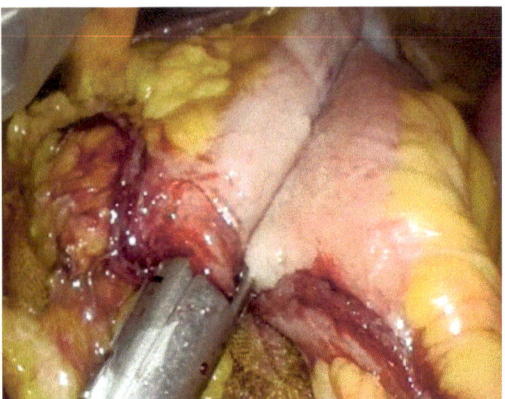

Fig. 8 Forming the intracorporeal antiperistaltic ileocolic anastomosis using a laparoscopic stapler

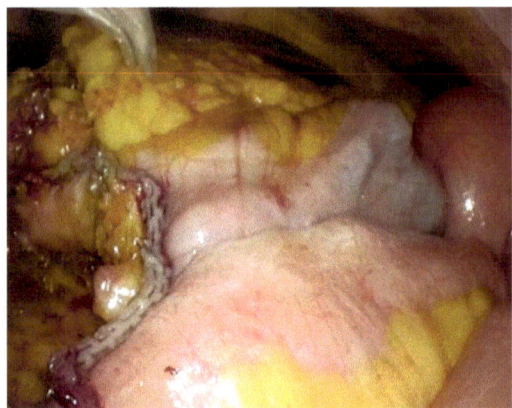

Fig. 10 The completed anastomosis

Alternatively, if the bowel ends are sufficiently mobile, they can be exteriorized via a mini midline laparotomy wound and anastomosed in the usual fashion as per open surgery. After the anastomosis is done, the remaining peritoneal attachments of the right colon are divided and the specimen is retrieved through a Pfannenstiel wound. The authors routinely place a drain adjacent to the anastomosis (Figs. 8, 9, and 10).

Complications and Management

The authors wish to highlight certain complications and pitfalls specific to the operation.

(a) Misidentification of critical vessels. While performing CVL, it is important to dissect the right colonic vessels adequately and demonstrate their take-off from the SM pedicle prior to ligation. Clear demonstration of vascular anatomy is a critical step in preventing a catastrophic ligation of the SM pedicle.

(b) Injury to SM vessels. Excessive counter traction, for example, from an inexperienced assistant tenting up tissues during CVL, may result in avulsion of the SM pedicle or its branches. The authors address this issue by routinely performing the operation without a surgical assistant. This means that counter traction is solely provided by the surgeon and makes it less likely for unintended tissue avulsion or trauma to happen. Also, by keeping the right colon's lateral attachments untouched till the specimen is ready to be extracted provides an additional degree of counter traction for the surgeon. However, in situations such as patients with copious visceral fat, the availability of another assistant is a significant benefit. When bleeding occurs around the SM pedicle region, it is imperative to (a) stop the bleeding, (b) assess where the bleeding is arising from, and (c) ensure the integrity of the SM vessels. For (a), initial compression using gauze combined with the use of an effective suction device to remove surrounding blood is useful in stopping/slowing bleeding as well as maintaining clear visualization of the surgical field. For additional hemostasis, adjuncts like surgicel may be considered. The 5 mm port in the right iliac fossa may be converted into a 12 mm port which can be used to facilitate gauze insertion. In (b) and (c), the surgeon should dissect carefully around the SM region to ascertain the exact point of bleeding. Most of the time, bleeding is from avulsion of small blood vessels contained within surrounding mesenteric tissues and will stop after a period of compression. Should bleeding from the main superior mesenteric vessels be confirmed or persistent bleeding which does not stop despite the aforementioned maneuvers, the authors advise calling for help from another surgeon. If there is injury to the main SM vessels, recommendation is for conversion to open and urgent on-table referral to a vascular surgeon for repair. Persisting with laparoscopic repair is futile unless skilled expertise is available.

(c) Injury to duodenum and pancreas. Prior to commencing CVL, it is necessary to achieve adequate medial mobilization of the right colonic mesentery. The authors' extent of medial dissection is when the pancreatic head and duodenum are exposed. Such an extensive medial mobilization ensures that the mesentery containing the SM branches is not attached to the pancreas or duodenum. While performing CVL around this area, the chances of injuring small vessels around the pancreas or duodenum, or even direct injury to these organs, is hence minimized if the mesentery is well mobilized.

(d) Intracorporeal anastomosis. Performing anastomosis this way has several advantages. Firstly, the surgeon will be able to avoid unnecessary traction onto the transverse colon when delivering it through a midline mini-laparotomy wound. This is particularly relevant in obese patients as well as those with shortened transverse colon mesenteries. An intracorporeal anastomosis provides the surgeon with superior visualization of the small bowel orientation prior to performing the anastomosis, mitigating the risk of small bowel torsion. Next, the surgeon has the option of extracting the tumor via a Pfannenstiel wound, which has clearly defined benefits over a midline wound in terms of incisional hernia and infection rates. A Pfannenstiel wound also provides improved cosmesis.

On the other hand, this technique has its problems. It requires a learning curve and is usually more time-consuming. When the ileotomy and colotomy are created, there is a potential for bowel content to leak out into the peritoneal cavity and result in contamination. As such, prior to making the ileotomy/colotomy, the authors routinely place chlorhexidine gauzes in the peritoneal cavity in advance. After creating the opening in the bowel, should there be bowel content leaking out, it can be quickly wiped away using the gauzes. After completing the anastomosis, the surgeons routinely place all gauzes in a laparoscopic bag which is subsequently extracted. An intracorporeal anastomosis also poses technical difficulty as it requires the surgeon to close the anastomosis via suturing. The authors mitigate this by using the laparoscopic stapler for anastomosis closure.

Postoperative Care

The nasogastric tube is removed immediately after the operation. Once awake, the patient is allowed oral fluids ad libitum and progressed to an oral diet from the first postoperative day. The urine catheter is removed on the first postoperative day and the drain is removed prior to discharge. Average length of hospital stay is 5 days.

References

1. Hohenberger W, Weber K, Matzel K, Papadopoulos T, Merkel S. Standardized surgery for colonic cancer: complete mesocolic excision and central liga-tion–technical notes and outcome. Color Dis. 2009;11(4):354–64.
2. West NP, Hohenberger W, Weber K, Perrakis A, Finan PJ, Quirke P. Complete mesocolic excision with central vascular ligation produces an oncologically superior specimen compared with standard surgery for carcinoma of the colon. J Clin Oncol. 2010;28(2):272–8.
3. Bertelsen CA, Neuenschwander AU, Jansen JE, Wilhelmsen M, Kirkegaard-Klitbo A, Tenma JR, et al. Disease-free survival after complete mesocolic excision compared with conventional colon cancer surgery: a retrospective, population-based study. Lancet Oncol. 2015;16(2):161–8.

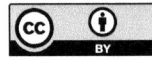

Laparoscopic Left Hemicolectomy

Ming-Yin Shen, Yeen Chin Leow,
and William Tzu-Liang Chen

Introduction

What is the clear definition of left colectomy? Unfortunately, the answer is not as clear as it is with a right colectomy. The resection can involve resection of the colonic segment anywhere between the left transverse colon and the upper rectum. For tumors involving the left transverse colon or splenic flexure, left hemicolectomy (LC) is the preferred operation. A LC is considered to be a resection of the mid-transverse colon to the descending/sigmoid junction. In complete mesocolic excision (CME) and central vascular ligation (CVL) for left transverse colon or splenic flexure colon cancer, ligation of the inferior mesenteric vein (IMV), left branch of the middle colic artery (lt-MCA), and left colic artery (LCA) at the root must be considered [1]. For resection of mid- or distal descending colon tumors, the oncological resection requires division of the inferior mesenteric artery at its origin. If the resection carried out involved the distal transverse colon up to the sigmoid-descending junction, it should be considered as a left segmentary colectomy [2].

The question of whether extended right colectomy (ERC) or LC should be more strongly indicated for the tumors involving the left transverse colon or splenic flexure remains open. The rate of R0 resection as well as long-term oncological outcomes are not different between ERC and RC [2–4]. Nevertheless, the concept has been proposed that synchronous liver metastases are associated with the risk of distal positive lymph nodes, and ERC should be considered for metastatic patients suitable for curative treatment to ensure R0 resection of both tumor sites [5].

The attempts at an anastomosis of LC may be difficult because of inadequate length and tension. Under these circumstances, total or subtotal colectomy is a reasonable alternative. The inverted right colonic transposition (the so-called Deloyers procedure) and trans-mesenteric colorectal anastomosis represent another alternative [6].

Minimal invasive approaches to colon and rectal resection have resulted in earlier tolerance of diet, accelerated return of bowel function, lower analgesia requirement, and shorter length of hospital stay. Large multicentre randomized trials have shown comparable disease-free and overall survival between open and laparoscopic approaches for colon cancer [7–9]. However, all these studies exclude patients with transverse colon and splenic flexure lesions, probably

M.-Y. Shen · W. T.-L. Chen (✉)
Division of Colorectal Surgery, Department of Surgery, China Medical University Hsinchu Hospital, Zhubei City, Hsinchu County, Taiwan
e-mail: wtchen@mail.cmuh.org.tw

Y. C. Leow
Colorectal Surgery Unit, Department of Surgery, Hospital Sultanah Bahiyah, Alor Star, Malaysia

Division of Colorectal Surgery, Department of Surgery, China Medical University Hospital, Taichung, Taiwan

because of technical difficulties specific to this location or the rarity of this condition. With the improvements in surgical techniques and instruments, increasing numbers of studies demonstrated that the laparoscopic LC is a feasible, safe, and effective procedure, as well as acceptable short-term and oncologic long-term outcomes [2, 10, 11].

Indications

The most common indication for LC is colon cancer (e.g., distal transverse colon cancer, splenic flexure colon cancer, proximal to mid descending colon cancer). Other indications include benign conditions such as diverticulitis, trauma, segmental Crohn's colitis, ischemic colitis, polyps unresected through a colonoscopy, and colonic volvulus. Diverticular disease, typically with sigmoid colon resection, may require a LC if the descending colon is unsuitable for an anastomosis due to active diverticulitis or muscular hypertrophy.

Contraindications

Contraindication often depends on the surgeon's level of expertise with less straightforward patients and diseases. Certainly, hemodynamically instability or cardiopulmonary disease that is severe enough to make peritoneal insufflation and Trendelenburg positioning dangerous represent a physiologic derangement that precludes the safe application of laparoscopy. Another relative contraindication includes large bowel obstruction. Depending on the degree of proximal intestinal dilatation present, the more limited volume of unencumbered working space, coupled with higher risk of bowel perforation during manipulation, may warrant an open approach. The application of self-expanding stents in obstructed colon as a bridge to laparoscopic surgery could be an alternative option. Severe adhesion due to previous surgeries pose a technical challenge to minimally invasive surgeons which may render patients not suitable for laparoscopic

colectomy. Phlegmonous tissue which is usually encountered in severe, complicated Crohn's disease or in diverticulitis may not also be resectable via laparoscopy due to the tissue friability, bleeding, and distortion anatomy that necessitates open exposure. Severe peritoneal carcinomatosis secondary to left-sided colon may also preclude laparoscopic LC. There are no common criteria to apply laparoscopic technique for combined resection for T4 colon cancer. Tumor invasion into other organs is not an absolute contraindication if en bloc resection could be achieved. However, laparotomic conversion is necessary if oncologically curative resection is not achieved laparoscopically. Significant intraoperative hemorrhage, in the presence of visceral lesion, incorrect dissection, all conditions that may affect the outcome, are contraindications of laparoscopy and the conversion is necessary.

Preoperative Assessment

All patients undergoing colonic surgery should have the same preoperative workup including anesthetic workup regardless of the surgical approaches. All patients should have a complete history and physical examination. Adjunct testing such as blood test, additional imaging (CT scan, barium enema), or cardiopulmonary testing is performed when indicated. The only special consideration for laparoscopic surgery is ensuring that the surgeon can identify the site of pathology at the time of operative intervention. The loss of tactile sensation in laparoscopic surgery stresses the importance of localizing techniques, especially for small lesions. These can be evaluated preoperatively by colonoscopy and tattooing of the lesion can be performed during the colonoscopy 1–2 days prior to the surgery especially for early colonic cancer which ensures the oncological safe margins. It is helpful to have flexible colonoscopy in the operating room as it may be needed intraoperatively to identify lesions if the location of the lesion remains doubtful. All elective colonic resections should follow ERAS preoperative protocol. The protocols include perioperative opioid-sparing analgesia, avoidance of nasogastric tubes and peritoneal drains, aggressive management of postoperative nausea and vomiting, and early oral feedings and ambulation. Mechanical oral bowel preparation is not needed for elective laparoscopic LC. An urinary catheter is placed at the beginning of the procedure and is removed on the first morning after the operation. Prophylaxis antibiotic and deep vein thrombosis (DVT) prophylaxis should be included.

OT Setup (Fig. 1a, b)

Authors routinely placed patients in lithotomy position with both arms tucked and the thighs positioned using stirrups at no more than a 10° angle to the torso. Lithotomy allows simultaneous access to the abdomen and perineum for colorectal anastomosis when using the circular stapler, as well as for intraoperative colonoscopy. It also provides additional space for a second assistant and an additional position for the operating surgeon when mobilizing the splenic flexure. The patient should be fixed securely on the table because the patient's position could be changed during the operation. A beanbag is used to secure the patient to the table, along with reinforcement by adhesive tapes wrapping the patient's chest to the table. The patient's position

can be adjusted intraoperatively at the stage of left flexure or rectal mobilization. The procedure is usually performed with one assistant. Surgeon will stand on the patient's right while the camera assistant on surgeon's right. During the approach of the middle colic artery, the surgeon may stand in between the patient's legs. The monopolar device with hook, spatula, or scissor or energy-based devices are adapted for the plane dissection, depending on the surgeon's preference. The adaptation of energy-based devices in laparoscopic colon cancer surgery could reduce chyle leakage, minimize bleeding on dissection planes, and facilitate complete plane dissection.

Surgical Techniques

Ports Placements (Fig. 2)

Four trocars are placed. By open technique, Camera port is inserted infra or supra umbilically using a balloon trocar. Pneumoperitoneum 12–15 mmHg is created and the abdomen is inspected for findings. A 12 mm port is placed in the right lower quadrant, for the operator's right hand. A 5 mm port is placed in the right hypochondrium for the operator's left hand. A second 5 mm port is placed over the left side abdomen.

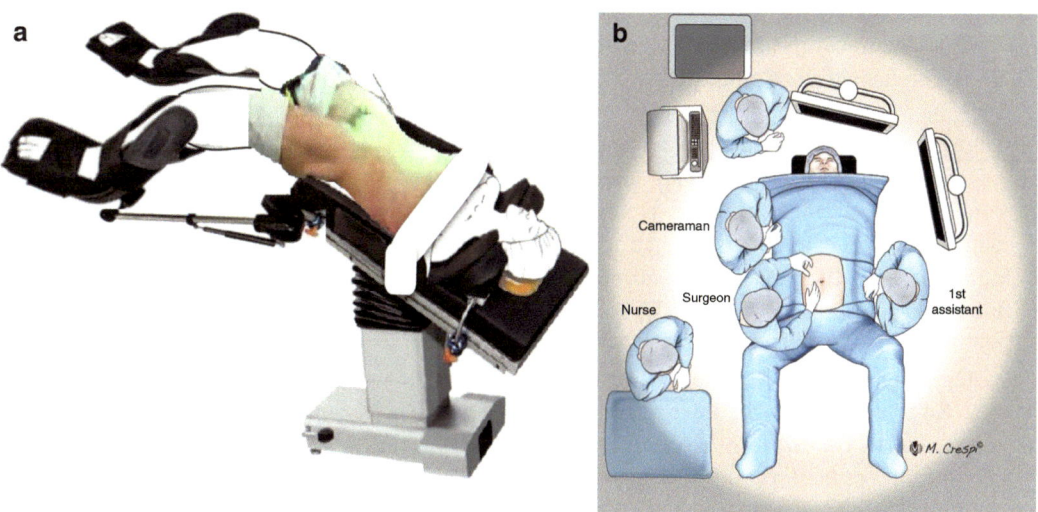

Fig. 1 (**a**) Patient positioning in Trendelenberg and right side down position. (**b**) Surgeon and assistants standing position

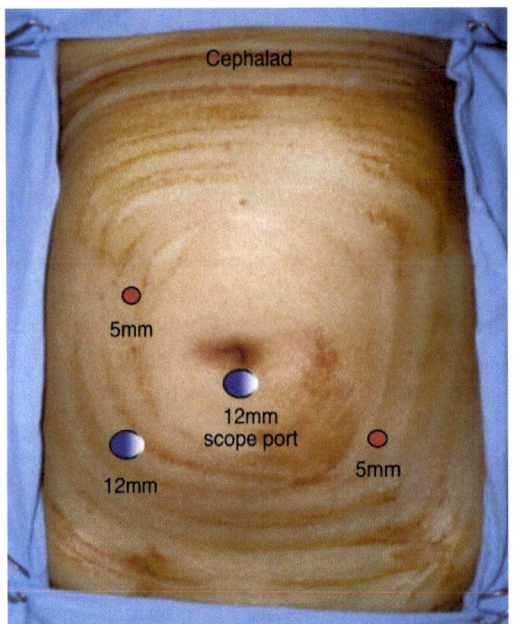

Fig. 2 Port placement for LC

Operatives Details

1. *Vascular Pedicle Isolation and Ligation* (Fig. 3a–f)

   Patient is tilted head down 15° (Trendelenberg) and right side down for gravitational drag of the small bowel to the right and omentum and transverse colon slightly to cephalad. Omentum is swept cephalad direction and the transverse mesocolon is lifted up to expose the cleavage plane of the pancreas. Incision of transverse mesocolon at the level below lt-MCA either by monopolar diathermy or energy device to enter the lesser sac (Fig. 3a). The Treitz ligament is dissected with maximum care not to damage the jejunum (Fig. 3b). The peritoneal layer medial to the inferior Mesenteric Vein (IMV) is incised paralleled to the vessel. The IMV is easily visualized, or in case of more obese patients, search for, right below the inferior margin of the pancreas. The IMV is dissected free and then divided at the level close to the inferior border of the pancreas (Fig. 3c).

   In order to perform central ligation of lt-MCA with a lateral-to-medial approach to the left-sided transverse mesocolon (TM), the posterior layer of TM is dissected along the pancreas and spread cephalad. The middle colic artery is identified from the superior mesenteric artery. Then the lt-MCA is dissected free and divided at the root (Fig. 3d).

   The medial-to-lateral (MTL) approach to the left mesocolon easily brings the inferior mesenteric artery (IMA) into view. The root of sigmoid mesentery is retracted up to create tension on the peritoneum which is then incised using monopolar diathermy from caudal to cephalad position starting from the sacral promontory. Pneumo-dissection might help to open up further the embryological plane. The mesentery of sigmoid can be retracted away from the retroperitoneum by performing a blunt and bloodless dissection using monopolar or advanced energy devices. Proper Medial-To-Lateral (MTL) dissection will not expose the left ureter, left gonadal vessel, and psoas muscle, which are left undisturbed retroperitoneally. The retracting instrument can be inserted into the plane between the mesentery and the retroperitoneum, lifting the mesentery toward the anterior abdominal wall without grasping and tearing tissue. Dissection carried on cephalad till the root of IMA with careful identification and preservation of hypogastric nerves, which control urinary and sexual function. With D3 lymph node dissection at the IMA root (Fig. 3e), the left colic artery (LCA) is ligated near the origin from IMA (Fig. 3f).

2. *Splenic Flexure Mobilization* (Fig. 4a, b)

   The splenic flexure of colon is mobilized using medial-to-lateral approach. After the procedures of central vascular ligation, the lessor sac has been entered through the TM window and the mesentery root of the left colon is incised. By insertion of retracting instrument and tenting of mesentery of both transverse and descending colon, the pancreatico-colonic ligament is divided using either monopolar diathermy or advanced energy devices (Fig. 4a). Lifting the IMV arch allows furthering MTL dissection by opening a window between the Toldt fascia anteriorly

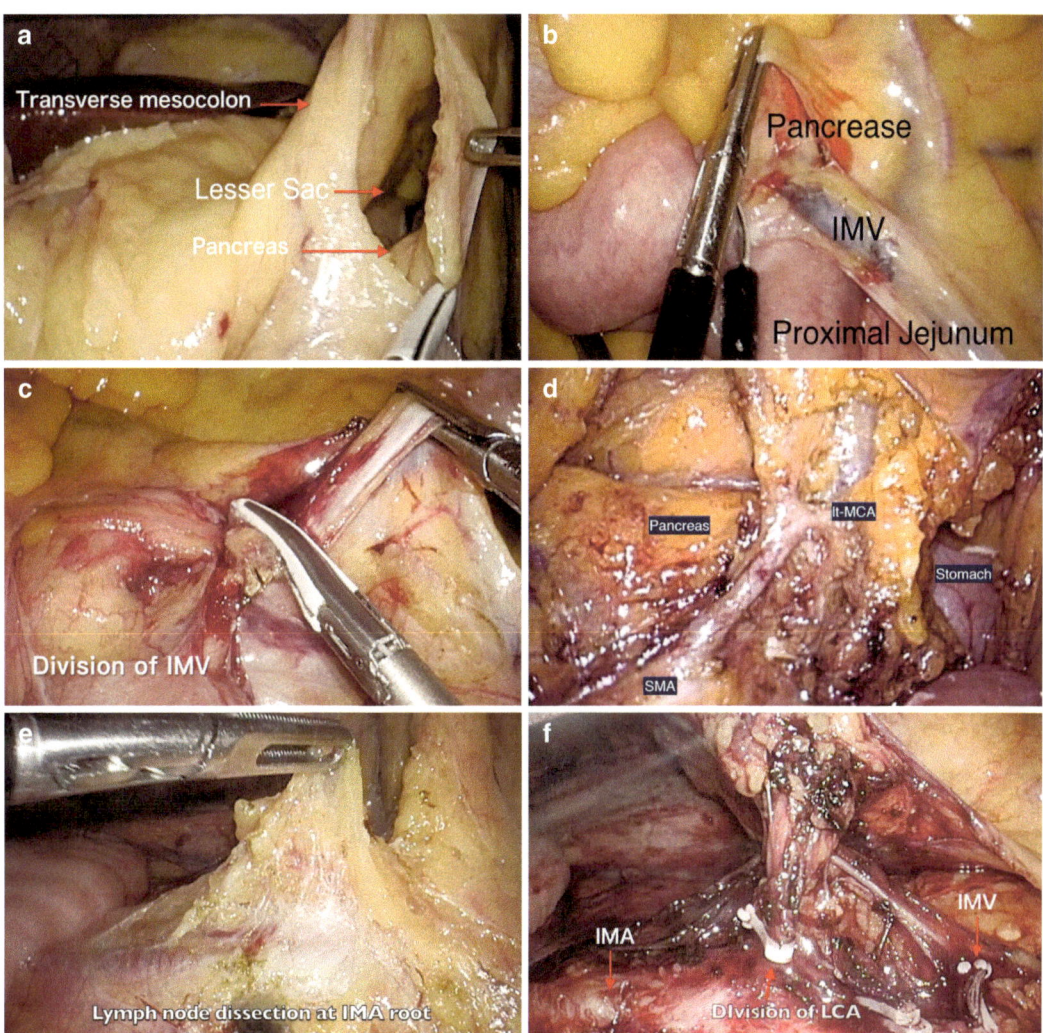

Fig. 3 (**a**) Incision of transverse mesocolon at the level below lt-MCA to enter the lesser sac. (**b**) The Treitz ligament is dissected with maximum care not to damage the jejunum. (**c**) The IMV is divided at the level close to the inferior border of the pancreas. (**d**) The lt-MCA is divided at the root. (**e**) D3 lymph node dissection at the IMA root. (**f**) LCA is ligated near the origin from IMA

and the Gerotal fascia posteriorly (Fig. 4b). The border between the two fascias, which indicates the embryonic plane of coalescence of posterior mesocolon and retroperitoneum is whitish, a clear sign of correct dissection plane (Fig. 4b). A tough elevation of mesocolon anteriorly toward the abdominal wall facilitates the dissection as far as the pericolic gutter, and downward to the level of sacral promontory.

3. *Mobilization of Colon* (Fig. 5a–c)

If the medial approach was done adequately, colon (descending and sigmoid) can be easily mobilized from the Toldt's fascia. Gently retract the descending colon medially, this thin Toldt's fascia is scored and divided using monopolar diathermy and advanced energy devices (Fig. 5a). The splenic flexure proper can then be dissected down by dividing the spleno-colic ligament (Fig. 5b). The greater omentum is separated from the gastric curvature. The gastrocolic ligament is also

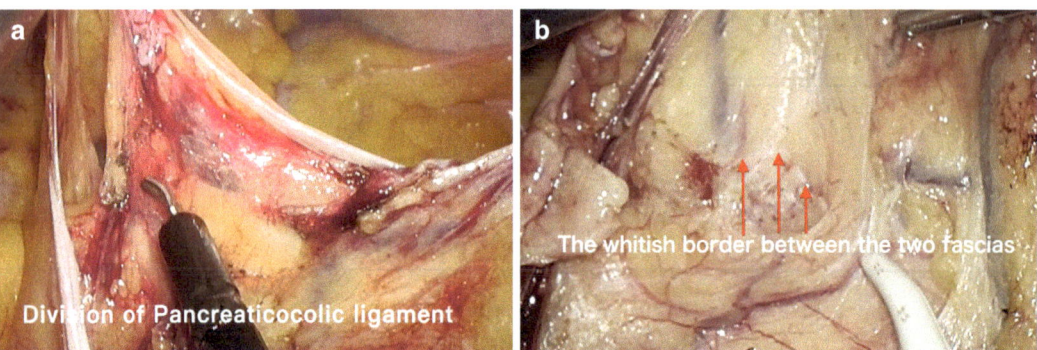

Fig. 4 (**a**) The pancreatico-colonic ligament is divided (**b**) Dissection between the Toldt fascia anteriorly and the Gerotal fascia posteriorly

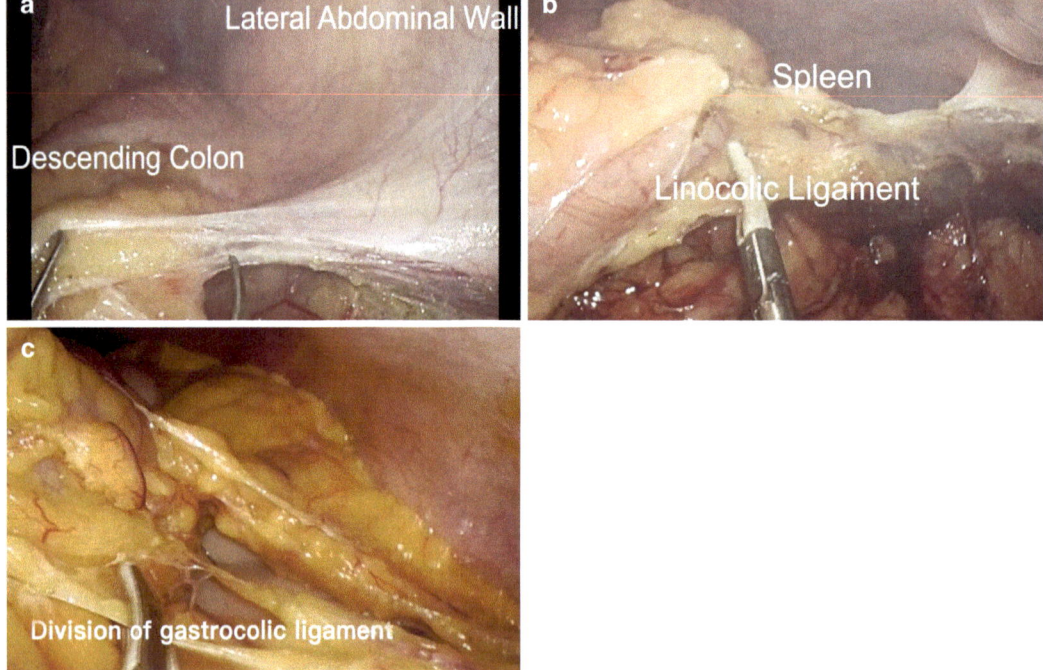

Fig. 5 (**a**) Gently retract the descending colon medially, the Toldt's fascia is divided (**b**) Division of the spleno-colic ligament (**c**) Division of the gastrocolic ligament

divided (Fig. 5c). The sigmoid and descending colon is fully mobilized until it is a midline structure. For a tension-free anastomosis, sometimes mobilization of hepatic flexure may be indicated.

4. *Construction of Anastomosis and Specimen Extraction* (Fig. 6a–e)

Authors prefer extracorporeal hand-sewn end-to-end colo-colonic anastomosis, which offers the advantages of tension-free anastomosis, and less risk of jejunum compression which results in postoperatively intestinal obstruction. The specimen is extracted through the umbilical port, which extended to about 3–6 cm. To avoid contamination, a wound protector is used. Care to be taken when extracting the colon with the lesion as too much of traction can disrupt the colonic wall and marginal artery which will jeopardize anastomosis. Excessive traction may also cause contamination, and in the worst scenario tumor cell seeding in colonic malignancies. After division of the mesocolon, routine Indocyanine Green (ICG) is used to assure good vasculature of the remaining colon before every transaction. After restoration of bowel continuity, the colon is placed back into the abdomen and insufflation is reestablished. Closure of the mesenteric gap is recommended to minimize the risk of internal herniation.

Alternatively, intracorporeal colocolic functional end-to-end anastomosis, which is technically a side-to-side approach, can be performed if adequate bowel is preserved in some of the cases. The superiority of side-to-side anastomosis compared with hand-sewn is having better blood flow and wider diameter thus reducing intraluminal pressure and proximal ischemia. Advantage of performing intracorporeal anastomosis is avoidance of bowel twisting in the wrong orientation and avoidance of excessive traction on bowel during anastomosis. A totally laparoscopic approach represents the better treatment particularly for obese patients, as it avoids the exteriorization of heavy and short mesenteries through much thicker abdominal walls and the risk of microlacerations which may affect the success of the anastomosis. The intracorporeal transections of the transverse and descending colon are accomplished using 60 mm/3.5 mm blue-load articulating linear endoscopic staplers. The specimen, completely separated from all attachments, is then kept aside in the abdominal cavity. The transverse and the left colon are lined up side to side (isoperistaltic manner), and a stapled side-to-side colocolic anastomosis (SSSA) is conducted with one fire of a 60 mm blue endostaper load (Fig. 6a). The enterotomy is closed using a 3–0 PDS double layer running suture (Fig. 6b). Antiperistaltic SSSA is also feasible; however, it may run higher risk of tensioned anastomosis. Antiperistaltic SSSA required more intestinal mobilization than isoperistaltic SSSA [12].

Extended right hemicolectomy (ERC) or subtotal colectomy has significant technical advantages over left colectomy, especially under the circumstances of obstructing tumors of the left colon, synchronous cancers in other segments, clinically evident diverticular disease, or inadequate remaining bowel length for anastomosis. Technically, it utilizes a highly mobile segment of the bowel, the ileum, to transpose it toward the left colon and perform the intracorporeal ileocolonic anastomosis without tension.

Trans-mesenteric colo-colonic or colorectal anastomosis are feasible laparoscopically and allow tension-free anastomosis in patients with a short proximal colonic segment after extended LH. The proximal colon is mobilized as completely as possible. The gastocolic ligament is divided and the second position of duodenum is exposed. An ileal mesenteric window is creased in the avascular area between the superior mesenteric and ileocolic pedicles (Fig. 6c). Then the proximal transverse colon is pulled through the mesenteric window to create a tension-free anastomosis (Fig. 6d). In most cases, division of the middle colic vessels is necessary for full mobilization; therefore, it is important to preserve the marginal vessels to avoid the risk of ischemia after middle colic vessel ligation.

If trans-mesenteric anastomosis is still not feasible, the inverted right colonic transposition procedure is an alternative salvage. After full mobilization and middle colic vessel ligation, the right colon is rotated 180^0 counterclockwise around the ileocolic vessel axis such that the cecum is cephalad while the hepatic flexure is caudal (Fig. 6e). The right colon can easily be anastomosed tension-free to the colonic or rectal stump. All patients undergoing the Deloyers procedure have routine appendectomy.

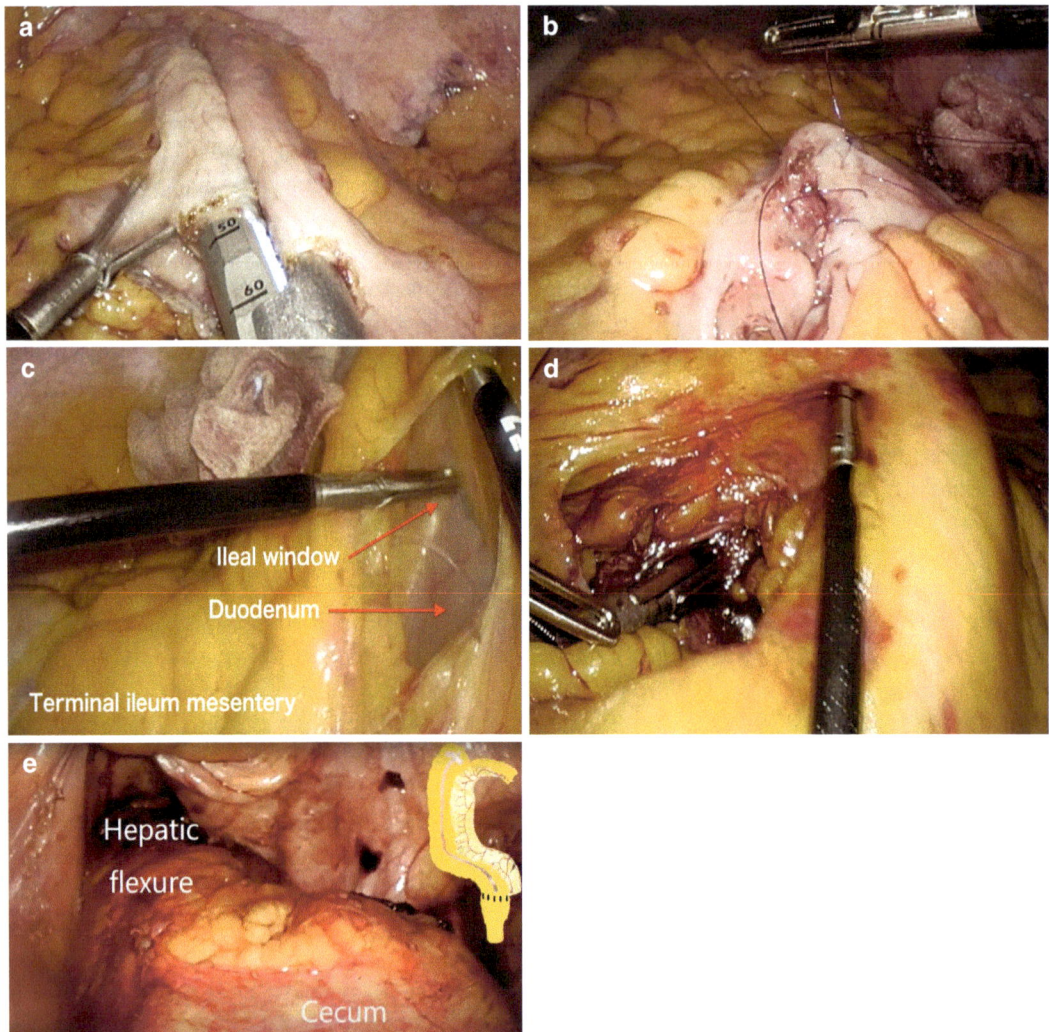

Fig. 6 (**a**) Isoperistaltic SSSA is conducted with one fire of a 60 mm blue endostaper load (**b**) The enterotomy is closed using a 3–0 PDS double layer running suture (**c**) An ileal mesenteric window is creased in the avascular area between the superior mesenteric and ileocolic pedi- cles (**d**) The proximal transverse colon is pulled through the mesenteric window (**e**) Deloyers procedure: the right colon is rotated 180⁰ counterclockwise around the ileoco- lic vessel axis such that the cecum is cephalad while the hepatic flexure is caudal

Postoperative Care

Authors follow postoperative ERAC protocol management. Postoperatively, the patients are placed on an enhanced recovery pathway. The orogastric tube is removed in the operating room prior to awakening from anesthesia. Following the operation, the patient is given oral fluid diet and progressed to an oral diet from the first post- operative day as long as patients tolerate well. The urine catheter is removed on the next day and if drain is inserted, the drain is removed prior to dis- charge. Postoperative analgesia as per pain team. The average length of hospital stay is 3–5 days.

References

1. Watanabe J, Ota M, Suwa Y, et al. Evaluation of lymph flow patterns in splenic flexure colon cancers using laparoscopic real-time indocyanine green fluorescence imaging. Int J Color Dis. 2017;32(2):201–7.

2. Martínez-Pérez A, Brunetti F, Vitali GC, et al. Surgical treatment of colon cancer of the splenic flexure: a systematic review and meta-analysis. Surg Laparosc Endosc Percutan Tech. 2017;27(5):318–27.

3. Secco GB, Ravera G, Gasparo A, et al. Segmental resection, lymph nodes dissection and survival in patients with left colon cancer. Hepato-Gastroenterology. 2007;54(74):422–6.

4. Gravante G, Elshaer M, Parker R, et al. Extended right hemicolectomy and left hemicolectomy for colorectal cancers between the distal transverse and proximal descending colon. Ann R Coll Surg Engl. 2016;98(5):303–7.

5. Manceau G, Mori A, Bardier A, et al. Lymph node metastases in splenic flexure colon cancer: is subtotal colectomy warranted? J Surg Oncol. 2018;118(6):1027–33.

6. Chen YC, Fingerhut A, Shen MY, et al. Colorectal anastomosis after laparoscopic extended left colectomy: techniques and outcome. Color Dis. 2020;22(9):1189–94.

7. Clinical Outcome of Surgical Therapy Study Group, Nelson H, Sargent DJ, et al. A comparison of laparoscopically assisted and open colectomy for colon cancer. N Engl J Med. 2004;350(20):2050–9.

8. Veldkamp R, Kuhry E, Hop WC, et al. Laparascopic surgery versus open surgery for colon cancer: short-term outcome of a randomised trial. Lancet Oncol. 2005;6(7):477–84.

9. Jayne DG, Thrpe HC, Copeland J, et al. Five-year follow-up of the Medical Research Council CLASICC trial of laparoscopically assisted versus open surgery for colorectal cancer. Br J Surg. 2010;97(11):1638–45.

10. Grieco M, Cassini D, Spoletini D, et al. Laparoscopic resection of splenic flexure colon cancers: a retrospective multi-center study with 117 cases. Updat Surg. 2019;71(2):349–57.

11. Okuda J, Yamamoto M, Tanaka K, et al. Laparoscopic resection of transverse colon cancer at splenic flexure: technical aspects and results. Updat Surg. 2016;68(1):71–5.

12. Matsuda A, Miyashita M, Matsumoto S, et al. Isoperistaltic versus antiperistaltic stapled side-to-side anastomosis for colon cancer surgery: a randomized controlled trial. J Surg Res. 2015;196(1):107–12.

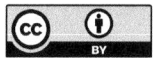

Laparoscopic Anterior Resection

Elaine Hui Been Ng, Yeen Chin Leow,
and William Tzu-Liang Chen

Introduction

The first radical rectal surgery was first performed by Sir William Ernest Miles with a permanent stoma in 1907 while restorative rectal resection was introduced in 1948 by Claude F Dixon. The evolution of using surgical staplers in 1972 by Mark Mitchell Ravitch, doubling stapling technique by Knight and Griffen in 1980 as well as the development of coloanal anastomosis, intersphincteric dissection, and colonic-pouch anal anastomosis by Parks, Larzothes, and Parc respectively between 1980 and 1986 allows more opportunities for restorative resections for low rectal tumors. The concept of Total Mesorectal Excision (TME) with sharp dissection under direct vision and gentle continuous traction by RJ Heald [1] heralded the major milestone in modern rectal cancer surgery in significantly reducing local recurrence and improving patient outcomes. Although laparoscopic surgery began in the 1980s, the first laparoscopic colonic surgery was only performed in 1991. Laparoscopic rectal resection according to the principles of TME has been performed increasingly since with a few randomized controlled clinical trials (CLASICC, COLOR II, ACOSOG Z6051, ALaCaRT) [2–7] demonstrating significantly better postoperative pain, shorter hospital stay, and improved quality of life with controversial but mostly comparable short- and intermediate-term oncological outcomes.

E. H. B. Ng
Colorectal Surgery Unit, Department of Surgery, Hospital Raja Permaisuri Bainum, Ipoh, Malaysia

Division of Colorectal Surgery, Department of Surgery, China Medical University Hospital, Taichung, Taiwan

Y. C. Leow
Division of Colorectal Surgery, Department of Surgery, China Medical University Hospital, Taichung, Taiwan

Colorectal Surgery Unit, Department of Surgery, Hospital Sultanah Bahiyah, Alor Star, Malaysia

W. T.-L. Chen (✉)
Division of Colorectal Surgery, Department of Surgery, China Medical University Hsinchu Hospital, Zhubei City, Hsinchu County, Taiwan
e-mail: wtchen@mail.cmuh.org.tw

Indications

The most common indication is for resection of sigmoid and rectal tumors as long as a negative distal resection margin and adequate postoperative anal sphincter integrity can be preserved. Other indications include large rectal polyps not amenable to other excisional techniques, severe pelvic inflammation or infection causing refractory rectal stricture, severe pelvic endometriosis, salvage prostectomy for benign causes (rectovaginal or rectourethral fistula) with failure of all other treatment modality, secondary tumor by direct invasion, presacral tumors, and rectal trauma.

© The Author(s) 2023
D. Lomanto et al. (eds.), *Mastering Endo-Laparoscopic and Thoracoscopic Surgery*,
https://doi.org/10.1007/978-981-19-3755-2_71

Contraindications

Absolute contraindications are inability to tolerate prolonged pneumoperitoneum in a Trendelenburg position especially for patients with cardiac failure or severe pulmonary disease, hemodynamic instability, or cases of compromised oncological safety (sphincter, pelvic floor, sacral, and/or pelvic side wall invasion). Relative contraindications would be dependent on the skills of the surgeon and patient characteristics that may prohibit a laparoscopic approach including bulky rectal tumors requiring en bloc multivisceral resection, morbid obesity, severe adhesions, pregnancy, and bowel obstruction.

Preoperative Assessment

Postoperative expectations of pelvic organ function including infertility and possibility of stoma must be discussed as anatomical restoration in low rectal resection may not be functionally acceptable for certain patients because of their lifestyle or occupation.

A routine anesthetic assessment is performed prior to surgery. Preexisting anal sphincter function and previous trauma including perianal surgery must be elicited. Digital rectal examination is mandatory to assess the preexisting anal tone, sphincter integrity, distal margin of rectal tumor focusing on proximity to the sphincters and pelvic floor muscles, and possibility of invasion to adjacent structures. A complete preoperative colonoscopy is mandatory to exclude synchronous proximal lesions and biopsy the tumor (tattoo if small). Complete TNM staging with appropriate locoregional imaging is necessary to guide the optimal treatment approach. Computed tomography (CT) is used for the assessment of distant metastases and magnetic resonance imaging (MRI) is the current gold standard for preoperative T- and N-stage evaluation for rectal tumors as well as assessment for invasion into sphincters and pelvic floor [8].

Preoperative oral bowel preparation for rectal surgery has been controversial but the current ASCRS recommendation for elective surgery is for preoperative oral antibiotics in combination with mechanical bowel preparation [9].

OT Setup and Techniques

The patient is placed in the modified lithotomy position with both legs on adjustable stirrups. Both arms are tucked in. A Trendelenburg position is utilized to gravitationally move the omentum and bowels cephalad for unobstructed access to the pelvis. Tilting the patient to the right allows unhindered access to the regions of the inferior mesenteric artery and vein, left mesocolon, left retroperitoneum, splenic flexure, and left colon (Fig. 1).

The surgeon (S) stands on the right side of the patient with the camera assistant (C) beside the surgeon. The first assistant (F) stands on the left side of the patient (Fig. 2). The monitor screens (M) are placed on the left side of the patient with flexible mobility between the cranial and caudal end as required.

(a) **Placement of Trocars**

We use an open technique to insert the 12 mm trocar for the telescope at the umbilical region, favoring the supraumbilical position. Additional varying number of working trocars are placed under direct visualization. We use the 5-trocar technique—Fig. 3. A high anterior resection may not require the fifth port. The second port at RLQ (two

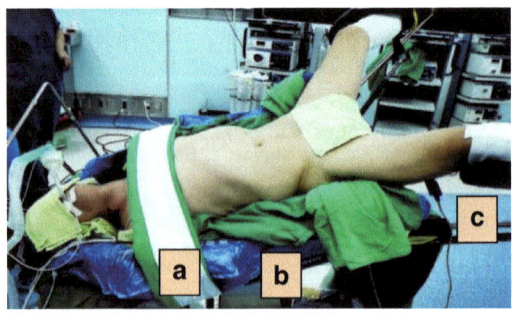

Fig. 1 Patient is strapped to the table with a chest strap (**a**) and mouldable bean bag (**b**), both legs in adjustable stirrups (**c**) to prevent truncal sliding in the Trendelenburg position with right table tilt

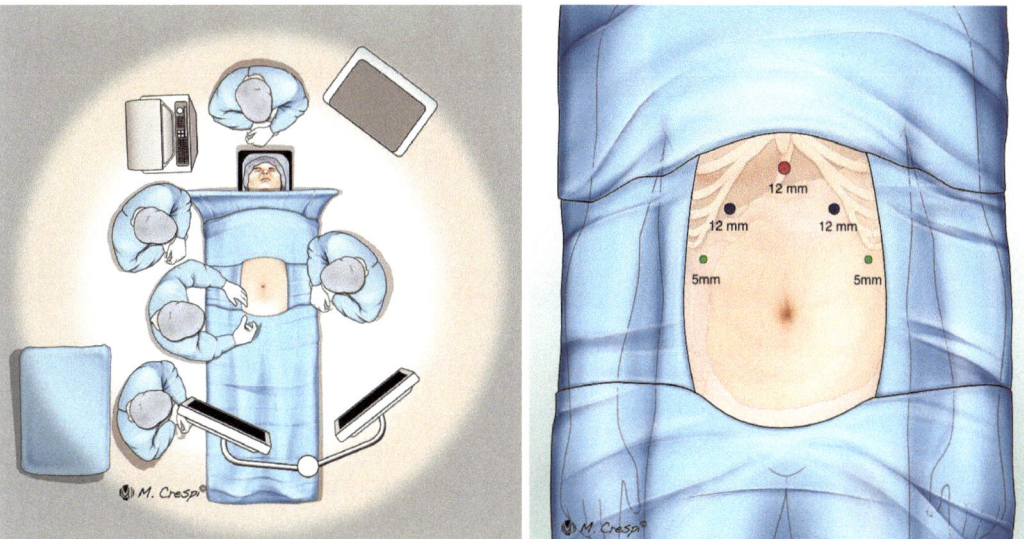

Fig. 2 OT setup and port placement

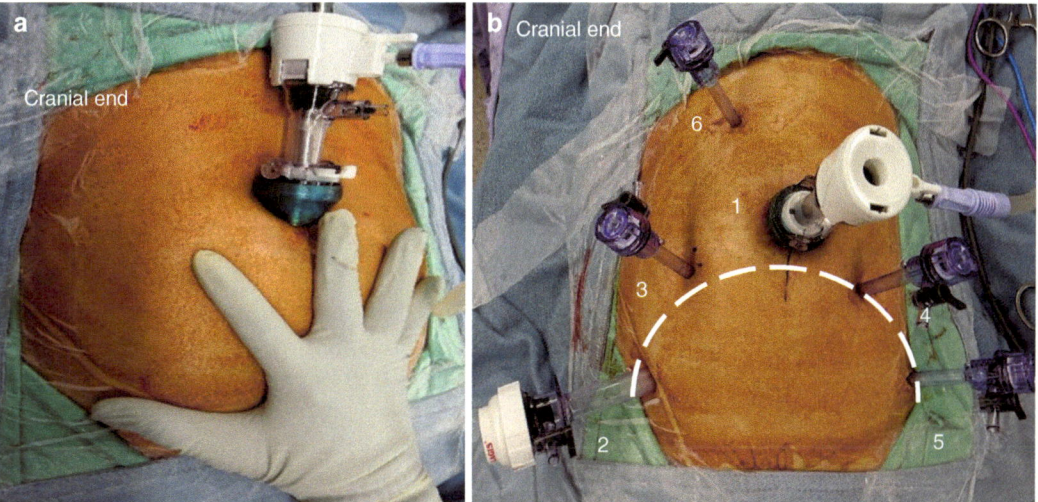

Fig. 3 Placing the palm with the wrist on the symphysis pubis and fingers spread open on an insufflated abdomen (**a**) can guide the positions of the trocars (**b**) placed on a semi-circular line with the left trocars as mirror trocars of the right

fingerbreadths anterior to the ASIS) is a 12 mm access port for the endoscopic stapler. The left-sided trocars are mirror trocars of the right. An additional sixth trocar at the RUQ is used to access the lesser sac and aid splenic flexure mobilization.

(b) **Medial-to-lateral mesocolic dissection, IMA division**

Pneumoperitoneum is created at 10–15 mm Hg and abdominal cavity is inspected for metastases. The sigmoid colon is retracted anteriorly out of the pelvis. Dissection begins at the level of sacral promontory and continued cephalad towards the ligament of Treitz, anterior to the aorta. An avascular plane is created beneath the SRA arch to separate the left mesocolon from the posterior retroperitoneal fascia in a medial-to-lateral fashion all the way to the left lateral peritoneal reflection (Fig. 4). An alternative

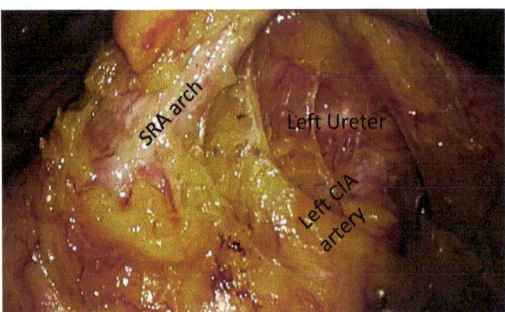

Fig. 4 Medial-to-lateral dissection (arrow) with the SRA arch being retracted anteriorly and the retroperitoneal fascia and structures being swept posteriorly

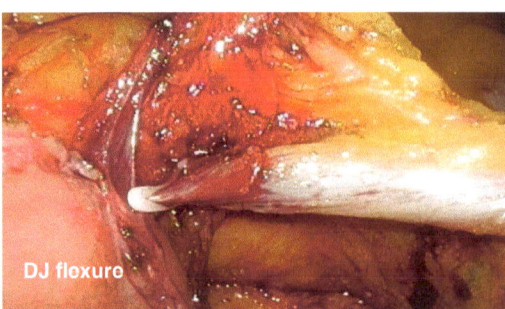

Fig. 6 IMV ligation, lateral to the ligament of Treitz, below the inferior border of the pancreas

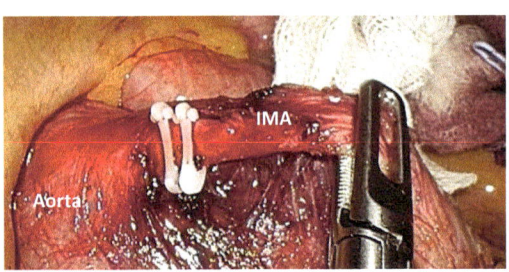

Fig. 5 IMA ligation—clips placed proximally at the root, 2 cm distal to the aorta, after adequate skeletonization

lateral-to-medial approach is used if this approach becomes difficult, especially in obese patients.

High ligation of the IMA requires exposure of the root of the IMA and ligating it at 1–2 cm from the aorta. The IMA can be divided between clips or with a linear vascular stapler/vessel-sealing device—Fig. 5.

(c) **Inferior Mesenteric Vein (IMV) Division and Access to Lesser Sac, Splenic Flexure, and Lateral Colonic Mobilization**

The dissection continues superiorly along this avascular plane all the way to the inferior border of the pancreas and ligament of Treitz with a high IMV ligation at this position (Fig. 6). Transverse colon is then retracted anteriorly adjacent to the ligament of Treitz to divide the root of the transverse mesocolon anterior to the pancreas to enter the lesser sac (Fig. 7a). Pancreaticocolic ligaments are divided, taking care to avoid

the marginal artery. Transverse colon is retracted caudally to divide the gastrocolic ligament (Fig. 7b) to meet the dissection plane in the lesser sac. Left colonic and splenic flexure mobilization is completed with the division of the remaining lateral peritoneal attachments and splenocolic ligaments (Fig. 7c, d).

Alternatively, a reversed lateral-to-medial splenic flexure mobilization can be used to enter the lesser sac but it is technically more difficult and has a higher chance of pancreatic injury.

(d) **Pelvic   Dissection: Total   Mesorectal Excision (TME) and Bowel Transection**

Sigmoid colon is retracted cephalad and anteriorly to identify the retrorectal space. The posterior rectal mobilization is carried out with sharp dissection preferably with monopolar electrocautery along the avascular areolar plane between the visceral and parietal endopelvic fascia while simultaneously maintaining gentle continued traction of the rectum anteriorly all the way to the pelvic floor (Fig. 8a, b). A tape can be used to aid rectal retraction during the TME (Fig. 8c). The dissection continues in the same plane bilaterally (Fig. 8d, e) and anteriorly along the Denonvillier's fascia (Fig. 8f) down to the pelvic floor. Be wary not to injure the parasympathetic nervi erigentes (S2 to S4) from overzealous lateral dissection beyond the mesorectal fascia. Coordinated planar tractions and counter tractions are needed for

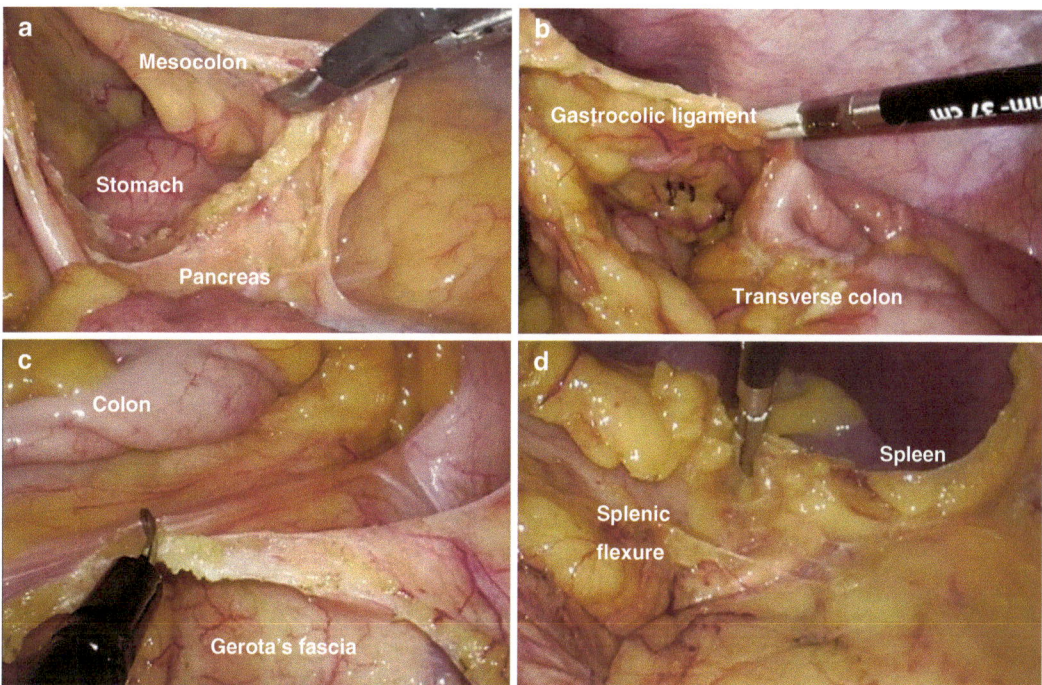

Fig. 7 (**a**) Entering lesser sac. (**b**) Division of gastrocolic ligament. (**c**) Dividing lateral peritoneal attachment. (**d**) Dividing splenocolic ligament

accurate TME dissection. The level of rectal transection is then confirmed by digital rectal and/or endoscopic examination after a complete circumferential TME. The rectum is irrigated, stapled, and divided with an endoscopic stapler (Fig. 9).

The mesocolon is divided intracorporeally. A grasper holding the proximal bowel presents the specimen at the extraction site for exteriorization (Fig. 10a). Anvil of the circular stapler (at least 28 mm) is anchored in the conduit with a purse-string suture after transection (Fig. 10b). The colon is returned to the abdomen and the extraction site is temporarily closed for re-pneumoperitoneum in preparation for intracorporeal anastomosis.

(e) **Anastomosis**

The rectal stump is transfixed with the tip of the head of the circular stapler while the posterior vaginal wall/prostate is retracted anteriorly to avoid inclusion into the stapler line. The colonic mesentery is checked for twisting before firing the stapler. The integrity of the anastomosis is assessed by visually verifying the completeness of the proximal and distal donuts, performing an air insufflation test and endoscopic evaluation of the anastomotic stapling line. Several intracorporeal stapled anastomotic techniques other than end-to-end anastomosis (ETE) can be used to reduce the incidence of low anterior resection syndrome (LARS) by creating a neorectal reservoir (Fig. 11). We do not routinely insert a drain in the pelvis. A temporary diverting stoma is constructed mainly in low anastomosis of immunosuppressed individuals and/or irradiated pelvis.

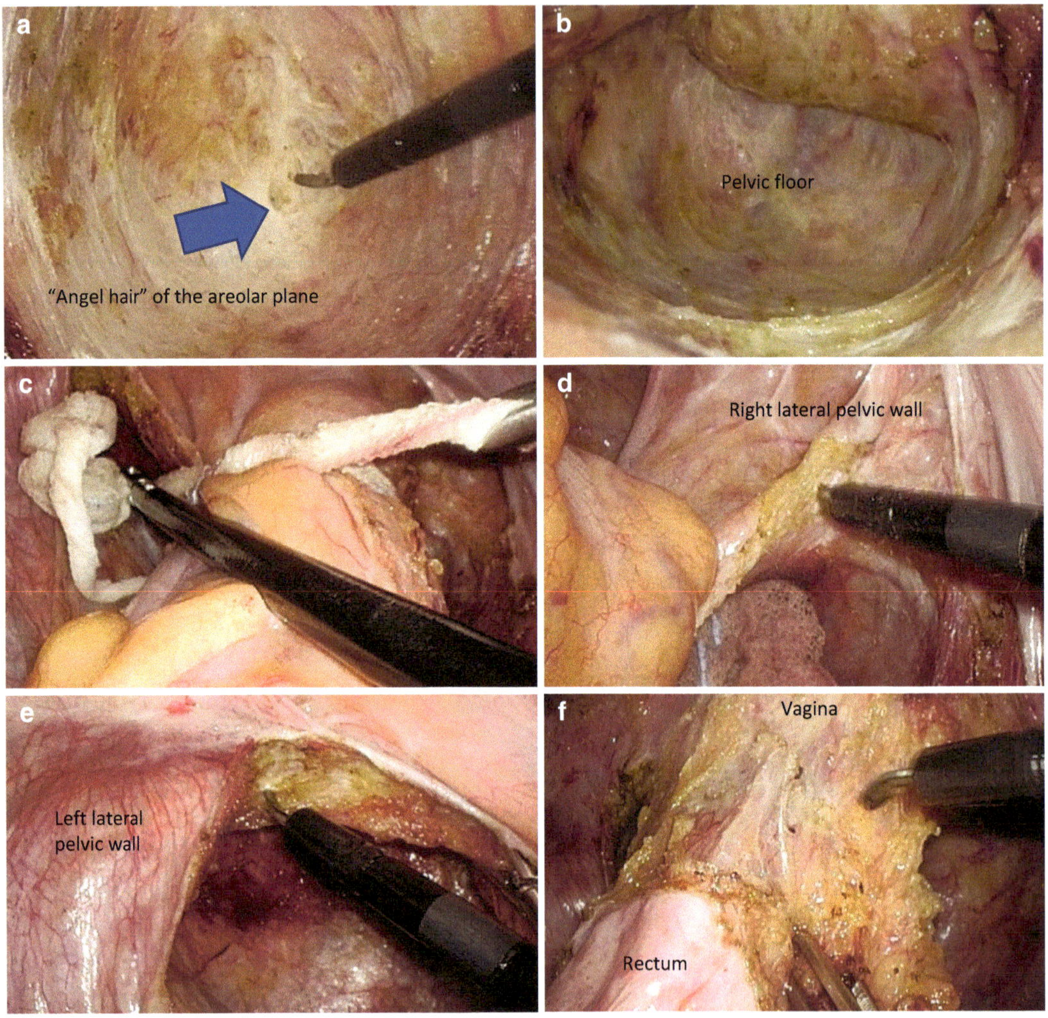

Fig. 8 (**a**) Posterior TME, sharp dissection at the avascular areolar plane; (**b**) complete posterior TME down to the pelvic floor; (**c**) cotton sling/tape to retract the rectum cephalad; (**d**) right lateral TME; (**e**) left lateral TME; (**f**) anterior TME

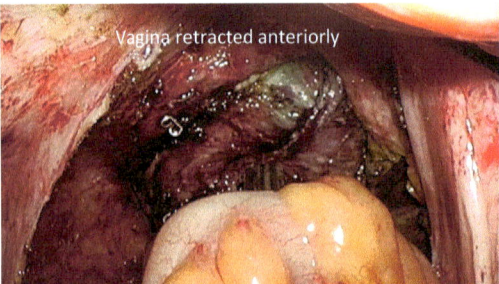

Fig. 9 Rectal transection with GIA, vagina retracted anteriorly by the first assistant

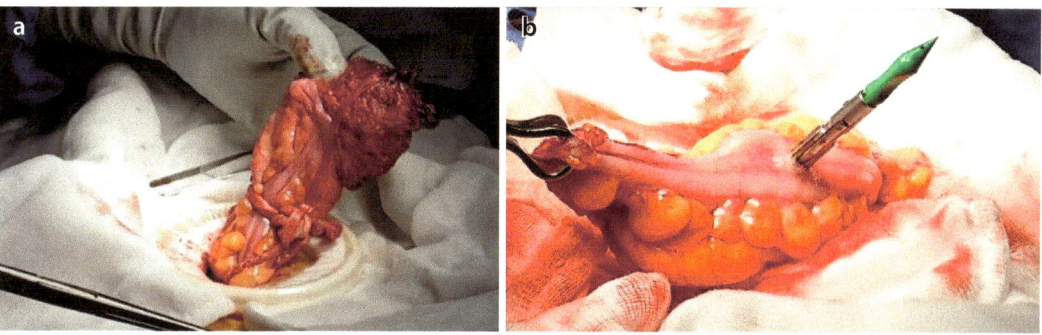

Fig. 10 (**a**) Specimen extraction. (**b**) Anvil inserted into the antimesenteric border of colonic conduit for side-to-end anastomosis

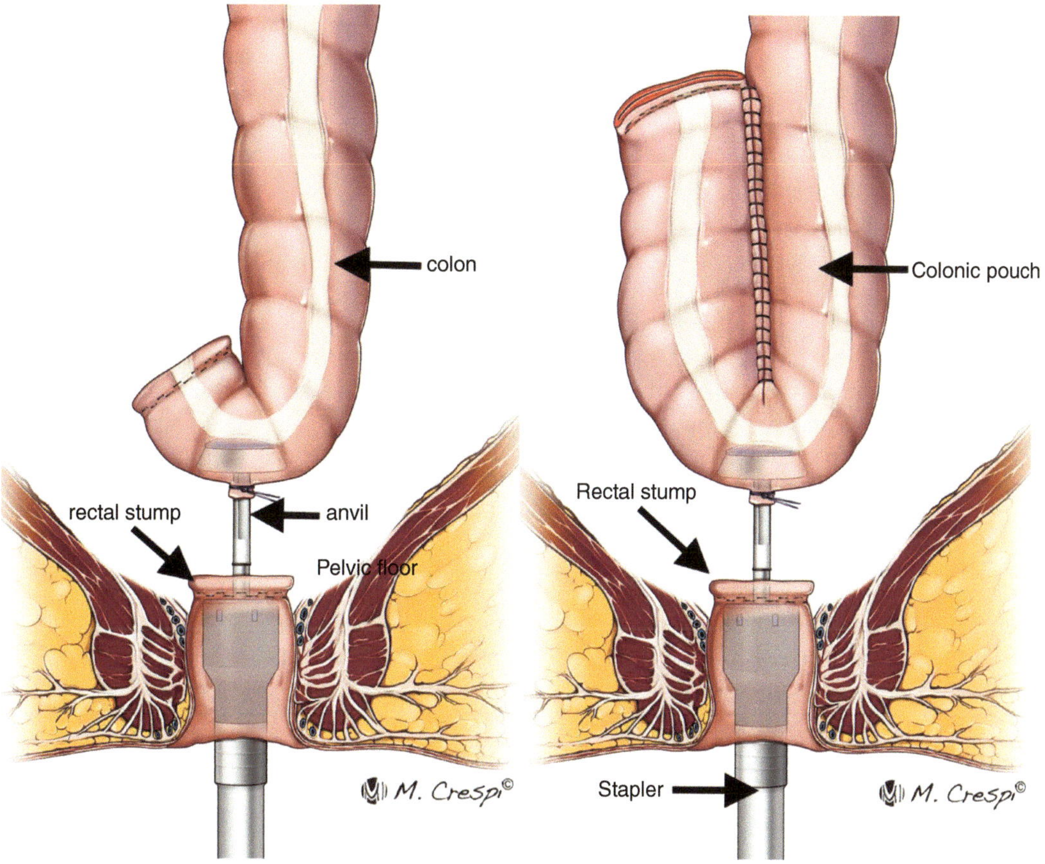

Fig. 11 Intracorporeal colorectal end-to-end (ETE) stapled anastomosis, side-to-end anastomosis, colonic J-pouch

Complications and Management

Ureteric and Bladder Injury

Adequate exposure in the correct dissection plane would avoid accidental injury. Inflammation, cancer infiltration, and adhesions can alter the regional anatomy and would require insertion of an intraoperative ureteric stent for identification. Repair is dependent on the location of injury and length of transected ureter. Bladder injury usually results from electrocoagulation tears during TME. Immediate suturing with postoperative bladder catheterization for 7–10 days is usually adequate.

Vascular Injury

Aggressive grasping or lifting of the vessels during mesenteric dissection can cause vessel tear. IMA and IMV must be adequately skeletonized with forceps in an alternating parallel and perpendicular direction to the vessel from its surrounding tissues at an appropriate exposure length before vascular clipping or sealing prior to division. Injury to the marginal artery and Arc of Riolan can occur during the medial dissection into the lesser sac and should be avoided to maintain collateral supply to the left colonic conduit. Bleeding from presacral venous plexus during TME may require second-look laparotomy after pelvic packing if conventional hemostatic methods fail. Iatrogenic splenic injury can occur from traction or capsular tear during splenic flexure mobilization.

Neurological Injury

Urinary and sexual dysfunction from damaged superior hypogastric plexus, the hypogastric nerves, the inferior hypogastric plexus, the pelvic splanchnic nerves, and the neurovascular bundle of Walsh from thermal injury, ischemia, tension, or inflammation during IMA dissection and TME can be avoided by careful sharp dissection with anatomical familiarization in these areas.

Anastomotic Leak

Any error during intracorporeal stapling anastomosis must be fixed immediately. A close-up visual inspection of the staple formation on the rectal stump should be undertaken after the firing of the endoscopic stapler and when the circular stapler is pushed up to the top of the rectal stump before anastomosis. Any incomplete donuts would require inspection of the anastomosis, leak test, and additional suturing of the defect. Recently, the use of indocyanine green (ICG) in the evaluation of perfusion for both proximal and distal stumps prior to anastomosis may reduce the risk of anastomotic leak from ischemia [10]. A tension-free anastomosis is essential. Proximal diverting stoma should always be considered in the presence of any doubt of the anastomotic integrity.

Low Anterior Resection Syndrome (LARS)

Alternative anastomotic techniques of STE, CJP, and TC create a neorectal reservoir to reduce the incidence of LARS, especially in young patients with irradiated pelvis. CJP has been demonstrated to provide better bowel function for up to 2 years compared to ETE but is technically limited by a narrow pelvis, insufficient colonic length, or colonic diverticulosis. STE seems to be functionally comparable to CJP in a limited literature review [11, 12].

Fistula

Although rare, rectovaginal fistula is caused more commonly by inadequate dissection and stapling error. One must carefully dissect between the rectal stump and posterior vaginal wall and introduce the circular stapler at a marked posterior angle in the rectal stump to avoid the inclusion of the vaginal wall in the tissue rings (donuts).

Incisional Hernia

Specimen extraction from the conventional left iliac fossa port or midline contributes to a higher incidence of incisional hernia. Moving the specimen extraction site to a Pfannenstiel incision reduces the incidence [13].

Postoperative Care

Nasogastric tube is removed at the end of surgery. Pelvic and peritoneal drains are not routinely inserted. Postoperative urinary drainage should be ideally ≤24 h for low-risk patients but those with extensive pelvic dissection may require catheterization up to 3 days after surgery. Early diet on the first day (liquids/low residue diet within 4 h) after surgery should be introduced. Early postoperative mobilization is encouraged as early as 2 h after surgery and 6 h thereafter.

References

1. Heald RJ, Moran BJ, Ryall RD, Sexton R, MacFarlane JK. Rectal cancer: the Basingstoke experience of total mesorectal excision, 1978–1997. Arch Surg. 1998;133:894–9.
2. Green BL, Marshall HC, Collinson F, Quirke P, Guillou P, Jayne DG, et al. Long-term follow-up of the medical research council CLASICC trial of conventional versus laparoscopically assisted resection in colorectal cancer. Br J Surg. 2013;100:75–82.
3. Bonjer HJ, Deijen CL, Abis GA, Cuesta MA, van der Pas MHGM, de ESM L-d K, COLOR II Study Group, et al. A randomized trial of laparoscopic versus open surgery for rectal cancer. N Engl J Med. 2015;372:1324–32.
4. Fleshman J, Branda M, Sargent DJ, Boller AM, George V, Abbas M, et al. Effect of laparoscopic-assisted resection vs open resection of stage II or III rectal cancer on pathologic outcomes: the ACOSOG Z6051 randomized clinical trial. JAMA. 2015;314:1346–55.
5. Stevenson AR, Solomon MJ, Lumley JW, et al. Effect of laparoscopic assisted resection vs open resection on pathological outcomes in rectal cancer: the ALaCaRT randomized clinical trial. JAMA. 2015;314(13):1356–63.
6. Stevenson ARL, Solomon MJ, Brown CSB, et al. Disease free survival and local recurrence after laparoscopic assisted resection or open resection for rectal cancer: the Australasian laparoscopic cancer of the rectum randomized clinical trial. Ann Surg. 2019;269(4):596–602.
7. Fleshman J, Branda ME, Sargent DJ, et al. Disease free survival and local recurrence for laparoscopic resection compared with open resection of stage II to III rectal cancer: follow up results of the ACOSOG Z6051 randomized controlled trial. Ann Surg. 2019;269(4):589–95.
8. MERCURY Study Group. Diagnostic accuracy of preoperative magnetic resonance imaging in predicting curative resection of rectal cancer: prospective observational study. BMJ. 2006;333:779.
9. Migaly J, Bafford AC, Francone TD, et al. The American Society of Colon and Rectal Surgeons clinical practice guidelines for the use of bowel preparation in elective colon and Rectal surgery. Dis Colon Rectum. 2019;62:3–8.
10. Gilshtein H, Yellinek S, Wexner SD. The evolving role of indocyanine green fluorescence in the treatment of low rectal cancer. ALES. 2018;3(10):1–4.
11. Huttner FJ, Tenckhoff S, Jensen K, et al. Meta-analysis of reconstruction techniques after low anterior resection for rectal cancer. Br J Surg. 2015;102:735–45.
12. Brown CJ, Fenech DS, McLeod RS. Reconstruction techniques after rectal resection for rectal cancer. Cochrane Database Syst Rev. 2008;2008(2):CD006040. https://doi.org/10.1002/14651858.CD006040.pub2.
13. Samia H, Lawrence J, Nobel T, Stein S, Champagne BJ, et al. Extraction site location and incisional hernias after laparoscopic colorectal surgery: should we be avoiding the midline? Am J Surg. 2013;205:264–7.

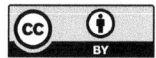

Laparoscopic Abdominoperineal Resection

Isaac Seow-En and William Tzu-Liang Chen

Introduction

A rectal cancer located within the narrow confines of the bony pelvis has for centuries been the bugbear of abdominal surgeons. Advances in operative technique, surgical technology, imaging methods, and multimodal therapies have dramatically improved the prospects of this once fatal disease. Despite the considerable progress, cancer of the rectum remains one of the most challenging conditions encountered by colorectal surgeons in present times.

Perhaps the most notable contribution of the twentieth century to the management of rectal cancer was that by Sir William Ernest Miles, who described abdominoperineal excision of the rectum and anal sphincter complex with a permanent colostomy in 1908 [1]. His groundbreaking notion of reducing recurrence by removing as much lymphatic drainage of the rectum as possible in a "cylindrical" concept formed the basis of modern rectal cancer surgery [2]. Miles' revolu-

tionary work is still the topic of vivid discussion more than 100 years later [3, 4]. For decades, abdominoperineal resection (APR) was the standard treatment for all rectal cancers, until anterior resection with a colorectal anastomosis was reported (in 1948) to be a safe and acceptable surgical therapy for lesions located in the upper half of the rectum [5]. From the late 60s to the early 70s, introduction of a transrectal circular stapling device [6], as well as the coloanal handsewn anastomotic technique [7] enabled surgeons to perform progressively more distal rectal resections while preserving the anal sphincter. In 1982, Bill Heald identified the "Holy Plane" of dissection between the mesorectal and presacral fascia for total mesorectal excision (TME) [8], which became the gold standard for oncologic resection of middle to low rectal cancers.

Still, it was recognized that TME alone provided insufficient local control for more advanced disease. A major milestone came in the form of combined chemoradiotherapy prior to surgery [9]. For the past 20 years, neoadjuvant chemoradiation therapy (NACRT) has been advocated for locally advanced, i.e., stage 2 and 3 cancers located in the mid to distal rectum, prior to surgical resection, followed by adjuvant chemotherapy for nodepositive disease. 50–60% of patients are downstaged after NACRT, with approximately one-fifth showing a pathologic complete response [10]. This approach, along with enhanced surgical techniques, has reduced the local recurrence rate to 5–10% at 5 years. Next,

I. Seow-En
Department of Colorectal Surgery, Singapore General Hospital, Singapore, Singapore

Division of Colorectal Surgery, China Medical University Hospital, Taichung, Taiwan

W. T.-L. Chen (✉)
Division of Colorectal Surgery, Department of Surgery, China Medical University Hsinchu Hospital, Zhubei City, Hsinchu County, Taiwan
e-mail: wtchen@mail.cmuh.org.tw

© The Author(s) 2023
D. Lomanto et al. (eds.), *Mastering Endo-Laparoscopic and Thoracoscopic Surgery*,
https://doi.org/10.1007/978-981-19-3755-2_72

the focus turned to improving systemic control [11]. Total neoadjuvant therapy, which provides all necessary chemotherapy and radiation prior to surgery, aims to deal with circulating micrometastases earlier for better systemic control and is now recognized as a valid treatment option for locally advanced tumors [10, 12].

With increasing acknowledgment of the effectiveness of adjunctive therapies, Habr-Gama and colleagues in the mid-2000s pioneered the "watch-and-wait" approach on the basis of an observed 26–27% rectal cancer pathological response rate to NACRT [13]. Organ preservation (of the rectum) thus emerged as a possible nonsurgical option in the management of rectal cancer [14]. A 2018 meta-analysis of 13 cohorts showed a complete clinical response rate of 22.4% with a 3 year cumulative local recurrence risk of 21.6%. Most of these patients underwent salvage surgery with a 79.1% R0 resection rate, 45.3% sphincter preservation rate, and 3-year overall survival and disease-free survival of 93.5 and 89.2%, respectively [15]. No randomized trial exists and substantial deficiencies in our knowledge of the organ-preserving approach prevent it from becoming mainstream therapy. Nonetheless, current evidence suggests that the watch-and-wait may be reasonable for selected, including high surgical risk patients, with locoregionally advanced mid to distal rectal cancers who demonstrate complete clinical response [11].

Surgical technique for rectal cancer has come a long way since Miles' seminal paper. The laparoscopic approach to APR has been proven to reduce postoperative complications and hasten recovery, without compromising oncologic outcomes, recurrence rates, and survival [16]. Moreover, the advantages of laparoscopic APR over open surgery are more pronounced than that of anterior resection as only small port scars remain without the need for abdominal specimen extraction. Robotic surgery and transanal total mesorectal excision are two newer methods that have been the focus of both retrospective research and prospective trials in recent years. A 2019 meta-analysis by Simillis et al. involving 6237 patients from 29 randomized trials compared the classic open versus laparoscopic versus robotic versus transanal TME; all methods appeared to have comparable morbidity rates and long-term outcomes. However, the laparoscopic and robotic methods appeared to improve postoperative recovery and the open and transanal approaches seemed to benefit oncologic resection [17].

Enhanced surgical techniques in the setting of effective multimodal adjunctive therapies for low rectal cancers have decreased the rates of APR. A pooled analysis of five large European trials suggests that the APR procedure itself was a predictor of increased local recurrence and death [18]. Compared to anterior resection, patients who undergo APR also report worse body image and sexual enjoyment at 1 year postsurgery [19]. Nonetheless, APR is still the requisite procedure in many circumstances and remains an essential component of the armamentarium of colorectal surgeons today. In this chapter, we will examine the use of the laparoscopic APR technique for low rectal cancer.

Indications

An individualized approach is mandatory in the management of patients with distal rectal cancer. Accurate systemic staging along with a dedicated multidisciplinary team discussion should be conducted as per existing clinical guidelines [10, 20]. The following should be considered when establishing the optimal surgical approach for each patient:

Tumor Characteristics

Location of the tumor and involvement of the anal sphincters can be determined by a digital rectal examination. Fixed tumors with sphincter or levator muscle invasion will necessitate an APR. Involvement of the prostate or anterior wall of the vagina may require pelvic exenteration. Magnetic resonance imaging (MRI) of the pelvis using a specific rectal cancer protocol is the modality of choice for locoregional staging. The MERCURY trial showed that MRI can predict surgical resectability, overall survival, and local recurrence through assessment of the MRI tumor regression grade [21]. The utility of endorectal ultrasound is limited to the differentiation of T1 and T2 tumors, the former of which may be amenable to local excisional procedures in the absence of high-risk MRI features. Locally advanced low rectal cancers should be referred for neoadjuvant radiation. We use a long course protocol of 45–50.4 Gy in 25–28 doses given in conjunction with chemotherapy, typically 5-FU. Surgery may be performed between 5 and 12 weeks following full dose 5.5 weeks NACRT [10], although the ideal timing remains the subject of controversy [20]. Posttreatment MRI is important to assess response and can be performed at the mid-way point between the end of treatment and intended timing of surgical resection.

Sphincter preservation may become possible in cases where initial tumor bulk prevented consideration of such surgery and the extent of the tumor is improved after neoadjuvant therapy. An APR is indicated where an R0 resection of the tumor would result in loss of anal sphincter function and incontinence [10]. The acceptable distal resection margin for low rectal cancers should be greater than 1 cm, although a < 1 cm margin has been shown not to compromise oncologic safety in selected patients [22]. Intersphincteric resection for very low locally advanced rectal cancer has also been found to have acceptable oncologic outcomes [23].

Sphincter Function

A thorough history and physical examination can determine the pretreatment baseline function. It would be pointless exercise to preserve a poorly functioning anal sphincter. A meta-analysis of 25 studies with 6548 patients demonstrated that NACRT negatively affected long-term anorectal function after surgery [24]. It is therefore advisable to repeat functional assessment following

neoadjuvant therapy. If available, objective measurement using anal manometric studies can be performed. For borderline cases, it is important to consider the high prevalence (of approximately 40%) and long-term persistence of bowel dysfunction, the so-called low anterior resection syndrome (LARS), following sphincter-sparing rectal surgery [25–27]. Patients with severe LARS symptoms may prefer a permanent stoma and would have benefited from an upfront APR. This possibility should be emphasized preoperatively to patients who are at higher risk for LARS, including those with a history of radiotherapy or in whom anterior resection would result in a low anastomotic height [26]. Overall functional status should also be taken into account.

Preoperative Preparation

Ostomy nurse counseling and stoma site selection for optimal positioning of the permanent colostomy are important to facilitate postoperative stoma care and function. The patient should be enrolled in an enhanced recovery after surgery (ERAS) program. We do not advocate mechanical bowel preparation before APR. Prophylactic intravenous antibiotics are given at anesthetic induction and throughout the duration of surgery. Pharmacological or mechanical venous thromboembolism prophylaxis should be instituted due to the high-risk nature of this surgery. The ureters can be stented prior to rectal resection to facilitate intraoperative identification, which may be advantageous in difficult cases with previous pelvic surgery. A urinary catheter must be inserted.

OT Setup

Abdominal Phase

Our patient position prior to draping can be seen in Fig. 1. The patient is placed in the modified Lloyd-Davis position with the lower limbs in

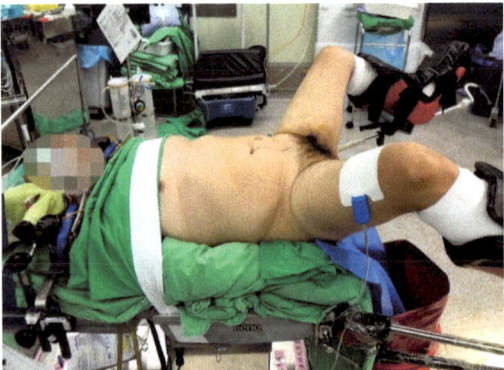

Fig. 1 APR abdominal phase standard positioning before draping

foot stirrups and the buttocks a few centimeters off the caudal edge of the operating table. Both arms are tucked in to facilitate positioning of the surgeon, camera operator, and assistant. A small sandbag (or folded drapes) is placed below the sacrum to elevate the pelvis, enabling better visualization of the deep pelvic structures during surgery. A steep Trendelenburg position is maintained for most of the abdominal phase. To stabilize the patient's position, we use fixed shoulder supports to absorb the patient's weight, with soft gel pads minimizing the risk of pressure injury. To provide additional support, a strip of strong adhesive tape is used to strap the patient's chest, just above the nipple line, to the sides of the table. Alternatively, an adjustable "bean bag" above a soft gel layer can be molded around the patient to prevent sliding. We use a soft elastic bandage, wrapped tightly around the lower limb, as a substitute for compression stockings. The lower limbs should be in a relaxed posture with the knees flexed at 45° to prevent overstretching of the peripheral nerves (Fig. 2).

Operating setup and ports are shown in Fig. 3. A 12 mm camera trocar is placed via an umbilical incision under direct vision. Working trocars consist of a 12 mm trocar placed two fingerbreadths medial to the right anterior superior iliac spine and a 5 mm trocar midway between

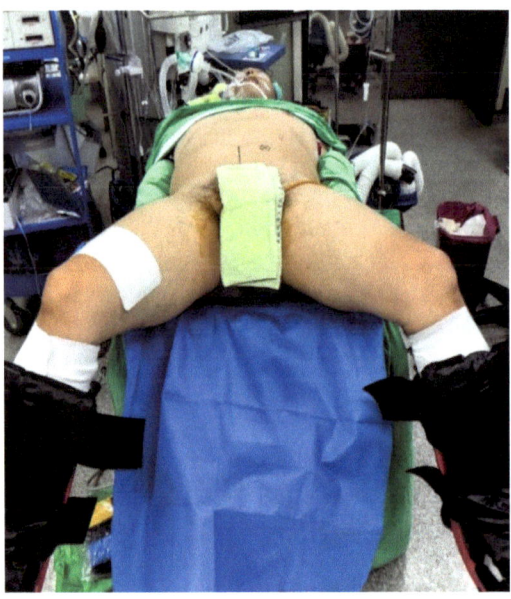

Fig. 2 The ideal position of the lower limbs during surgery

the right iliac fossa trocar and the umbilical trocar. In our experience, this port position provides the best ergonomics for deep pelvic dissection. The assistant ports are a right-to-left mirror image of the working ports, using two 5 mm trocars. One assistant trocar can be placed at the intended (and preoperatively marked) colostomy site to minimize operative incisions. A single assistant trocar may be sufficient in straightforward cases.

Perineal Phase

Upon completion of the abdominal phase, the patient is transferred to a trolley and the operating table is prepared for the prone jackknife (Kraske) position as shown in Fig. 4. The leg boards are reattached. A donut head pad is used for facial support. It is necessary to provide adequate padding for the colostomy and drain site while the patient is prone to prevent pressure injury. The knees are kept in slight flexion on a separate cushioned cardiac trolley

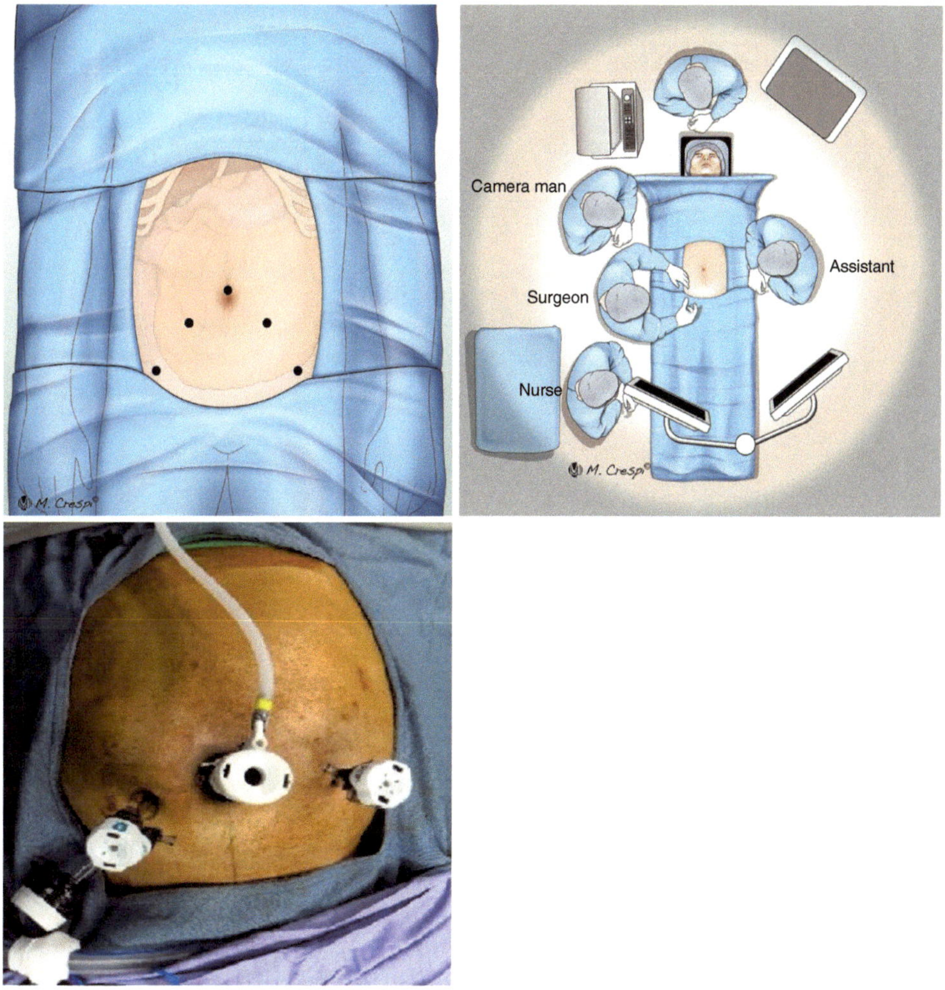

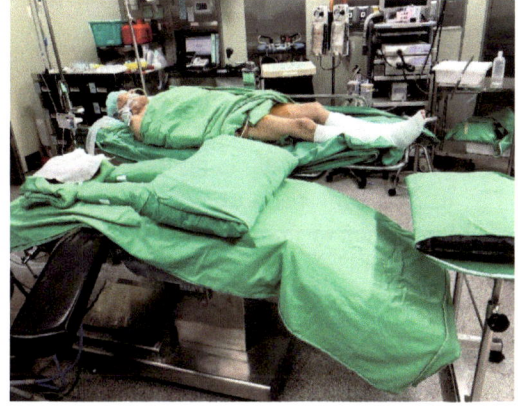

Fig. 3 (*Above*) Schematic of operating setup and port placement for laparoscopic APR. (*Below*) Left-sided assistant trocar can be placed at the intended end colostomy site

Fig. 4 Preparing the operating table for the prone jack-knife position

(Fig. 5), to prevent stretch of the lower limb nerves.

Adhesive tape is used to splay the buttocks apart and anchored to the table frame on each side (Fig. 6). The anus is sutured shut to prevent leakage of stool during the procedure. For the perineal skin incision, the posterior extent should be midway between the tip of the coccyx and the anus, the anterior extent at the perineal body, and the lateral extent midway between the ischial tuberosities and the anus. Operative landmarks as well as the elliptical skin incision are shown in Fig. 6.

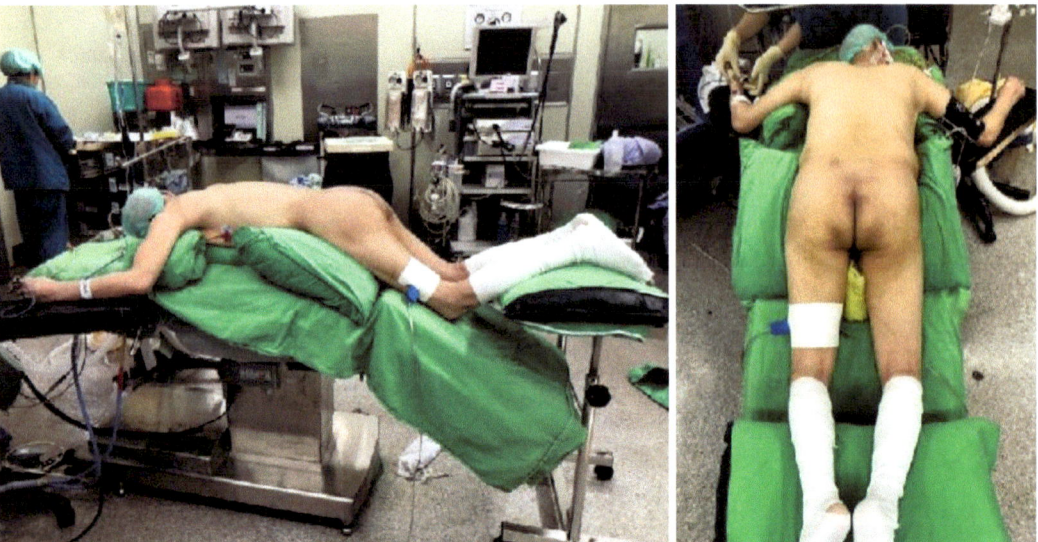

Fig. 5 The prone jackknife position for the APR perineal phase

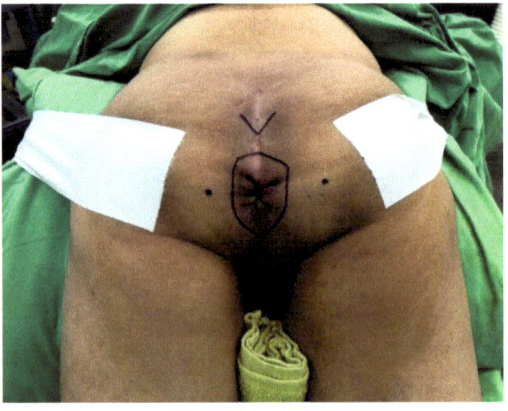

Fig. 6 Preparing the perineum for the perineal phase. The downward arrow marks the coccygeal location and the points on either side of the anus indicate the position of the ischial tuberosities. Using these landmarks, the skin incision is delineated as shown

Surgical Technique

Abdominal Phase Essential Steps

1. Medial to lateral colonic mobilization
2. Inferior mesenteric artery ligation
3. Rectal mobilization pelvic floor
4. Proximal bowel transection
5. End colostomy creation

Abdominal Phase Technique

The initial approach to the APR abdominal phase is not unlike that for a low anterior resection (see chapter on Anterior Resection). A splenic flexure takedown is unnecessary, and the proximal colon is mobilized just enough to allow the exteriorization of an end colostomy following bowel resection. TME dissection and rectal mobilization should be progressed as distally as possible to facilitate the subsequent perineal phase. A cotton tape tie at rectosigmoid junction is useful to provide traction of the rectum out of the pelvis (Fig. 7). The knot is grasped by the surgical assistant for retraction and manipulation of the rectum during TME. For females, the uterus can be temporarily hitched to the anterior abdominal wall using a Prolene 2–0 straight needle passed through the uterine fundus or the broad ligaments (Fig. 8). This provides visualization without the need for traction by the assistant. Following adequate colon and rectal mobilization, the proximal colon is transected with an appropriate oncologic margin using an endoscopic linear stapler. A drain is placed in the pelvis prior to closure. The sigmoid colon is exteriorized via a left-sided skin incision and the abdominal wounds are closed before the end colostomy is matured.

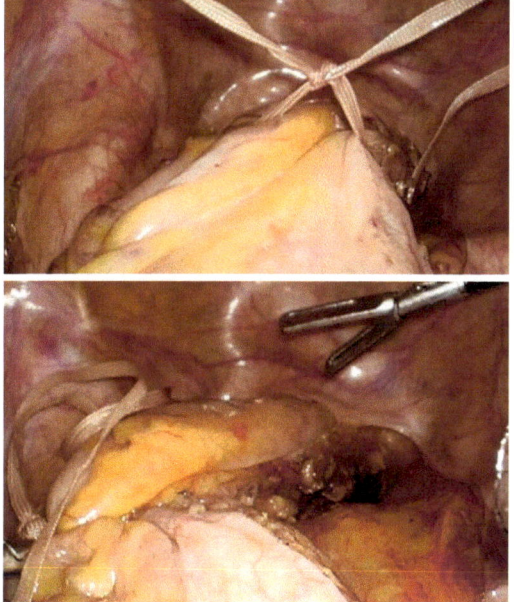

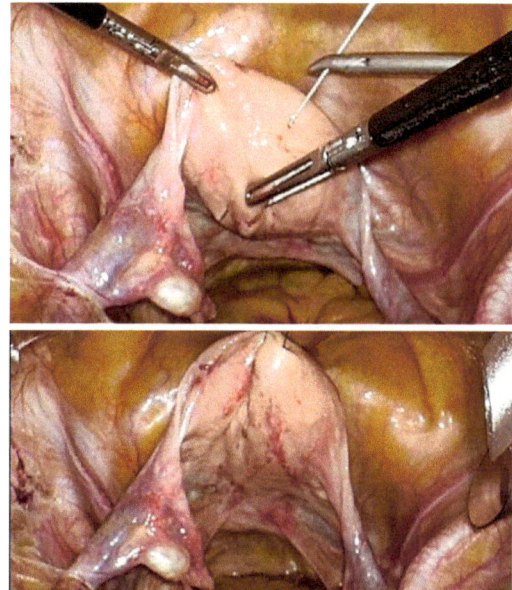

Fig. 7 (*Above*) A cotton tape is tied around the upper rectum. (*Below*) The knot is grasped by the surgical assistant for retraction and manipulation of the rectum

Fig. 8 (*Above*) A straight needle is passed from the skin through the fundus of the uterus. (*Below*) The uterus is hitched to the anterior abdominal wall to provide better access to the deep pelvis

Perineal Phase Essential Steps

1. Extra-sphincteric incision
2. Entry into abdominal cavity via anococcygeal ligament
3. Division of lateral levator attachments
4. Exteriorization of proximal end of the specimen
5. Division of the anterior attachments (to the prostate/vagina)
6. Wound closure (with mesh or flap reconstruction if necessary)

Perineal Phase Technique

A 2018 meta-analysis of 1663 patients found that the prone approach for APR is associated with decreased blood loss and operative time, with no differences in the incidence of postoperative wound infection or intraoperative rectal perforation (IOP). Positioning also did not affect circumferential resection margin (CRM) positivity or local recurrence rates [28]. We favor a prone position for APR for anteriorly based tumors for the superior visualization of the anterior plane between the tumor and the prostate or vagina. For cases in which the dissection is potentially difficult due to anatomical constraints, bulky tumors, or previous radiation, the lithotomy position allows a combined abdominal and perineal approach which may be useful to establish an accurate plane of dissection, although pneumoperitoneum will be lost once the abdominal cavity is entered from below.

The objective of the perineal phase of an APR for low rectal cancer is to excise the anal canal with a wide margin. The initial elliptical incision is deepened past the ischiorectal fat circumferentially until the levator muscles are encountered. The optimal location for entry into the abdominal cavity is through the anococcygeal ligament posteriorly (Fig. 9). The coccyx can be excised to facilitate entry or a margin-negative resection [4]. The St. Marks perineal retractor or the Lone Star retractor may also be used during the perineal phase of surgery.

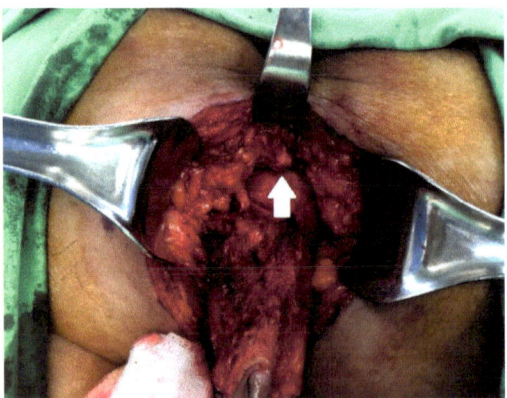

Fig. 9 Traction on the anus with the arrow showing the position of the coccyx

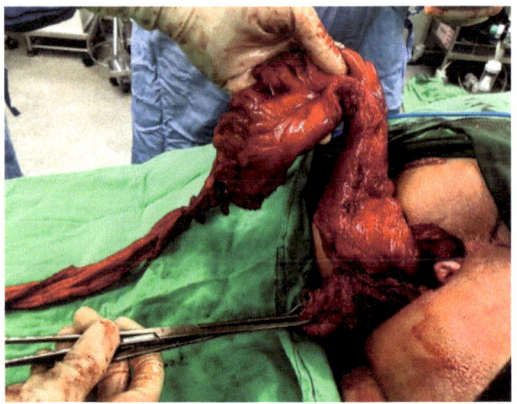

Fig. 10 Traction on the mobilized anus and exteriorization of the proximal end of the specimen

In a conventional APR (CAPR), the lateral attachments of the levators to the distal rectum/upper anal sphincter are divided close to the bowel. This type of dissection frequently produces a "waisted" specimen where the abdominal and perineal dissections meet. This was reported to increase the rate of IOP, CRM positivity, and local recurrence. The extralevator abdominoperineal excision (ELAPE) approach, described by Holm et al. in 2007 [29], produces a more "cylindrical" specimen by avoidance of dissection of the mesorectum off the levators during the abdominal phase and complete (wide) excision of the levators during a prone perineal phase. A recent meta-analysis shows that ELAPE reduces IOP and local recurrence rates, without increasing perineal wound complication rates, when compared with CAPR [30]. The RELAPe randomized trial also showed no difference in complications with ELAPE, and in addition found a statistically significant reduction in CRM positivity rates, compared to non-ELAPE [31]. We recommend the extralevator approach for locally advanced tumors involving the levators or external sphincters and tumors with a threatened CRM following NACRT.

Following division of the posterior and lateral attachments, the proximal end of the specimen can be exteriorized (Fig. 10). A method to facilitate the proximal exteriorization is to

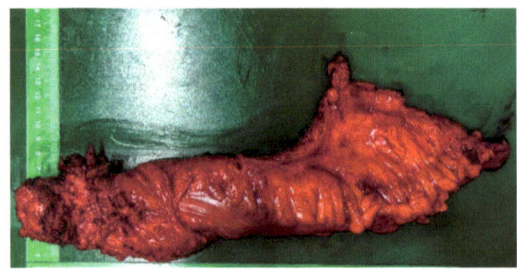

Fig. 11 APR specimen

suture a gauze to the staple line during the abdominal phase; the gauze is then inserted into the presacral space and can be easily identified upon entry into the abdominal cavity during the perineal phase. With the proximal and distal ends of the bowel already mobilized, the specimen can be dissected off the prostate or vagina anteriorly. The ideal APR specimen should have an intact mesorectum without "waisting" (Fig. 11). The wound is cleansed thoroughly before the transabdominal drain is located and appropriately positioned within the pelvis prior to closure (Fig. 12).

The perineal wound can be closed primarily or using a mesh or flap. If a mesh is used, the edges are sutured to the insertions of the excised levator muscles to close the tissue defect at the level of the pelvic floor, providing support and theoretically reducing the risk of perineal herniation.

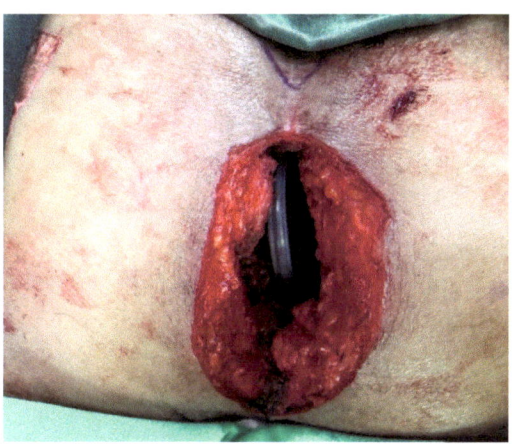

Fig. 12 The perineal wound is closed over the drain in the pelvis

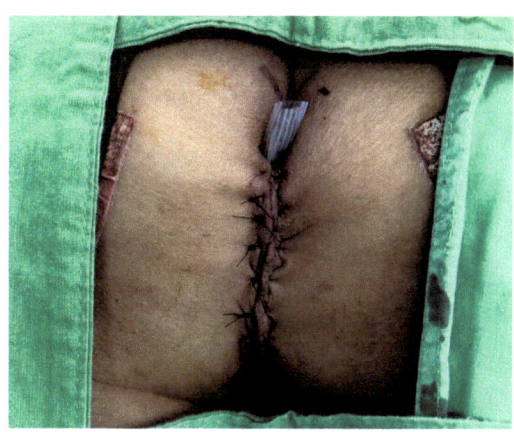

Fig. 13 Closure of the perineal wound using interrupted mattress suture and a subcutaneous drain

Biologic mesh is preferred over synthetic due to reduced adhesions with small bowel, as well as the better infection risk profile in a contaminated field.

The 2017 Association of Coloproctology of Great Britain and Ireland (ACPGBI) Position Statement on the closure of the perineal defect after APR for rectal cancer makes the following relevant recommendations/findings [32]:

- Primary closure of the perineum can be used following CAPR (strong recommendation)
- Mesh closure has rarely been used for perineal wound closure following CAPR (moderate quality evidence)
- When concerns regarding perineal wound healing exists, myocutaneous flap closure may be considered as an alternative method (weak recommendation)
- Primary perineal wound closure following ELAPE has been reported and appears to be feasible (weak evidence)
- Biologic mesh has been used to reconstruct the perineal defect after ELAPE (moderate quality evidence)
- Perineal wound complications are significantly increased when neoadjuvant radiotherapy is delivered, regardless of whether CAPR or ELAPE is performed (moderate quality evidence)
- There is insufficient evidence to recommend one particular method of perineal closure over another following neoadjuvant radiotherapy
- There is insufficient evidence to support a particular method of perineal wound closure following laparoscopic approach to APR

In a CAPR, the remnant levator muscles should be used to reconstruct the perineal defect. The subcutaneous tissue is then approximated in multiple layers. A subcutaneous drain may reduce the risk of infection (Fig. 13).

Complications and Management

During deep pelvic surgery, injury to the ureters, prostate, seminal vesicles, vagina, autonomic nerves, sacral venous plexus, and internal iliac vessels can occur. Membranous urethral injury is a risk during the anterior portion of the perineal dissection; this risk can be possibly reduced with prone positioning and exteriorization of the proximal end of the specimen after distal, posterior, and lateral mobilization as previously described.

While current evidence is inconclusive, ELAPE surgery is theoretically at higher risk for perineal wound complications due to the larger perineal defect and lack of muscle closure. A 2014 meta-analysis of 32 studies reported that the pooled percentage of perineal wound complications in patients who did not undergo neoadjuvant radiotherapy was 15.3% after CAPR versus 14.8% after ELAPE. After neoadjuvant radiotherapy, perineal wound problems occurred in 30.2% of CAPR versus 37.6% following ELAPE [33]. Data from the 2015 English Low Rectal Cancer Abdominoperineal Excision (LOREC APE) registry recorded overall perineal complications in 21% of patients, with the majority being infective [34]. Infective complications include cellulitis, abscess formation, wound dehiscence, and chronic sinus formation. Avoiding fecal contamination, meticulous hemostasis, and closed-suction drainage of the pelvis can reduce infective complications.

Perineal herniation, defined as a palpable perineal bulge on standing or straining, is a possible complication following APR. Following primary wound closure, the pooled incidence of perineal hernias was 1.8% and 2.0% after CAPR and ELAPE, respectively [33]. Surprisingly, perineal hernias after biological mesh closure following ELAPE had a meta-analysis pooled incidence of 8.2%, which the authors suggested may be a result of a learning curve issue or a longer follow-up period for mesh studies [33]. Omentoplasty is the transposition of a pedicled omental flap, which can be used to fill the presacral space or sutured to the pelvic inlet during the abdominal phase. There is some evidence showing that omentoplasty, in conjunction with primary closure or a biological mesh, may reduce wound-related complications and herniation, by occupying the pelvic dead space rather than fluid or small bowel [35]. This technique is limited by the amount of omentum available. Repair of a perineal hernia may be difficult and generally involves the use of a combined abdominal and perineal approach with mesh or flap reconstruction of the pelvic floor.

Postoperative Care

The postoperative management of APR patients follows that of colorectal enhanced recovery protocols. In our experience, no particular posture is necessary to facilitate healing but the patient is advised to avoid squatting for 3 weeks as this position may increase tension on the perineal wound closure. The perineal wound must be examined for possible complications prior to discharge.

References

1. Miles WE. A method of performing Abdominoperineal excision for carcinoma of the rectum and of the terminal portion of the pelvic colon (1908). CA Cancer J Clin. 1971;21(6):361–4.
2. Miles WE. The radical abdomino-perineal operation for cancer of the rectum and of the pelvic colon. Br Med J. 1910;11:941–3.
3. Campos FG, Habr-Gama A, Nahas SC, Perez RO. Abdominoperineal excision: evolution of a centenary operation. Dis Colon Rectum. 2012;55(8):844–53.
4. Hawkins AT, Albutt K, Wise PE, Alavi K, Sudan R, Kaiser AM, Liliana BL. Continuing education committee of the SSAT abdominoperineal resection for rectal cancer in the twenty-first century: indications, techniques, and outcomes. J Gastrointest Surg. 2018;22(8):1477–87.
5. Dixon CF. Anterior resection for malignant lesions of the upper part of the rectum and lower part of the sigmoid. Ann Surg. 1948;128(3):425–42.
6. Rygick AN, Juchvidova GM, Rivkin VL, Gureeva CF, Militarev JM. Colo-rectal anastomosis with a suturing apparatus in resection of the rectum and colon. Gut. 1967;8(2):189–91.
7. Parks AG. Transanal technique in low rectal anastomosis. Proc R Soc Med. 1972;65(11):975–6.
8. Heald RJ, Husband EM, Ryall RD. The Mesorectum in Rectal Cancer Surgery–The Clue to Pelvic Recurrence? Br J Surg. 1982;69(10):613–6.
9. Minsky BD, Cohen AM, Kemeny N, Enker WE, Kelsen DP, Reichman B, Saltz L, Sigurdson ER, Frankel J. Enhancement of radiation-induced Downstaging of rectal cancer by fluorouracil and high-dose Leucovorin chemotherapy. J Clin Oncol. 1992;10(1):79–84.
10. Benson AB 3rd, Venook AP, Al-Hawary MM, et al. Rectal cancer, version 2.2018, NCCN clinical practice guidelines in oncology. J Natl Compr Cancer Netw. 2018;16:874–901.
11. Lawson EH, Melvin JC, Geltzeiler CB, Heise CP, Foley EF, King RS, Harms BA, Carchman EH. Advances in the Management of Rectal Cancer. Curr Probl Surg. 2019;56(11):100648.
12. Ludmir EB, Palta M, Willett CG, Czito BG. Total neoadjuvant therapy for rectal cancer: an emerging option. Cancer. 2017;123(9):1497–506.
13. Habr-Gama A, Perez RO, Nadalin W, Sabbaga J, Ribeiro U Jr, Silva e Sousa AH Jr, Campos FG, Kiss DR, Gama-Rodrigues J. Operative versus nonopera-

tive treatment for stage 0 distal rectal cancer following Chemoradiation therapy: long-term results. Ann Surg. 2004;240(4):711–7. discussion 717-8.

14. Perez RO, Habr-Gama A. Putting down the scalpel in rectal cancer management–a historical perspective. Color Dis. 2018;20(Suppl 1):12–5.

15. Dattani M, Heald RJ, Goussous G, Broadhurst J, São Julião GP, Habr-Gama A, Perez RO, Moran BJ. Oncological and survival outcomes in watch and wait patients with a clinical complete response after neoadjuvant Chemoradiotherapy for rectal cancer: a systematic review and pooled analysis. Ann Surg. 2018;268(6):955–67.

16. Zhang X, Qingbin W, Tao H, Chaoyang G, Bi L, Wang Z. Laparoscopic versus conventional open abdominoperineal resection for rectal cancer: an updated systematic review and meta-analysis. J Laparoendosc Adv Surg Tech A. 2018;28(5):526–39.

17. Simillis C, Lal N, Thoukididou SN, Kontovounisios C, Smith JJ, Hompes R, Adamina M, Tekkis PP. Open versus laparoscopic versus robotic versus Transanal Mesorectal excision for rectal cancer: a systematic review and network meta-analysis. Ann Surg. 2019;270(1):59–68.

18. den Dulk M, Putter H, Collette L, Marijnen CAM, Folkesson J, Bosset JF, Rödel C, Bujko K, Påhlman L, van de Velde CJH. The abdominoperineal resection itself is associated with an adverse outcome: the European experience based on a pooled analysis of five European randomised clinical trials on rectal cancer. Eur J Cancer. 2009;45(7):1175–83.

19. Russell MM, Ganz PA, Lopa S, Yothers G, Ko CY, Arora A, Atkins JN, Bahary N, Soori GS, Robertson JM, Eakle J, Marchello BT, Wozniak TF, Beart RW Jr, Wolmark N. Comparative effectiveness of sphincter-sparing surgery versus abdominoperineal resection in rectal cancer: patient-reported outcomes in National Surgical Adjuvant Breast and bowel project randomized trial R-04. Ann Surg. 2015;261(1):144–8.

20. Glynne-Jones R, Wyrwicz L, Tiret E, Brown G, Rödel C, Cervantes A, Arnold D. ESMO guidelines committee rectal cancer: ESMO clinical practice guidelines for diagnosis, treatment and follow-up. Ann Oncol. 2017;28(suppl_4):iv22–40.

21. Patel UB, Taylor F, Blomqvist L, George C, Evans H, Tekkis P, Quirke P, Sebag-Montefiore D, Moran B, Heald R, Guthrie A, Bees N, Swift I, Pennert K, Brown G. Magnetic resonance imaging-detected tumor response for locally advanced rectal cancer predicts survival outcomes: MERCURY experience. J Clin Oncol. 2011;29(28):3753–60.

22. Bujko K, Rutkowski A, Chang GJ, Michalski W, Chmielik E, Kusnierz J. Is the 1-cm rule of distal bowel resection margin in rectal cancer based on clinical evidence? a systematic review. Ann Surg Oncol. 2012;19(3):801–8.

23. Park JS, Park SY, Kim HJ, Cho SH, Kwak SG, Choi GS. Long-term oncologic outcomes after neoadjuvant Chemoradiation followed by Intersphincteric resection with Coloanal anastomosis for locally advanced low rectal cancer. Dis Colon Rectum. 2019;62(4):408–16.

24. Loos M, Quentmeier P, Schuster T, Nitsche U, Gertler R, Keerl A, Kocher T, Friess H, Rosenberg R. Effect of preoperative radio(chemo)therapy on long-term functional outcome in rectal cancer patients: a systematic review and meta-analysis. Ann Surg Oncol. 2013;20(6):1816–28.

25. Chen TYT, Wiltink LM, Nout RA, Kranenbarg EMK, Laurberg S, Marijnen CAM, van de Velde CJH. Bowel function 14 years after preoperative short-course radiotherapy and Total Mesorectal excision for rectal cancer: report of a multicenter randomized trial. Clin Colorectal Cancer. 2015;14(2):106–14.

26. Croese AD, Lonie JM, Trollope AF, Vangaveti VN, Ho YH. A meta-analysis of the prevalence of low anterior resection syndrome and systematic review of risk factors. Int J Surg. 2018;56:234–41.

27. Pieniowski EHA, Palmer GJ, Juul T, Lagergren P, Johar A, Emmertsen KJ, Nordenvall C, Abraham-Nordling M. Low anterior resection syndrome and quality of life after sphincter-sparing rectal cancer surgery: a long-term longitudinal follow-up. Dis Colon Rectum. 2019;62(1):14–20.

28. Mesquita-Neto JWB, Mouzaihem H, Macedo FIB, Heilbrun LK, Weaver DW, Kim S. Perioperative and oncological outcomes of abdominoperineal resection in the prone position vs the classic lithotomy position: a systematic review with meta-analysis. J Surg Oncol. 2019;119(7):979–86.

29. Holm T, Ljung A, Häggmark T, Jurell G, Lagergren J. Extended abdominoperineal resection with gluteus Maximus flap reconstruction of the pelvic floor for rectal cancer. Br J Surg. 2007;94(2):232–8.

30. Qi XY, Cui M, Liu MX, Xu K, Tan F, Yao ZD, Zhang N, Yang H, Zhang CH, Xing JD, Su XQ. Extralevator abdominoperineal excision versus abdominoperineal excision for low rectal cancer: a meta-analysis. Chin Med J. 2019;132(20):2446–56.

31. Bianco F, Romano G, Tsarkov P, Stanojevic G, Shroyer K, Giuratrabocchetta S, Bergamaschi R. International rectal cancer study group Extralevator with vs Nonextralevator abdominoperineal excision for rectal cancer: the RELAPe randomized controlled trial. Color Dis. 2017;19(2):148–57.

32. Foster DJ, Tou S, Curtis NJ, Smart NJ, Acheson A, Maxwell-Armstrong C, Watts A, Singh B, Francis NK. Closure of the perineal defect after abdominoperineal excision for rectal adenocarcinoma–ACPGBI position statement. Color Dis. 2018;20(Suppl 5):5–23.

33. Musters GD, Buskens CJ, Bemelman WA, Tanis PJ. Perineal wound healing after abdominoperineal resection for rectal cancer: a systematic review and meta-analysis. Dis Colon Rectum. 2014;57(9):1129–39.

34. Jones H, Moran B, Crane S, Hompes R, Cunningham C. LOREC group the LOREC APE registry: operative technique, oncological outcome and perineal wound healing after abdominoperineal excision. Color Dis. 2017;19(2):172–80.

35. Butt HZ, Salem MK, Vijaynagar B, Chaudhri S, Singh B. Perineal reconstruction after extra-Levator abdominoperineal excision (eLAPE): a systematic review. Int J Color Dis. 2013;28(11):1459–68.

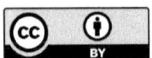

Laparoscopic Total Colectomy

Mina Ming Yin Shen and William Tzu-Liang Chen

Introduction

Total colectomy (TC) with ileorectal (IRA) is frequently performed for colorectal cancer, familial adenomatous polyposis, unidentified bleeding from the lower GI tract, inflammatory bowel disease, and sometimes for extended diverticulosis or colonic inertia. Minimally invasive approaches to total colectomy have significantly lower morbidity compared to open approach, with significantly shorter hospitalization length [1].

Contraindications

The most common relative contraindications to laparoscopic procedures are preoperative abdomens caused by adhesion formation, coagulopathy, cirrhosis, aberrant anatomy, small bowel obstruction, disseminated abdominal cancer, pulmonary compliance and cardiovascular issues, and intracranial disease. Certainly, hemodynamical instability or cardiopulmonary disease that is severe enough to make peritoneal insufflation and Trendelenburg positioning dangerous represent a physiologic derangement that precludes the safe application of laparoscopy. Phlegmonous

tissue which is usually encountered in severe, complicated Crohn's disease or in diverticulitis may not also be resectable via laparoscopy due to the tissue friability, bleeding, and distorted anatomy that necessitates open exposure. There are no common criteria to apply laparoscopic technique for combined resection for T4 colon cancer. Tumor invasion into other organs is not an absolute contraindication if en bloc resection could be achieved. However, laparotomic conversion is necessary if oncologically curative resection is not achieved laparoscopically. Significant intraoperative hemorrhage, in the presence of visceral lesion, incorrect dissection, all conditions that may affect the outcome, are contraindications of laparoscopy and the conversion is necessary.

Preoperative Assessment

All patients undergoing colonic surgery should have the same preoperative workup including anesthetic workup regardless of the surgical approaches. All patients should have a complete history and physical examination. Adjunct testing such as blood test, additional imaging (CT scan, MRI), or cardiopulmonary testing is performed when indicated. The only special consideration for laparoscopic surgery is ensuring that the surgeon can identify the site of pathology at the time of operative intervention. The loss of tactile sensation in laparoscopic surgery stresses the impor-

M. M. Y. Shen · W. T.-L. Chen (✉)
Division of Colorectal Surgery, Department of Surgery, China Medical University Hsinchu Hospital, Zhubei City, Hsinchu County, Taiwan
e-mail: wtchen@mail.cmuh.org.tw

© The Author(s) 2023
D. Lomanto et al. (eds.), *Mastering Endo-Laparoscopic and Thoracoscopic Surgery*,
https://doi.org/10.1007/978-981-19-3755-2_73

537

tance of localizing techniques, especially for small lesions. These can be evaluated preoperatively by colonoscopy and tattooing of the lesion can be performed during the colonoscopy 1–2 days prior to the surgery especially for early colonic cancer which ensures the oncological safe margins. It is helpful to have flexible colonoscopy in the operating room as it may be needed intraoperatively to identify lesions if the location of the lesion remains doubtful. All elective colonic resections should follow ERAS preoperative protocol. The protocols include perioperative opioid-sparing analgesia, avoidance of nasogastric tubes and peritoneal drains, aggressive management of postoperative nausea and vomiting, and early oral feedings and ambulation. Mechanical oral bowel preparation is not needed for elective laparoscopic TC. A urinary catheter is placed at the beginning of the procedure and is removed on the first morning after the operation. Prophylaxis antibiotic and deep vein thrombosis (DVT) prophylaxis should be included.

OT Setup (Fig. 1a–c)

Authors routinely placed patients in lithotomy position with both arms tucked and the thighs positioned using stirrups at no more than a 10° angle to the torso. Lithotomy allows simultaneous access to abdomen and perineum for ileorectal anastomosis when using the circular stapler, as well as for an intraoperative colonoscopy. It also provides additional space for a second assistant and an additional position for the operating surgeon when performing D3 dissection at the superior mesenteric artery (SMA) and superior mesenteric vein (SMV) root. The patient should be fixed securely on the table because the patient's position could be changed during the operation. A beanbag is used to secure the patient to the table, along with reinforcement by adhesive tapes wrapping the patient's chest to the table. The patient's position can be adjusted intraoperatively at the stage of splenic flexure, hepatic flexure, or rectal

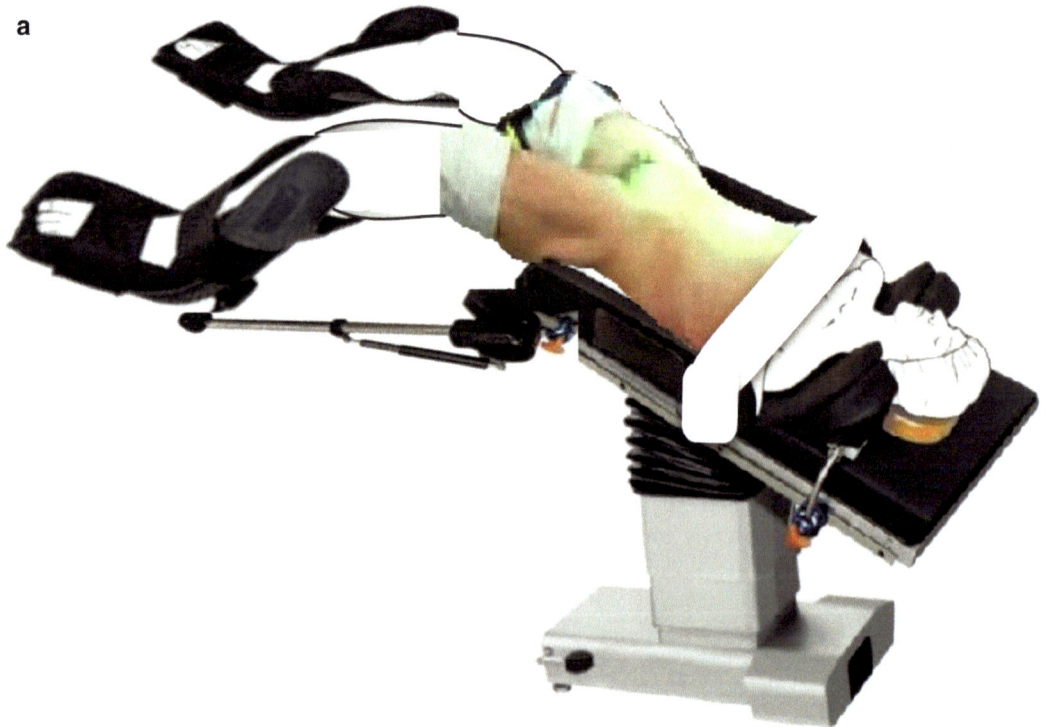

Fig. 1 (**a**) Patient positioning in Trendelenberg position (**b**) Surgeon and assistants standing position during approach of left side colon (**c**) Surgeon and assistants standing position during approach of right side colon

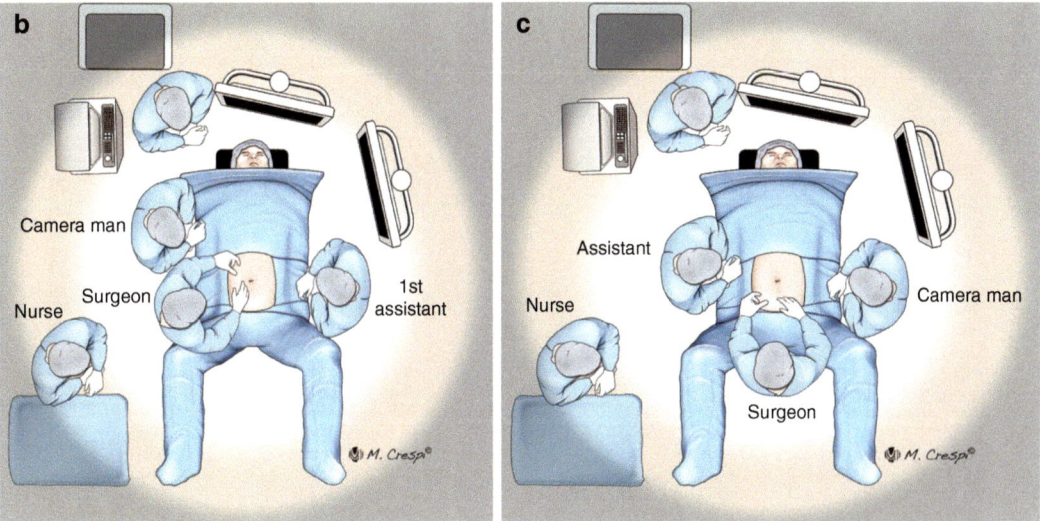

Fig. 1 (continued)

mobilization. The procedure is usually performed with one or two assistants. During the procedure of central vascular ligation (CVL) from SMA and SMV, the surgeon may stand in between the patient's legs. When mobilizing from splenic flexure to rectum, the surgeon will stand on the patient's right while the camera assistant on the surgeon's right. The monopolar device with hook, spatula, or scissor or energy-based devices are adapted for the plane dissection, depending on the surgeon's preference. The adaptation of energy-based devices in laparoscopic colon cancer surgery could reduce chyle leakage, minimize bleeding on dissection planes, and facilitate complete plane dissection.

Surgical Techniques

Port Placements (Fig. 2)

Five trocars are placed. By open technique, Camera port is inserted infra or supra umbilically using balloon trocar. Pneumoperitoneum 12–15 mmHg is created and abdomen is inspected for findings. Two 12 mm ports are placed in the right lower quadrant and 2 cm superior to the pubic symphysis at the midline. A 5 mm port is placed in the right hypochondrium and a second 5 mm port is placed over left-sided abdomen.

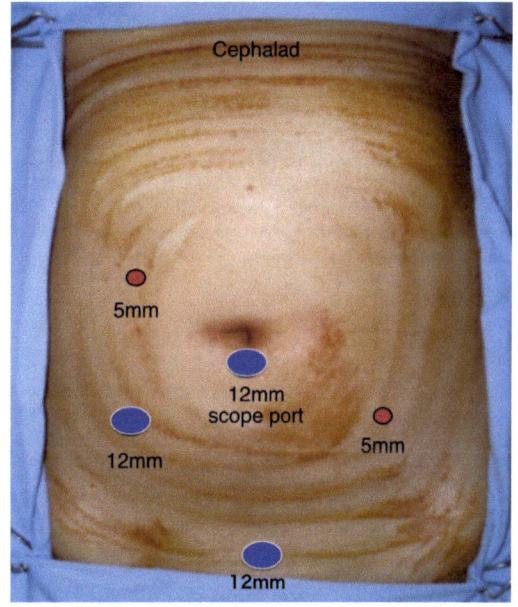

Fig. 2 Port placement for TC

Operatives Details

Approach of Right Side Colon

Colon Mobilization (Fig. 3a–d)
Once the patient is positioned in a Trendelenburg position with the left side down, the omentum, small bowel, and transverse colon are swept in a cephalad direction. The terminal ileum is lifted

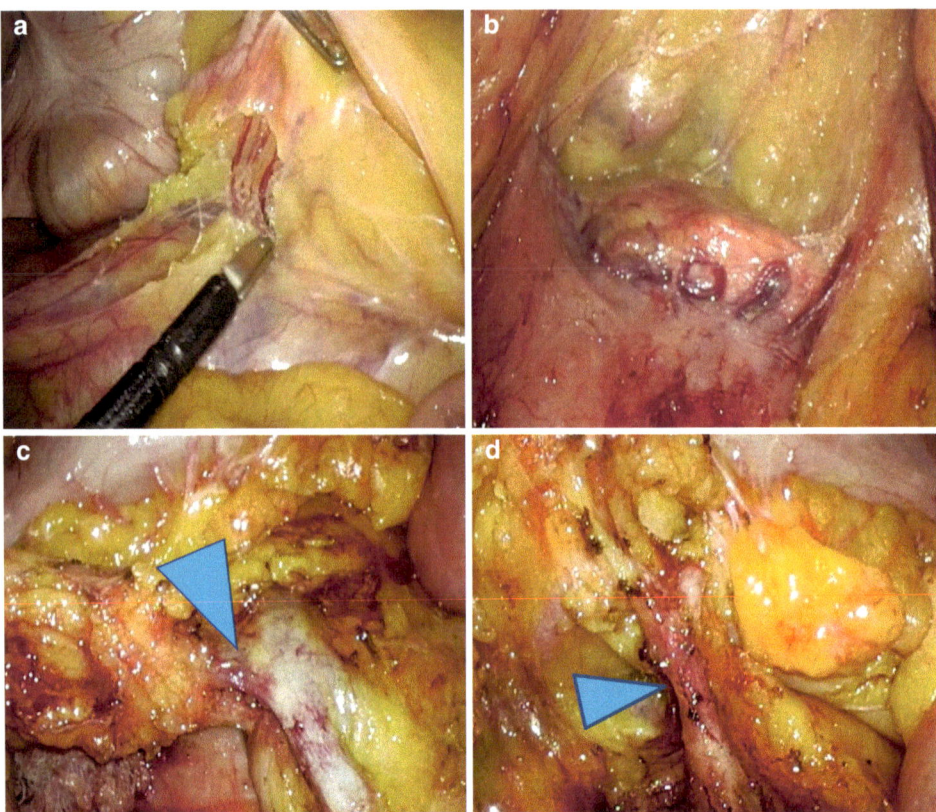

Fig. 3 (**a**) Tenting the terminal ileum mesentery and mobilization of the retroperitoneum using monopolar cautery (**b**) At the medial extent of mobilization, the duode-num and pancreatic head are exposed (**c**) Ileocolic artery and vein (arrowed) take-off from SM pedicle (**d**) Middle colic artery (arrowed) branching off from SMA

anteriorly toward the abdominal wall (refer to Fig. 3a), exposing the cleavage plane between ileal mesentery and retroperitoneum. Peritoneum overlying this plane is scored with either monopolar diathermy or an advanced energy device. As dissection proceeds along Toldt's fascia, the ileal mesentery and posterior aspect of the right colon are mobilized off the retroperitoneum. The authors routinely leave the lateral attachments of the colon untouched, as this helps to provide additional counter traction.

During dissection in the superior direction, it is important to look out for the duodenum and subsequently dissect anterior to it. In the author's practice, the medial extent of dissection is reached when the duodenum and pancreatic head are exposed (refer to Fig. 3b). Further mobilization is performed in toward the direction of Morrisons' pouch until the dissection plane is separated from Morrisons' pouch by a layer of peritoneum. A gauze is placed at the dissected area to demarcate the dissected plane.

CVL

Prior to commencing the CVL, the mesentery of the ascending and transverse colon is spread out to visualize the location of the ileocolic (IC), middle colic (MC), and superior mesenteric (SM) pedicles. The peritoneum overlying the pedicles is scored. Next, the terminal ileum is located and the proximal transection point is decided. Using an energy device, a mesenteric window is created adjacent to the proximal transection point. A laparoscopic stapler is introduced through this window to transect the ileum. The ileal mesentery is divided using an energy device in the direction of the SMA pedicle.

At the junction of the IC and SM pedicles, fine dissection is performed to skeletonize the vessels and demonstrate the take-off of the IC from the SM vessels (refer to Fig. 3c, d). Failure to demonstrate this could lead to inadvertent ligation of the SM vessels, resulting in excessive small bowel ischemia. In the event that initial vessel identification is in question, it is advised that dissection continues along the SM pedicle in the cephalad direction; dissected vessels subsequently arising from the SM pedicle will provide more information on vascular anatomy.

After ligation of the IC pedicle, the next vessel to be ligated is the right colic artery should it be present. Approximate location of the middle colic (MC) pedicle can be located via inspection of the transverse colonic mesentery. The main MC vessels are dissected free and ligated. The gastrocolic trunk is usually identified and preserved.

Approach of Left Side Colon

Vascular Pedicle Isolation and Ligation
(Fig. 4a–e)

Patient is tilted head down 15° (Trendelenberg) and right side down for gravitational drag of

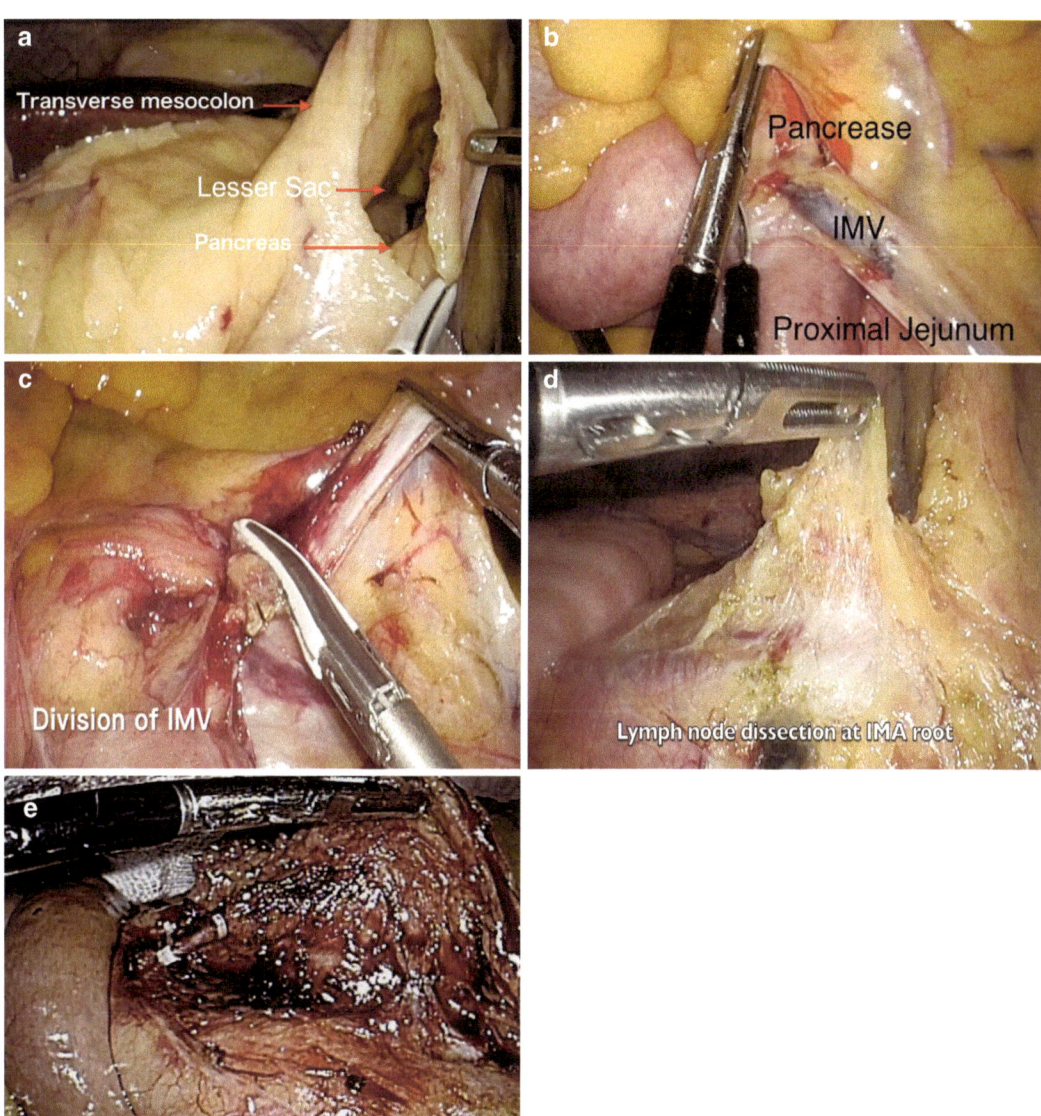

Fig. 4 (**a**) Incision of transverse mesocolon at the level below lt-MCA to enter the lesser sac (**b**) The Treitz ligament is dissected with maximum care not to damage the jejunum (**c**) The IMV is divided at the level close to the inferior border of the pancreas (**d**) D3 lymph node dissection at the IMA root (**e**) IMA is divided near the origin from abdominal aorta

small bowel to the right and omentum and transverse colon slightly to cephalad. Omentum is swept cephalad direction and transverse mesocolon is lifted up to expose the cleavage plane of the pancreas. Incision of transverse mesocolon at the level below lt-MCA either by monopolar diathermy or energy device to enter the lesser sac (Fig. 4a). The Treitz ligament is dissected with maximum care not to damage the jejunum (Fig. 4b). The peritoneal layer medial to the inferior Mesenteric Vein (IMV) is incised paralleled to the vessel. The IMV is easily visualized, or in case of more obese patients, search for, right below the inferior of the margin of the pancreas. The IMV is dissected free and then divided at the level close to the inferior border of the pancreas (Fig. 4c).

The medial-to-lateral (MTL) approach to the left mesocolon easily brings the inferior mesenteric artery (IMA) into view. The root of sigmoid mesentery is retracted up to create tension on the peritoneum which is then incised using monopolar diathermy from caudal to cephalad position starting from the sacral promontory. Pneumodissection might help to open up further the embryological plane. The mesentery of the sigmoid can be retracted away from the retroperitoneum by performing a blunt and bloodless dissection using a monopolar or advanced energy device. Proper Medial-To-Lateral (MTL) dissection will not expose the left ureter, left gonadal vessel, and psoas muscle, which are left undisturbed retroperitoneally. The retracting instrument can be inserted into the plane between the mesentery and the retroperitoneum, lifting the mesentery toward the anterior abdominal wall without grasping and tearing tissue. Dissection carried on cephalad till the root of IMA with careful identification and preservation of hypogastric nerves, which control urinary and sexual function. With D3 lymph node dissection at the IMA root (Fig. 4d), the IMA is divided near the origin from abdominal aorta (Fig. 4e).

Splenic Flexure Mobilization (Fig. 5a, b)

The splenic flexure of colon is mobilized using medial-to-lateral approach. After the procedures of central vascular ligation, the lessor sac has been entered through the TM window and the mesentery root of left colon is incised. By insertion of retracting instrument and tenting of mesentery of both transverse and descending colon, the pancreatico-colonic ligament is divided using either monopolar diathermy or advanced energy devices (Fig. 5a). Lifting the IMV arch allows furthering MTL dissection by opening a window between the Toldt fascia anteriorly and the Gerotal fascia posteriorly (Fig. 5b). The border between the two fascias, which indicates the embryonic plane of coalescence of posterior mesocolon and retroperitoneum is whitish, a clear sign of correct dissection plane (Fig. 5b). A tough elevation of mesocolon anteriorly toward the abdominal wall facilitates the dissection as far as the pericolic gutter, and downward to the level of the sacral promontory.

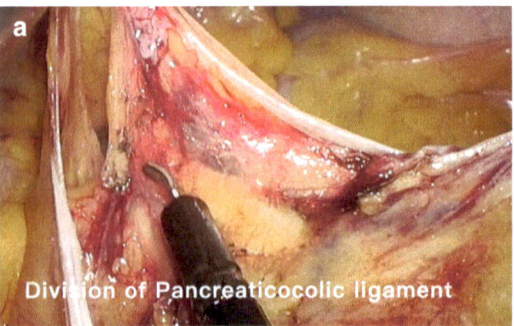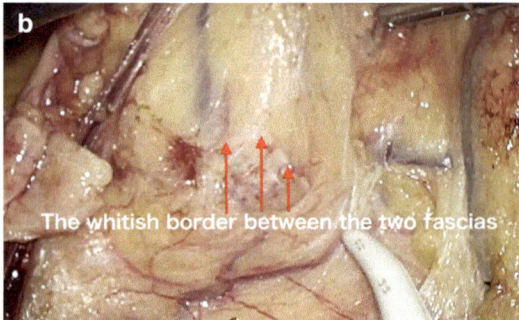

Fig. 5 (**a**) The pancreatico-colonic ligament is divided (**b**) Dissection between the Toldt fascia anteriorly and the Gerotal fascia posteriorly

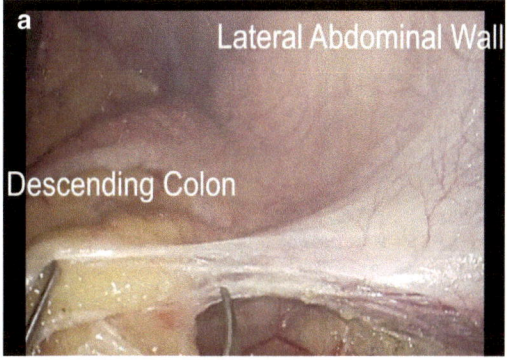 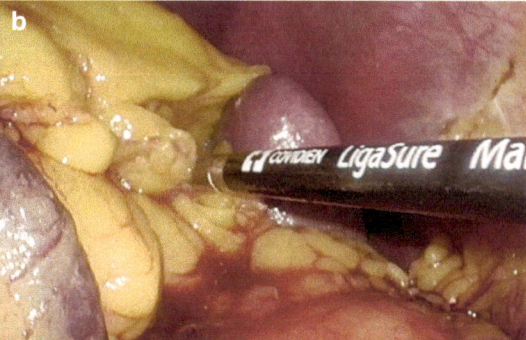

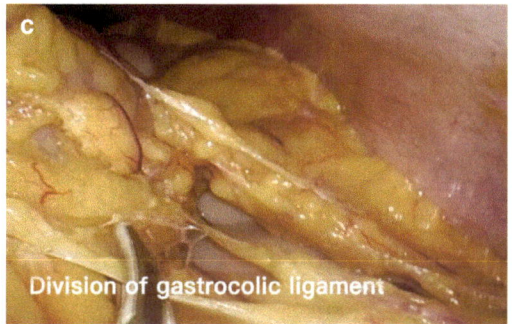

Fig. 6 (**a**) Gently retract the descending colon medially, the Toldt's fascia is divided (**b**) Division of the spleno-colic ligament (**c**) Division of the gastrocolic ligament

Mobilization of Colon (Fig. 6a–c)

If the medial approach was done adequately, colon (descending and sigmoid) can be easily mobilized from the Toldt's fascia. Gently retract the descending colon medially, this thin Toldt's fascia is scored and divided using monopolar diathermy and advanced energy devices (Fig. 6a). The splenic flexure proper can then be dissected down by dividing the spleno-colic ligament (Fig. 6b). The greater omentum is separated from the gastric curvature. The gastrocolic ligament is also divided (Fig. 6c). The sigmoid, descending colon, and transverse colon are fully mobilized.

Construction of Anastomosis and Specimen Extraction (Fig. 7a–c)

Following this, the entire colon and the terminal ileum are mobilized and freed. The initial dissection plane at the level of the upper rectum is identified, at the level of the promontory where the posterior mesorectal plane is identified and the initial "holy plane" is dissected using monopolar scissors. Once the distal extent of resection is

identified, the rectal wall is dissected circumferentially. Transanal distal rectal washout is introduced, and then the section of the distal margin is performed with laparoscopic linear staplers. A suprapubic Pfannenstiel mini-laparotomy without muscles division is carried out and, after placing a wound protector, the specimen is retrieved. The terminal ileum is exteriorized and the staple line is resected. The anvil of a circular stapler is inserted through the end of the ileum, and perforates the anti-mesenteric border, leaving 5 cm of the terminal ileum distal to the anastomosis. The rod of anvil is fixed to the ileum bowel wall by a purse-string suture (Fig. 7a). The end of the ileum is closed using a mechanical stapler or manual suture. Then the bowel is placed back into the abdomen and pneumoperitoneum is reestablished. The correct position of the ileum is checked to eliminate any eventual twisting of the mesentery (Fig. 7b). The circular stapler is introduced through the anus and assembled with its head to perform side-to-end ileorectal anastomosis at the level of the promontory under laparo-

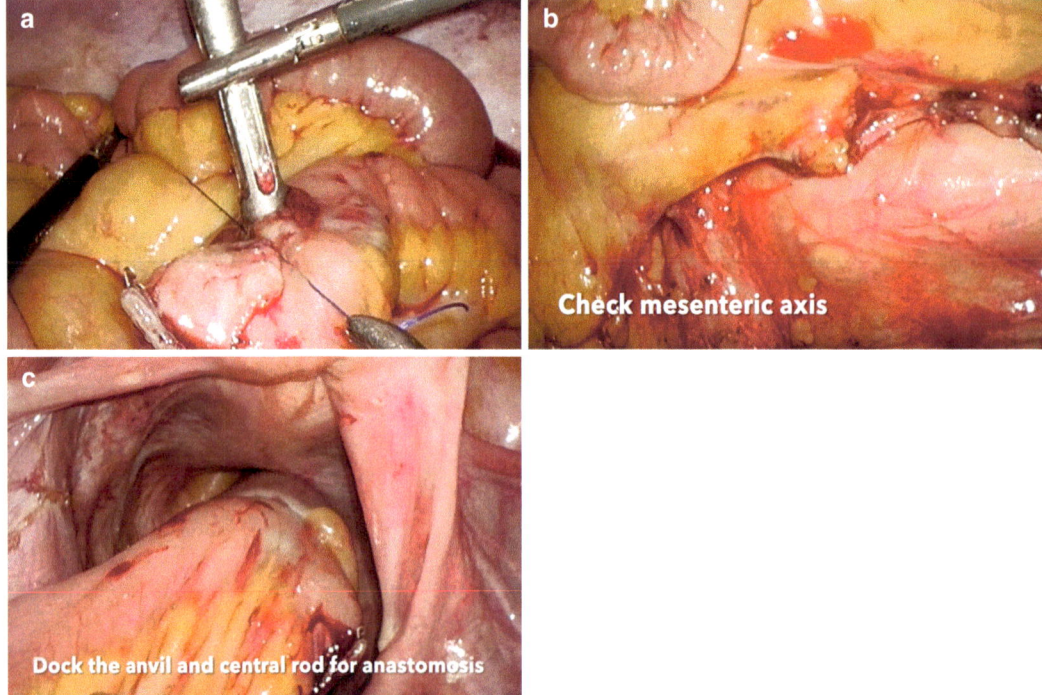

Fig. 7 (**a**) The rod of anvil is fixed to the ileum bowel wall by a purse-string suture (**b**) Check the correct position of the ileum (**c**) Side-to-end ileorectal anastomosis

scopic control (Fig. 7c). The donuts must be evaluated to ensure that they are complete. Intraoperative colonoscopy is performed to check the completeness of the anastomosis or anastomosis site bleeding. In some cases, a drain is placed for postoperative surveillance.

Reference

1. Moghadamyeghaneh Z, Hanna MH, Carmichael JC, Pigazzi A, Stamos MJ, Mills S. Comparison of open, laparoscopic, and robotic approaches for total abdominal colectomy. Surg Endosc. 2016;30(7):2792–8.

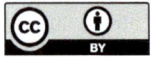

Laparoscopic Ventral Mesh Rectopexy

Isaac Seow-En, EmileTan Kwong-Wei,
and WilliamTzu-Liang Chen

Introduction

Rectal prolapse (RP) is a disabling condition and can range from internal rectal prolapse (IRP) or rectal intussusception to full-thickness external rectal prolapse (ERP). RP occurs in 0.5% of the general population, with a higher incidence in females and the elderly [1].Intellectual disability and psychiatric conditions are a risk factor for RP in younger patients. Patients with an IRP usually experience functional symptoms of obstructed defecation (OD) or fecal incontinence (FI), while patients with ERP suffer from pain, rectal bleeding, and FI [2].Two recent guidelines have been published on the management of rectal prolapse, the 2017 American guidelines [1] and the 2017 Dutch guidelines [2].The recommendations in this chapter are summarized from these sets of guidelines as well as additional up-to-date evidence.

The evaluation of a patient with suspected RP should include a thorough history and physical examination. Bowel symptom severity should be graded using validated questionnaires for constipation or fecal incontinence. Up to a third of patients with RP have concomitant symptoms of anterior compartment prolapse, including urinary incontinence and vaginal vault prolapse. Decreased anal sphincter tone is often present, and proctoscopy may show an anterior solitary rectal ulcer in 10–15% of cases. Straining in the squatting position may be required to induce ERP.

If the diagnosis of IRP is uncertain, fluoroscopic or MRI defecography should be performed. A transit marker study can be considered to assess symptoms of slow transit constipation, which is a relative contraindication to surgery. Anorectal function tests including manometry and anorectal physiology studies may be useful if IRP is suspected based on bowel symptoms, and results may alter management. In patients with OD, pelvic floor muscle dyssynergia is a contraindication to rectopexy. ERP is an absolute indication for surgery; therefore, imaging and anorectal function tests generally do not add any further value to management. Patients with various functional symptoms arising from multicompartment prolapse should be discussed in a multidisciplinary setting to achieve optimal decision-making. For selected patients, psychiatric evaluation may be necessary to exclude a psychosomatic origin of symptoms. Endoscopic colonic evaluation should be performed to rule out malignancy. Patients with functional symptoms from IRP must be considered for

I. Seow-En
Department of Colorectal Surgery, Singapore General Hospital, Singapore, Singapore

Division of Colorectal Surgery, China Medical University Hospital, Taichung, Taiwan

E. Kwong-Wei · W.-L. Chen (✉)
Division of Colorectal Surgery, Department of Surgery, China Medical University Hsinchu Hospital, Zhubei City, Hsinchu County, Taiwan
e-mail: wtchen@mail.cmuh.org.tw

conservative therapy, including lifestyle modification, pharmacological treatment, pelvic floor physiotherapy, and retrograde colonic irrigation, if available.

Choice of Surgery

Although associated symptoms can be alleviated with conservative management, RP cannot be corrected without surgery. Surgical intervention should be tailored to the patient's overall health status, concomitant pelvic organ prolapse, and history of previous procedures. A host of different techniques have been described in the literature, with two main approaches, perineal versus transabdominal. The choice between the two is usually determined by the surgeon's preference and experience as well as the patient's comorbidities and bowel function. The most performed perineal methods are the perineal rectosigmoidectomy (Altemeier procedure) and perineal mucosal sleeve resection with muscular plication (Delorme procedure). The most common transabdominal techniques are the anterior rectopexy with or without sigmoid resection, and the ventral mesh rectopexy.

Previous evidence reported that transabdominal approaches resulted in lower recurrence rates and better functional outcomes compared to a perineal approach [1]. However, a 2015 Cochrane review of 15 randomized trials involving 1007 patients was unable to demonstrate a significant difference in the recurrence rate between an abdominal or perineal technique [3]. A 2015 randomized trial comparing laparoscopic ventral mesh rectopexy versus the Delorme procedure similarly did not show a statistically significant difference in the incidence of recurrence or complication rates [4].

Open rectopexy is associated with higher postoperative morbidity compared to laparoscopic or perineal surgery. The well-documented advantages of minimally invasive surgery in the early postoperative period also make laparoscopy preferred over open rectopexy. Laparoscopic ventral mesh rectopexy (LVMR) was described by D'Hoore et al. in 2004; [5] this technique was

autonomic nerve-sparing, addressed the anterior lead point of an IRP, and corrected a concomitant rectocele, resulting in significant improvement in postoperative constipation and no incidence of de novo constipation.

A recent 2018 meta-analysis [4] of 17 studies (13 retrospective studies, three randomized trials, and one prospective cohort study) with 1242 patients undergoing LVMR for ERP showed a mean complication rate of 12.4%, with a mean ERP recurrence rate of 2.8% over a median follow-up duration of 23 months, and mean rates of improvement in fecal incontinence and constipation of 79.3% and 71%, respectively. Median operating time was about 120 min and conversion to open surgery was necessary in 1.8% of patients. Acceptable long-term outcomes have also been published; the 10 year recurrence rate following LVMR was 8.2% with a 4.6% mesh-related complication rate (1.3% vaginal mesh erosion) in 919 patients [6]. 76% of patients reported subjective functional symptom relief at a median follow-up time of 44 months from surgery [7].

In view of these findings, the LVMR has become the most popular laparoscopic technique for RP, particularly in Europe. The 2017 Dutch guidelines recommend the LVMR as the first-choice procedure for ERP as well as IRP with an indication for surgery [2]. Although resection rectopexy is thought by some to improve symptoms of constipation in patients with a redundant sigmoid colon, there is no evidence favoring it over LVMR and the risk of an anastomotic leak must be considered. The robotic-assisted LVMR is similar to LVMR in terms of functional outcome, complication, and recurrence rates, although it requires a longer operative time and increased costs [8, 9]. Further evidence is required to determine if the potential technical benefits of robotic surgery translate to better clinical outcomes.

OT Setup

Bowel preparation using 2 L polyethylene glycol is used. Below-knee compression stockings are applied and a urinary catheter is inserted. The patient is placed in the modified Lloyd-Davis

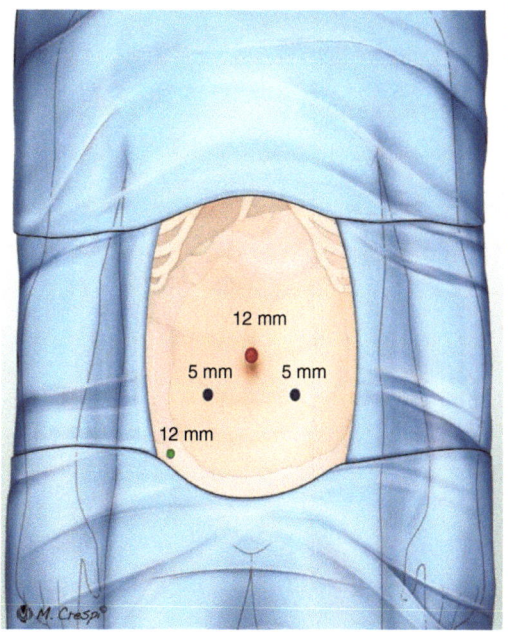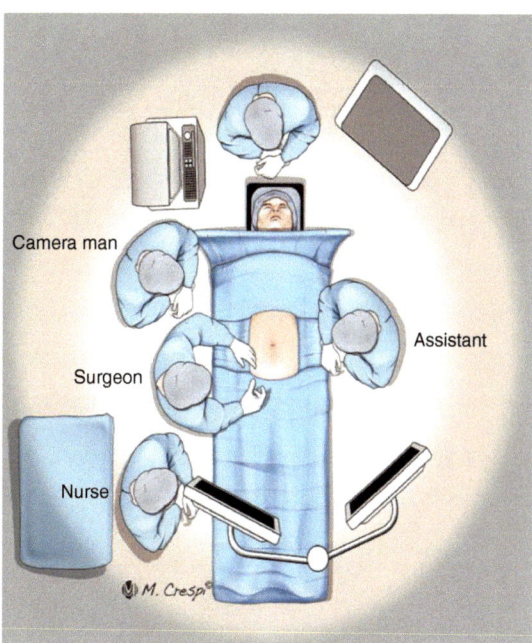

12 mm

5 mm   5 mm

12 mm

Camera man

Surgeon

Assistant

Nurse

Fig. 1 OT setup and port placement

position with the lower limbs in foot stirrups. Both arms are tucked in to facilitate positioning of the surgeon, camera operator, and assistant. A small sandbag (or folded drapes) is placed below the sacrum to elevate the pelvis approximately 4–5 cm anteriorly to enable better visualization of the deep pelvic structures during surgery. A single dose of prophylactic intravenous antibiotics is given at anesthetic induction. A schematic of the operating setup and port positioning is shown in Fig. 1. A 12 mm camera trocar is placed at the umbilicus. A 12 mm trocar is placed at the right iliac fossa and two 5 mm trocars are placed at the right and left flanks.

Surgical Technique

Essential steps and technique
1. Dissection
2. Mesh fixation
3. Vaginal fornix fixation
4. Neo-Douglas formation

We use the technique as described by D'Hoore for LVMR in 2006 [10]. With the patient in a

steep Trendelenburg position, the uterus is temporarily hitched to the anterior abdominal wall using a Prolene 2–0 straight needle passed through the uterus fundus or broad ligaments (Fig. 2). With the surgical assistant providing traction on the sigmoid out of the pelvis and to the left, the peritoneum is incised from the sacral promontory to the pouch of Douglas (Fig. 3). The rectum is not mobilized laterally or posteriorly, and the right hypogastric nerve is preserved, decreasing injury to the parasympathetic and sympathetic rectal innervation. The rectovaginal septum is carefully opened down to the pelvic floor, avoiding injury to the rectum (Fig. 4).

Choice of mesh is an important consideration. In D'Hoore's original description, a 3 × 17 cm polypropylene mesh was used [10]. A 2017 systematic review of eight studies from 2004 to 2015 compared 3517 patients using synthetic mesh and 439 patients using biological mesh for LVMR, with the rates of mesh-related erosion at 1.9% and 0.2%, respectively [11]. The largest series of biological mesh used with the longest follow-up was published in 2017 [12]. Of 224 patients who underwent LVMR using Permacol™ biological mesh, mesh-related morbidity was

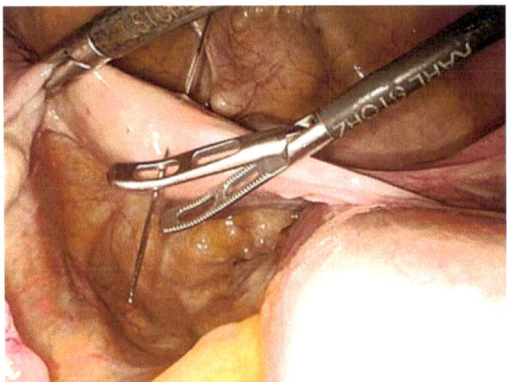

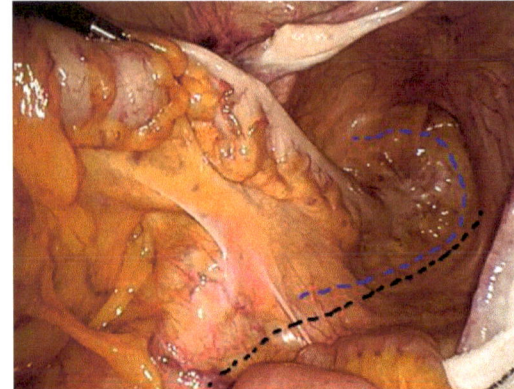

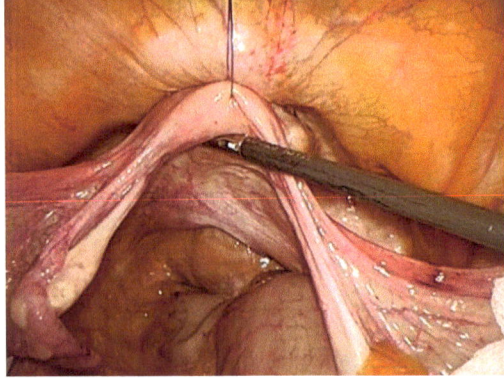

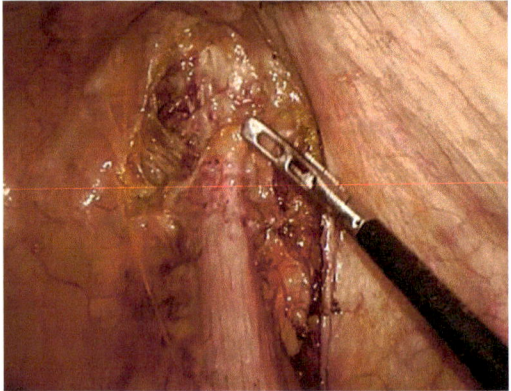

Fig. 2 (Above) A straight needle is passed from the skin through the fundus of the uterus. (Below) The uterus is hitched to the anterior abdominal wall to provide better access to the deep pelvis

Fig. 3 (Above) Blue line shows the extent of peritoneal incision from the sacral promontory to the pouch of Douglas. Black line shows the position of right hypogastric nerve. (Below) The incision is carried to the left-most edge of the pouch of Douglas

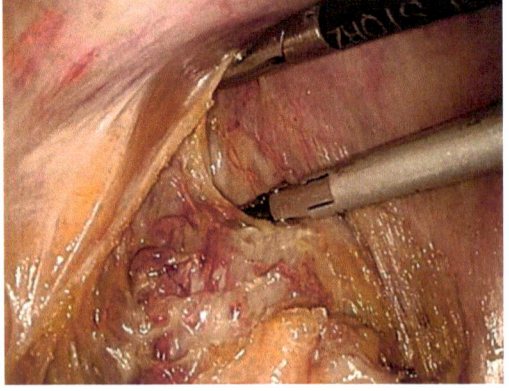

Fig. 4 The rectovaginal septum is opened down to the pelvic floor

0.5%, with a 11.4% recurrence rate. There was significantly improved constipation, fecal incontinence, quality of life outcomes, and associated improvement in urogynecological symptoms.

We use a 10 × 10 cm, 1 mm thick Permacol mesh, cut and stitched together using Prolene 2–0 sutures to fashion a [3, 13] × (15–20) cm strip of mesh. The mesh must be long enough to allow the distal end to reach the anterior rectal pelvic floor and the proximal end to be secured to the sacral promontory. If available, the 4 × 18 cm 1 mm thick Permacol mesh will be better suited for this purpose. The mesh is sutured to the distal rectum using Prolene 2–0, with four sutures on

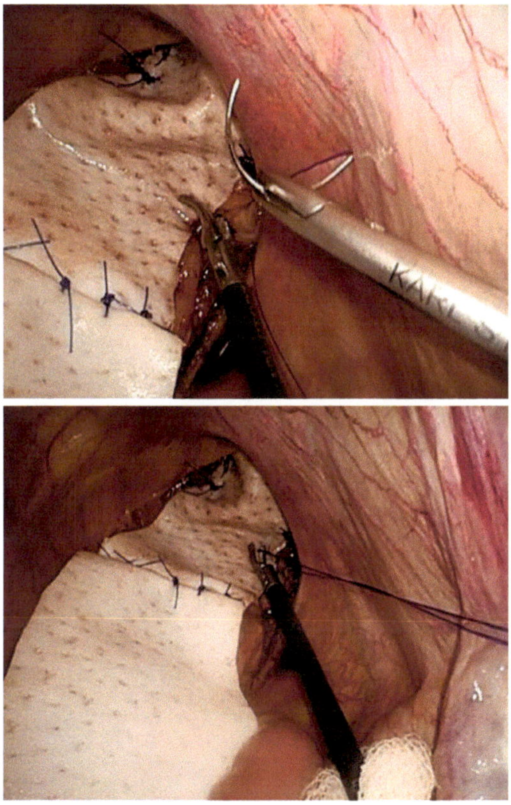

Fig. 5 Interrupted Prolene 2–0 sutures are placed on either ventrolateral edge of the distal rectum. The row of sutures can be seen where the square mesh was divided and fashioned into a single strip

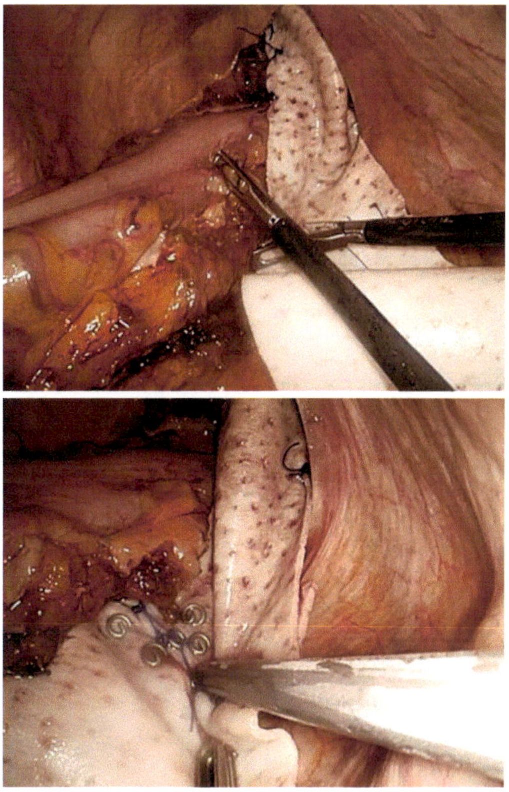

Fig. 6 The mesh is secured to the sacral promontory using laparoscopic tacks

each ventrolateral edge of the rectum (Fig. 5). The sutures are applied with the aid of a knot-pusher from distal to proximal at approximately 1 cm intervals, beginning at the level of the pelvic floor. Although the RP should be reduced at the time of mesh fixation, no traction should be exerted on the rectum, which remains along the curve of the sacrococcygeal hollow [10]. The mesh is fixed onto the sacral promontory using a laparoscopic tacker (Fig. 6). Next, the posterior vaginal fornix is sutured onto the distal aspect of the mesh. This closes the rectovaginal septum and corrects a rectocele (Fig. 7). Excess proximal mesh is trimmed following fixation (Fig. 8).

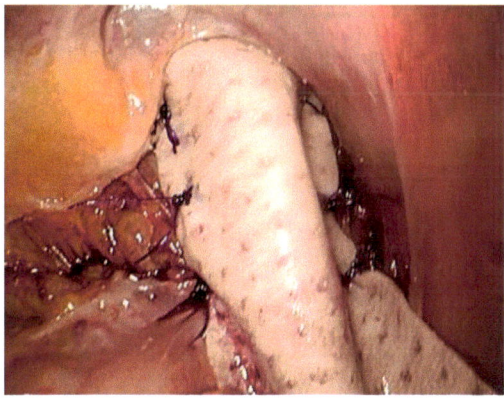

Fig. 7 The rectovaginal septum is recreated by suturing the vaginal fornix to the ventral aspect of the mesh

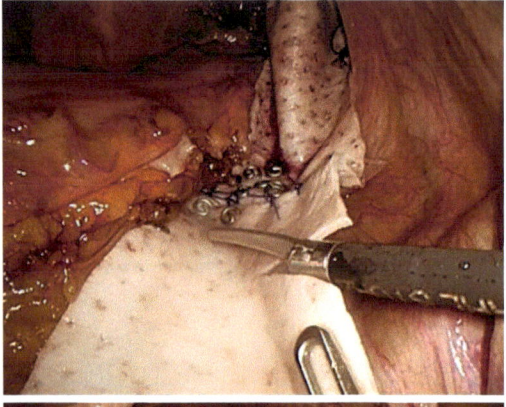

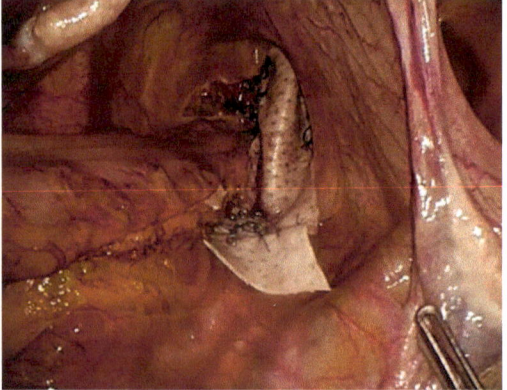

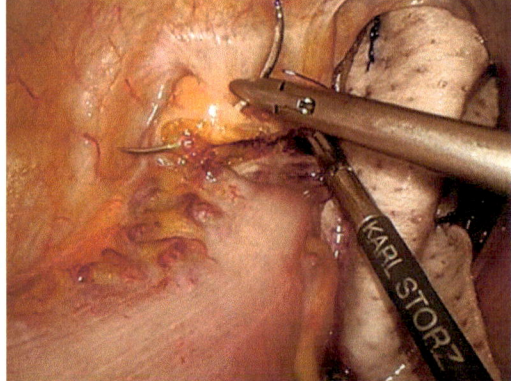

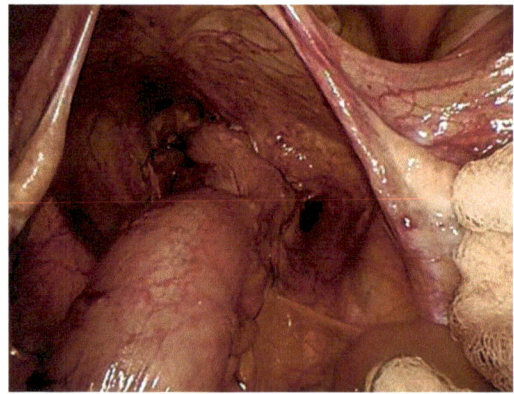

Fig. 8 The mesh is trimmed after fixation

Fig. 9 The peritoneum is closed from the left lateral incised edge to the sacral promontory, completely covering the mesh

The peritoneum is closed over the mesh using a continuous PDS 2–0 suture, commencing from the left lateral edge of the peritoneal incision to the sacral promontory (Fig. 9). The pouch of Douglas is recreated by approximating the peritoneum to the rectal serosa above the rectovaginal colpopexy. In this manner, the entire mesh is covered, preventing future adhesion to the small bowel (Fig. 9). The uterine hitch is removed. No abdominal drain is placed. Finally, the abdominal wounds are closed, concluding the surgery.

Complications and Management

A 2015 study looked at data from 2203 patients from five centers undergoing LVMR from 1999 to 2013 [14]. Synthetic mesh was used in 80% of patients versus biological mesh in 20%. Non-mesh morbidity occurred in 11% (including pain, port site complications, urinary retention, or infection). The overall rate of mesh erosion was 2.0% (2.4% synthetic mesh and 0.7% biologic mesh), including 20 vaginal, 17 rectal, 7 rectovaginal fistula, and 1 perineal, at a median time to erosion of 23 months. Of patients who suffered mesh erosion, 50% required treatment for minor erosion morbidity including local excision of stitch or exposed mesh. 40% underwent intervention for major erosion morbidity including operative mesh removal, colostomy creation, and anterior resection of rectum.

Postoperative Care

No further antibiotics are given beyond the induction dose. The urinary catheter can be removed on postoperative day 1 or 2, and the patient is discharged following bowel motion. The patient is advised to avoid excessive straining, and a course of stool bulking agents may be required.

References

1. Bordeianou L, Paquette I, Johnson E, Holubar SD, Gaertner W, Feingold DL, Steele SR. Clinical practice guidelines for the treatment of rectal prolapse. Dis Colon Rectum. 2017;60(11):1121.
2. van der Schans EM, Paulides TJC, Wijffels NA, Consten ECJ. Management of patients with rectal prolapse: the 2017 Dutch guidelines. Tech Coloproctol. 2018;22(8):589–96.
3. Tou S, Brown SR, Nelson RL. Surgery for complete (full-thickness) rectal prolapse in adults. Cochrane Database Syst Rev. 2015;2015(11):CD001758.
4. Emile SH, Elfeki H, Shalaby M, Sakr A, Sileri P, Wexner SD. Outcome of laparoscopic ventral mesh rectopexy for full-thickness external rectal prolapse: a systematic review, meta-analysis, and meta-regression analysis of the predictors for recurrence. Surg Endosc. 2019;33(8):2444–55.
5. D'Hoore A, Cadoni R, Penninckx F. Long-term outcome of laparoscopic ventral rectopexy for total rectal prolapse. Br J Surg. 2004;91(11):1500–5.
6. Consten EC, van Iersel JJ, Verheijen PM, Broeders IA, Wolthuis AM, D'Hoore A. Long-term outcome after laparoscopic ventral mesh Rectopexy: an observational study of 919 consecutive patients. Ann Surg. 2015;262(5):742–7; discussion 747-8
7. Mäkelä-Kaikkonen J, Rautio T, Kairaluoma M, Carpelan-Holmström M, Kössi J, Rautio A, Ohtonen P, Mäkelä J. Does ventral Rectopexy improve pelvic floor function in the long term? Dis Colon Rectum. 2018;61(2):230–8.
8. Ramage L, Georgiou P, Tekkis P, Tan E. Is robotic ventral mesh rectopexy better than laparoscopy in the treatment of rectal prolapse and obstructed defecation? A meta-analysis. Tech Coloproctol. 2015;19(7):381–9.
9. Albayati S, Chen P, Morgan MJ, Toh JWT. Robotic vs. laparoscopic ventral mesh rectopexy for external rectal prolapse and rectal intussusception: a systematic review. Tech Coloproctol. 2019;23(6):529–35.
10. D'Hoore A, Penninckx F. Laparoscopic ventral recto(colpo)pexy for rectal prolapse: surgical technique and outcome for 109 patients. Surg Endosc. 2006;20(12):1919–23.
11. Balla A, Quaresima S, Smolarek S, Shalaby M, Missori G, Sileri P. Synthetic versus biological mesh-related erosion after laparoscopic ventral mesh Rectopexy: a systematic review. Ann Coloproctol. 2017;33(2):46–51.
12. McLean R, Kipling M, Musgrave E, Mercer-Jones M. Short- and long-term clinical and patient-reported outcomes following laparoscopic ventral mesh rectopexy using biological mesh for pelvic organ prolapse: a prospective cohort study of 224 consecutive patients. Color Dis. 2018;20(5):424–36.
13. Emile SH, Elbanna H, Youssef M, Thabet W, Omar W, Elshobaky A, Abd El-Hamed TM, Farid M. Laparoscopic ventral mesh rectopexy vs Delorme's operation in management of complete rectal prolapse: a prospective randomized study. Color Dis. 2017;19(1):50–7.
14. Evans C, Stevenson AR, Sileri P, Mercer-Jones MA, Dixon AR, Cunningham C, Jones OM, Lindsey I. A multicenter collaboration to assess the safety of laparoscopic ventral Rectopexy. Dis Colon Rectum. 2015;58(8):799–807.

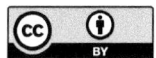

Robotic Surgery: Operating Room Setup and Docking

Sajid Malik

Introduction

Robotic surgery (RS) continues to impart its role in minimally invasive surgery (MIS) since its first emergence. It has rapidly been adopted by different specialties including general surgery, urology, gynecology, and orthopedic surgery, and now is becoming a mainstay of MIS technique around the globe [1–3]. During the last 30 years, many different robotic systems came into surgical practice but the da Vinci® is currently the most commonly utilized and is available in four different models (standard, streamlined, streamlined High definition, S-integrated). Despite its enhanced view of 3D system and angulations of instruments, its practical application for training surgical residents is less emphasized and addressed [4, 5]. This chapter will guide in the basic principles of setting operating room and equipments for da Vinci®. It is further emphasized that hands-on training on simulators and in operating rooms under a trained mentor is highly suggestive of learning robotic skills.

Practical Applications

Robotic surgery has successfully made it possible to complete complex and advanced surgical procedures with precision while staying with the promises of minimally invasive techniques [5]. Many surgeons around the globe have already been practicing RS in all specialties and disciplines like urology, general surgery, pediatric surgery, neurosurgery, gynecology, cardiac, and orthopedic surgery. It has been further applied to subspecialties of general surgery like colorectal, hepatobiliary, bariatric and antireflux surgery, gastric oncology, endocrine, hernia, and complex abdominal wall reconstruction [1, 5, 6].

In contrast to 2D view of laparoscopic surgery, operating surgeon is sitting comfortably on consol with physical ease, enjoying 3D view with depth perception. Robotic arm manipulation and 360 articulation is the beauty of RS which allows the surgeon to perform a more complex procedure without much strain [5–7].

Limitations

RS has few limitations despite rapidly developing technique. Cost and safety always remained questionable in this technique [8, 9]. Human error along with mechanical failures of RS component like robotic arm, lens, camera, and instruments can completely halt the procedure. Extreme

S. Malik (✉)
Department of Surgery, National University Hospital, Singapore, Singapore

Department of Surgery, Allama Iqbal Medical College, Jinnah Hospital, Lahore, Pakistan

© The Author(s) 2023
D. Lomanto et al. (eds.), *Mastering Endo-Laparoscopic and Thoracoscopic Surgery*,
https://doi.org/10.1007/978-981-19-3755-2_75

body positions can cause nerve palsies in inexperienced hand [1, 8, 9].

Bulkiness of RS set may be overcome in large institute with dedicated RS operation suite but lack of tactile sensations and force feedback are still a major drawback of this technique [9–11].

Surgical Team

Minimum surgical team required to run RS setup is surgeon, surgical assistant, circulating nurse, and surgical technician. All surgical staff should be trained in robotic surgery and must have basic knowledge of it which must be gained by proper training. This team should be persistent and dedicated for RS cases to achieve a good learning curve. Surgeon and assistant must not only have mastering skills in operating Da Vinci but also have basic knowledge of RS system and also be aware of troubleshooting the system. Surgical assistant play a vital role and should be efficient enough in trocar placement, draping, docking,

irrigation, retraction, changing instruments, and must have basic laparoscopic skills [12].

Basic Requirements for Robotic Surgery

The basic system for robotic surgery consists of three components: Vision Cart, Patient Cart, and Surgeon's Cart (Console) (Fig. 1). Other requirements are according to the type of surgery. This chapter will try to include the basic minimum requirements for any robot-assisted surgical procedure.

Minimum Personnel Required

- Trained robotic surgeon
- Anesthesia Team trained to conduct robotic surgery
- Trained surgical assistant(s)
- One/two trainees or residents

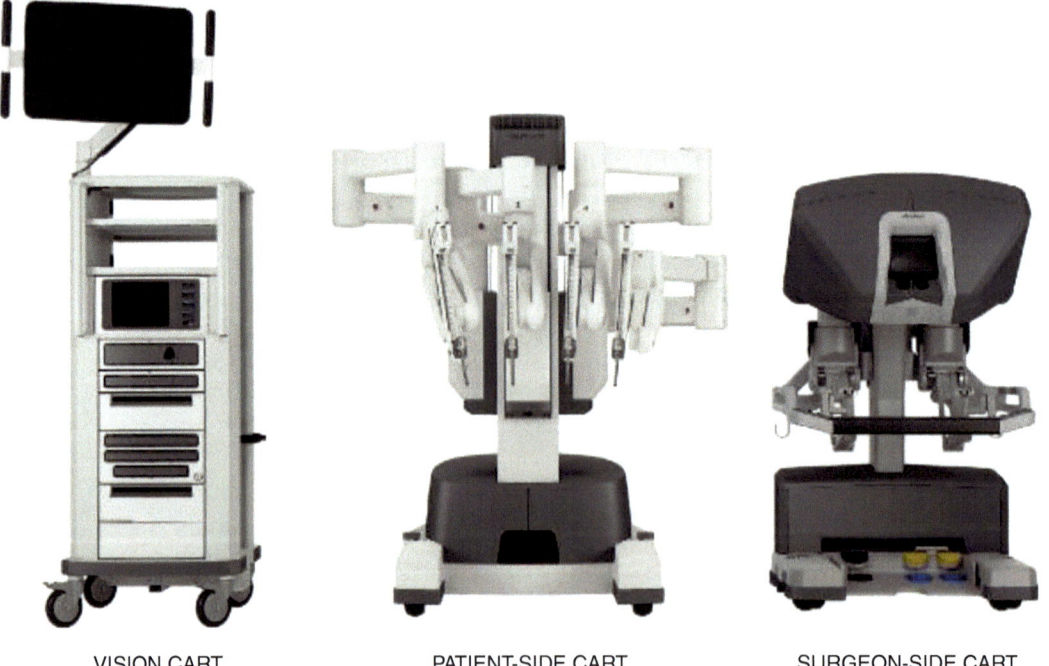

VISION CART   PATIENT-SIDE CART   SURGEON-SIDE CART

Fig. 1 Vision cart, Patient-side cart, and Surgeon-side cart

- Circulating nurse
- OR technicians

Laparoscopic Instruments

- Veress needle (optional)
- 12 mm × 1 Optiview Visiport for camera port
- 12 mm Xcel port × 2
- 6 mm port × 2
- Metzenbaum scissors
- Hook cautery, Maryland dissector, Needle driver
- 5 mm × 1 Hem o lok clips and its applicator
- 10 mm × 1 Hem o lok clips and its applicator
- 0 and 30° scopes
- Suction irrigation setup

Robotic Instruments

- da Vinci robotic system (Intuitive surgical, CA, US)
- 8 mm robotic trocar × 2
- 5 mm robotic trocars × 3
- Camera adapter
- Sterile camera trocar mount and drapes
- Sterile drapes for camera and instrument arms
- Sterile camera mount and instrument adapter
- Endowrist instruments

Operating Room Configuration

Operating Room Setup

Conventional operating room (OR) can be used to set up RS system but, due to its size and extra component, it is advised to have a dedicated RS room to accommodate not only the system and also to allow free movement of OR personnel. It will further allow docking of the robot from different angles depending on the type of surgery. Availability of space could be a major issue for already established OR setups but this problem can be overcome by restructuring operating room according to the need. Some of the components may be placed on vision cart. Ceiling-mounted

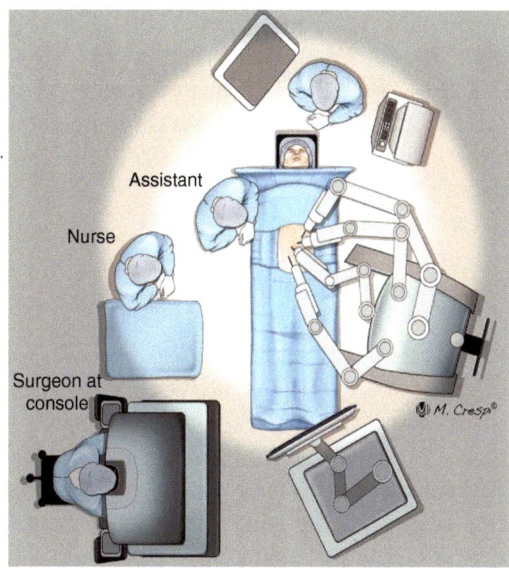

Fig. 2 Operating room setup

booms can harbor insufflators, electrosurgical units, camera, and light source equipment. Operating room should be arranged in a fashion that surgeon has a clear view of the patient from console with a clear pathway for OR staff to move around (Fig. 2).

Patient Position and Preparation

In contrast to conventional laparoscopic surgery, extreme positioning is required in order to achieve optimized exposure for robotic surgery procedures and often requires a strong teamwork to ensure patient safety [13]. Patient safety concerns during RS are to maintain circulation, nerve protections, and pressure injuries to bony prominences. Every effort should bring in consideration to provide proper exposure of surgical site, adequate room for anesthetists to proceed. Another main concern regarding positioning is the safe docking of robot and safe access for bedside surgeon to the surgical ports [14].

For ventral hernia, patients are directly moved onto OR table in supine position with both arms tucked in by the side of body. Arms can be placed in a sling or arm boards to optimize the access of da Vinci arms. All the bony prominences and pressure areas should be covered with a gel pad. Patient cart approach side should be lifted up. The patient is then exposed in a way that he could be prepped from xiphoid to perineum and can be approached from any side if needed [15].

Patient Cart Position

Patient cart should be sterilized and draped before bringing into surgical field. Once the patient positioning is set and cart itself is draped, it should be moved in by using motor drive. Patient cart brakes are designed by default to stop if it is not in use, but it is advised to refer to the manual setting for safety concerns [14, 15].

Patient cart for standard systems has camera and instrument arms. Each arm has several joints and clutches for gross movements and also to insert and withdraw instruments. These arms have two clutch buttons. One dedicated to free gross movement and the other to adjust final trajectory of arm for final docking. The author advises to refer to the system manual for clutch settings as wrong movements can lead to a major disruption. Third arm is in alignment with camera arm therefore care must be taken into account to avoid sword fighting of arms. It is further rec-

ommended to refer to manual for color coding and numbering of arms for standard or S model. (Fig. 3).

An extra and very useful feature of Touch screen monitor is to use it to draw real-time images on monitor. This feature is very useful for teaching and training surgical residents and should be emphasized to use it during surgery to let them know about surgical steps and techniques.

Vision Cart Position

The vision cart should be next to patient cart in order to visualize the component display and also to prevent uninterrupted and free movement of camera cable during surgery. It contains many storage areas to harbor different equipment. It typically contains light source, video processor, and camera control. It can further house insufflators, DVD recorders, and electrosurgical units. Light source is connected with endoscope by a single cable and the endoscope comes in 0°and 30° lense and further has a right and left optical channel to record images. While the standard or S type higher robotic systems endoscopes are connected with higher magnification of 15× with 45° view or wider view of 60° with 10× magnifica-

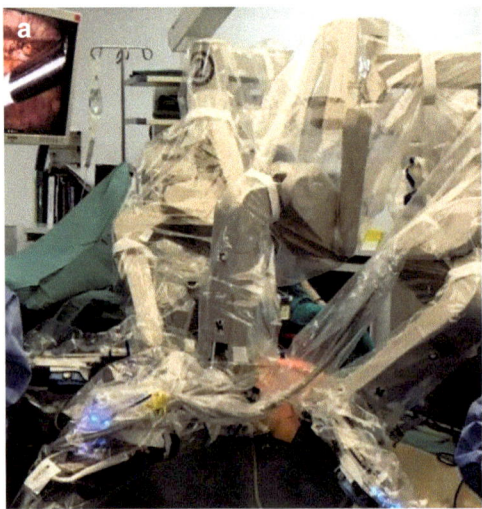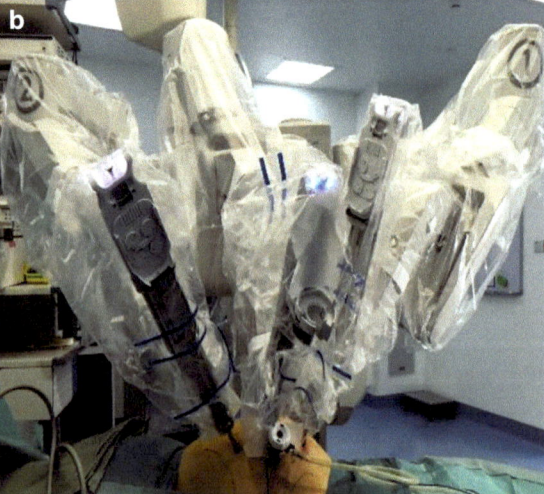

Fig. 3 Position of patient cart on patient for docking (**a, b**)

tion. Resolution and aspect ratio of images can be set from manual and new systems are designed with higher resolutions and AR.

Steps of Docking

Abdominal Access and Port Placement

Abdominal access and port placement are very crucial to start RS. Pneumoperitoneum can be created using either open or closed technique, the author was working with MIS team and recommends to proceed with open technique to better avoid injury. Once peritoneum is accessed, 12 mm visiport for da Vinci endoscope must be introduced and secured in place.

Positions of various ports could vary from patient to patient according to the procedures and is also depended upon the surgeon's preference (Fig. 4). In order to have optimum working conditions, the following principles should be kept in mind.

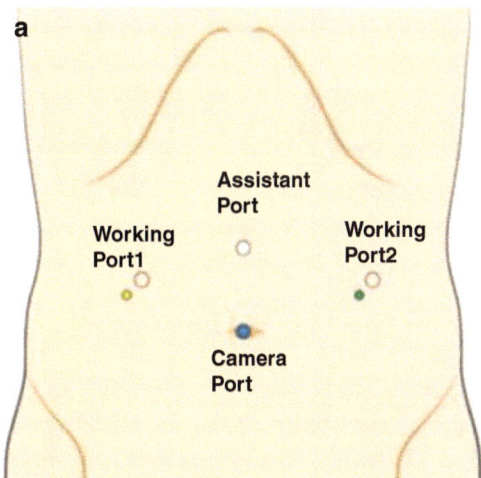
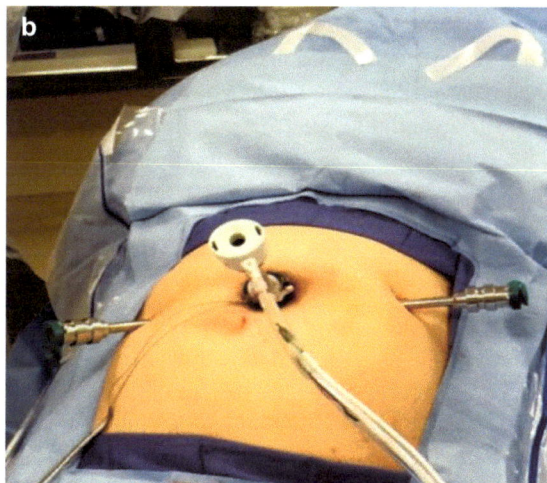
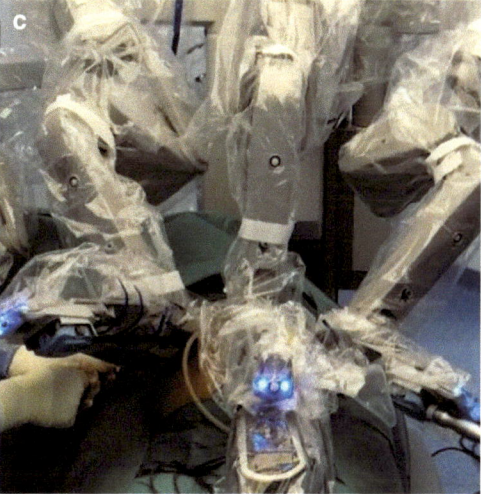

Fig. 4 Port placement (**a**), Position (**b**), and Docking with an extra assistant port (**c**)

- Camera port should be in the same line as surgical target area
- Target area should not be more than 20 cm from camera port
- Working ports should be at least 8 cm form camera port on each side
- Assistant port, if needed, should be atleast 4 cm from camera port

Ports placement in robotic complex ventral or lateral hernia is a critical step and patient factors and anticipated docking should be kept in mind before this step. Patient BMI, body habitus, previous surgery, defect orientation, and its size may affect port positioning and minor amendments can be done accordingly. Port should be placed as much laterally as possible and after insufflations up to 15 mmHg. Assess defect orientation and mark the site. Consider additional 3–5 cm for mesh placement around the defect. Mark the anticipated mesh perimeter at which fixation will be considered latterly. Draw a semicircular line around the mesh perimeter marking, 10–12 cm away from mesh perimeter. Camera port should be placed on this line exactly opposite to anticipated patient cart. Two working arms ports should be placed on each side of camera port almost 8 cm away and on semicircular line. It is better to place assistant port at this stage if needed. Later, once docking is done, we cannot move the patient or patient cart afterward. Assistant port is placed almost 4 cm from camera port and at least 6 cm away from the semicircular line. These port placements are critical for surgery because this will ultimately bring optimal triangulation [15].

Preparing da Vinci

Operating room preparation should be started well before patient's arrival in preoperative area. Surgical team can follow steps that should be considered while setting up system for surgery.

- Before turning on the system, it is advised to connect all cables necessary to run it and do not manipulate system until it is on and self-testing is done.

- Camera arm and other instruments should be positioned in ways that smooth functioning and movements can be observed during procedure.
- After initiating homing sequence, camera, endoscope, instruments, and touch screen are draped and locked.
- Similar to laparoscopic setting, proceed with white balance.
- Align camera port towards targeted anatomical area and surgical cart center column.
- Lock the wheels once cart is in position.
- "Sweet spot" (arrow is pointing towards thick blue line) of camera arm should be set by bringing the trocar mount in alignment with the center of the patient cart column and also by simultaneous extension of camera arm.
- Check the set up joint angles to minimize the potential collision. The angle at the second joint should be 90°.
- System is ready to use and is docked (Fig. 5).

Console Function and Terminology

Surgeon should be aware of the console's different part and terminology being used. Basic terminology according to the site is mentioned in the picture (Fig. 6).

- Clutch plate
- Camera peddle
- Focus bar
- Cautery peddle

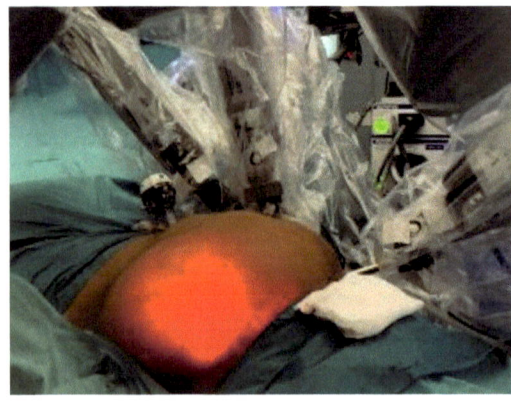

Fig. 5 Docked system

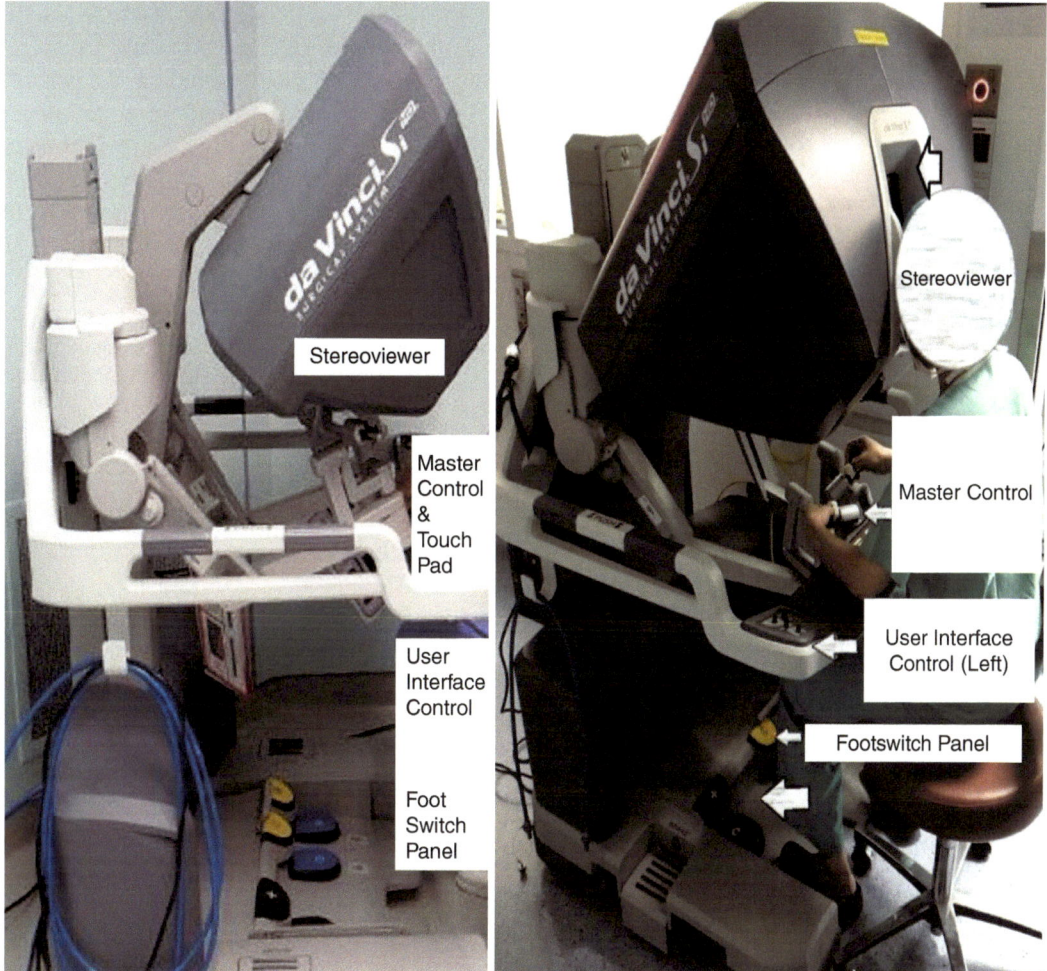

Fig. 6 Surgeon's Cart/Console and its various parts

Left Side

Left side of console bears the following buttons and controls

- Stop angle button
- Console height adjustment button
- Fault reset button

Right Side

- On/Off button
- Ready button
- Emergency stop button

Inserting/Changing Instruments

Always start by straightening the instrument tip and slide it to port to bring under vision. Push the instrument into surgical area by pressing the arm clutch button. If any resistance is felt during this manure, stop and check to identify the problem and address it accordingly. Surgeon should only proceed to drive once the LED light indicator is "ON" (Fig. 7).

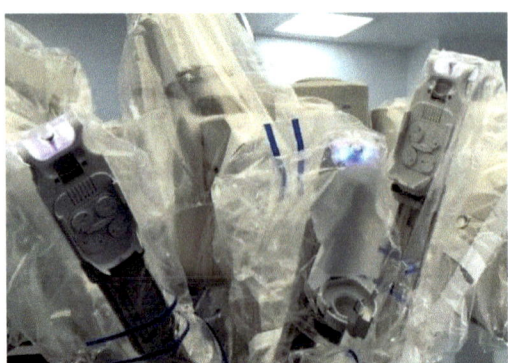

Fig. 7 Control and Clutch with LED indicator ON to proceed

Instruments Removal

Instruments being removed should be straightened and jaws should be visualized. Before proceeding with instrument removal, make sure that no tissue is being held in the jaws of instruments. Simply press the release lever on instrument housing and take out the instruments.

System Shutdown

Once the surgery is completed, all the instruments are removed first same as laparoscopic surgery, followed by endoscope removal. Arms are disconnected from the trocars and patient cart is undocked from the patient. New system does not allow undocking by no activation of motor drive system until the instruments and camera are removed and undocked. 12 mm trocar incision or any other incision more than 12 mm should be considered for fascial closure. 8 mm or 5 mm trocar incision is not required to be closed. All sterilized drapes or clothes used should be removed and system can be switched off. If there is any subsequent case, it is better to keep the system on.

Conclusion

Limitations of conventional laparoscopy like 3D visualization and good ergonomics have been overcome by the use of technology of robots. Robotic surgery procedure has dramatically increased during the last decade. Complete understanding of instrumentation, knowledge of robotic system, and robotic program hinges on a proper OR is a mainstay for successful outcome. Well trained, enthusiastic, dynamic, and knowledgeable surgical team is a key for OR dynamics to provide excellent quality care to patients.

Acknowledgments Professor Davide Lomanto.
Professor of Surgery, National University of Singapore.
Senior Consultant & Director, Advance Surgical Training Centre.
National University Hospital, Singapore.

References

1. Palep JH. Robotic assisted minimally invasive surgery. J Minim Access Surg. 2009;5(1):1–7.
2. Sudan R, Desai SS. Emergency and weekend robotic surgery are feasible. J Robot Surg. 2011;6(3):263–6.
3. Farivar BS, Flannagan M, Leitman IM. General surgery residents' perception of robot-assisted procedures during surgical training. J Surg Educ. 2015;72(2) article no. 990:235–42.
4. Ghezzi TL, Corleta OC. 30 years of robotic surgery. World J Surg. 2016;40(10):2550–7.
5. Moorthy K, Munz Y, Dosis A, et al. Dexterity enhancement with robotic surgery. Surg Endosc. 2004;18:790–5.
6. Marescaux J, Rubino F. The ZEUS robotic system: experimental and clinical applications. Surg Clin North Am. 2003;83:1305–15.
7. Tholey G, Desai JP, Castellanos AE. Force feedback plays a significant role in minimally invasive surgery: results and analysis. Ann Surg. 2005;241:102–9.
8. Townsend CM Jr, Beauchamp RD, Evers BM, Mattox KL. Sabiston textbook of surgery E-book. Elsevier Health Sciences; 2016.
9. Morgan JA, Thornton BA, Peacock JC, et al. Does robotic technology make minimally invasive cardiac surgery too expensive? A hospital cost analysis of robotic and conventional techniques. J Card Surg. 2005;20:246–51.
10. Camarillo DB, Krummel TM, Salisbury JK. Jr robotic technology in surgery: past, present, and future. Am J Surg. 2004;188:2S–15S.
11. Hubens G, Ruppert M, Balliu L, Vaneerdeweg W. What have we learnt after two years working with the da Vinci robot system in digestive surgery? Acta Chir Belg. 2004;104:609–14.
12. Gettman MT, et al. Current status of robotics in urologic laparoscopy. Eur Urol. 2003;43(2):106–12.

13. Guideline for positioning the patient. In: Guidelines for perioperative practice. Denver, CO: AORN, Inc; 2014. p. 563–81.
14. Molloy BL. Implications for postoperative visual loss: steep Trendelenburg position and effects on intraocular pressure. AANA J. 2011;79:115–21.
15. Lomanto D, Malik S. Robotic repair of ventral hernias. Ann Laparsc Endosc Surg. 2019;4:61. https://doi.org/10.21037/ales.2019.05.13.

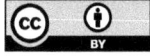

Part XXII

Other Laparoscopic Procedures

Laparoscopic Varicocelectomy

Rakesh Kumar Gupta

Introduction

Varicocele is defined as dilated and tortuous veins of the pampiniform plexus of scrotal veins. Varicocele occurs in approximately 15% of the male population [1] and 21–39% of infertile men [2].

Clinically, there are three grades for varicocele [3].

- Grade I. The patient is standing and varicocele appears while the scrotum is palpated and Valsalva maneuver is done.
- Grade II. Varicocele appears while the scrotum is palpated without Valsalva maneuver.
- Grade III. Varicocele appears as a "bag of worms" while the patient stands, without Valsalva and palpation.

Despite extensive information being available on varicoceles and many studies on different surgical solutions, the ideal method of varicocele ligation is still a matter of controversy. The ideal technique would have low recurrence and complication rates [4].

Different approaches have been applied for the treatment of varicocele, including open surgery, sclerotherapy, and, recently, laparoscopy [5–7]. The Palomo technique was associated with a relatively high incidence of postoperative discomfort [8] and for this reason the modified Palomo procedure was often preferred [9].

Ivanissevich described a procedure where the testicular vein is tied at the inguinal ring and the testicular artery is spared [8]. In 1991 Aaberge et al. introduced laparoscopic varicocelectomy as the new and less invasive treatment for varicocele [10].

In recent years laparoscopic varicocele ligation (LV) had been popularized and had gained growing acceptance. The built-in magnification of the laparoscope facilitates identification of the spermatic veins and artery, potentially reducing the risk of recurrence of the varicocele and of ischemic damage to the testis. Magnification also allows the surgeon to preserve lymphatics and the genital branches of the genitofemoral nerve that runs along the spermatic vessels, which may reduce lymphocele formation and postoperative pain [11].

Laparoscopic management of varicoceles in adults may reflect the excellent visibility of the posterior abdominal wall achieved using the laparoscope, which allows a thorough search of sites known to be responsible for recurrent varicoceles, viz., renal, vas associated, pelvic, and retropubic cross-over veins [11].

The conventional technique of laparoscopic varix ligation is to ligate the vessels with clips and then transect them in between the clips [12–14]. Sasagawa reported that they successfully transected the internal spermatic vessels purely using a harmonic scalpel, which comes only in diameters of 5 and 10 mm [15].

R. K. Gupta (✉)
GS & MIS Unit, Department of Surgery, B.P. Koirala
Institute of Health Sciences, Dharan, Nepal

D. Lomanto et al. (eds.), *Mastering Endo-Laparoscopic and Thoracoscopic Surgery*,
https://doi.org/10.1007/978-981-19-3755-2_76

Indications

American Urological Society recommends that varicocele treatment should be offered to the male partner of a couple attempting to conceive when all of the following are present.

1. A varicocele is palpable.
2. The couple has documented infertility.
3. The female has normal fertility or potentially correctable infertility.
4. The male partner has one or more abnormal semen parameters or sperm function test results.

The indications in adolescents—presence of significant testicular asymmetry ($< > 20\%$) demonstrated on serial examinations, testicular pain, and abnormal semen analysis results. Very large varicoceles may also be repaired; however, in the absence of atrophy, this indication is relative and controversial.

Preoperative Assessment

A proper history regarding the onset of symptoms to its presentation is important. General physical examination followed by a proper clinical examination of external genitalia, groin, and the testis.

Once the clinical diagnosis of varicocele is made, routine preoperative investigations were done, for fitness of general anesthesia.

Ultrasonographic examination can be done for the evaluation of:

(a) Enlarged veins along the spermatic cord and epididymis.
(b) Diameter of the largest vein while the patient performed a Valsalva maneuver in a standing position.
(c) Reflux in the veins during the Valsalva maneuver.
(d) Grade of the varicoceles.
(e) Detect other pathologies in the right or left retroperitoneum that might have caused a varicocele.

Preoperative semen analysis should be carried out in all patients aged 18 years and above. Pre-anesthetic checkup was done. After the patients were considered fit for surgery, they were informed in their native language about the nature of the disease process, the procedure, the possible complications of the procedure, the possibility of conversion of laparoscopic surgery to open in cases of difficulty and about the hematoma, wound infections, pneumoscrotum, hydrocele, prolonged pain, and recurrence.

Surgical Technique

Operation theater setup is done as shown in Fig. 1. The procedure is performed under general anesthesia. A prophylactic intravenous antibiotic (third generation cephalosporins IV) is given at induction prior to the incision. The patient is placed in a supine position.

Once painting and draping are done pneumoperitoneum is created either by open or closed technique, depending upon the surgeon's preference. In Open technique, 10 mm transverse infra-umbilical port is made and pneumoperitoneum is created with CO_2 at 2–3 liters/minute and an intra-abdominal pressure of 10–12 mmHg is

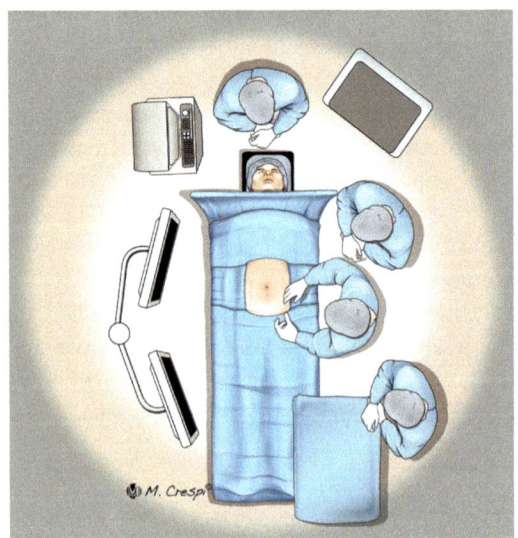

Fig. 1 Operative Setup

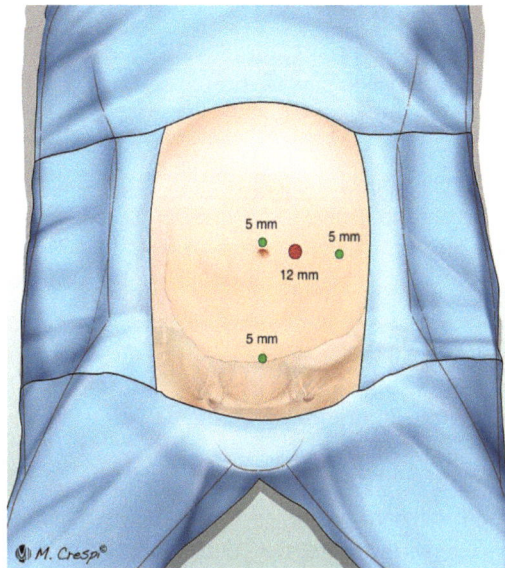

Fig. 2 Landmarks with trocar sites

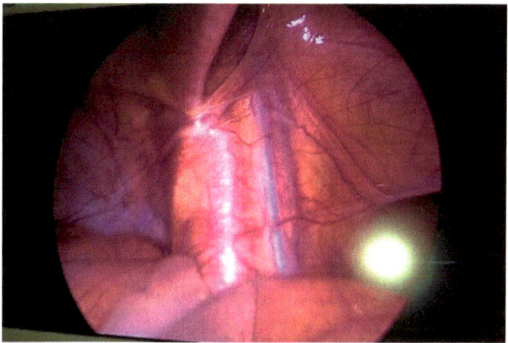

Fig. 3 Laparoscopic view of right spermatic vessels

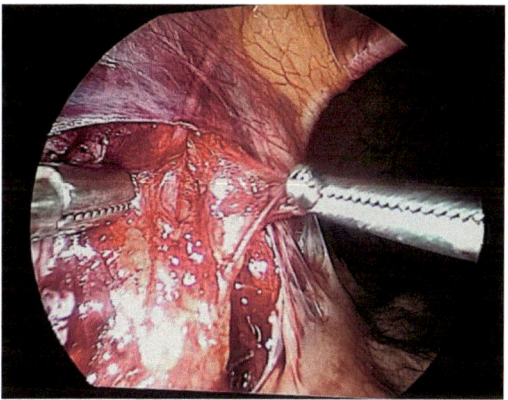

Fig. 4 Dissection of parietal peritoneum exposing right spermatic vessels

obtained. A 30° laparoscope is then inserted and the abdominal cavity was evaluated. Two 5 mm trocars were inserted as in Fig. 2.

Landmarks: pubic symphysis, anterior superior iliac spines. Surgical preparation field: well above umbilicus, lateral to iliac spines, penis and scrotum.

Trocar placement left side
- • 5 mm supra-umbilical trocar for camera and insufflation
- 5 mm trocar halfway to two-thirds between the umbilicus and pubic symphysis in the midline (for unilateral case)
- 5 mm trocar on ipsilateral side of the varicocele, lateral to the epigastric vessels around the line of the umbilicus (for bilateral cases two 5 mm trocars on each side).

Patient is then placed in a slight reverse Trendelenburg position and tilted to the opposite side of the operative field (10–15°). Abdominal organs are assessed. Internal spermatic vessels are identified (Fig. 3).

Peritoneum overlying the left or right internal spermatic veins are opened (Fig. 4).

Veins are dissected, testicular artery, artery o vas deference must be identified and preserved.

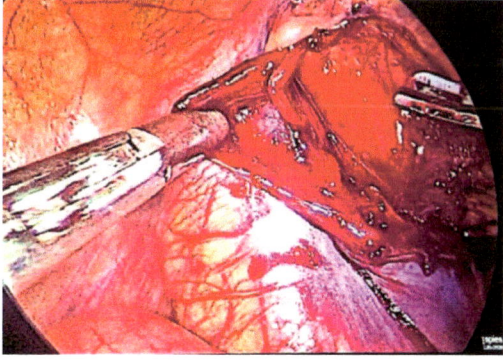

Fig. 5 Dissection and identification of gonadal vessels and vas

The testicular veins are sealed with suture/clips/harmonic scalpel (depends upon the surgeon's preference). Hemostasis is secured and confirmed (Figs. 5, 6).

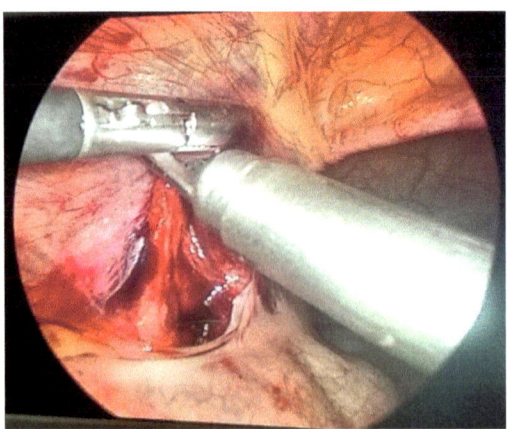

Fig. 6 Ligation and division of right spermatic vessels

Skin is closed with skin staplers and a sterile dressing is applied.

Troubleshooting in identifying testicular artery:

1. For identification of the internal spermatic artery, use of a laparoscopic Doppler is helpful, especially as often the artery will stop pulsating after manipulation.
2. Papaverin injection can also be used to differentiate artery and veins. The Doppler probe used to identify pulsation also helps with dissection.

Complications and Management

- **Intraoperative complications**
  - Damage to the vessels in the area (inferior epigastric artery, inferior mesenteric vein, spermatic vessels).
  - Injury to the vas.
  - Transection of the genitofemoral nerve.
- **Immediate complications**
  - Port site Hematoma
  - Wound complications (2%)
  - Subcutaneous emphysema (20%)
  - Pneumo-scrotum (15%)
  - Postoperative pain
- **Long-term complications**
  - Testicular atrophy (3%)
  - Genitofemoral nerve injury

- Hydrocele (5%)
- Epididymo-orchitis
- Prolonged pain (5–6%)
- Recurrence (5–20%)

Laparoscopic ligation is an effective and safe approach to achieve pain relief in varicocele patients [16].

Postoperative Care

After the surgery, they are shifted to the wards for postoperative care.

- A standard analgesic regimen was administered (intramuscular Diclofenac 75 mg 8 hourly and on demand).
- Pain measurement was done using Visual Analog Scale (VAS score).
- Antibiotics were not used beyond the intraoperative period.
- Feeding was resumed as soon as there was a full regain of consciousness.

Patients were discharged on the following day after assessment with proper medical advice including the date of suture removal and they received similar instructions to return to normal activity.

References

1. Hopps C, Lemer M, Schlegel P, Goldstein M. Intraoperative varicocele anatomy: a microscopic study of the inguinal versus subinguinal approach. J Urol. 2003;170(6):2366–70.
2. Greenberg SH, Wallach E. Varicocele and male fertility. Fertil Steril. 1977;28(7):699–706.
3. Itoh K, Suzuki Y, Yazawa H, Ichiyangi O, Miura M, Sasagawa I. Results and complications of laparoscopic Palomovaricocelectomy. Arch Androl. 2003;49(2):107–10.
4. Hassan J, Adams M, Pope J, Demarco R, Brock J. Hydrocele formation following laparoscopic Varicocelectomy. J Urol. 2006;175(3):1076–9.
5. Kocvara R, Dvoracek J, Sedlacek J, Dite Z, Novak K. Lymphatic sparing laparoscopic varicocelectomy: a microsurgical repair. J Urol. 2005;173(5):1751–4.
6. Misseri R, Gershbein A, Horowitz M, Glassberg K. The adolescent varicocele. II: the incidence of

hydrocele and delayed recurrent varicocele after varicocelectomy in a long-term follow-up. BJU Int. 2001;87(6):494–8.

7. Palomo A. Radical cure of varicocele by a new technique: preliminary report. J Urol. 1949;61(3):604–7.

8. Ivanissevich O. Left varicocele due to reflux; experience with 4,470 operative cases in forty-two years. J Int Coll Surg. 1960;34(12):742–55.

9. Link BA, Kruska JD, Wong C. Two trocar laparoscopic varicocelectomy: approach and outcomes. JSLS. 2006;10(2):151–4.

10. Donovan J, Winfield H. Laparoscopic Varix Ligation. J Urol. 1992;147(1):77–81.

11. Franco I. Laparoscopic varicocelectomy in the adolescent male. Curr Urol Rep. 2004;5(2):132–6.

12. Matsuda T, Ogura K, Uchida J, Fujita I, Terachi T, Yoshida O. Smaller ports result in shorter convalescence after laparoscopic Varicocelectomy. J Urol. 1995;153(4):1175–7.

13. Pianalto B, Bonanni G, Martella S, Renier M, Ancona E. Results of laparoscopic bilateral varicocelectomy. AnnaliItaliani di Chirurgia. 2000;71(5):587–91.

14. Huscher C, Lirici M, Di Paola M, Crafa F, Corradi A, Amini M, et al. Laparoscopic cholecystectomy by ultrasonic dissection without cystic duct and artery ligature. Surg Endosc. 2003;17(3):442–51.

15. Sasagawa I, Yazawa H, Suzuki Y, Tateno T, Takahashi Y, Nakada T. Laparoscopic varicocelectomy in adolescents using an ultrasonically activated scalpel. Arch Androl. 2000;45(2):91–4.

16. Maghraby HA. Laparoscopic varicocelectomy for painful varicoceles: merits and outcomes. J Endourol. 2002;16(2):107–10.

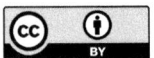

Laparoscopic Pediatric Inguinal Hernia Repair

Hrishikesh Salgaonkar and Rasik Shah

Inguinal hernia repair is one of the commonest elective surgical procedure performed in the pediatric age group. The incidence of inguinal hernia in children varies between 1 and 5% and is more commonly seen in premature infants. Similarly, it is more common in boys as compared to girls. Almost always clinically diagnosed by a palpable reducible lump in the inguinal region, the mere presence of an inguinal hernia in children is an indication of surgical repair. Traditionally, pediatric inguinal hernias are repaired by an open technique which involves high ligation of the hernial sac at the level of the internal ring. Laparoscopy is a safe, easy, and reproducible technique in the hand of an experienced surgeon with similar results. In this chapter, author discusses the details of the technique of laparoscopic inguinal hernia repair.

Introduction

Pediatric inguinal hernia repair is a commonly performed procedure by pediatric surgeons. It is due to the persistent processus vaginalis. Standard open repair involves ligation of the hernial sac at

the deep or internal inguinal ring after reduction of contents. In girls, the hernial sac is transfixed and divided at the level of the internal ring along with the round ligament [1, 2]. With the advent of minimally invasive surgery, many pediatric surgeons repair the inguinal hernia laparoscopically to achieve the same results. The main advantages are visualization of the opposite internal ring, decrease in the incidence of injury to vas and vessels, and esthetic small scars.

Anesthesia, Preoperative Evaluation, and Counseling

While open repair of inguinal hernia can be performed under caudal block or laryngeal mask anesthesia, laparoscopic repair is performed under controlled general anesthesia with endotracheal intubation. Also, during the learning curve, laparoscopic repair takes more time compared to open repair. Always counsel the parents and get consent for possible bilateral repairs, which is not uncommon to encounter.

Theater Setup and Patient Position

The patient is placed in a supine position and properly secured to the operating table. The monitor is placed at the foot end of the operating table. The first port is inserted by an open technique while the surgeon is standing on the left

H. Salgaonkar (✉)
Department of Bariatric and Upper GI Surgery,
University Hospitals North Midlands,
Stoke-on-Trent, UK

R. Shah
SRCC Children's Hospital, Narayana Health,
Mumbai, India

© The Author(s) 2023
D. Lomanto et al. (eds.), *Mastering Endo-Laparoscopic and Thoracoscopic Surgery*,
https://doi.org/10.1007/978-981-19-3755-2_77

side of the operating table and then the surgeon inserts the remaining ports and then he moves to the head end of the operating table to carry out the surgery.

Port Placement

The first port (5 mm) is inserted at the superior aspect of the umbilicus using an open technique and a 5 mm 30^0 telescope is inserted (alternatively even 3 mm telescope gives good view while using HD camera). Pneumoperitoneum of 8 mm of water is achieved by CO_2 insufflation, with a flow of 1–2 liters per minute. General examination of the entire abdominal cavity is performed and then the preliminary examination of both internal inguinal rings is carried out to check for their patency. Two additional (3 mm) working ports are inserted under laparoscopic guidance on either side of the umbilicus in the midclavicular line in bilateral disease. This is to maintain at least 8–10 cm distance between the entry site of the port and the internal ring. In case of unilateral hernia, the 3 mm port on the opposite side of the hernia can be placed a little lower and closer to the internal ring so as to achieve better triangulation.

In newborns and infants, the ports can be inserted at a higher level to maintain adequate working distance from the internal ring. Once the port placement is accomplished, the patient is placed in a Trendelenburg position. Visual examination of internal genitalia should be carried out to rule out disorders of sexual differentiation (DSD).

Hernia Repair

Peritoneal Incision

Author prefers to repair symptomatic side first in case of a bilateral inguinal hernia. The peritoneal lining at the internal ring is marked with diathermy on a hook or scissors. Then the perito-

neum is incised at the level of the internal ring. The authors being right-handed surgeons, prefer to start the incision from lateral to the medial direction for the right-side hernias and medial to lateral for the left-side hernia.

Dissection of Hernial Sac

Identify the cord structure (Vas and vessels in the male) or round ligament (in females). Dissect carefully, with minimal handling of cord structures to reduce damage due to tissue handling. Continue dissection posterior to the deep ring to gradually isolate the hernial sac. Continue dissection of the sac into the inguinal canal for only up to 2 cm to avoid unnecessary muscle damage (Fig. 1). The dissected sac is excised using diathermy. In female children, if meticulous care is taken, the sac can be safely dissected off the round ligament upto the level of the internal ring, avoiding the need for dividing the round ligament.

Assessment of the Myo-Pectineal Orifice

At this point assess the approximation of the conjoint muscle with the inguinal ligament (internally identified as the Ilio-pubic tract) at the internal ring. In case of poor approximation, suture the conjoint muscle with the ilio-pubic tract lateral to the inferior epigastric vessels using 3–0 absorbable or nonabsorbable suture (better to use permanent suture like 3–0 polyester instead of polyglycolic) on a round body needle [3]. Too tight approximation is avoided and usually 1–2 interrupted sutures are sufficient.

Closure of Peritoneal Defect

In children, it is easy to introduce the needle transabdominally as the abdominal wall is relatively thin. The peritoneum in children at the

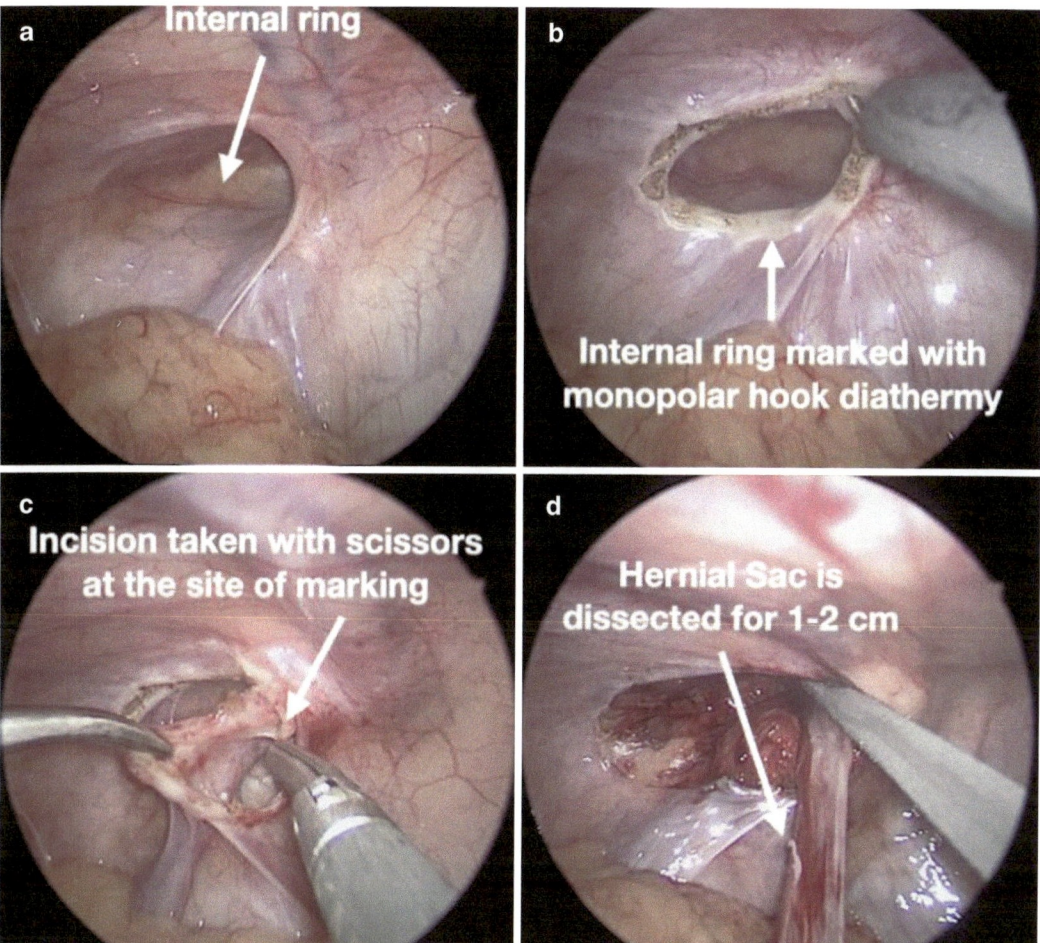

Fig. 1 Steps of hernia repair (**a**) Identification of hernia (**b**) Marking of the peritoneal incision (**c**) peritoneal incision (**d**) dissection of sac into the inguinal canal

internal ring is very thin and loose and it can be easily closed by a purse-string suture. As the peritoneum is loose, it can be easily fed on the tip of the needle instead of taking a bite with the needle. This avoids any chance of injury to the surrounding structures (Fig. 2). After closing the peritoneal defect, the needle is removed along with the port by holding the suture 1 cm away from the swaged end of the needle. Even the hernial sac is then removed along with the trocar. The 3 mm port sites are closed with steristrips,

and 5 mm supra-umbilical incision is closed with 3–0 polyglycolic acid suture.

Postoperative Care and Follow-Up

Feeding is resumed 3–4 h after the procedure and patients are discharged on the same day or the next day morning. All patients are evaluated after 1 week, 1 month, 6 months, and then annually if feasible.

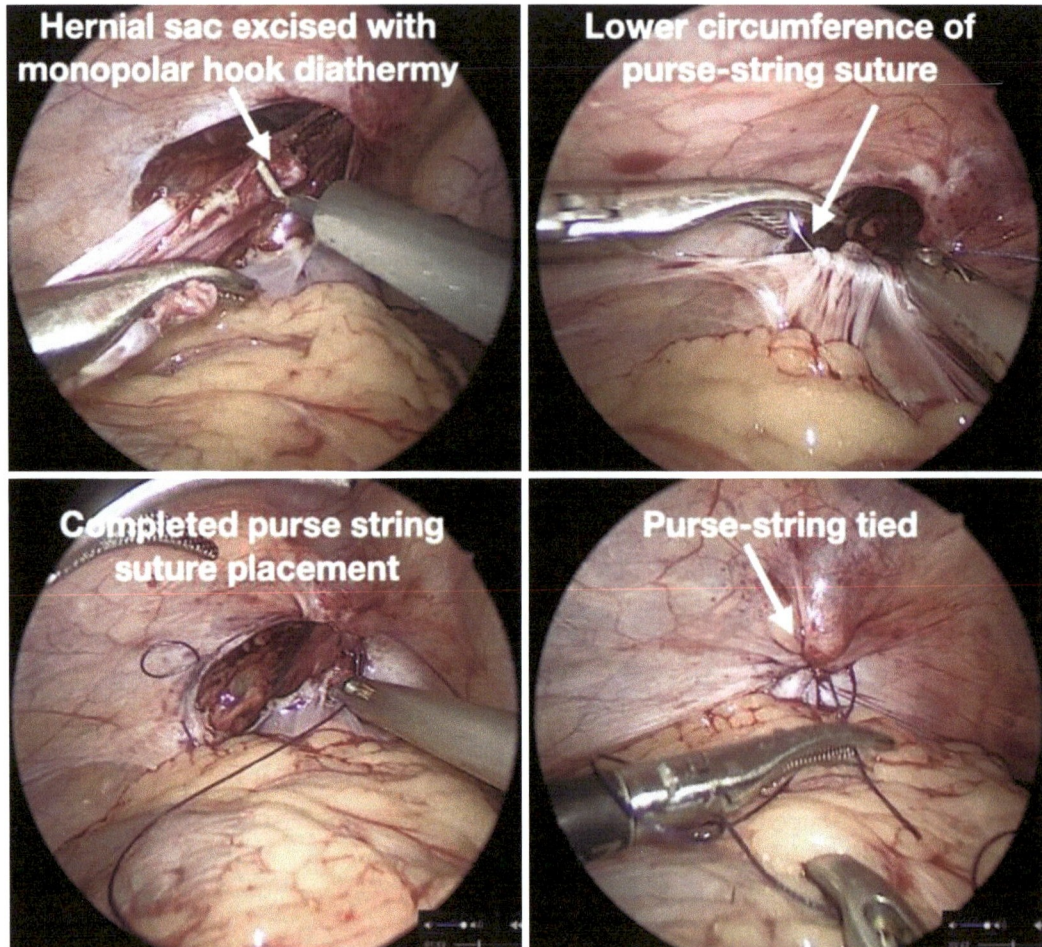

Fig. 2 Excision of the hernial sac and purse-string closure of the internal ring

Other Techniques

The author prefers the abovementioned technique of laparoscopic sac resection and peritoneal closure with an intracorporeal suture. There are multiple techniques of direct internal ring suture closure without sac dissection and excision. This may be achieved by intracorporeal or extracorporeal suturing.

Laparoscopic Intracorporeal Purse String

In this technique, sac dissection is avoided. After incising the peritoneum around the internal ring,

using an absorbable or nonabsorbable suture a purse-string stitch is taken around the internal inguinal ring to approximate the crural arch and conjoined tendon. In larger hernias, one or more interrupted stitches are made.

Laparoscopic Percutaneous Extracorporeal Closure

Under laparoscopic vision using a suture passer device transabdominally, a suture is passed through a 2 mm stab incision and guided around the lateral half of the circumference of the internal inguinal ring. Through the same skin cut, pass the suture passer device around the medial half of the internal ring to withdraw the suture out creating a loop and tie the suture extracorporeally. Care is taken to avoid damaging the vas deferens and testicular vessels. Based on surgeon preference different devices may be used to form a loop and close the internal inguinal ring with an extracorporeal knot under laparoscopic vision, e.g., hollow bore needle—18 G, LPEC needle with a special wire loop at the tip, Reverdin needle, herniotomy hook.

Complications

Complications in pediatric inguinal hernia are similar to standard laparoscopic inguinal hernia repair. Whether we perform an open or laparoscopic hernia repair, every surgeon should follow the basic principles of good surgical practice. It is paramount to handle tissues carefully, perform a meticulous dissection, have a good understanding of the anatomy of the groin, safe use of energy device, and secure hemostasis. If care is not taken complications like bleeding, hematoma, wound infection, bowel/bladder injury, injury to vas or gonadal vessels can occur. Injury to gonadal vessels may lead to testicular atrophy. In girls damage to fallopian tubes is a possibility with future implications of infertility, so care should be taken to minimize handling. Post-op hydrocoele, scrotal edema/erythema, chronic pain, port site hernias are not unheard of. Excessive dissection of the inguinal canal, tight sutures approximating conjoint muscle with ilio-pubic tract, inability to excise the hernia sac can all lead to recurrence. Meta-analysis comparing laparoscopic vs open pediatric inguinal hernia repair has not shown any conclusive superiority of one over the other with similar operative times, perioperative results, and complication rates including recurrence [4]. In fact, laparoscopy has been proven to be better for bilateral hernias and meta-chronic contralateral hernias [5]. The recurrence rates for uncomplicated inguinal hernia repair in children range between 1.2 and 2.8%, regardless of the child's gender. This rate increases in premature infants and those with an incarcerated hernia [6, 7]. Laparoscopy offers us all the proven benefits of minimally invasive surgery, e.g., better cosmesis, lesser pain, etc. By allowing us a visualization of contralateral groin it offers us the advantage of simultaneous repair. Young surgeons and trainees should not hesitate to call for help from seniors as the safety of patients is paramount and should never be compromised.

Conclusion

Surgeons well versed in both open or laparoscopic approaches can utilize the benefits of either procedure. Laparoscopy offers more peroperative information of both groins as compared to open, and hence offers an advantage in case of uncertain diagnosis, especially for infants or prematurely born neonates. It also seems better in those with recurrent hernias. In experienced hands, laparoscopic inguinal hernia repair in children is a safe and feasible procedure.

References

1. Glick PL, Boulanger SC. Inguinal hernias and hydroceles. In: Grosfeld JL, O'Neill Jr JA, Coran AG, Fonkalsrud E, editors. Pediatric surgery. 6th ed. Philadelphia: Mosby; 2006. p. 1172–9.
2. Levitt MA, Ferraraccio D, Arbesman MC, Brisseau GF, Caty MG, Glick PL. Variability of inguinal hernia surgical technique: a survey of north American pediatric surgeons. J Pediatr Surg. 2002;37(5):745–51.
3. Shah R, Arlikar J, Dhende N. Incise, dissect, excise and suture technique of laparoscopic repair of paediatric male inguinal hernia. J Minim Access Surg. 2013;9:72–5.
4. Dreuning K, Maat S, Twisk J, van Heurn E, Derikx J. Laparoscopic versus open pediatric inguinal hernia repair: state-of-the-art comparison and future perspectives from a meta-analysis. Surg Endosc. 2019;33(10):3177–91.
5. Yang C, Zhang H, Pu J, Mei H, Zheng L, Tong Q. Laparoscopic vs open herniorrhaphy in the management of pediatric inguinal hernia: a systemic review and meta-analysis. J Pediatr Surg. 2011;46(9):1824–34.
6. Ein SH, Njere I, Ein A. Six thousand three hundred sixty one pediatric inguinal hernias: a 35 year review. J Pediatr Surg. 2006;41(5):980–6.
7. Zendejas B, Zarrouq AE, Erben YM, Holley CT, Farley DR. Impact of childhood inguinal hernia repair in adulthood: 50 years of follow up. J Am Coll Surg. 2010;211(6):762–8.

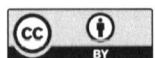